10/97

The Fabric of the Body

The Fabric of the Body

European Traditions of Anatomical Illustration

K. B. Roberts and J. D. W. Tomlinson

CLARENDON PRESS · OXFORD · 1992

Oxford University Press, Walton Street, Oxford OX2 6DP

Oxford New York Toronto
Delhi Bombay Calcutta Madras Karachi
Petaling Jaya Singapore Hong Kong Tokyo
Nairobi Dar es Salaam Cape Town
Melbourne Auckland
and associated companies in
Berlin Ibadan

Oxford is a trade mark of Oxford University Press

Published in the United States
by Oxford University Press, New York

A catalogue record for this book is available from the British Library

Library of Congress Cataloging in Publication Data
Roberts, K. B.
The fabric of the body: European traditions of anatomical
illustrations/K. B. Roberts and J. D. W. Tomlinson.
p. cm.
Includes index.
1. Medical illustration—History.   I. Tomlinson, J. D. W.
II. Title.
R836.R63   1990   611'.0022'2—dc20   90–7650
ISBN 0–19–261198–4

Typeset by Butler & Tanner Ltd
Printed in Great Britain by
Butler & Tanner Ltd, Frome and London

Contents

Preface

THIS book is an anthology of anatomical illustration from the medieval period to the present day. The plates have been chosen to demonstrate the European tradition as it developed on the Continent, in Britain, and in North America. It is a collection of representative examples, not a comprehensive treatise or encyclopedia. The anatomy we illustrate and discuss is the anatomy of the human body studied by dissection and observed with the naked eye. Illustrations to comparative and pathological anatomy, embryology, and microanatomy have not been included. There are close interrelationships of art and anatomy; we hope that this book will assist those who are considering such things.

The text is about anatomists, their collaborators, and their books, but is also about the contexts in which anatomical illustrations were prepared and distributed. We have included extensive quotations from anatomical atlases that throw light on these questions.

During our search through illustrated works of anatomy we came to realize the intriguing complexities inherent in each picture. What was shown, and the way it was shown, depended on the anatomist's and the artist's didactic intentions, and on their understanding of anatomical science. But it depended also on so much else: the training they received; the society, and the professional milieu, in which they worked; the technology used; the economic and administrative arrangements made to produce and sell the work; the anatomist's and artist's attitude to the living and the dead human body ... We hope that this anthology may assist historians of medicine, science, and art by providing a well-illustrated narrative about anatomical atlases; some of the themes that have emerged may lead to more detailed, specific study.

Each plate chosen has a commentary, essentially in the form of a critique of the anatomy illustrated, its felicities and its short-comings. These comments, not intended as a comprehensive review of all the anatomy shown, will be of particular interest to students of medicine and anatomy.

One author (KBR) has written the text, the other (JDWT), the anatomical commentary on the plates. We have assisted each other in preparing our respective sections.

We have confined ourselves to works on paper, and have not considered any form of anatomical model. We selected the plates, by consensus, from books in private and academic libraries. Many have been called from the stacks, but few have been chosen.

The primary sources of this book are thus illustrated works of anatomy, consulted in libraries in Canada, Britain, Continental Europe, and the United States of America. References to many of these books occur in appropriate places in the text. At the end of each chapter we have included a *Selected Reading* list to indicate some of the secondary sources that have proved useful. We hope readers may find in these lists an introduction to the relevant literature. By judicious use of the references cited in the text and of the *Selected Reading* lists, it is possible to investigate the original sources for quotations. In this way we have avoided intrusive footnoting, and provided for the general reader an uninterrupted narrative.

A few key books have been consulted frequently. To these authorities we wish to acknowledge our particular indebtedness. We are delighted to call our reader's attention to these by listing them at the end of the Preface. We have benefited particularly by consulting the erudite writings of the late Robert Herrlinger and of K. F. Russell of Melbourne.

For the names of the older anatomists and their collaborators, we have usually employed the vernacular rather than the Latin form. However, the author of the *Fabrica* is so well known in the English-speaking countries as Andreas Vesalius, rather than André Vésale, Andres Vesalio, Andres van Wesale, or Wesal, and his publisher as Oporinus, and not Herbst, that in these and in some other cases we have retained the Latin usage. We have had to decide arbitrarily on the spelling of other personal names—Platter rather than Plater, for instance. For place names we have generally followed Moore's *Penguin encyclopedia of places*.

In 1852 in Leipzig, the scholar and physician Ludwig Choulant published an excellent treatise on the history and bibliography of anatomical illustration, whose full title was: *Geschichte und Bibliographie der anatomischen Abbildung nach ihrer Beziehung auf anatomische Wissenschaft und bildende Kunst*. Around 1915 Mortimer Frank, an ophthalmological surgeon and medical historian from Chicago, began a translation of Choulant's book. It was published, posthumously, in 1920 by the University of Chicago Press, and reprinted in revised form by H. Schuman in New York,

1945, with essays by F. H. Garrison, E. C. Streeter, C. Singer, and Mortimer Frank himself.

Before we started this present book we read Frank's expanded English language edition of Choulant's work on anatomical illustration. However, in order not to be influenced unduly, we laid it aside when we came to write our first drafts; it has certainly not been our purpose to rewrite or update Choulant–Frank, though a modern reference work, along the lines of that book, would be invaluable to students of anatomy, medical illustration, and art history. When completing our draft manuscript we returned, with benefit, to Choulant–Frank.

In the early days of research into our subject we visited libraries in Canada, particularly the Osler Library at McGill University, the Woodward Biomedical Library at the University of British Columbia, and the Fisher Rare Book Library at the University of Toronto. We were then privileged to be allowed to search through the practically inexhaustible collections at the Library of the Wellcome Institute in London, the Countway Library of Medicine in Boston, and the Cushing Collection of the Yale Medical Historical Library. More recently we have relied heavily on the holdings in the Cambridge University Library, the Library of Gonville and Caius College, Cambridge, the Bodleian Library of Oxford University, and, in London, the Libraries of the Royal Society of Medicine, the Royal College of Surgeons, the Royal College of Obstetricians and Gynaecologists, and the British Library. The fine collection first assembled in the eighteenth century by William Hunter, and housed, since his death, in Glasgow University, provided a rich source of books, manuscripts, and drawings. We were grateful to have been allowed to see at Leiden University the anatomical drawings that Wandelaar made for Albinus. The anatomical sketches of Stubbs were examined at the Yale Centre for British Art, New Haven.

We owe a large debt of gratitude to these and other libraries; without the knowledge and co-operation of their librarians, and the skill of their photographers, our work would not have been possible.

We have had access on a continuing basis to a private collection of anatomical atlases purchased from the Anatomy Department of the London Hospital Medical College in 1965 by May Roberts, then of The Bookshop, Blackheath, London, now of Cambridge. It was her enterprise which sowed the seeds of our endeavour; her help and encouragement have continued since.

In 1981 one of us prepared an exhibition of anatomical illustrations under the title *Maps of the Body*. It was shown at the Art Gallery of Memorial University of Newfoundland (MUN), and toured a number of Canadian cities. The favourable response of the general public, as well as of artists and members of the health professions, encouraged us to explore the subject more widely.

Many in the Medical School of MUN have given us help, at much cost to their time. Without the assistance of the Deans, and the facilities of the Health Sciences Library, and Medical Audio-Visual Services, we would not have been able to prepare our book.

Mimi Cazort, Curator of Prints and Drawings at the National Gallery of Canada; John Ryder, who knows so much about books and their design; Sir James Gowans; Jane Lewis of the London

School of Economics; Jim Hansen and Marlene Creates, artists; Monique Kornell of the Warburg Institute, London; and Sandra Raphael, authority on botanic illustration, have each educated us and given us encouragement and valued support.

The commentary to each of our plates begins by acknowledging the source of the original illustration from which our photograph was taken. For the most part we have used the earliest edition available to us. We are grateful to the owners for giving us permission to reproduce these illustrations. Acknowledgements are made on p. xix with respect to the plates and text figures.

We wish to thank particularly Philip Teigen, Marilyn Fransiszyn, and Faith Wallis at the Osler Library; Lee Perry at the Woodward Library; Richard Wolfe at the Countway Library; Ferenc Gyorgyey and Susan Alon at Yale; Eric Freeman, William Schupbach, and the late Renate Burgess at the Library of the Wellcome Institute; H. J. Heaney and P. K. Escreet at Glasgow University Library; Brian Jenkins at Cambridge University Library; Alison Sproston at Gonville and Caius College Library; and Catherine Quinlan at the Health Sciences Library, MUN. We would like to acknowledge Caroline Stone's permission to expand her succinct account of printing techniques, which appeared first in a catalogue by Sylvia Bendzsa of our exhibition *Maps of the Body*. Albert Cox, long-term Dean of Medicine at MUN, supported our work throughout.

Brian Payton has been an unfailing help, personally with advice and support and also as Director of Medical Audio-Visual Services at MUN.

Without the skill of photographers at the institutions listed in the attributions to each plate we could not have collected together this anthology of illustrations. In this regard we would particularly like to acknowledge the forbearance and professional excellence of Eugene Ryan and his colleagues, MUN, who photographed the plates and figures from volumes in a private collection. Also at MUN, Cliff George and Sylvia Ficken have drawn the maps and John Bear has assisted us by reading critically drafts of early chapters.

Our manuscript, as it has been produced and then modified time after time, has over the years been entered into the word-processor by Barbara Ryder, Beatrice Schinagl, June Vallis, Sharon Brenton, but principally Mary Fennessey. We value their friendship and acknowledge their patience, skill, and hard work.

In so many ways we have been indebted to the support of Jane Tomlinson, and we have valued throughout the practical encouragement of our friends Deborah Hyam and Penny Hansen.

We have also received help and advice from many other people in addition to those named above, to all of whom we extend our thanks. We are, of course, solely responsible for errors incorporated into our book.

It may be noted here that the original size of each anatomical illustration reproduced as a plate is given in centimetres, height first and width second. In intaglio prints, here referred to under the generic, common name of engravings (see p. xvii), the size of the blind impression of the metal plate is noted, in relief and lithographic plates, and those originally produced photographically, the given dimensions are those of the image itself.

We wish to end these introductory remarks by recognizing the immense labours of those who have produced complex works of scientific anatomy. For example, to illustrate the *Fabrica*, 1543, the artists who made the woodcuts must have utilized around 400 precise drawings, some simple, many complex. The finished drawings were probably preceded by an anatomical sketch made by Vesalius himself or by an artist under his supervision. Again under his scrutiny, the drawing was reproduced in relief on the surface of a woodblock. Vesalius started these tasks soon after the publication of the *Tabulae anatomicae* in 1538; he completed them within four years, for the finished woodcuts were transported to Basle before Vesalius made the same journey to oversee the printing of his book. On average then, through four years, a new anatomical drawing was made every four days.

There are many books of anatomy that are as fully illustrated as the *Fabrica*, but few where so much was accompanied within the lifetimes of the anatomist and artist. The dedication of such persons to this precise task, and the excellence of the extraordinary and moving images that so often resulted, excites our admiration and gratitude.

August, 1990   KBR
                                                                               JDWT

Select bibliography

Bayle, A. L. J. and Thillaye, A. J. (1855). *Biographie médicale* ... A. Delahaye, Paris. (Reprinted, B. M., Israel, Amsterdam, 1967.)

Bynum, W. F., Browne, E. J., and Porter, R. (ed.) (1983). *Dictionary of the history of science.* The Macmillan Press, London.

Choulant, L. (1945). *History and bibliography of anatomic illustration.* Ed M. Frank. Schuman, New York.

Clair, C. (1976). *A history of European printing.* Academic Press, London.

Clarke, E. and Dewhurst, K. (1972). *An illustrated history of brain function.* Sandford, Oxford.

Clendening, L. (1960). *Source book of medical history.* Dover, New York. (Reprint of 1942 edition.)

Cole, F. J. (1975). *A history of comparative anatomy. . . .* Dover, New York. (Reprint of 1949 edition.)

Cushing, H. W. (1943). *A bio-bibliography of Andreas Vesalius.* Schuman, New York.

Febvre, L. and Martin, H. J. (1984). *The coming of the book: the impact of printing 1450–1800,* (trans. D. Gerard). Verso, London.

Gillispie, C. C. (Editor in Chief) (1970 etc). *Dictionary of scientific biography.* C. Scribner's Sons, New York.

Godfrey, R. T. (1978). *Printmaking in Britain: a general history. . . .* Phaidon, Oxford.

Herrlinger, R. (1970). *History of medical illustration from antiquity to AD 1600* (trans. G. Fulton-Smith). Pitman, London.

Herrlinger, R. and Putscher, M. (1972). *Geschichte der medizinischen Abbildung: Vol. 2, Von 1600 bis 1972.* Heinz Moos, Munich.

Hind, A. M. (1963). *A history of engraving and etching. . . .* Dover, New York. (Reprint of 1923 edition.)

Hind, A. M. (1963). *An introduction to a history of woodcut. . . .* Dover, New York. (Reprint of 1935 edition.)

McEvedy, C. (no dates). *The Penguin atlases of history: ancient, medieval and modern.* Penguin, Harmondsworth.

Mayor, A. H. (1971). *Prints and people: a social history of printed pictures.* The Metropolitan Museum, New York.

Mayor, A. H. (1984). *Artists and anatomists.* The Metropolitan Museum of Art, New York.

Moore, W. G. (1971). *The Penguin encyclopedia of places.* Penguin, Harmondsworth.

Morton, L. T. (1970). *A medical bibliography (Garrison and Morton)....* Andre Deutsch, London.

Munk, W. (1878 and later). *The role of the Royal College of Physicians of London: comprising biographical sketches....* Royal College of Physicians, London.

O'Malley, C. D. (ed.) (1970). *The history of medical education.* University of California Press, Berkeley.

Premuda, L. (1957). *Storia dell'iconografia anatomica.* Aldo Martello, Milan.

Russell, K. F. (1963). *British anatomy 1525–1800....* Melbourne University Press. (Reissued: St Paul's Bibliographies, Winchester, 1987.)

Stillwell, M. B. (1970). *The awakening interest in science during the first century of printing 1450–1550....* The Bibliographical Society of America, New York.

Thornton, J. L. (1966). *Medical books, libraries and collectors....* Andre Deutsch, London.

Notes on printing techniques

The transmission of anatomical knowledge depends on an ability to produce many precisely-identical images. This is only possible through some form of printing; the main methods used to print anatomical illustrations up to 1850 are the following:

WOODCUT.   A relief process. A block of wood is carved so that the artist's image stands in relief. The surface parts of the block are rolled with ink, and paper pressed down upon it to receive the image.

This method was used in pre-Vesalian printed anatomy books and by Vesalius' block-makers in Venice during the sixteenth century. For book production, the woodcut's advantage was that both illustration and text could be incorporated and printed together.

For a woodcut, the planed face of a piece of wood, such as pear, is cut away leaving a relief surface to be inked and printed. In the technique of *wood engraving*, developed in the late eighteenth century, the sawn end surface of very hard wood, such as box, is prepared using a graving tool, or burin. The outstanding unengraved surface is again inked and printed, but sometimes the artist works in 'negative' with the drawing showing white in the print on a black background.

ENGRAVING.   An intaglio process. Using a gouging tool known as a burin or graver, the artist cuts lines into a metal printing plate. Ink is applied to the plate, then wiped off the unengraved surfaces so that some ink remains in the grooves formed by the engraved lines. Paper is laid on the plate, pressure applied by means of 'wringer-type' or roller press so that it is forced down to pick up the ink in the grooves, and the image is transferred. The anatomists

Woodcut

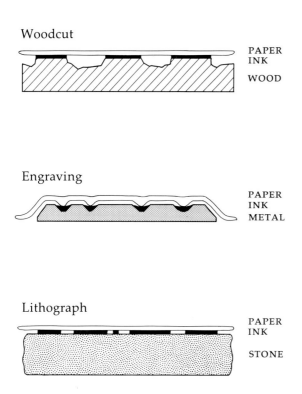

PAPER
INK
WOOD

Engraving

PAPER
INK
METAL

Lithograph

PAPER
INK

STONE

Bidloo and Albinus employed this method in their finely detailed illustrations during the seventeenth and eighteenth centuries. However, unlike woodcuts, engraved plates could not be printed at the same time as book text.

In this book, all intaglio prints have been called 'engravings', even though in some the grooves in the metal plate that retain the ink may have been made not by a burin but by acid etching. Intaglio prints may be prepared by etching the main outlines and then finishing the details with the burin. Since we have no expertise in this field, we decided that it would divert us from our main purposes if we attempted to define each intaglio print reproduced in our anthology in terms of the relative contributions of engraving and etching.

LITHOGRAPHY. A planographic process. Invented in 1798, this printing process is based on the fact that grease and water repel each other. Marks are applied to a limestone or metal printing plate with a lithographic grease crayon or liquid 'tusche'. After chemically fixing the drawing, the stone is moistened with water which settles on the unmarked areas. Ink is rolled over the whole; it adheres where the grease drawing has been. In traditional lithography, paper is laid on the plate, pressure applied by a flat-bed scraper press, and the image printed. This process permitted faithful reproduction of a lifelike drawing. The Victorian Maclise and many others made anatomical illustrations in this way.

Acknowledgements for the illustrations

We wish gratefully to thank all who have allowed us to reproduce, either as plates or text figures, the majority of the illustrations in this book.

By gracious permission of Her Majesty Queen Elizabeth II, Plates 22–27 and text figures 4.1–4.5, from the Leonardo collection in the Royal Library, Windsor.

By courtesy of the Wellcome Institute Library, London, Plates 7, 9,12–20, 21(b), 29, 33, 36, 51, 52, 54, 60, 65–69, 80–82, 84–91, 99, 101, 109–111, 113–117, 119, 120, 125, and 126 and text figures 1.3, 3.1, 3.2, 3.4–3.8(b), 3.9(a & b), 6.1(b), 6.2–6.5, 7.7(b), 7.9, 8.4, 8.10, 10.1–10.5, 11.2, and 12.4.

By permission of the Syndics of Cambridge University Library, Plates 10, 11, 28, 30–31, 35, 39–45, 53, 55–57, 59, 70–73, 79, 83, 93–94, 100, 104–105, 108, 127–129 and text figures 2.17, 5.13, 6.8–6.9, 6.12, 8.5, 8.8(b), 8.14, 9.2–9.3, 12.1, and 12.3.

By courtesy of the Librarian, Glasgow University Library, Plates 58, 97, 98 and text figures 1.2, 5.7, 6.10–6.11, 7.5, 7.6(a & b), 7.7(a), 11.7, 11.15, and 12.2.

By courtesy of the Bodleian Library, Oxford, Plates 1, 2 and text figures 2.3–2.8.

By courtesy of the Francis A. Countway Library of Medicine, Boston MA, Plates 106, 112 and text figures 11.10–11.11, 11.16 and 13.3–13.5.

By courtesy of Yale Medical Historical Library, New Haven CT, Plates 21(a), 37, 38 and text figures 8.6 & 8.7.

By courtesy of Pitman Publishing, London, text figures 2.10, 2.12, and 2.16.

By permission of the Master & Fellows of Gonville and Caius College, Cambridge, Plate 3.

By courtesy of the British Library, London, Plate 8.

By courtesy of Professor R. M. H. McMinn & Mr R. T. Hutchings, Plate 134.

By courtesy of the University of Basle Library, Plate 4.

By courtesy of the Bibliothèque royale Albert 1er, Bruxelles, text-figure 2.18.

By courtesy of the Royal Library, Stockholm, Plate 5(a & b).

By courtesy of the Metropolitan Museum of Art, New York, text figure 5.8.

By courtesy of Williams & Wilkins, Baltimore, Plate 132.

By courtesy of W. B. Saunders Company, Baltimore, Plate 131

By courtesy of Amsterdam Historisch Museum, text figure 8.3.

By courtesy of the Woodward Biomedical Library, University of British Columbia, Vancouver, text figure 8.8(a).

By courtesy of Urban & Schwarzenberg GmbH, München, Plate 130.

By courtesy of Cornell University Press, text figure 6.13, from Howard B. Adelmann: The Embryological Treatises of Hieronymus Fabricius of Aquapendente, copyright 1942.

By courtesy of CIBA–GEIGY Corporation, copyright 1971. Reproduced with permission from the *Ciba collection of medical illustrations* by Frank H. Netter, MD. All rights reserved.

Anatomists, scribes, and printers

1

*I*N THIS chapter, we outline the development of scientific anatomy in the Alexandrian medical schools, the subsequent work of synthesis by Galen in the second century A D, and the preservation of ancient anatomical knowledge in Byzantine, Arabic, and Renaissance writings. The uses made of illustrations in anatomical manuscripts are compared with the purposes served by the woodcuts found in early printed books.

The beginnings of scientific anatomy

To understand human anatomy it is necessary to dissect, to cut apart and show the intricate patterns and relationships of the body's structures.

For a period around 300 B C human dissection was first practised, and the study of anatomy flourished, at the periphery of the ancient classical world. Alexander the Great of Macedonia had laid out a new city on the Mediterranean near the delta of the Nile. When he died in 323 B C, one of his generals, Ptolemy Soter, made Alexandria the centre of his empire. Greek scholarship was encouraged, and a school of medicine was founded that emphasized anatomy as studied by dissection of the human body. There is insufficient evidence to support the

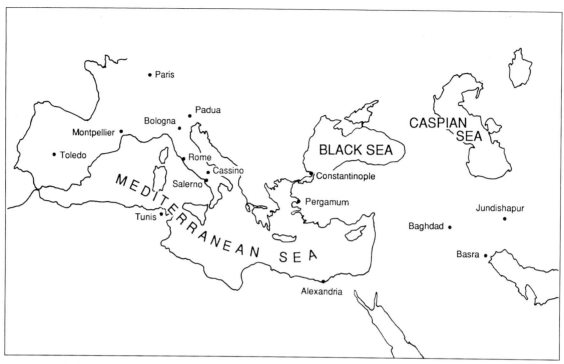

1.1 Map of The Mediterranean and Middle East showing places mentioned in this chapter.

scurrilous accusations of Celsus and St Augustine, made centuries later, that dissection of live human beings was practised at Alexandria. Although this city remained a centre for medical study for centuries, human dissection there had certainly lapsed by the time Egypt finally came under direct Roman rule following the death in 30 BC of Cleopatra, the last of the Ptolemies.

In the second century after Christ, the Greek physician Galen (c.129–199) codified what was known of anatomy—much from Alexandrian sources—and formulated a theoretically coherent system to explain the workings of the structures he described. Galen came from Pergamum in Asia Minor, another centre of Greek learning since the second century BC, which at one time had possessed a great library. He travelled throughout the eastern Mediterranean, making a visit to Alexandria, where he studied a human skeleton remaining from an earlier period. Galen spent much of his professional life in Rome, serving as physician to Marcus Aurelius and other emperors. In Galen's anatomical writings each structure has a described purpose; form and function are both related to that end—the whole demonstrates 'infinite wisdom'. In this Galen supported the Aristotelian view that all animals have been fitly equipped with the best possible bodies. He described the body, in his book *On the usefulness of parts*, as a 'sacred discourse [composed] as a true hymn of praise to our Creator'. Such views endeared him to later religious authorities, both Christian and Islamic. Galen did not dissect humans, but he had learnt much from careful dissection and study of animals, particularly pigs and Barbary 'apes'. The information gained was applied to human anatomy, sometimes, of course, erroneously.

Much of the scholarship and knowledge of the Greeks was preserved in the post-classical period at various centres in the eastern Mediterranean, including Alexandria, where an amended and edited collation of Galen's works was produced—the *Summaria Alexandrinorum*. The Arabs captured Alexandria in AD 642, during the period of rapid expansion when they established their religion and influence over Syria, Egypt, and Mesopotamia. Many Greek texts came into their hands. A more important way in which Greek texts were preserved for the Arabs was through the intermediary of the Nestorian Christians, whose language, Syriac, is still used in the liturgy of some churches in the Middle East, but is otherwise virtually extinct. Greek medical texts were translated into Syriac in the Nestorian cultural centre of Jundishapur in Persia in the periods before, and, more particularly, after its conquest by the forces of Islam in the seventh century AD. Prominent among the Jundishapur Christian translators was Hunayn ibn-Is'haq, known in the west as Johannitius (*c.*809–*c.*877). Successive caliphs in Baghdad supported Hunayn in his scholarly endeavours to compare and translate the best available Greek medical manuscripts. It is to Hunayn that we owe the annotated list of 129 books of Galen known in the ninth century. Sometimes he translated directly from Greek to Arabic—he had visited Byzantium, possibly Greece and Basra in order to perfect his knowledge of these languages; sometimes he appears to have put the Greek text into Syriac, leaving his nephew to prepare the Arabic version.

Galen's work of anatomy, *On anatomical procedures*, is known today in part through manuscripts in Greek; however, the last third of the work is available only through a thousand-year-old Arabic translation. The anatomical texts were preserved and discussed by the Arabic physicians, but not significantly added to; there were strong objections to human dissection in Islam.

Contact between Italy and the Arabic settlements in Sicily and the eastern Mediterranean increased from the ninth century onwards. From the eleventh century, the works of Galen became more widely known in western Europe through translations from the Arabic into Latin. About 1080, Constantine the African (d. 1087) composed *Liber pantegni* (The whole art), based on *Kitab al-malaki* ('The royal book'), written by Ali ibn al Abbas al-Majusi, a scholar known to the Christian world as Haly Abbas (d. 994). Constantine is thought to have been born a Muslim in Tunis—even perhaps to have studied in Baghdad—but to have spent the last years of his life as a Benedictine monk in Italy at Monte Cassino. In *The royal book* al-Majusi had attempted to present medicine, including anatomy, in its entirety, his compilation being based extensively on Galen.

Constantine's book circulated at the medical school at Salerno, not far from Naples. This centre had developed under the influence of Islamic, Jewish, and Christian—both Italian and Greek—scholars. By the beginning of the twelfth century systematic anatomical dissection was practised there; but the subjects were pigs, not humans. Nevertheless, actual exploration of anatomical structures was being regularly employed, both for investigation and for the training of medical students, for the first time since the Alexandrians fifteen hundred years previously.

The work describing the procedures used, *Anatomia porci*, was later mistakenly attributed to Copho of Salerno, who remains otherwise unidentified. This, and the handful of other anatomy texts known from the twelfth and thirteenth centuries, was influenced not only by Constantine's translations but also by those of Gerard (Gherardo) of Cremona (1114–87). He worked in Moorish Toledo, and translated into Latin the Arabic texts of Abu Ali ibn-Sina (Avicenna) (d. 1037) and Muhammad ar-Razi (Rhazes) (d. 923).

In the early fourteenth century, Galen's book of functional anatomy *On the usefulness of parts* was translated from Greek directly into Latin—a translation perhaps by Nicolo da Reggio that was to survive to be the basis for many printed versions. But Galen's *On anatomical procedures* was not translated into Latin until the sixteenth century.

At the beginning of the thirteenth century four major medical centres in Europe were Salerno and Bologna in Italy, and Montpellier and Paris in France. Anatomy was taught from Arabic sources, which were, in turn, almost exclusively dependent on Galenic originals; recourse was sometimes made to dissections of the pig. By the end of the century, however, human dissections were being carried out at Bologna. In 1302 a post-mortem examination was recorded as a not unusual happening; and, by 1316, Mondino de' Luzzi (Raimondino, Mundinus: *c.* 1275–1326) had written what was essentially a dissection manual, *Anatomia* (or *Anothomia*) *corporis humani*, a text that was to influence anatomy for more than two hundred years. There were, prior to 1550, thirty or more printed editions of Mondino's anatomy; further editions included this manual together with the printed works of Ketham.

The French surgeon, Guy de Chauliac (*c*1300–1368), who studied at Bologna as well as Montpellier and Paris, has left a succinct description of the way in which anatomies were performed (the word *anatomy* has been used not only for the study of the structure of the body but also for the performance of an actual dissection):

Having laid the dead body on the table, [the anatomist] made four lessons on it. In the first the digestive members were treated since they decay the soonest. In the second the spiritual members, in the third, the animal organs and in the fourth the extremities were treated. And following the commentary ... [by Galen] there are nine things to see: that is to know the situation, the substance, the constitution, the number, the figure, the relations of connections, the actions and the uses and the diseases which affect them. Thus from anatomy the physician may gain assistance and aid in the knowledge of diseases, in the prognosis and in the cure. We make anatomies also on bodies dried in the sun, or consumed in the earth, or immersed in running or boiling water. This shows us the anatomy at least of the bones, cartilages, joints, large nerves, tendons, and ligaments. By these two means we must teach anatomy on the bodies of men, apes, pigs, and many other animals, and not from pictures as done by Henri [Henri de Mondeville], who had thirteen pictures for the demonstration of anatomy.

There are illustrations of dissections in miniatures, painted at a somewhat later date, that give vivid impressions of academic dissections. The scene included in one fifteenth-century manuscript shows a pedestalled dissecting table set outside Renaissance buildings (Fig. 1.2). Flowering plants are on the ground. On the table is the naked corpse of a woman. Incisions

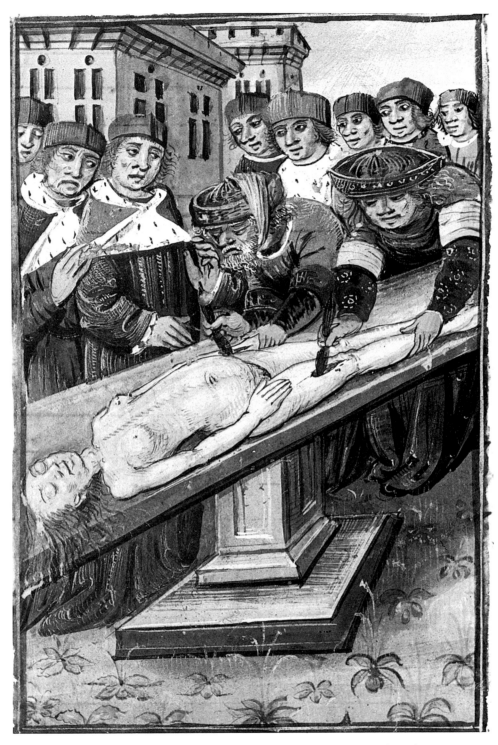

1.2 Dissection scene, fifteenth century. The original miniature is brightly coloured.
(Hunterian MS G, fo. 22, recto. University of Glasgow Library.)

are being made in the thigh and forearm by two sumptuously clothed laymen, while academics, some with ermine capes, crowd around the dissection, which, as was not uncommon, was carried out in the open air and not in a specifically built demonstration theatre. It should be remembered that, at the time of Mondino, universities had no permanent buildings.

The frequency of anatomical demonstrations at Bologna is not known; but Mondino writes that he dissected two female subjects in 1315, and probably more males were used than females. Some of the cadavers were obtained after execution by hanging or beheading. Later, in the fourteenth and fifteenth centuries, dissection at some centres was a rare, perhaps only an annual, event, or one carried out every second, third or fourth year; thus, each student might see only one anatomy during his training. Even in Padua in the mid-sixteenth century, when it was pre-eminent in anatomy, there was a gap of two or three years when no anatomical demonstrations were given.

Dissections were performed in order to demonstrate Galen's veracity—the Arabs and their translators had relied on his texts—much as a present-day student might dissect, placing reliance on the accuracy of anatomical textbooks. Where there were obvious differences between what the dissection revealed and the text, then the latter was suspected of having been erroneously copied or translated from the original authority; undoubtedly this was sometimes true.

Anatomists and humanists

Until the invention of printing, books were disseminated by making manuscript copies—and scribes could miscopy. Words, written in a language known to literate copyists, have a certain inherent resistance to misreading or mistranscription, even when the redundancy which assists accurate identification is reduced by the use of abbreviations. But when the subject matter was unfamiliar to the scribe, and especially when translations were made from Greek to Arabic to Latin, errors could be perpetuated and texts corrupted. Since dissections were not performed in the Arabic world, words necessarily became divorced from structures; there was no agreed nomenclature, and medieval terminology included terms in all three languages.

In the thirteenth century there was a stronger growth of classical scholarship in Italy, and, beginning in the fifteenth century, a particular study of Greek works, which was assisted by an influx of Greek scholars following the fall of Constantinople in 1453. Some of these Renaissance humanists concerned themselves with Greek anatomical texts, and faced directly the problems presented by their ambiguities, in a determination to recover, through intensive study of the written language and by comparisons between many texts, the purity of the Greek originals. The recovery of the learning of the Greeks was the major academic work of many university teachers of anatomy throughout the fifteenth and into the sixteenth centuries—a valid, scholarly approach if one could accept the premise that the Greeks had discovered all, or nearly all, things. Günther of Andernach in Paris, John Caius in England, and even, in a small way, Vesalius in Padua contributed to re-establishing authentic Greek texts.

However, new knowledge of anatomy could be acquired only by reference to actual human bodies, not to Greek manuscripts. During the fourteenth and fifteenth centuries some anatomists, for the first time, became willing to point out differences between the actual anatomy seen in dissections and that which Galen had described and recorded, even in the best available texts. In this they were, perhaps, encouraged by what Galen himself had written:

[The student must] learn thoroughly all that has been said by the most illustrious of the Ancients. And when he has learnt this, then, for a prolonged period, he must test and prove it, observing what part of it is in agreement, and what is disagreement with obvious fact; thus he will choose this and turn away from that. [*On the natural faculties,* **3**, 10.]

If anyone wishes to observe the works of nature, he should put his trust not in books on anatomy but in his own eyes and either come to me, or consult one of my associates, or alone by himself industriously practise exercises in dissection. [*On the usefulness of parts,* **2**, 3.]

Anatomy and illustrations

The knowledge gained by dissection had to be transmitted to others, but the complexities of anatomy were (and still are) difficult to describe and remember. At Salerno, medical practice had been systematized in the form of verses—more easily memorable than prose; but this method was not easily adaptable to anatomy. Words alone, especially as there was no agreed nomenclature, were tedious and difficult to memorize, often obscure in meaning, and called to mind but an uncertain recollection of the actual anatomical appearances of dissections made months or years previously. Between such dissections only the skeleton was available for reference; other parts could not be studied, for it was not until the late seventeenth century that adequate methods of preservation began to be used. The situation around 1500 was described by Leonardo da Vinci in his notebooks, and his views are just as relevant today as when they were written:

I counsel you not to cumber yourself with words unless you are speaking to the blind ... How in words can you describe this heart without filling a whole book? Yet the more detail you write concerning it the more you will confuse the mind of the hearer.

What could be done to make the subject more intelligible and memorable? During anatomical dissection and in the schoolroom the professor could attempt to resolve complex anatomical structures by simple analogies with reference to common objects, or to simple geometrical or architectural figures. These would in turn appear in notes as words, or—and here a new element is introduced—as simple diagrams. Diagrams could indicate topology even if they did not convey the dimensions, proportions, or appearances of the parts being considered. Such diagrams are found in books of anatomy from medieval times to the present day.

It is also possible to attempt to reproduce not only the pattern but also the actual appearance of the organs as revealed by dissection: to represent in two dimensions what can be seen in the round. The word *image* may be used to indicate such representation; this word can also embrace the pictorial translation of structures seen during dissection into a representation of those of a supposed living person. Anatomical images can, therefore, represent either the actual appearance of a dissection, or alternatively the make-believe appearance of a living being as that person might appear had dissection been performed without the loss of life (or indeed loss of *sang-froid* or even *sang-chaud*)—in this way evincing at the same time both a stoicism and a miraculous physiology: a remarkable conceit.

Scribes and printers

When anatomical images were attempted in the years before 1500, two great problems required resolution.

First, the difficulty of representing what was revealed by dissection when presented with different anatomical arrangements from those described in the Galenic texts. Whereas a diagram can more readily accommodate expected forms, representational images cannot easily do so; however Leonardo da Vinci, for example, drew non-existent, but textually required, structures on images of dissections.[1]

Secondly, when copied, images readily degenerate, but the essential aspects of diagrams may remain intact. Images copied by scribes, who probably knew little or nothing of anatomy, would be debased, and quite without the didactic significance of a diagram prepared by an anatomist. When copied, true anatomical diagrams, like words in a known language, can correct themselves, and may preserve their form; but attempts at representation, the images of anatomy, are doomed to alteration and debasement every time a copy is made, and every time a copy is made of a copy the mistakes are perpetuated and multiplied.[2]

Printing with movable type, an invention of the mid-fifteenth century, had spread to many European countries twenty-five years later. Although this has long been recognized as one of the turning points in human history, the precise impact of printing has only recently begun to be studied. In anatomy, there was little initial advance in substance, but much advance in scholarship and in the dissemination of authoritative texts. The first printed Greek edition of Galen's collected works came from the Aldine Press in Venice in 1525, and the first Latin *Opera* of Galen had been published in Venice in 1490.

---

[1] More modern examples of failures of perception might be given: microscopists had looked at microscopical preparations of the pancreas without seeing the islets until Langerhans perceived them; and until the 1950s haematologists had observed, described, and pictured neutrophil polymorphonuclear leucocytes without noticing the sex chromatin drumsticks that were present in such cells only when they belonged to females.

[2] In the trenches of the First World War, messages were whispered from one soldier to another along the line. A message, it was said, started as 'we are going to advance, send reinforcements', but reached the end as 'we are going to a dance, send three and fourpence'.

It now became worth while to add images to texts of anatomy, since it is a characteristic of printed illustrations that they are reproduced identically, or very nearly identically, each time an impression is taken. Once the publishers could make identically-printed illustrated anatomical works available simultaneously in Bologna, Padua, Paris, and other centres, then it became much easier to appraise excellence and criticize error. Alterations could be made in later editions; succeeding writers could retain good points and correct mistakes when preparing new illustrated texts.

The first great impetus to anatomical knowledge in early Renaissance Europe was the recognition that much could be learnt from the writings of the Greeks and Arabs. The second was public and scholastic recognition that human dissection was an activity proper to medical schools. The multiple error-free reproduction of images may be regarded as the next, and possibly the most important, step in anatomical studies. Once this was possible the subject was able to develop largely by the accretion of new or more accurate facts.

In an image of human anatomy, the complicated pattern of any system (of the heart and blood-vessels, for example), or of any region (the axilla, for example) appears to a newcomer to be muddled; images are not as easily memorized as diagrams. They can, however, be readily

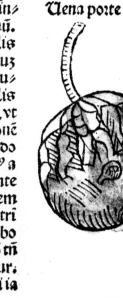

1.3 Liver diagram from Hundt *Antropologium*, Leipzig, 1501. Woodcut.

used for reference when a human corpse is not available for anatomizing. In periods when the supply of cadavers did not meet the demands of medical students, illustrated anatomical books were used extensively; when cadavers were available and when there was a universally accepted terminology which enabled unambiguous descriptions, then illustrations were used for different purposes. When the subject of anatomy extends to *function* and to *development* then new methods of communication become more useful—and diagrams, in new forms, come into their own again. For example, computer-derived video images may be used to demonstrate the complex anatomy of the brain, or animated cartoons to show embryological development.

A sequence has been suggested, and will be described further, whereby anatomical texts were supplemented by diagrams, and then, with the onset of printing, by representational images. As in every historical change, this sequence is only discernible by analysis of selected examples; in the transitional period the two traditions overlap. *Figure* 1.3 shows a woodcut diagram of the liver from Hundt, *Antropologium* ..., 1501, which is in the same style as many simple diagrams of organs found in manuscripts two hundred years or more earlier. As we shall see, some fine printed illustrations of the early sixteenth century, including Vesalius' early work, perpetuate the older schematic drawing; some anatomical drawings of Leonardo da Vinci combine realistic representations with elements derived from earlier diagrams.

With these general comments as background, we can return to the medical centres of Europe to consider the role of illustration in early anatomical texts.

Chapter 1: Selected reading

Galen

Brock, A. J. (1963). *Galen: On the natural faculties.* Harvard University Press, Cambridge, MA.

Christie, R. V. (1987). Galen on Erasistratus. *Perspect. Biol. Med.,* **30,** 440–9.

Duckworth, W. L. H. (ed.) (1962). *Galen: On anatomical procedures.* Cambridge University Press.

Hoolihan, C. (1986). The transmission of Greek medical literature from antiquity to the renaissance. *Med. Heritage,* **2,** 430–42.

Lloyd, G. E. R. (1973). *Greek science after Aristotle.* Chatto and Windus, London.

May, M. T. (ed.) (1968). *Galen: On the usefulness of the parts of the body.* Cornell University Press, Ithaca, N.Y.

Singer, C. (ed.) (1956). *Galen: On anatomical procedures. . . .* Wellcome Historical Medical Museum, London.

Temkin, O. (1973). *Galenism: Rise and decline of a medical philosphy.* Cornell University Press, Ithaca.

Arabic medicine

Anawati, G. C. and Iskander, A. Z. (1978). Hunayn ibn 'Ishaq. *Dict. sci. Biog* **15,** 230–49.

Campbell, D. (1973). *Arabian medicine and its influence on the middle ages.* Kegan Paul, Trench, Trubner, London. (1926, reprinted by AMS, 1973.)

Elgood, C. (1979). *A medical history of Persia and the eastern Caliphate.* APA-Philo Press, Amsterdam. (Reprint of 1951 edn).

Ullmann, M. (1978). *Islamic medicine.* Edinburgh University Press.

Weitzmann, K. (1952). The Greek sources of Islamic scientific illustrations. In *Archaeologica orientalia* in memoriam *Ernst Herzfeld* (ed. G. C. Miles). J. J. Augustin, Locust Valley, NY.

Middle Ages

Clark, J. M. (1950). *The dance of death in the middle ages and the renaissance.* Jackson, Glasgow.

Corner, G. W. (1927). *Anatomical texts of the earlier middle ages.* Carnegie Institution, Washington.

Crombie, A. C. (1969). *Augustine to Galileo. 1: Science in the middle ages 5th to 13th centuries.* Penguin, Harmondsworth.

Jones, P. M. (1984). *Medieval medical miniatures.* The British Library, London.

Lindberg, D. C. (1978). The transmission of Greek and Arabic learning to the west. In *Science in the middle ages* (ed. D. C. Lindberg). University of Chicago Press.

Singer, C. (1955). A study in early renaissance anatomy. In *Studies in the history and method of science.* Dawson, London. (Reprint of 1917 edn.)

Sudhoff, K. (1964). *Anatomie im Mittelalter* ... Georg Olms, Hildesheim. (Reprint of 1908 edn.)

Weitzmann, K. (1959). *Ancient book illumination.* Harvard University Press, Cambridge, MA.

Weitzmann, K. (1977). *Late antique and early Christian book illumination.* George Braziller, New York.

Dissection

Alston, M. N. (1944). The attitude of the church towards dissection before 1500. *Bull. Hist. Med.,* **16,** 221–38.

Brown, E. A. R. (1981). Death and the human body in the later middle ages: the legislation of Boniface VIII on the division of the corpse. *Viator,* **58,** 977–86.

Edelstein, L. (1967). The history of anatomy in antiquity. In *Ancient Medicine* ed. O. and C. L. Temkin. The Johns Hopkins Press, Baltimore.

O'Neill, Y. V. (1976). Innocent III and the evolution of anatomy. *Med. Hist.,* **26,** 429–33.

Pouchelles, M. C. (1976). La prise en charge de la mort: médecine, médecins et chirurgiens devant les problèmes liés à la mort à la fin du Moyen Age (XIII–XVe/s). *Arch. europ. Sociol.,* **17,** 249–78.

Streeter, E. C. (1968). Fifteenth century miniatures of extramural dissections in *Essays on the history of medicine* ... ed. C. Singer and H. E. Sigerist. Books for Libraries Press, Freeport, N.Y. (Reprint of 1925 edn.)

Printing and illustration

Eisenstein, E. L. (1979). *The printing press as an agent of change.* Cambridge University Press.

Febvre, L. and Martin, H. J. (1984). *The coming of the book: The impact of printing 1450–1800.* Verso, London.

Ivins, W. M. (1978). *Prints and visual communication.* The MIT Press, Cambridge, MA. (Reprint of 1953 edn.)

Ivins, W. M. (1958). *How prints look. . . .* Beacon Press, Boston.

MacKinney, L. C. (1962). The beginnings of western scientific anatomy ... *Med. Hist.,* **6,** 233–9.

Sarton, G. (1962). *On the history of science,* (ed. D. Stimson) [see p. 111]. Harvard University Press, Cambridge, MA.

Stillwell, M. D. (1970) *The awakening interest in science during the first century of printing 1450–1550. . . .* The Bibliographical Society of America, New York.

2

Pre-scientific anatomical illustration

ALTHOUGH ancient pictures and sculptures of naked men and women may still be seen both at their sites of origin and in museums and libraries, no images of human anatomy survive from European antiquity. The attempted representations of human skeletons were produced for other purposes than to illustrate osteology. What might be judged anatomical illustrations can be found in some surviving manuscripts from the ninth century onwards. There was much repetition, but little scientific development until around 1500, with the private work of Leonardo da Vinci and the publication of printed illustrated anatomies.

It has been suggested that some of the illustrations made during the Middle Ages derived from figures prepared in the Alexandrian schools during the years when human dissection was practised, about 300 BC. Such illustrations would, in this case, have been copied from these supposed earlier ones, none of which have survived. Medical teaching at Alexandria continued for centuries after the practice of human dissection had lapsed. If there were illustrations, made originally with reference to an actual dissection, they would be uninterpretable hundreds of years later. If there were successive copies made they would have been without value as an aid in teaching actual anatomy, that is, the structure of the body seen when a dissection is made. As we have seen, texts have inbuilt mechanisms for self-correction, if words and sentences can be understood and if the scribe is intent on preserving the original. Such resistance to degradation does not exist in representations of complex biological forms.

Fine original pictures of plants accompany some Byzantine and Arabic manuscript herbals based on texts and, possibly illustrations of Dioscorides (Dioskurides), a Greek physician who travelled extensively in the Roman world as a military man in the years around AD 60. If the illustrator knew the particular plant that Dioscorides had named then he had the opportunity of picturing it naturalistically from an actual botanic specimen, and this sometimes he did. However, the plant may have been unknown to the illustrator or scribe. So some of these herbal illustrations appear to us to be lifelike, others purely diagrammatic, and still others, wholly imaginary.

Anatomical illustrations can only be constructed with reference to the actual object. Before the revival of dissection, illustrations were often fanciful; some were diagrams based on textual descriptions transmitted, sometimes accurately, from times when anatomical specimens were available. Others were debased copies of figures that might possibly have been used to illustrate the original texts; whatever the situation with other sciences, there is no certain indication that classical or Alexandrian anatomy texts were illustrated. It should be recalled, however, that the body of manuscript illustration extant from late antiquity and the earlier centuries of the Christian era represents only a very small proportion of the work produced during that time. 'All that is left is comparable to a few islands in an ocean reaching farther than the eye can see . . .' (Weitzmann). There were also many lost texts. There are no surviving books by the chief Alexandrians who wrote on anatomy; the work of Herophilus and Erasistratus is known because Galen and others discussed and criticized it.

If there were Alexandrian illustrations, they would have been on papyrus sheets some ten metres in length, rolled into scrolls. Egypt controlled the production of papyrus, obtainable principally in the region of the Nile. There may have been half a million scrolls in the libraries at Alexandria at the time of Cleopatra. The introduction of the codex, or book with leaves bound together, occurred in the first century AD; by the fourth century, codices had largely replaced scrolls. This made possible painted and decorated illustrations to written texts, for the leaves of a book, not being rolled, could preserve even a thickly painted image decorated with gold leaf; the paintings remained undamaged when the leaves were turned. Vellum and other animal-derived materials were used in codices; but by the early fifteenth century books were more often made of paper. Originating in China, where it had been in use since at least the second century BC, paper made of vegetable fibre was introduced into the Arabic Middle East by the ninth century, and thence into Europe around the eleventh century.

Many of the earliest surviving anatomical illustrations were simple diagrams. The liver was usually illustrated as a five-lobed structure—as Galen had taught, having dissected animals, where the liver is often multilobed; the oesophagus and stomach were indicated by diagrams which some scribes copied so carelessly that the gullet either showed no opening into the stomach or an opening into the liver. These designs conveyed an idea, sometimes erroneous, of number or relationship, but not of shape or relative size. In addition to these simple diagrams there were also more complex ones—schemata of the female and of the male genito–urinary tract, of the intestines, and of the eye and brain.

Gravida figures

Little more than symbolic were anatomical illustrations, dating from the ninth century, of babies in the womb—although 'babies' is an inappropriate term for these miniature adults, who stand on their feet or their heads, or pose as if dancing or diving, within a commodious uterus. This organ was pictured, in some of these illustrations, as having two upwardly-directed lateral prolongations—the uterine horns of cattle and other species, erroneously transferred to women. The illustration of one such figure drawn in the ninth century derives from a sixth-century codex, itself derived from a second-century work by Soranus (*Fig. 2.1*). Similar illustrations—which were no better than symbolic—are to be found in thirteenth-century manuscripts (*Plate 1*). By the fifteenth century, many of these *gravida* figures had further stylizations which have nothing to do with anatomy; for example, the hair of the mother was shown covered by a snood (*Fig. 2.2*).

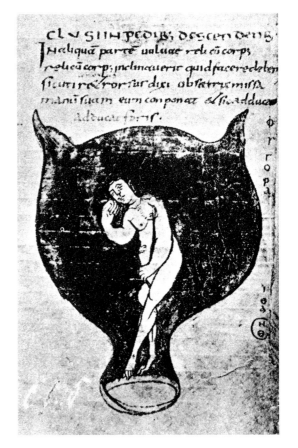

2.1   The fetus *in utero*. One of a series from a ninth-century MS of Maschion's works, which is itself based on the writings of Soranus of Ephesus (MS 3714, in Royal Library, Brussels. From Sudhoff, 1908.)

Similar images, both of fetuses *in utero* and of pregnant women, persisted in appearing, for example, in a book on midwifery by Jakob Rueff, *De conceptu . . .*, (originally in German) printed in a number of editions in the second half of the sixteenth century. In many homes in Britain earlier in our present century figures not too dissimilar could be found, crudely printed in red, in a home, marriage, and sex advice book, namely *Aristotle's masterpiece*, a work (*not* by that natural scientist) that had been popular since the seventeenth century. The stylized figures had been in existence for more than a thousand years.

In some of these *gravidae* the frog-like stance and the purely symbolic diagrams of internal organs contrast with realistic representations of the face and hands. The illustration in *Fig. 2.2*,

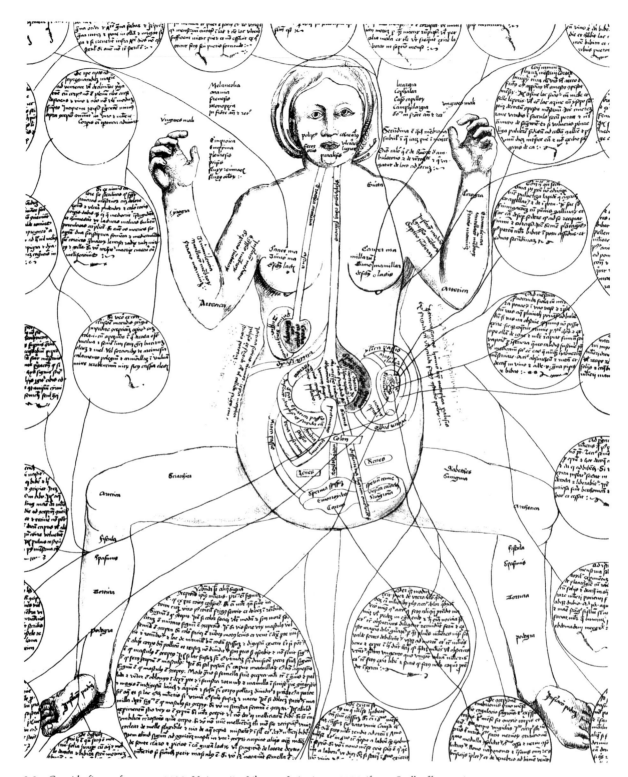

2.2 *Gravida* figure from MS 1122, University Library, Leipzig, *c.* 1400 (from Sudhoff, 1907).

and many like it in manuscripts up to the late fifteenth century, did not attempt to represent anatomical structures in any way naturalistically. This very large drawing succeeds in attracting our attention to the figure, and thence secondarily to the surrounding medical (rather than anatomical) text. The *gravida* figure justified itself perhaps by being the framework on which a medical text was organized and summarized. Even if the artist may not have realized that the aorta and the trachea were separate tubes anatomically, he must have known that a woman's heart was not in the lower right chest; he knew that a newly-born child has to come out of the womb *per viam naturalem* in spite of the fact that, in his drawing, there is no possible exit for this fetus from this uterus. The kidneys were not shown even as bean-shaped symbols; the word 'renes' appears in each of two boxes, unconnected with other structures in the lower abdomen.

Frog-like figures

Figures of pregnant women are sometimes to be found in medieval manuscripts in association with a series of anatomical schemata, each figure illustrating a major body system, so that there are artery-men, muscle-men, nerve-men, and so on. The figures of such series were usually placed in frog-like postures (*Plate 2*). Such illustrated manuscripts may be seen in many libraries. The German medical historian Karl Sudhoff travelled throughout Europe before and after the First World War comparing various series. Many interrelationships are discernible; the figures were sufficiently interesting to medieval persons for copies to have been made, largely for readers in religious orders, and also copies of those copies. Early examples of such series that have been preserved were drawn in the twelfth century; but they were probably copied from even earlier figures, said by some to be Alexandrian in origin. There were usually five frog-like figures; to these were added diagrams of other systems. A representative series is to be found in a late-twelfth- or early-thirteenth-century manuscript belonging to the library of Gonville and Caius College in Cambridge (*Plate 3*). In this there are the following figures: veins; arteries; bones; nerves; muscles; along with diagrams of the male organs; female organs; abdominal organs; and the brain and eyes. In the Bodleian Library of the University of Oxford, there is a volume of seventy-three vellum leaves (Ashmole manuscript 399) containing the text of eighteen or nineteen books of medicine, obstetrics, astrology, palmistry, and physiognomy, the fifth of which is an illustrated work on anatomy. Associated with this book are five full-page human figures in frog-like posture, each drawn, painted, and illuminated very carefully. The first of these is shown in *Fig. 2.3* and the second in our *Plate 2*. On the facing page of the latter there is a well-lettered text, with a gold-illuminated initial letter, stating that the figure shows the arteries which emerge from the heart. ('Hec est historia arteriarum que procedunt ex corde ...'. Many early anatomical illustrations, printed as well as drawn, begin their captions with 'Hic est historia ...', where 'historia' means the results of enquiry.)

Somewhat confusingly to a modern reader, what are probably meant to be the veins are

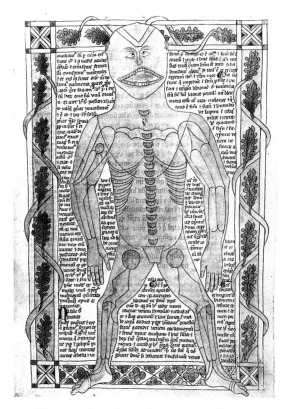

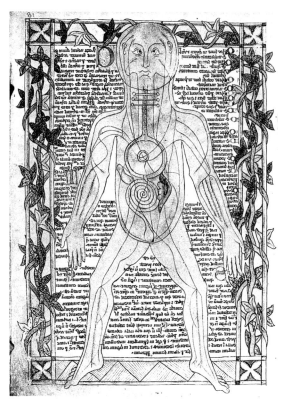

2.3 Vein man from Ashmole MS 399, Bodleian Library, Oxford, thirteenth century.

2.4 Skeletal figure from Ashmole MS 399, thirteenth century.

coloured red, and what are meant to be the arteries are blue. The other three highly-finished figures which make up the sequence of five show the bones (*Fig. 2.4*), the nerves, and the muscles. A noticeable feature of these illustrations is that each face shows a pronounced internal squint. On other pages of this manuscript there are precise, coloured, elaborate diagrams of the male (*Fig. 2.5*) and of the female genitalia, and of the eyes, and optic nerves proceeding to what is presumably the brain (*Fig. 2.6*). In a different style, there are a few pages containing more or less realistic diagrams of the visceral organs as they would be seen as removed at autopsy or during an anatomical dissection. One of these latter diagrams (*Fig. 2.7*) pictures the heart, with auricular appendices, lungs, and trachea. On the same page there is a diagram of a vertically-placed stomach, with an oesophagus entering horizontally; the pyloric exit is below. Closely applied to the stomach is a five-lobed liver, coloured brown, with a symbolic gall-bladder, coloured green. In a manuscript in the University of Pisa Library (Codex Roncioni 99) there is a similar diagram, but in this the copyist has drawn the gullet entering the liver rather than the stomach!

Other manuscripts of the twelfth to fourteenth centuries, scattered in many European libraries,

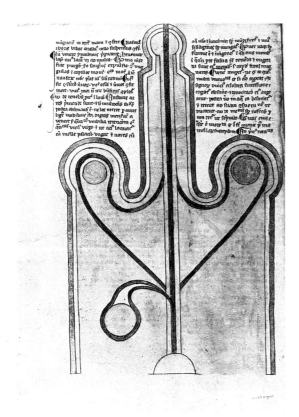

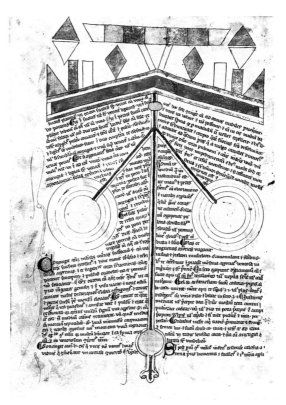

2.5 Diagram of male urogenital system from Ashmole MS 399, thirteenth century.

2.6 Diagram of eyes, optic nerves, nose, olfactory nerve and (?) brain from Ashmole MS 399, thirteenth century.

contain similar examples of the five-figure series in their frog-like poses; they are sometimes accompanied by elaborate diagrams of female and of male urogenital tracts and of the eye, and by simpler diagrams of viscera. The Caius and the Bodleian manuscripts are obviously indebted ultimately to similar sources; the Caius manuscript is the more hurriedly drawn and is less precise. The Bodleian manuscript contains other illustrations; there are figures of fetuses, in flask-shaped rather than bicornuate uteruses—the babies are again miniature adults, this time with attractive curly hair (*Plate 1*)—and there is a sequence of illustrations related to clinical medicine, one of which shows an autopsy in progress (*Fig. 2.8*). This latter figure includes diagrams of viscera removed which are similar to those depicted earlier in the book.

The frog-like series had a wide distribution and persistence, being found for instance in Arabic, Persian, and Indian manuscripts up to the nineteenth century; it has also been suggested that their origins were Arabic, or Indian, rather than Alexandrian. The characteristic frog-like stance has received no satisfactory explanation. The similar squatting figures of the Egyptian dwarf god Bes, a deity associated with fertility, may be fortuitous. The Bodleian manuscript we have been discussing, in common with others of the same kind, contains works on sexuality

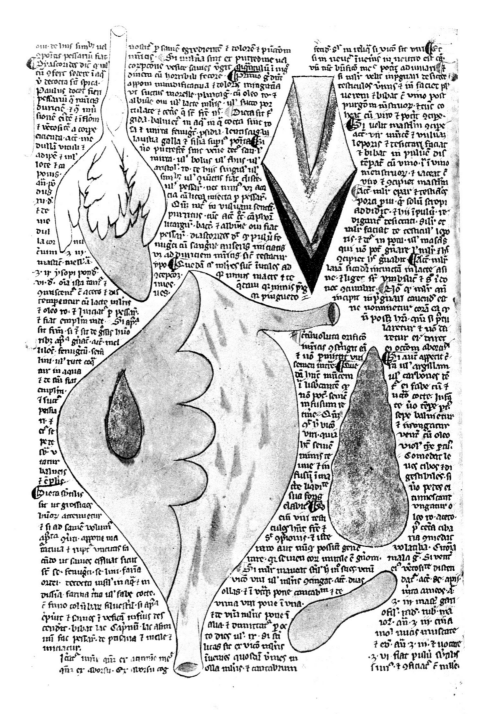

2.7 Figure of viscera from Ashmole MS 399, thirteenth century.

and obstetrics, such as Constantine the African's *De coitu*.

An interesting variant of some of the figures in such frog-like series was to depict both the back view of the head *and* the face; the head was shown, as it were, spread out, with the face upside-down—an attempt, one supposes, to represent a complete rounded structure on the plane surface of the paper (*Plate 4*).

One early-fifteenth-century anatomical illustrator, who would by this date probably have been familiar with human dissection, attempted to resolve similar problems. In 1400, as now, the internal organs of the human body were explored by carrying the dissection from the front to the back, starting with a mid-line incision in the abdomen. The reverse procedure, starting in the midline of the back, is hindered by the presence of the backbone— just as it is harder to open a herring from the dorsal than from the ventral surface. (There have been exceptional illustrations from time to time, such as that by Kilian in the nineteenth century, showing a child's thorax and abdomen in posterior view, see *Plate 120*, p.

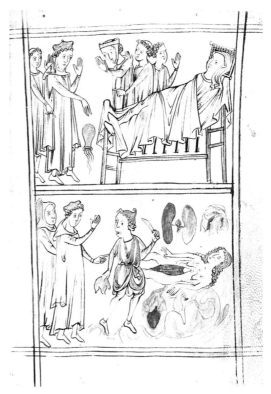

2.8 Two illustrations from Ashmole MS 399, thirteenth century: in the upper one, the patient's prognosis is regarded as poor by the physician, who upends the urine flask; in the lower, an autopsy on a woman is performed. The organs removed are figured.

557.) In this manuscript, dated about 1412, two companion figures attempted to show the internal organs from the front and from the back; with great boldness the artist conveyed also the lateral symmetry of some structures—the backbone and the male genitalia, for example; and the asymmetry of others—the heart, liver, etc. (*Plate 5*). The body is shown incompletely split vertically in the mid-sagittal plane. These extraordinary attempts at two-dimensional representation of a complex solid object are among the most original of anatomical illustrations. They successfully recall structures seen during a conventional dissection, and are at the same time complex teaching aids, though they place a considerable burden of comprehension on the student.

Most medieval illustrations were derived from anatomical texts and the illustrations of earlier periods, not directly from observation of dissections; they usually did not represent even those elements of anatomy which must have been well known to contemporary physicians and even to lay persons. At a time in the fifteenth century, when the skeletal figures of a series showed purely diagrammatic ribs and only one bone for the forearm, some Gothic artists were illustrating somewhat more accurately, in crucifixions and the Dance of Death, the thoracic cage of emaciated Christs, and the forearm bones of figures of Death.

The series of frog-like figures were hardly intended to convey precise information: their use was more that of a logo, symbolically indicating the characteristics of the subject matter of the various systems in the body.

1   Figure of the gravid uterus to be found on fo.14^r of MS Ashmole 399, probably late thirteenth century. Coloured manuscript drawing on vellum (Bodleian Library, Oxford). Page size: 26.8 × 19.1 cm

It is of interest to compare these thirteenth-century drawings of adult manikins, masquerading as fetuses 'bottled-up' inside the uterus, with *Fig. 2.1* (see p. 15), one of a series of drawings representing the same condition, but produced some four hundred years earlier.

Here two (why only two?) of the 'fetuses' possess an umbilical cord, whereas none of the ninth-century drawings feature such a structure. Here also the uterus is represented as a smooth-contoured inverted flask shape, while the uterus in the *Fig. 2.1* drawing sports two 'horns' springing from its upper corners—structures which, in diverse forms and flitting from place to place on the uterus (sometimes even the vagina) bedevilled illustrations of female reproductive anatomy for hundreds of years.

14

Sunt pedibus descendit aliqua parte
matris reliquum corpus inclinauerit
qui facere debemus sicuti diximus su
perius obstetrix imista manu eum
componat et deinde adducat.

Si diuisis pedibus duabus parti
bus uulue plantas intingat quid
faciemus inmista manu obstetrix
eos ligat et ad orificium matricis
eos componat et sic adducat.

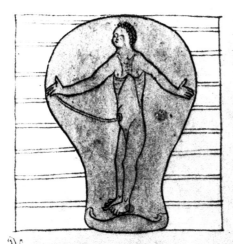 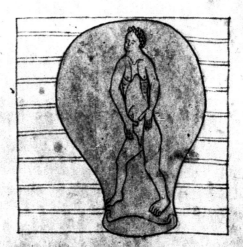

Si unum pedem foras habuit que cunque in
uideatur nunquam eum obstetrix teneat
et conet ne reliquo corpore infantis pl
mater claudat. Sed paruus infantis digi
tis ad unguem infantis tali reuocet
imista manu pede altum colligat et
apprehensis pedibus foras adducat.

Si genu ostenderit et sic cona
exire quid faciemus retrorsum
inpelendus est et correctis pedibus
est adducendus.

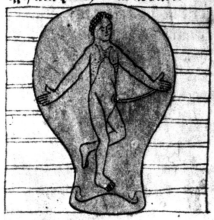 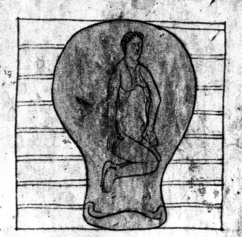

PLATE 1

2 The arterial figure of fo. 19ʳ of MS Ashmole 399, thirteenth century. Coloured manuscript drawing on vellum (Bodleian Library, Oxford). Page size: 26.8 × 19.1 cm

3 The venous figure on fo. 14ᵛ from Caius College, MSS 190/223, thirteenth century (By permission of the Master and Fellows of Gonville and Caius College, Cambridge). 20.7 × 16.0 cm.

Plate 2 and *Plate 3* are considered together. *Plate 2* is of folio 19 recto in the Ashmole manuscript. On the opposite page, folio 18 verso, is an explanatory text for the figure, beginning *Hec est historia arteriarum*—in other words this drawing purports to represent the arterial system. It should be mentioned that the succeeding frog-like drawings of the bones (20 recto), nerves (21 recto), and muscles (22 recto) are similarly arranged, that is, with the drawing on the right-hand page, and the text opposite it on the left. *Plate 3* is from the manuscript in the library of Caius College. It is headed *historia arteriarum*, but we believe this attribution to be in error, since this drawing is in essence the same as other venous figures, including that in the Ashmole manuscript considered below.

When *Plates 2 and 3* are compared they are obviously very different. On examination of the only other Caius manuscript drawing representing blood-vessels, one finds many points of similarity with our *Plate 2*. The other Ashmole 'vessel-man' (folio 18 recto, reproduced here as *Fig. 2.3*) is closely similar to our *Plate 3*, from Caius. Unfortunately the leaf that should precede Ashmole folio 18 is missing; it presumably would have consisted of the explanatory text of our *Fig. 2.3*.

We strongly incline to the view that *Plate 2* (Ashmole) is of the arteries: it shows a simple pattern (just two vessels on each side of the head and neck); the vessels mainly arising from a single locus in the heart; and a *rete mirabile* in the head. From the above we believe that *Plate 3* (Caius) and *Fig. 2.3* (Ashmole) are drawings representing the venous system. *Plate 3* is a more primitive drawing than *Fig. 2.3* with regard to the representation of the trachea (just two parallel lines); the faint pear-shaped spleen (seen on the left side of the abdomen); and the intestines. When one considers these two illustrations together—the five-lobed livers, each with a gall-bladder superimposed; the heart–lung complexes; and the similar pattern and number of blood-vessels—one must surely conclude that the Caius drawing was a rather crude copy of the Ashmole figure, or that both were copied from another, unidentified, source.

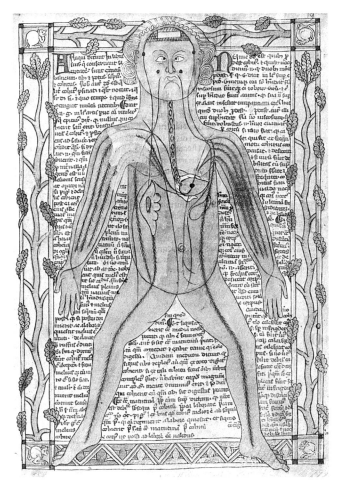

PLATE 2

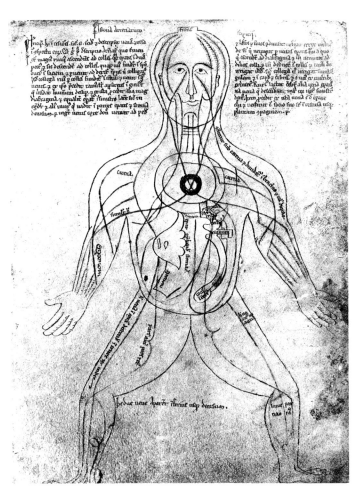

PLATE 3

4   The skeletal figure on fo. 169ᵛ from University Library, Basle, ᴍꜱ D.11.II, thirteenth
     century. Coloured manuscript drawing (Basle University Library).

This drawing schematically represents portions of the human skeletal system. Twenty-four
vertebral bodies are (correctly) featured (but with thirteen ill-positioned ribs), together with the
sacrum.

The skull is represented from the back, and no attempt thas been made to show the facial
skeleton: the face is shown turned upside-down (it is coloured red in the original). The 'papilla
capi ...?' may refer to the external occipital protuberance, and the inverted V-line the lambdoid
suture of the skull; but the rest of the skull parts shown do not lend themselves to easy
interpretation.

The bilateral curved structures in the upper chest and arm are coloured red in the original,
and most probably represent a blood-vessel, perhaps the subclavian artery and its continuation.
However, its quality of delineation makes it likely that it was added to the main drawing at a
later date. Interestingly the head, trunk, and upper limbs are viewed from the back, while the
lower limbs are clearly viewed from the front.

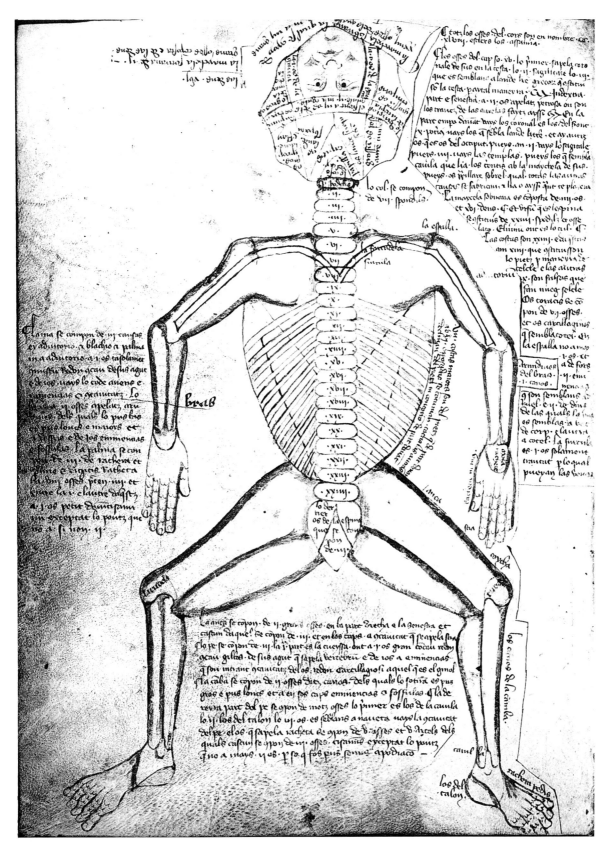

PLATE 4

5 a and b. Incomplete mid-line sagittal sections carried through from the back and from the front. Two figures included in a manuscript (MS x.118), from about 1412, of a work of John Ardene. Manuscript drawing; original coloured (Royal Library, Stockholm).

As if 'normal' anatomy were too simple to draw, these two illustrations present the human and trunk partially sectioned in the mid-sagittal plane.

In the former, viewed from in front, one can make out the vertebral column, the brain and the upper part of the spinal cord, the oesophagus, and the trachea; but the heart and lungs are a fudged *mélange*. Below the diaphragm, which is shown with the inferior vena cava piercing it, can be recognized the liver and stomach; but the intestines are schematized. Two ovals, rather low down, represent the kidneys. The penis and its opened urethra lead from the bladder; but there is a strange absence of a scrotum.

The drawing of the posterior aspect does feature two halves of the scrotum, and also a very wide penile urethra. Again the intestines are a mess, but the two dark kidneys are better positioned. The two halves of the hemisected vertebral column and spinal cord are clear. The ribs also, though only nine are featured. No diaphragm is seen, though the heart and lungs are now obvious. A hemisected trachea is present, but although part is seen leading to the right lung, there is a long offshoot to the left side that defies identification, and the trachea appears to continue downwards into the liver–stomach complex.

Two halves of the jaws are clearly shown, with possibly a narrow split oesophagus leading from the back of the mouth space. The dark mid-line structure is probably the unsplit tongue. Centrally, above the upper jaw, can be seen the two sides of the nasal cavity. Exactly what the four 'spiders' (two on each side, beneath the halved three-celled brain) represent is diffcult to determine—most probably 'nerves' going to or from the brain 'cells', that is, the stylized brain ventricles.

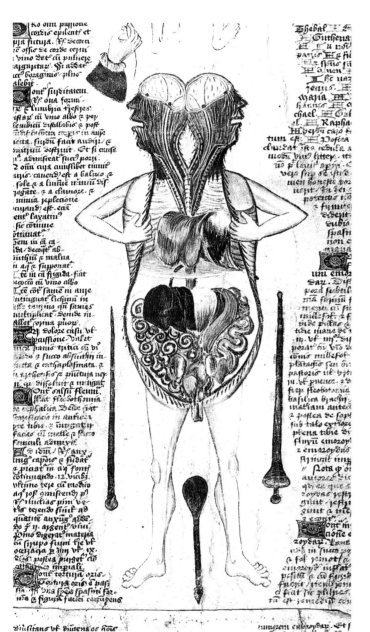

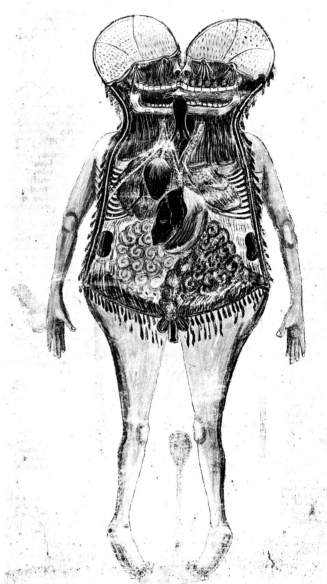

PLATE 5   (a)   (b)

Upright figures

The frog-like series was not the only way of portraying anatomical figures. The French surgeon and anatomist, Henri de Mondeville, after study in Montpellier, Bologna, and Paris lectured at Montpellier in 1304 and again in Paris in 1306 using original anatomical illustrations. The illustrations were of two kinds: first, figures of individual organs, such as we have seen in the Oxford Ashmole MS 399 series, and secondly, upright figures of a new type. These were illustrations made for didactic anatomy; they were the product of the renewed interest in the fourteenth century in human anatomy, and the return to the practice of pig and human dissection. From the viewpoint of a present-day anatomist, the illustrations seem trivial, even absurd. But we know from Guy de Chauliac, his pupil, that figures were used as an integral part of Mondeville's lectures at Montpellier—these may have been the sketches of individual organs rather than the upright figures. In the full-length figures used in the lectures in Paris, the subjects were mostly shown standing in natural, graceful postures, although one is frog-like. Perhaps the most striking and beautiful of the standing dissection pictures derived from Henri de Mondeville's series are those included in a 1345 manuscript *Anothomia* by Guido da Vigevano (*Plate* 6). This manuscript carries forward the teaching of Mondino (see Chapter 1); in it the author claims to have himself dissected human subjects. In one of his eighteen figures the cadaver is seen standing as if it were a living man, with the anatomist removing the skull cap with a mallet and chisel. Even if, as undoubtedly occurred, dissection were performed on suspended corpses, the painting was not intended to show realistically an actual dissection. Its purpose was to indicate the subject matter, not details of anatomy.

Related pictorially to some manuscript illustrations of anatomy were the cautery figures of the twelfth to the fifteenth centuries. Spots were placed on drawings and paintings of nude, or partially nude, men; in some drawings physicians were shown standing by with pointers indicating the sites propitious for cautery in particular diseases. The indicator lines of modern anatomical illustration are in the tradition of such medieval precursors.

In a printed book of natural philosophy written by Johannes Peyligk: *Philosophie naturalis compendium* ..., Leipzig, 1499, an anatomical figure exhibits a new convention of abstraction, for it represents a head, neck, and trunk, but no arms or legs. The figure was copied and changed in another philosophical and encyclopaedic printed work by Magnus Hundt, *Antropologium de hominis dignitate* ..., Leipzig, 1501 (*Plate* 7). Many of the illustrations in this book were simplified diagrams, not realistic images. At the turn of that century, when dissection had been practised in Europe for about two hundred years, anatomical illustrations were still not intended to have a direct relationship to reality. The figures were not drawn as if the artist were present at a dissection; they were devices for listing the main organs, much as a table in a modern monograph might indicate relationships. In other subjects, too, it was not always regarded as important to have figures correspond at all closely to actual appearances. In manuscripts and in early printed works on geography and travel, illustrations of towns bore little or no relationship to reality.

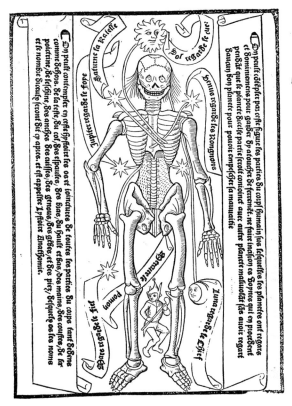

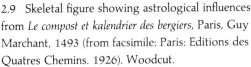

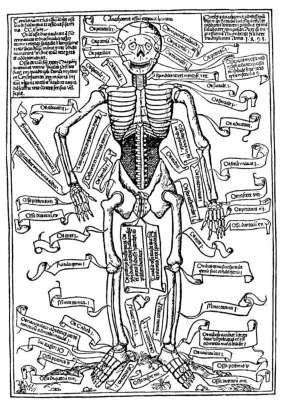

2.9 Skeletal figure showing astrological influences from *Le compost et kalendrier des bergiers*, Paris, Guy Marchant, 1493 (from facsimile: Paris: Editions des Quatres Chemins. 1926). Woodcut.

2.10 Skeletal figure, with bones named. Broadsheet published in Nuremberg, Richard Helain, 1493. Woodcut.

The same woodcut sometimes accompanied descriptions of quite different cities, hundreds of miles apart. Topographical maps, whether drawn or printed, were until the sixteenth century almost always produced without attempt at scale; they merely listed pictorially geographical features in some sort of order.

In manuscripts from the thirteenth to the sixteenth century, and in early printed illustrated books, skeletons are to be found drawn as viewed from the front, with legs hanging straight down, not bent into the frog-like position, and frequently—a persistent convention—with the abdominal region indicated in black.

The figure illustrated in *Fig. 2.9* has been taken from a printed book *Le compost et kalendrier des bergiers*.... Paris, 1493. This almanac includes woodcuts likely to appeal to all tastes: shepherds with bagpipes, men being broken on wheels, persons drowning in a flood, massacres, plagues of snakes, hell ... There is one of a naked man with pointers indicating areas to be used for venesection; the veins are not shown. The skeleton reproduced here has labelling describing astrological influences on the body: for instance, *Jupiter regarde le foye,* with a starred ribbon going to the site of the liver at the right costal margin. This obviously was a book intended for the general public. Very similar figures appear not only in nearly contemporary manuscripts but also in printed work aimed at a more professional readership. A very large skeletal woodcut, this time with a black abdomen (*Fig. 2.10*), was published by Richard Helain at Nuremberg in 1493, with the names of the bones, in Latin, contained in ribbons connected to the bone in question. This figure was cut on the basis of French models similar to that of the *Kalendrier*.

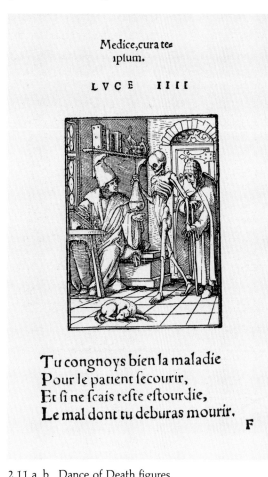

Medice, cura te=
ipsum.

LVCE   IIII

Tu congnoys bien la maladie
Pour le patient secourir,
Et si ne scais teste estourdie,
Le mal dont tu deburas mourir.

F

2.11 a, b   Dance of Death figures.
a. Death take the physician. Woodcut by Hans Holbein the younger, 1538.

The German figure, intended presumably for surgeons or barbers to nail to the wall, may be seen to be, in many ways, even less realistic than the popular French version.

The later Middle Ages were preoccupied with death; it is not surprising, therefore, that the skull, Death's trademark, and the articulated skeleton, Death's personification, appear in different guises in many drawings, paintings, sculptures, embroideries, stained glass panels, and—after about 1460—prints. In those times an artist portraying a hermit contemplating a skull, and hence mortality, might draw that skull with greater fidelity than a contemporary anatomical illustrator. And the skeletons of the Dance of Death were often no more anatomically incorrect than the skeletal figures in a late copy of the 'frog-like' or the 'black abdomen' series. It might be noted however that some of Holbein's skeletons seem to have two bones in the upper arm and only one in the forearm. Death may be represented not by a skeleton, but by a *lemur*, a spirit of the dead, which more resembles an extremely emaciated, decaying corpse, with a sunken and sometimes black abdomen, often shown with a mid-line incision through which the rapidly-decomposing intestines had been removed.

The tragi-comic strip of the Dance of Death, a mortality and morality show, may picture a skeleton—Death—challenging a warrior, whilst in the background another skeleton beats a drum with osteological drum-sticks. 'No man knoweth the hour of his death . . .': this is the text for these pictorial sermons—and no class, no station in life, no office is immune from Death's attentions. The origins of the Dance include, certainly, the great pestilence (later called the

Black Death)—the epidemic of bubonic plague which reached Europe in 1347, and spread over the entire continent within four years. Perhaps a fifth or more of Europe's population died. The plague, spread by rat fleas, affected particularly the ill-housed, but it was no respecter of persons; sovereigns and cardinals, as well as printers, soldiers, and poor friars, and even physicians were snatched away by death (*Figs 2.11a and b*).

Another most fearful tradition represented, in realistic three-dimensional images, the decay of the body after interment. In elaborate tombs of renowned clerics and temporal rulers, a stone canopy protects a life-like sculpture, clothed in a manner appropriate to sex and rank; underneath—placed so that one has to bend down to see it—lies a sculpture of

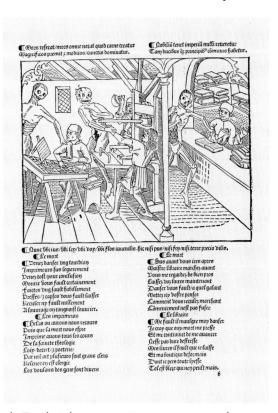

the body eaten away by worms and decayed almost to a skeleton. again, paintings of elegant young men and women may have companion pictures, where their corpses are shown similarly eaten and corrupted.

Such intimations of mortality have, since the early sixteenth century, often been included in illustrations of anatomy. In Dryander's *Anatomia capitis humani*, Marburg, 1536, a skull rests on a board inscribed *inevitabile fatum* (see *Plate 19*, p. 89); in Vesalius' *Fabrica*, Basle, 1543, a skeleton contemplating a skull leans on a tomb whose engraved message reads: *Vivitur ingenio, caetera mortis erunt* ('Genius lives on, all else is mortal'); accompanying Ruysch's (1638–1731) illustrations of his cabinet such remarks as *Ah fata, ah aspera fata* comment on anatomical preparations. These are but a few examples associating anatomical illustrations of skulls and skeletons with moral sermons on the omnipresence of death and the inevitable Judgement that follows.

b. Deaths take a compositor, a pressman, and a bookseller. Woodcut in *La grant danse macabre*. Lyons, M. Husz, 1499. Woodcut.

Early Renaissance anatomy

In various parts of Europe, and particularly in some cities of Italy and Germany, a different way of looking at the human body helps to define the advent of the Renaissance. Artists and medical men from the early fifteenth century onwards were prepared to regard the human body as of objective interest. This interest did not necessarily conflict with medieval religious sentiment. As St Thomas Aquinas (1225–74) writes in the *Summa theologica* (Question 93):

Now it is manifest that in man there is some likeness to God, copied from God as from an exemplar; yet this likeness is not one of equality, for such an exemplar infinitely excels its copy. Therefore there is in man a likeness to God; not, indeed, a perfect likeness, but imperfect.

There were also philosophical, or metaphysical, reasons for interest in the human frame. The microcosm of the body represented analogously the macrocosm of the Universe—and as the heavens were shown to have a degree of order, so order, proportion, and measure were looked for in human beings, and such study came to be a central concern for many inquiring minds.

It was not therefore fortuitous, but appropriate, even inevitable, that in such circumstances, during the fifteenth century, representations of the Christ-child with his mother became lifelike; that perspective was understood and used in painting; that Dürer spent so long in attempting to define human proportions geometrically; that Leonardo and others tried to solve the humanistic, Vitruvian problem of placing a man's figure within a square and a circle; that artists such as Donatello, Antonio Pollaiuolo, and Michelangelo concentrated their efforts on the appearance of perfect young male bodies, with muscles and bones perceived clearly and realistically under the skin.

Nor was it surprising that medieval ideas on the influence of the macrocosm, as represented by the planets, should still be accepted in Renaissance times as affecting profoundly the microcosm, as represented by the human body—a concept possibly Persian in origin. To demonstrate these ideas, there were zodiacal figures in which the signs of the planets were placed around a human figure, with each sign connected with a bodily part (*Fig. 2.12*). Figures based on the same plan, with indicator lines, have already been noted in medieval maps of cautery points; and there were parallel disease figures and skeletal figures, where diseases, or names of bones, were written around the figure, and connected by lines to appropriate parts.

To illustrate the ancestry of such figures, we may take one early printed text, Johannes de Ketham's *Fasciculus medicinae*, 1491. This compilation of medical knowledge was possibly made by a German-speaking physician (Johann von Kirscheim) earlier in the century. The enterprising Venetian firm of Johannes and Gregorius de Gregoriis issued the work in Latin; the volume also included a short treatise on the plague. There were six large full-page woodcut illustrations, including a *gravida* in a frog-like stance (*Fig. 2.13*), two figures combining venesection and zodiacal information, a wound-man, a disease-man, and a circle of urine glasses. Most of these illustrations were similar to those of earlier manuscripts: the potentiality of printing had not

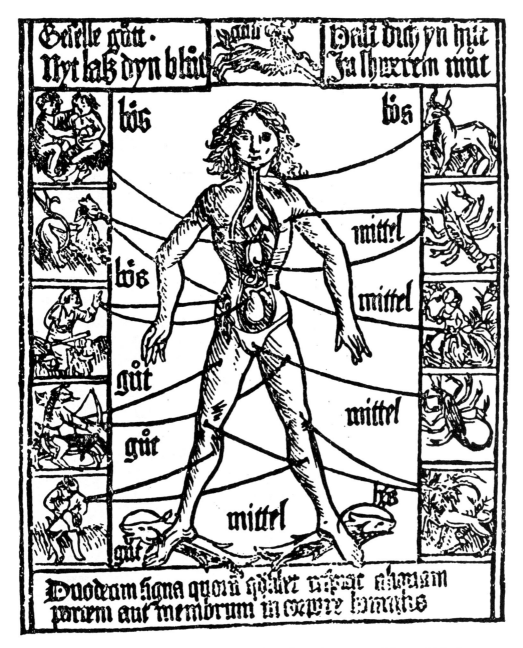

2.12   Figure correlating anatomical structures and astrological signs. Broadsheet published *c.* 1480 (from Herrlinger 1970). Woodcut.

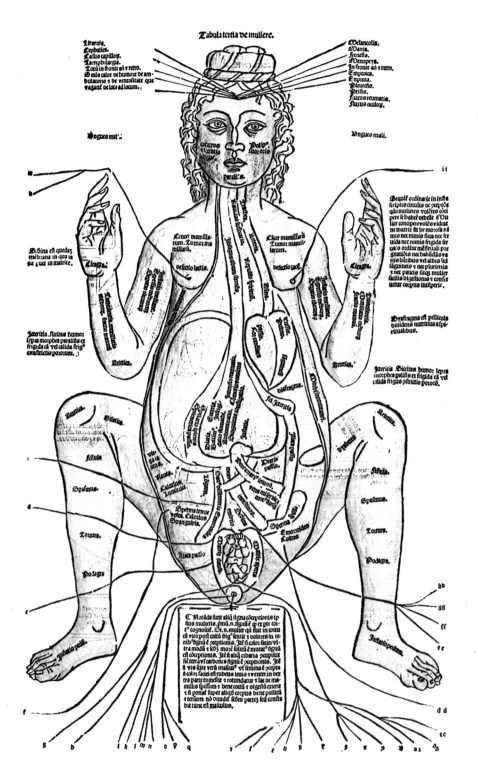

2.13 *Gravida* figure from Ketham *Fasciculus medicinae*, Venice, 1491. Woodcut.

yet been realized. In 1493 the work was reissued as *Fasciculo de medicina*, in the Italian language, along with a reprint of Mondino, by the same publishers, with slightly smaller but more sophisticated illustrations—drawn this time by Gentile Bellini or his brother-in-law Andrea Mantegna, or by an artist directly influenced by one or the other. The figures can be seen to have many of the characteristics of medieval anatomy figures, but drawn with much greater assurance and sophistication. The *gravida* particularly is improved (*Plate 8*). The frog-like position of the 1491 figure achieves a certain amount of justification, for in this 1493 edition the woman is seated with her thighs apart so as to show the dissected reproductive tract; the uterus is not bicornuate—a probable indication that the artist had seen a dissection or had been directed by someone who had been present at one, though it is to be noted that some earlier manuscripts had pictured the uterus in this more correct manner (see *Plate 1*, p. 23). A fine woodcut, also added to this edition, shows an anatomical dissection in progress (*Fig. 2.14*). This

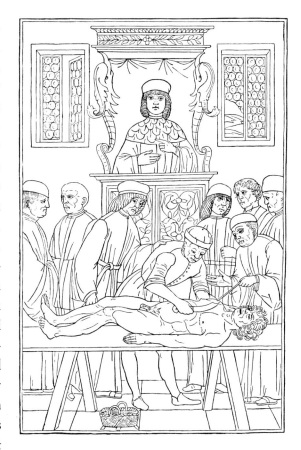

2.14   Dissection scene from [Ketham] *Fasciculo de medicina*, Venice, 1493. Woodcut.

dissection scene has been widely reproduced as an illustration of great character that shows how dignified was the ideal conduct of an anatomy in the late fifteenth century. In some copies of this work the illustrations are imaginatively coloured, probably by the use of stencils rather than by direct hand-painting or multiple woodcut printing. In these Venetian woodblocks—perhaps the finest up to that period—the figures were cleanly cut, without attempts at shading.

Medical illustration was benefiting by the skill of Renaissance artists and wood-cutters, but the anatomical figures were still largely determined by medieval ideas. Beautiful though they are, the illustrations hardly advanced anatomical science.

6   The visceral figure from Guido da Vigevano, *Anothomia*, 1345, a manuscript (MS 334, ex. 569) in the Musée Condé, Chateau Chantilly. Coloured manuscript drawing (taken from Wickersheimer 1926).

The widely-opened thorax and abdomen are separated by a very thick diaphragm, over-labelled very faintly 'dyafragma', which is shown as being concave upwards. The banded trachea, with a mid-point dilatation, is seen merging into a three-lobed lung. The small 'heart-shaped' heart is shown overlying the left lobe, receiving, or giving off, descending vessels as well as ones to the head, neck, and shoulder region. The oesophagus pierces the diaphragm centrally to enter the stomach, which exits to the intestine on the left side. The intestines themselves are layered, with no differentiation as to large or small; they terminate seemingly to the left of the mid-line. A globular liver (there is a possible representation of the portal vein, but no gall-bladder), the urinary bladder, the kidneys, and the spleen are portrayed, with various ducts or vessels. The penis and scrotum are minuscule; the artist concerned would, of course, have been aware of the ludicrous nature of this representation, even if ignorant of the form and positioning of the thoracic and abdominal contents. When the completely fanciful limb-joints are also taken into consideration, it is obvious that this illustration is very largely symbolic in nature, and is based on written, not visual, anatomy.

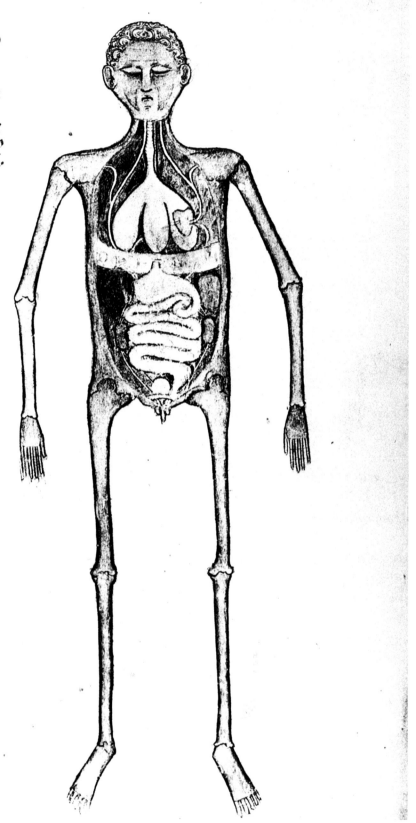

hec est figura
octaua anoto
mie in qua de
monstrantur
ota membr cor
pis compositi
que sit i corpe
a capite inferi
us ad uesica.

PLATE 6

7 Visceral figure from Magnus Hundt, *Antropologium* ... Leipzig, Wolfgang Stöckel, 1501. Woodcut (Wellcome Institute Library). 13 × 8 cm.

In this unlabelled head, neck, and trunk illustration the thorax and abdomen are widely opened.

The two strap-like structures extending from the lower jaw to the thorax appear more like the ends of a tape tied under the chin than any anatomical structures, though the one on the right represents the trachea, that on the left the oesophagus. The thoracic 'crazy paving', to which the trachea leads, represents the lungs. Something like a heart is shown on the left side of the thorax; from its shading it presumably was considered to be three-chambered. It is shown surrounded by a very thick pericardium and has two vessels—'vene arteriales'—attached to it, though it is not clear with which chambers of the heart they are associated.

The diaphragm is a bar of tissue separating the thoracic from the abdominal structures. The vast liver (? with gall-bladder) lies sideways, with six left-facing tongues. The intestines are portrayed as a thin, looped tube, literally knotted in many places.

The lower left structures are open to interpretation. Perhaps the upper bar is indicative of a blood-vessel suspending the kidneys. The latter are connected with the bladder by two ducts (the ureters). The other tube-like structures, lying lateral to the ureters, end inferiorly in round blobs; these may possibly be representative of the gonadal vessels and gonads.

The stomach lies to the left of the liver, with the presumed oesophagus above and to the left. The large structure on the left between the intestines and the stomach possibly represents the spleen and a splenic vessel (this seems more likely than the pancreas): but where fantasy reigns reality is difficult of discernment.

Figura de situ viscerum.

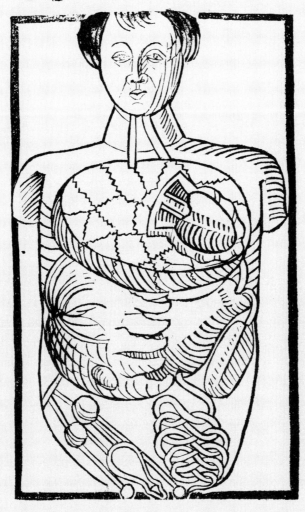

PLATE 7

8 Gravida figure from *Fasciculo de medicina*. Translation by Sebastiano Manilio of Rome. Venice: J. & G. di Gregorii, 1493–4. Woodcut (British Library). 30.0 × 19.7 cm.

This illustration, of a pregnant woman seated on a chair with her abdomen opened so as to show the uterus and other viscera, is a great improvement on the similar but far more crudely-drawn illustration in the 1491 Latin version.

It has been suggested by Singer that the wood-cutter reversed the original drawing—this is perhaps tenable with regard to the double parallel lines shown crossing in the abdomen (see later), and could also account for the right kidney's being represented as lying at a higher level than the left. However, as this latter representation was not uncommon in the sixteenth century, in itself it probably is not a signficant argument for reversal.

Inferiorly the vagina is laid wide open, with the cervix projecting into it from the body of an approximately five-month pregnant uterus. Most commonly, before the date of this illustration, the uterus was depicted as being bicornuate, and often, in addition, as having a septum dividing the body. From each side of the mid-point of the vagina two large curved 'horns' project laterally—structures much favoured both at this time and for a good while afterwards, for example in the *Tabulae* (1538) of Vesalius. It has been suggested that these result from misconstruction of the upper portion of the vagina when it was opened. This explanation certainly requires a considerable stretch of the imagination to be acceptable; if it was artistic misrepresentation, why was it not corrected?

In this plate it is a pity that the appropriate indicator line has no explanatory text attached to it. Projecting from the sides of the uterus are thick bands, then swellings with two divergent curving horns. The swellings could represent the ovaries, and perhaps the upper horn the Fallopian tube, whilst the lower could be the attachment of the broad ligament, or, less likely, the round ligament of the ovary. The thick band possibly represents the mythical duct (that is, the *ductus testium* of Vesling or the *vasa seminarium* of Mondino and others) said to connect the 'testiculum' (ovary) to the uterus, or, on occasions, to both the uterus and vagina. Perhaps nowadays it could be interpreted as being a large ligament of the ovary.

The two oval-shaped structures represent the kidneys and the other medially-directed oblique lines the ureters, here shown disappearing posterior to the uterus, as they may well be depicted during pregnancy.

The two curving lines, which cross the above-mentioned oblique lines, lead to the ovaries, and probably represent the ovarian vessels: the lines from which *they* 'arise' are possibly the renal veins, draining 'upwards' into the inferior vena cava, represented by the single line shown entering the liver which peeps out beneath the *left* costal margin. As, of course, the liver is predominantly a right-sided structure it is not unreasonable to assume that the wood-cutter *did* in fact reverse the original drawing. (By 1509, Milan edition, this *situs inversus* had been corrected.) This would indeed explain the liver being on the left (is the little structure to its left meant as the gall-bladder?), and also the relative position of the kidneys, as well as the interpretation of the parallel lines as representing the cut root of the mesentery (although they are too long, and the idea is far-fetched, nothing else springs to mind).

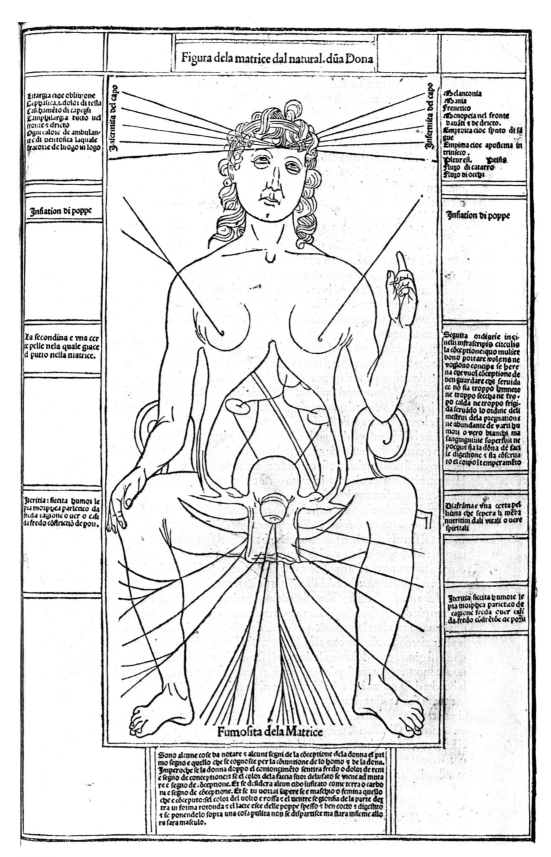

Figura dela matrice dal natural. dũa Dona

Litargia cioe oblinone
Cephalica.i.dolor di testa
Cascham̃eto di capegli
Zamphilargia tucto nel
fronte z drieto
Ogni calore de ambulan
re e di ventrofita laquale
fracorre de luogo in logo

Infermita del capo

Infermita del capo

Melanconia
Mania
Frenetico
Scuopeia nel fronte
danati z de drieto.
Emptoica cioe spnto di sã
gue
Empima cioe aposema in
trinseco.
Pleuresi.   Ptisis.
Fluxo di catarro
Fluxo di occhi

Infiation di poppe

Infiation di poppe

La secondina e vna cer
te pelle nela quale giace
il putto nella matrice.

Seguita ordiarie inci
nelli infrascripto circulis
la cõceptione:iquão mulier
bono portare volens ne
vogliono concape se here
na che vuol cõception de
ben guardare che seruida
ce nõ sia troppo humore
ne troppo seccha ne tro
po calda ne troppo frigi
da seruãdo lo ordine deli
mestrui dela pregnatione
ne abundante de varii hu
mori o vero bianchi ma
sanguinitne superflui ne
pocqui sia la dõna de faci
le digestione z sia cõseru
to el corpo li temperam̃eto

Iteritia: siccita humor le
pra morphea parietico da
freda cagione o ver o cal
da fredo cõstrictiõ de por

Diafrãma e vna certa pel
licina che sepera li mẽbra
nutritiui dali vitali o uere
spirituali

Iteritia siccita humore le
pra morphea parietico de
cagione freda ouer cali
da fredo cõstretõe de poẽ

Fumosita dela Matrice

Sono alcune cose da notare z alcuni segni de la cõceptione dela donna et pri
mo segno e quello che se cognosce per la congiuntione de lo homo z de la dona.
Imperoche se la donna doppo el contengimẽto sentira fredo z dolor de reni
e segno de conceptione: se el color dela faccia fuor delusato se viene ad mata
re e segno de cõceptione. Et se desidera alcun abo insitato come terra o carbo
ni e segno de cõceptione. Et se tu vorrai sapere se e masch[i]o o femina quello
che e cõceputo: sel color del volto e rossa z el ventre se gionsa de la parte dex
tra in forma rotonda z el lacte esce delle poppe spesso z ben cocto z digestiro
z se ponendelo sopra una cosa pulita non se dispartisce ma stara insieme allo
ra sara masculo.

PLATE 8

Venesection diagrams

Some of the plates in the 1493 *Fasciculo ...* could be considered to be professionally useful. There were both uroscopy and venesection plates; both techniques were needed in practical medicine, for looking at the characteristics of urine in a flask was thought to be a most important diagnostic procedure carried out by physicians, and bleeding by opening a vein, often carried out by surgeons or barbers, was one of the more important of therapeutic procedures—providing it was performed at the correct astrological moment, a consideration that explains the labelling of figures with details both of venous anatomy and astrological signs. Every time a patient's body was bled (and was therefore touched with iron) the surgeon or barber had to know the position of the moon and other astrological information. Venesection diagrams—often in a debased and quite useless form (*Fig. 2.15*)—can be seen in medieval manuals of surgery; printing allowed such figures to be reproduced, as in the *Shepherds' calendar* (*Fig. 2.9*). Even though some of these printed woodcuts of vein-men were crude, falling greatly from the standard set in the Ketham work, they showed more accurately than did manuscript equivalents which veins were available for opening. These diagrams could also be printed and published separately from any book, possibly being intended for display on the walls of barbers' shops to impress customers and to be an *aide mémoire* to the bloodletter.

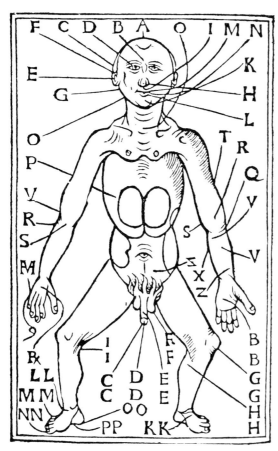

2.15 Venesection diagram still in use in Aberdeen in 1620. From *Articella*, Lyons, 1525.

Fugitive sheets

Not only would venesection figures be useful to surgeons, but also sheets containing other anatomical information. So that, in place of the frog-like series, there would be a requirement for more modern illustrations of the body systems. Such printed sheets are known to many who have written on early anatomy as 'fugitive' sheets; they may also be called broadsides, or broadsheets. Since printing produced large numbers of identical images, it was possible to convey information as to the actual form of body structure to a large number of persons. In these sheets the anatomist, artist, and publisher did not immediately make full, or elegant, use of the possibilities; but some of the figures were intended to be more realistic than the symbols of anatomy in medieval manuscripts. Many of the broadsides were hand-coloured, either before or after sale.

A remarkable German woodcut illustration of the abdominal and thoracic viscera was included in a book by Lorenz Fries published in 1518 (*Fig. 2.16*). The author's name was spelt variously as Phryesen, Phries, Frisius, Friesz . . . He was born about 1485, studied at Padua and Montpellier, and then became a physician at Metz, in Lorraine. He died in 1531. He wrote on a number of medical subjects, on Avicenna, on syphilis, and on medical nomenclature. The 1518 book was *Spiegel der Artzny* [that is, Looking-glass of medicine; *Speculum medicinae*]; it was published by Johann Grüninger, or Grieninger, whose firm was active in Strasburg 1483–1531. The book was obviously popular. The chief interest in the 1518 edition lies in a fine folio-size woodcut representing, more or less realistically, a cadaver with thorax and abdomen widely opened to show the internal organs. On the same page are six equally realistic dissections of the head, many showing the brain, and one picturing the tongue. The principal figure was based on an actual dissection of a hanged man, performed in Strasburg by Dr Wendelin Hock von Brackenau; this is stated in the original printing. The drawing was in the current north European tradition, probably the work of Hans Baldung Grien; Baldung painted and drew Deaths and *lemures* in a number of works. The wood-blocks were cut by Hans Wächtlin (Ulrich Pilgrim) of Basle, a master of chiaroscuro work. The paper on which the illustration is printed is larger than the book, and has had to be folded; the back of the sheet accommodates part of the text. There is a second folded illustration, of a skeleton, but this is undistinguished anatomically—which is not surprising, since it appears to have been copied from an inscribed gravestone, there being no skeleton in Strasburg at that time. The book contains other smaller woodcuts, inserted in the text and of little anatomical interest.

This remarkable visceral figure may well have been the first published illustration to have been drawn directly from an actual anatomical dissection. It was, however, not produced only for this book, but was first issued as a fugitive sheet and only secondarily incorporated in the Fries volume. The visceral and the skeletal woodcuts were published by Johann Schott, also in Strasburg; these are self-contained fugitive sheets where the visceral figure has the parts identified in German, with seven accessory figures and a series of verses ('I am a mirror, skilful physician . . .'), with the publisher's device and the date 1517. The visceral woodcut was included in Fries's book, and also in Hans von Gersdorff's *Feldtbüch der Wundartzney*, published by Schott in Strasburg in 1517. When Grüninger incorporated the woodcut in Fries's *Spiegel der Artzny* he did not include the verses. It was not unusual for valuable woodcuts to be passed from one printing-house to another, and blocks were used in more than one context, often appearing in a number of works issued from the same firm. In 1519, Grüninger reissued Fries's book with the original figure completely re-cut (*Plate 9*).

This much used and copied figure, taken at least in part from a dissection, and drawn somewhat realistically, can exemplify the beginning of modern anatomy; such figures—reproduced by

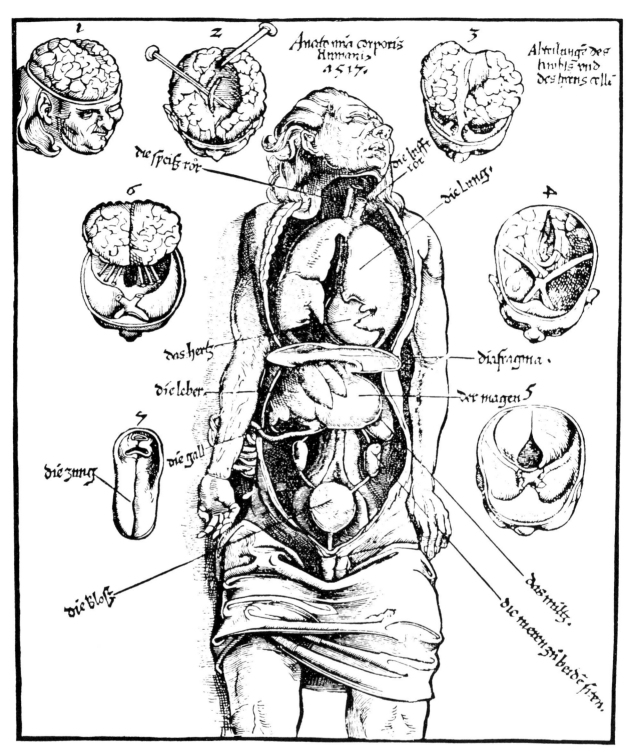

2.16 Viscera figure and associated figures showing brain dissections, etc., from Fries, *Spiegel der Artzny*, Strasburg, 1518. Woodcut made in 1517.

printing—could be improved, mistakes (of which there were many) could be corrected, and new figures could be prepared which were, as time went on, increasingly true to the actual appearance of the dissected subject.

The Fries visceral figure was reproduced with various modifications in the next decade, appearing, for example, in a book by Walther Hermann Ryff published in Strasburg in 1541 (*Plate 10*). In Ryff's woodcut the male figure is seated, on a classically pedimented stool, with knees apart, in a pose unlike that adopted in the Fries woodcut, but which calls to mind earlier frog-like figures.

Ryff was a medical man who has had a consistently bad press; his contemporaries Vesalius, Fuchs, and Gesner were highly critical; and, in recent times, Lynn Thorndike and Harvey Cushing have had little good to say about him. He wrote books (Cushing counted 65 works) on a wide variety of medically-related subjects, including a recipe book for sweetmeats, herbal remedies, and suchlike. He can have had little time for the practice of surgery. His work was based directly on that of others. In particular he frequently used figures from other books, copied with little modification and no acknowledgement. It was this that provoked Andreas Vesalius to call him the 'Strasbourg plagiarist'; Ryff had taken figures from the Vesalian fugitive sheets published in 1538 (see below). The three skeletal tables were copied direct on to the wood-block, keeping the same lettering; the skeletons therefore appear reversed in Ryff's book. The copying was done crudely, so that hands and feet appear absurdly large, every detail being coarsened and simplified. Another woodcut used two Vesalian illustrations of the veins and of the arteries; but in this case diagrams of the vessels have also been placed together within a seated figure—a modest contribution. Ryff also plagiarized, without acknowledgement, the 1517–18 Schott–Fries visceral figure (as we have seen); figures from Röslin's work on obstetrics, 1513; and illustrations from Dryander's book on the anatomy of the head, 1536. Ryff's *Omnium humani corporis partium descriptio . . .*, 1541, included however a woodcut of the base of the skull and the mandible (*see Plate 11*), and this remarkably accurate depiction appears to have been prepared specifically for this book. An even earlier, and again remarkable, illustration of the base of the skull was included in a Latin translation by Ferdinando Balamio of Galen's *De ossibus . . .*, Basle, 1538 (*Fig. 2.17*). The translation forms part of the Cratander edition of Galen (the other books are in Greek). The only other illustrations in this book are of two skeletons; these are more crudely drawn, resembling somewhat the skeletons in Berengario (1521).

Ryff (or was it his Strasburg publisher, Beck?) had the sense to employ Hans Baldung Grien to make many of the illustrations. The Dryander figures were re-drawn with skill and flourish. It seems probable that the ill-copied skeletal woodcuts were cut on to the wood-blocks directly from the Vesalian prints, without being redrawn by Baldung. (That German wood-cutters were up to Venetian standards is shown by the work of Jobst de Negker, who had cut and issued in 1539 from Augsburg what amounts to a true-facsimile of the figures of the Vesalian *Tabulae anatomicae*.) In Ryff's cookery book, published years later, the illustrations were made by another German 'little master', Jost Amman.

Ryff was a hard-working entrepreneur, often using the books and illustrations of others to produce many readily saleable works. He was commissioned and abetted by his publishers, specifically Beck and Egenolff, both famous throughout Europe. The wood-blocks of Ryff's book were used again in a collection of broadsides, ten large annotated pages which were issued the same year by the same publisher in a German, and also in a Latin, edition. Later the blocks were acquired by a Parisian printer, Chrestien or Chrétien Wechel. He published editions (1543, etc.) of Ryff's *Anatomica omnium* ... and the broadsides in Latin and French, and used the blocks in a popular work on surgery by Jean Tagault (1543). Ryff was aesthetically and technically well served not only by his artists but also by his printers, for the Strasburg and the Paris editions are elegant volumes.

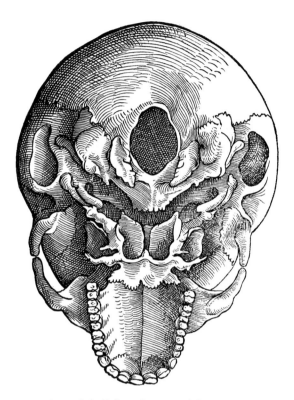

From the above we can conclude, first, that claims to copyright did not stand up internationally in the mid-sixteenth century; secondly, that wood-blocks passed from publisher to publisher and from city to city to be reused in various contexts; thirdly, that anatomy books were important and profitable enough to attract and retain the practical interest of distinguished printers and artists; and, finally, that work issued in one city was soon copied in others. The book trade a century

2.17 Base of skull, from fo. 727^v of the Cratander edition of Galen's *De ossibus*, 1538.

after the invention of printing can be seen to recognize few barriers, moral, geographical, or political, in the pursuit of the profit to be obtained from anatomy books.

In 1538, an innovative set of fugitive sheets were issued in Venice by the anatomist, Andreas Vesalius of Brussels, a young teacher at the medical school in Padua. Three of the figures in these untitled sheets, now known as *Tabulae anatomicae* or *Tabulae sex*, were drawn by Vesalius himself; the remaining three were by his fellow-countryman Jan Stevenszoon Van Calcar. Calcar had sponsored or arranged the publishing venture, and probably expected to profit by it. In Chapter 5 there will be occasion to put these into the context of Vesalius' later work, the *Fabrica* and the *Epitome*, 1543. The *Tabulae* also have their place here among the fugitive sheets and broadsides (*Plates 12 and 13*). The diagrams that Vesalius drew and the extensive text arranged around them were designed for students of anatomy and surgery—Vesalius had just started teaching both subjects at Padua in 1538. They are large; to study them a table must be cleared, or they may be fixed to the wall. The intended purchaser was an academic student, not an apprentice; the text is mostly in Latin. In places Vesalius claims, and ostentatiously displays, more scholarship than can be substantiated, for some Hebrew anatomical terms were reproduced, but misplaced. Greek words were included also; it is not now certain how much of a Greek scholar Vesalius was, but he was certainly within the medical humanistic movement intent on bringing the works of Galen, particularly, to the centre of medical studies. Even so Vesalius did not wish to reject what was valuable in the Arabic writers: he edited some Latin translations from Galen, but he also published a paraphrase of some translations from ar-Razi (Rhazes).

The text for these broadsheets is much concerned with nomenclature, an important matter at the period when the naming of anatomical parts was influenced variously by Greek, Latin, Arabic, and Hebrew terms. The second century AD scholar Julius Pollux had included a glossary of anatomical terms in the *Onomasticon*. This became known to medical people in 1502 when his work was printed at Venice. Vesalius' efforts were but one attempt to refine and fix the jargon of anatomy—a process that cynics have said, quite falsely, has been the chief work of gross anatomists in the last century or so. But nomenclature is not a trivial matter; anatomists of whatever nationality need to know unambiguously the names of identified structures.

Vesalius' precisely drawn three figures are just what teaching aids should be: a student may see immediately the main point of each diagram. The structures, though complex, can be taken in at a glance, yet there is sufficient detail in figure and text to be investigated by closer scrutiny. The anatomy was laid out in relation to function, both figures and text combining to this end. Since Galen had not fully understood the ways in which the anatomy of the human and that of the pig and monkey could differ, and since Vesalius' physiology was Galen's, the anatomy and physiology shown in the three Vesalian tables is in some major respects badly mistaken. For example, Vesalius drew a multilobed liver, a venous system without showing its relationship to the heart, and an arterial system in which a plexus of vessels at the base of the brain (the *rete mirabile*), non-existent in humans, is present. Smaller diagrams indicate supposed correspondences between the reproductive tracts in men and women which have no basis in reality.

As Vesalius described in the dedication printed on the first broadsheet, he had prepared an articulated skeleton 'which I had set up to the gratification of the students . . .'. The three skeletal figures were 'rendered from the three standard viewpoints by the distinguished contemporary artist, John Stephen [Calcar]. They will satisfy those who hold it fitting, fair, profitable, indeed essential, to contemplate the skill and craftsmanship of the Great Artist Himself and to peer into the 'house of the soul' as Plato has it'. Vesalius thus displayed his classical scholarship and demonstrated his religious orthodoxy; heresy in matters of faith might coexist with unorthodox medical views.

On the sixth and final broadsheet there is to be found a colophon which, translated, reads: 'Printed at Venice by B. Vitali of Venice at the cost of Stephen Calcar. For sale in the shop of

Signor Bernardo, Anno 1538'. This is followed by a warning: 'By decree of Pope Paul III and of His Sublime Imperial Majesty, and of the Most Illustrious Senate of Venice: Let no one either print or retail or hawk separately these plates of Andreas Vesalius of Brussels, under the heavy penalties set forth in the copyright'. This warning was ignored. Three years later Vesalius wrote in a letter to his Basle publisher, Oporinus: 'These privileges are often not worth the paper they cover, as I know but too well, from what happened to my *Anatomical Tables* published at Venice …'. He complains of plagiarists in Augsburg, Cologne, Paris, Strasburg, Marburg, and Frankfurt. This shows that copies of his woodcuts were distrbuted through a wide area beyond Padua and Venice. How many copies of the *Tabulae anatomicae* were printed is not known; many must have been so well-used that they disintegrated and were discarded. Probably only three complete copies survive.

We may add a footnote to this account of the *Tabulae*. Among the diagrams that Vesalius drew was one of the brain and nerves; this became the basis for a broadsheet published at Cologne by Aegidius Macrolios with effusive praise to Vesalius, who notwithstanding complained—in a letter to his publisher Oporinus—that this had been deplorably copied from a rough sketch made for one or two friends pending publication by himself. This 'seventh' *Tabula anatomica* (*Fig. 2.18*) was later much improved by Vesalius, and appears, on page 319 of his *Fabrica*, 1543.

An enquiring anatomist who taught vigorously with the aid of diagrams, a skilled artist with experience in Titian's workshop, highly able technicians to cut the wood-blocks—all these, associated with the mercantile city of Venice and its flourishing international school of medicine at nearby Padua, were the background from which emerged the six figures of Vesalius' fugitive sheets, the *Tabulae anatomicae.* These large pages obviously have an important place in the history of anatomical illustration. In 1946, Charles Singer and C. Rabin published 'a discussion of the history, sources and circumstances of the *Tabulae anatomicae sex* of Vesalius', entitled *A prelude to modern science.* Anatomy, when consolidated and advanced by illustrated printed work, was indeed a forerunner of modern observational science. The publication of Vesalius' broadsheets was one of a number of similar ventures; the first steps were taken within fifty years or so of the advent of printing. Anatomists, artists, and printers after the 1490s became increasingly aware that such illustrations were didactically useful, more effective than words alone, and profitable. The 1517 broadsheet of Schott (the Fries figure) and the publications of Berengario (1521, etc.), and Dryander (1536, etc.) precede Vesalius' *Tabulae,* and lead on to the independent contributions, of, among others, Canano, Estienne, and Eustachio—and, of course, to Vesalius' *Fabrica,* all of which we shall discuss later.

By 1550 anatomical science had set out on the straightforward path of descriptive science; other observational sciences, such as botany and geography, were taking the same route for similar reasons. This was before the work of Galileo, Harvey, and others in establishing quantitative and experimental sciences. Anatomy of the early sixteenth century, with the *Tabulae anatomicae* as one of its main elements, may indeed be thought of as a prelude to modern science.

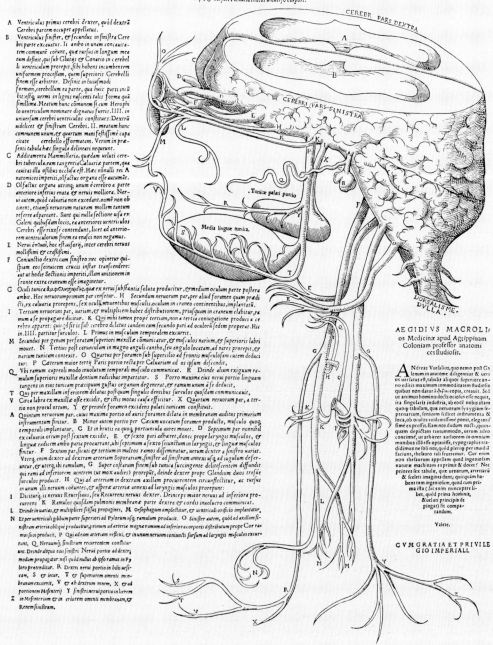

2.18 The brain. A broadsheet by A. Macrolios, published *c.* 1539 in Cologne: L. Molendinus. Copyright Bibliothèque royale Albert Ier, Bruxelles. Cabinet des Estampes, s.v.90092.

Flap-anatomies

Vesalius included in his *Epitome*, 1543, a series of woodcut prints from which composite pictures could be prepared. Illustrations of separate organs could be cut out with scissors and superimposed on a full-length anatomical illustration, and pasted so that, when completed, the figure would have flaps suggesting the three-dimensional, relative positions of internal organs. The technique of multilayered flap illustration had been used earlier in astrological works in the incunabula period (that is, that of printing before 1500). By 1543, when Vesalius issued his *Epitome*, other flap-anatomies were circulating, particularly in Germany and France, as broadsheets. Among the earliest of these appears to be the so-called 'Eve' figure by Jobst de Negker, 1538. The usual figures were a male and a female, both seated, with knees often spread apart—which brings them into the ancient tradition. The scene was sometimes made more plausible by being placed in Eden; the location in others was a bath-house—men and women bathing without clothes brought together a medieval practice and a health-related, sexually intriguing, situation, quite appropriate for public display in a barber-surgeon's establishment.

The males of a set of three fugitive sheets published at Wittenberg in 1573 have the head of a young, vigorous, bearded man, probably intended to represent Vesalius himself—the anatomist anatomized! In other flap-anatomies illustrating the female figure, a flap has to be lifted to expose a loin-cloth, which when turned down, shows the abdomen and gives a superficial view of the external genitalia—by which time the intrusive hand hesitates to go further, yet there are more layers, revealing the pudenda, a pregnant uterus (the position of the woman is similar to that of the Ketham *gravida*, and hence relates to the frog-like series), the fetus and its blood-vessels ... Although Germany was the origin of many of these works (for example a flap anatomy of the eye by G. Bartisch, *Ophthalmoduleia ...*, Dresden, 1583), derivative sheets were published in other countries—France, England, Italy, and Holland. With use the delicate, movable flaps become damaged or detached, so it is uncommon to find perfect examples. The technique of illustrating anatomy by multi-layered flaps has continued to the present time, reaching high levels of sophistication in the nineteenth centuries with the work of the Scottish-American, Alexander Ramsay, and the Englishman, Tuson. But the sixteenth- and seventeenth-century examples were, with some exceptions, essentially intended for barber-surgeons and lay-persons, having the vigour and naïvety of popular art. The most important figures in this tradition were those produced by Johann Remmelin (born 1583), a doctor of Ulm, a city on the Danube. There were three complex, full-page folio sheets of illustrations: the figures showed Remmelin a better anatomist than draughtsman (*Plate 14*). An unauthorized edition of the drawings was published in 1613; the authorized issue was *Catoptrum microcosmicum ...*, Ulm, David Franck, 1619. The engraving was done by Lucas Kilian. There was an accompanying text, indexes, and a portrait of Remmelin, aged thirty-five. The work was reproduced, with varying degrees of skill, a number of times and in other countries until 1754; a London edition was corrected by Clopton Havers: *A survey of the microcosme: or, the anatomy of the bodies of man and woman: useful for all physicians chyrurgeons, statuaries, painters . . .*, London, James Moxon, 1695 (second edition, 1702).

The diagrams and images of human anatomy to be found in surviving manuscipts and in early printed books convey only a portion of the information present in the accompanying text.

Just as the early printed page was an imitation of a manuscript, so early anatomical woodcuts were constructed on the basis of often-copied manuscript examples. A tradition was thereby established of debased, often merely talismanic, anatomical figures. This tradition may be seen in some broadsheets and in encyclopaedic and populist works; it continued long after academic images of anatomy had been refined into science and put to use to convey detailed information.

As anatomists and artists grew more confident in the use of anatomical illustration, the texts of academic anatomies became less important, even taking a secondary place to the figures. In the next chapter the early stages of this development are discussed.

9 Visceral figure (on page facing fo 9ʳ) from Lorenz Phryies [Fries], *Spiegl der Artzny*, Strasbourg, J. Grieninger, 1519. Woodcut (Wellcome Institute Library). 19.3 × 13.8 cm.

The central figure, with a rather piggish face, displays the thoracic and abdominal viscera; surrounding it are dissections showing skull contents and the tongue.

Sparse German labelling identifies the lungs, the liver, the horizontal diaphragm, the large and globular stomach, the spleen, the urinary bladder, the gall-bladder, the kidneys, the heart, the trachea, the thin oesophagus, and the intestines.

The lungs are lobed, and the heart is placed entirely on the left side, rather too upright. The liver is four-lobed, and barely reaches to the left of the mid-line. The urinary bladder is very large, with an enormous urethra; no prostate is seen. The displaced intestines look rather like rope; there is a large spleen, and small and very unkidney-shaped kidneys. Very short ureters are shown emerging from the lower pole of the kidneys and passing to the bladder.

About the only structures recognizable in the skull/brain drawings are the two cerebral hemispheres and the optic nerves, chiasm, and tracts. His figure five would seem to indicate that the optic nerves and tracts were considered to be hollow tubes. The drawings do, however, demonstrate an orderly progression of dissection to expose the intracranial structures.

The superscription to the plate indicates that it was based on an actual dissection. This must be true; despite crudities of position and form, it marks the transition in published anatomical illustrations from the symbolic or conceptual to the more factual. Modifications of several of the brain illustrations were employed by Dryander some twenty-five years later.

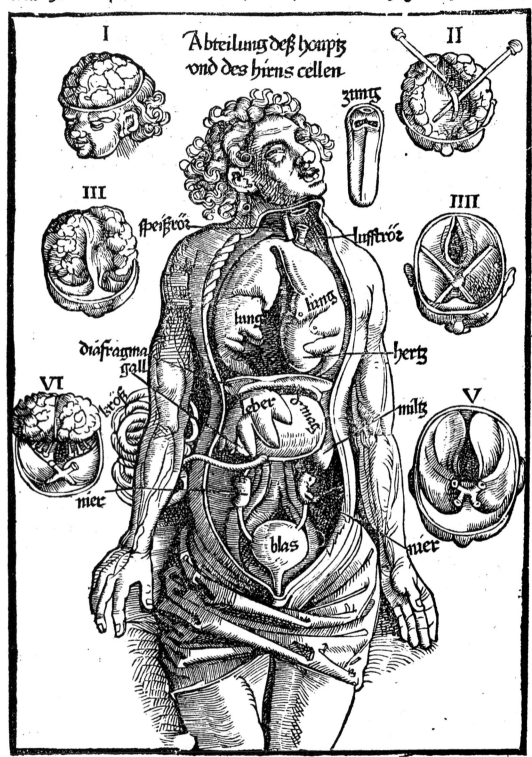

PLATE 9

10 Visceral figure from page 9 of W. H. Ryff, *Anatomica omnium humani corporis partium descriptio* ..., Paris, C. Wechel, 1543. Woodcut (Cambridge University Library). 20.7 × 14 cm.

This is an anterior view of a male figure with the thorax and abdomen widely opened; the enclosed structures are formally placed and indicated by letters. This illustration first appeared in 1541 publications by Ryff. In those copies of this date that were available to us the figure was not suitable for photography. However, the same wood-block was used in the 1543 Paris edition, from which our plate is taken.

The trachea (B) is shown entering the lungs, which are joined together superiorly. There is a suspicion of a cardiac notch on the right lung rather than on the left one. The heart is shown partially covered by both lungs, and is opened to show the right (E) and left (F) ventricles. The œsophagus (A) is seen passing behind the heart and lungs and appearing inferiorly, where it can be seen to pierce the diaphragm (I). It then enters an odd-shaped stomach which possesses no fundus. The liver is very small, turned on its side, and lobulated; the gall-bladder is indicated by (D). A tube issues from the lower right side of the stomach and then expands into the intestines, which are arranged on the arm of the chair. Here the rectum is shown as a straight tube, removed from the body and cut across, just below the caecum and appendix. With the exception of the latter and the ascending colon the guts are poorly drawn.

The kidneys are small, the right one being slightly higher than the left. The vena cava (no aorta is shown) has steeply inclined renal veins (which are rather too small) and testicular veins (which are rather too large) draining into it. The ureters are short and the vasa deferentia ('venae albae') hook round them. The latter arise from a recognizable epididymis, lying medial to the testis. The bladder is large, and a representative prostate is shown lying between it and the root of the penis. The left renal vein is shown communicating with the ureter; but this does not obtain on the right side.

The vena cava would, of course, have 'divided' before reaching the bladder, even if this were distended. The tributaries of the inferior vena cava are rather fanciful.

Ryff was something of an anatomical opportunist, and, as we have seen, Vesalius complained about his re-engraving and also embellishing his plate of the veins: some of Ryff's plates even employ the identical lettering that was used by Vesalius. The illustration shown here is obviously indebted to the Fries figure (*Plate 9*).

OMNIVM HVMANI CORPORIS INTE-
riorum membrorum feu vifcerum
ocularis defcriptio.

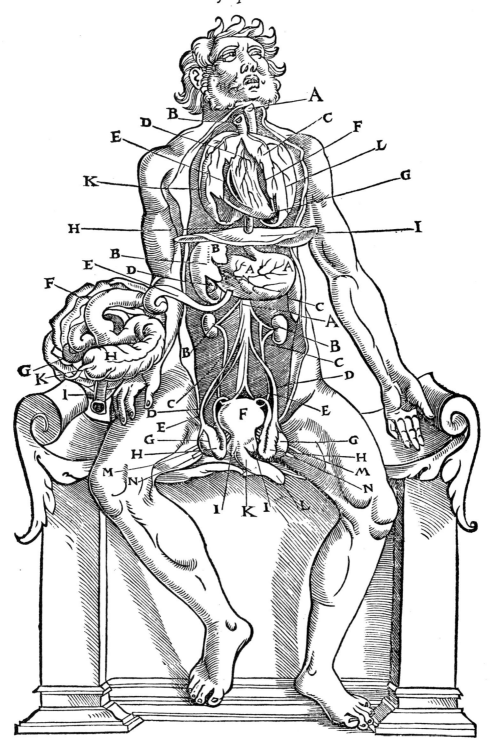

PLATE 10

11 Base of skull and lower jaw from page 35 of W. H. Ryff, *Anatomica omnium humani corporis partium descriptio ...*, 1543, Paris, C. Wechel. Woodcut (Cambridge University Library). 20.3 × 13.4 cm.

This drawing, of the base of the skull, together with a mandible viewed from the front, *pace* Cushing, is quite striking, particularly when the date of its original woodcut, 1541 (two years prior to the publication of Vesalius' *Fabrica*), is considered. The artist has been at pains to convey to the viewer as true an impression of the complex structural appearance of the skull base as lay within his power. Indeed, it may well be considered to succeed rather better in this regard than the skull-base illustration in Cratander's *Opera Galeni*, 1538 (*Fig. 2.17*), stated by Singer and Rabin (1946) to be 'The best printed figure of a skull, and perhaps of any bone, before the *Fabrica*.'

Though the remaining teeth are rather poorly drawn, the hard palate is particularly pleasing. In the Latin edition of his book Ryff terms the palatal portion of the maxilla (B) the 'os palati', and the horizontal plates of the palatine bones (DD) the 'colatoria'.

The foramen magnum (G), the occipital condyles (FF), and the unlabelled pterygoid plates are nicely drawn: the mastoid processes (H), the skull foramina, and the sockets for the heads of the mandible are less good.

It must be admitted that the representation of the mandible does not approach the quality of the skull drawing, quite apart from the oddly different scale employed.

This should not, however, detract from the fact that this pre-Vesalian illustration, inaccurate though it is in some respects, succeeds in portraying what a human skull does indeed look like when viewed from below.

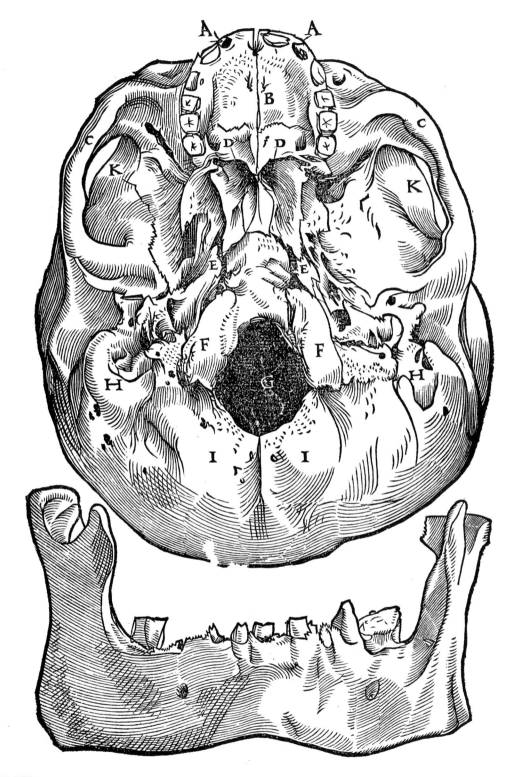

PLATE 11

12 The venous system, Tabula II from A. Vesalius, [*Tabulae anatomicae sex*], Venice, 1538. (Taken from the facsimile issued by Stirling-Maxwell, 1874.) Woodcut (Wellcome Institute Library). 45.8 × 33.5 cm., including text.

This illustration, almost certainly drawn by Vesalius himself, was produced in order to 'assist very greatly' both professors and students to follow his discourses on, and also his dissections of, the venous system.

It contains numerous errors, many of which are repeated later in the *Fabrica*. These include very small internal jugular veins (D), excessively large external jugulars (E), non-human brachiocephalic veins and superior vena cava, a single caval 'trunk' with the right atrio-ventricular orifice (C) opening into it, together with an enormous azygos vein.

The multilobed liver is in accordance with Galenic teaching; other mistakes and misconceptions abound, but as an attempt visually to present the human venous system this was an immense advance on anything that had appeared before.

TABULA II

ϘVENÆ CAVÆ, IECORARIÆ, ΚΟΙΛΗΣ, האורטי HA=

NABVB DESCRIPTIO, QVA SANGVIS OMNIVM PARTIVM NVTRIMENTVM PER
VNIVERSVM·CORPVS·DIFFVNDITVR.

A Vena post aures, et ad tempora.
B Ad nares, frontem et superiorem maxillam.
C Ad linguam, laryngem, fauces et palatum.
D Internæ iugulares, Apopleticæ, Profundæ.
E Iugulares externæ, Guidez, quas etiam Apople
ticas vocant.
F Ad colli musculos posteriores.
G Per transfersos vertebrarum ceruicis processus,
in spinalem medullam et cerebrum excurrunt.
K Ad scapularum gibbum et loca contermina.
L Humeraria, cubiti exterior, Chephalica, Capitis.
M Ad anteriora pectoris et mamillas.
N Ad musculos thoracis superiores.

Quemadmodum iugularis internæ, ac eæ quæ per
transfersos vertebrarum ceruicis processus propaga
tur, in cerebrum eiusq́; membranas et ventriculos
excurrunt, hic delineari nequit.

Hæc venæ in glandiu bifurcatio, nonnunquá pauló
inferius apparet, sic ut ab altero ramo axillaris, quem
admodum modo humeraria deduci uideatur. Præterea
pectoris venæ quæ ad mamillas quoque diffunduntur
ab axillaribus interdum propagatæ apparent. Adde
externas etiá iugularias subinde geminas vtrimque
in collo conspici.

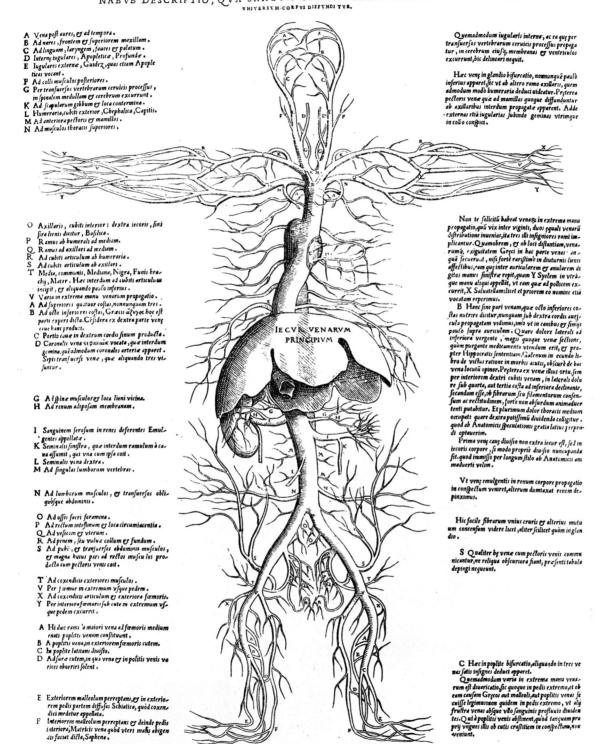

IECVR VENARVM
PRINCIPIVM

O Axillaris, cubiti interior: dextra iecoris, sini
stra lienis dicitur, Basilica.
P Ramus ab humerali ad mediam.
Q Ramus ad axillaris ad mediam.
R Ad cubiti articulum ab humeraria.
S Ad cubiti articulum ab axillari.
T Media, communis, Mediana, Nigra, Funis bra-
chy, Mater. Hæc interdum ab cubiti articulu us
incipit, et aliquando paulo inferius.
V Varia in extrema manu venarum propagatio.
A Ad superiores quatuor costas, nonnunquam tres.
B Ad octo inferiores costas, Græcis ἄζυγος hoc est
paris expers dicta. Cősidera ex dextra parte venæ
ecue hanc producti.
C Portio cauæ in dextrum cordu sinum producta.
D Coronalis vena σφφανιαλ vocata, quæ interdum
gemina, quædmodum coronales arteriæ apparet.
Septi transuersi venæ, quæ aliquando tres vi-
suntur.

G Ad spinæ musculos et loca lieni vicina.
H Ad renum adiposam membranam.

I Sanguinem serosum in renes deferentes Emul-
gentes appellatæ.
K Seminalis sinistra, quæ interdum ramulum à ca-
ua assumit, qui vna cum ipsa coit.
L Seminalis vena dextra.
M Ad singulas lumborum vertebras.

N Ad lumborum musculos, et transfersos obli-
quosque abdominis.

O Ad ossis sacri foramina.
P Ad rectum intestinum et loca circumiacentia.
Q Ad vesicam et vterum.
R Ad penem, seu vuluæ collum et fundum.
S Ad pubé, et transfersos abdominis musculos,
et magna huius pars ad rectos musculos pro-
ducta cum pectoris venis coit.

T Ad coxendicis exteriores musculos.
V Per fœmur in extremum vsque pedem.
X Ad coxendicis articulum et exteriora fœmoris.
Y Per interiora fœmoris sub cute in extremum vs-
que pedem excurrit.

A Hi duæ rami à maiori vena ad fœmoris medium
enati poplitis venam constituunt.
B A poplitis vena, in exteriorem fœmoris cutem.
C In poplite latitans diuisio.
D Ad suræ cutem, in qua vena et in poplitis venis va
rices oboriri solent.

E Exteriorem malleolum perreptans, et in exteriorem pedis partem diffusa: Schiatica, quòd coxen-
dici medetur appellata.
F Interiorem malleolum perreptans et deinde pedis
interiora, Matricis vena quòd vteri malis abigen
dis faciat dicta, Saphena.

Non te solicitú habeat venæq̃; in extrema manu
propagatio, quú vix inter viginti, duas equali venorú
distributione inuenias, ita tres illis insigniores rami im-
plicantur. Quamobrem, et ob loci distantiam, vena-
rumq̃; exiguitatem Grẹci in hac parte venæs ali-
quá secuerunt, nisi forté rarissimè in diuturnis lienis
affectibus, eam quæ inter auricularem et anularem di
gitos manus sinistræ repit, quam Y Syelem in vtrá-
que manu aliqui ad pollicem ex-
currit, X Saluatella: licet et priorem eo nomine etiá
vocatam reperimus.

B Hanc sine pari venam, quæ octo inferiores costas nutrire dicitur, nunquam sub dextra cordis auri-
cula propagatam vidimus, imò vt in canibus et simijs
pauló supra auriculam. Quare dolore laterali ad
inferiora vergente, magis quoque venæ sectione,
quàm purgante medicamento vtendum erit, et prop-
ter Hippocratis sententiam. Galenum in ecundo libro de victus ratione in morbis acutis, obscurè de hac
vena locutú opinor. Præterea ex venæ illius ortu, sem
per interiorem dextri cubiti venam, in lateralis dolo
re sub quarta, aut tertia costa ad inferiora declinante,
secandam esse, ob fibrarum seu filamentorum consen
sum ac rectitudinem, forté non absurdum animaduer
tenti putabitur. Et plurimum dolor thoracis medium
occupat quare dextra potissimú dividenda colligitur
quod ab Anatomicis speculationis gratia latius perpen
di optauerim.
Prima venæ cauæ diuisio non extra iecur est, sed in
iecoris corpore, si modo propriè diuisio nuncupanda
sit, quod immisso per longum stilo ab Anatomicis ani
maduerti velim.

Vt venæ emulgentis in renum corpore propagatio
in conspectum veniret, alterum dumtaxat renem de-
pinximus.

Hic facile fibrarum vnius cruris et alterius mutu
um concensum videre licet, aliter scilicet quàm in glen
dio.

S Qualiter bẹ venæ cum pectoris venis commu
nicantur, ne reliqua obscuriora fiant, præsenti tabula
depingi nequeunt.

C Hæc in poplite bifurcatio, aliquando in tres ve
nas satis insignes deduci apparet.
Quemadmodum varia in extrema manu vena-
rum est diuaricatio, sic quoque in pedis extremo, et ob
eam causam Grẹcos aut malleoli, aut poplitis venas se
cuisse legimus non quidem in pedis extremo, vt alij
frustra venas absque vllo sanguinis profluuio dividen
tes. Qui à poplitis venis abstinent, quod tanquam pro
prij vngues illis ob cutis crassitiem in conspectum, non
veniunt.

ALIQVI VENAE CAVAE RAMOS INSIGNIORES CENTVM ET SEXAGINTA OCTO POSVERVNT.

PLATE 12

13 Skeleton from front, Tab. IV from A. Vesàlius, [*Tabulae anatomicae sex*], Venice, 1538. (Taken from the facsimile issued by Stirling-Maxwell, 1874.) Woodcut (Wellcome Institute Library). 47.8 × 35 cm., including text.

This drawing, by Joannes Stephanus of Calcar, although crude when compared with the skeleton plates of the *Fabrica*, was at the same time a great improvement on those that had previously appeared.

Poorly portrayed, from an anatomical standpoint, are the wide skull; the sterno-clavicular joint and coracoid processes; the seven-piece sternum and lower costal cartilages; the pelvic girdle and the vertebral column in general; sinuous long limb bones with misshapen extremities, absent lesser trochanters, and an erroneous inclination of the femoral neck relative to the shaft.

From the presence of what are presumably representations of epiphyses (for example, of the radius, femur, tibia, and fibula) the skeleton would appear to be that of a person approximately eighteen years old at the time of death. It has been suggested (Saunders and O'Malley, 1950) that he (less likely, she) must have suffered from rickets during life, which could explain some of the unusual features mentioned above. If a different skeleton was employed for the *Fabrica* plates, Vesalius would seem to have had remarkable access to, or a predilection for, skeletons of young adults.

At the foot of this figure Vesalius expressed his opinion that the adult skeleton is composed of 246 bones (excluding sesamoids), which is somewhat of an over-estimate.

HVMANI CORPORIS OSSA PARTE ANTERIO-
RIEXPRESSA.

Foramina quæ in harum triũ chartarum delineatione conspici possunt, sunt in temporum osse auditorius meatus: post mamillarem processum vnum, per quod interna iugularis in cerebrum mergit:in facie circa oculorum sedem quatuor, primum ad frontem, secundum ad nares, tertium ad maxillam superiorem, quartum ad temporalem musculũ:duo quoq, in maxilla inferiori. Et per hæc singula ramulus tertij paris neruorum excidit.

Obsrnæ, dentes, שינים scinaim,plurimum triginta duo. רמאה ,incisorij,כזחחה mecbathcim, octo : כלב sorn,canini, כלב calbym quatuor,מלתא molares , maxillares,מחנ thochnim viginti. omnes disparibus radicibus suos aluçolos subeunt.

B Clauiculæ, κλμέσ, claues,iugula, תרקוה tharkuha,Furculæ: vtrumq, os literam.ſ.refert, figura inæquabili.

C Ακρώμιον , summus humerus, processus superior scapulæ, à Galeno in lib.de vsu par.κεραικι δ́σ ad rostri coruini similitudinem nominacu , כחף סח alzegam charton,huius appendix cuius principio claues per arthrodian dearticulantur, proprie κατακλειδ̀κ quasi ad clauiculas dicitur, R ostrum porcinum.

D Processus scapulæ interior inferiórque ab anchoræ similitudine ἀνκυροειδ̀ισ dictus,ex hunc sæpe κορωνοειδ́ια ex signonæle Gale. vocaut. כף עין hacatheph , Oculus scapulæ.

E Pectoris os, स́गνου,חזה bechaseh , Cassos, septem constat ossibus, sicuti costæ quæ illi alligantur,per vnionem potius,quàm per coarticulationem,parte inferiori iunctis:id ab vtroq, latere lunatum est.

F Cartilago ξιφοειδ́ισ, ensiformis, quo nomine totum os quoque dicitur, אלחנגרי alchangri,Ensifoidis,Malum granatum, Epiglottalis cartilago .

G Βραχίων, brachium,humerus Celso ex C.sari, זרוצ Zeroach, Adiutorium brachij, Aseth: hoc tile osse minus est.

H Sinus,humeri caput veluti in duo tubercula diuidens.

I Humeri orbita trochleis similis.

K Cubitus,ππίχυσ, קנה b kaneh, Asaid,quibus nominibus etiam tota hæc pars dicitur ,vlna. Focile maius, זנד אליון zenad elion , huius acutus processus ad brachiale συλcαδ́κ nominatur

L Radius, κερκίσ זנד תחתהון zenad tbachtbon, Focile minus brachy.

N Brachiale, κκρπόσ, רשג reseg,Raseta,Rasceba,ossibus disparibus octo ex duplici ordine distinctis constat,in superiori tribus, in inferiori quatuor:hæc simul figuram intrinsecus cauam, ex extrinsecus gibbam constituunt:istorum cum Celso non incertus numerus est.

O Μετακάρπιον, palma , pecten , משרק masrek, Postbrachiale ossibus quatuor Galeno , non quinque, vt alijs cunplurimis ,conformatum est.

P Δάκτυλοι , digiti, אצבעות esbaoth singuli ex ternis ossibus conformantur,priori semper interno dio in subsequentis sinum subeunte .

Q Μύλη, επιγουατίσ, patella , rotula genu, מגן הרקוב magen harcubach, scutum genu, Aresfatus os rotundum breuis scuti instar.

R Ασραγαλοσ,talus, כרסול karsul,Balistæ os,Cauilla,Chabab,Alsuchi:aliqui malleolum hodie ma̅e vertunt .

S Nauiforme, σκαφοειδ́ισ , nauiculare, כורכי zorki .

T τάρσος, רשג reseg,Raseta pedis,quatuor ossibus constat,quorum maximum extrinsecus situm à cuis figura dicitur κυβοειδ̀ισ,tesseræ os , תרדי thardy , Exagonon , Grandinosum, Nerdi.R eliqua tria nominibus carent,sed κυλλοαδ́κ nonnullis nominantur. Bis vidimus dextrum pedem vno abundare.

V Planta, planum , πεδίον, pecten משרק masrek, ossibus quinque constructum est, cui succedunt pedis digiti, X qui omnes ex ternis internodys cōstant,magno tantũ excepto,qui inter alios ex du plici osse constructus est.
Osticulum illud quod ad primum pollicis articulum apparet,vnum ex sesaminis ossibus est: ex in illo duntaxat loco duo in vtroq, pede obseruauimus .

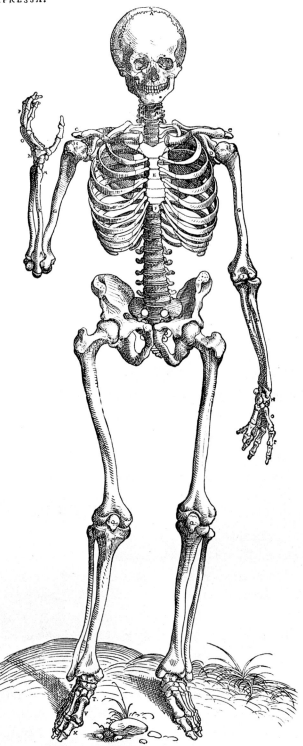

HVMANI CORPORIS OSSA NONNVLLI IN DVCENTA QVADRAGINTA OCTO, ALIQVI VERO, in alium numerum redigunt , ego excepto hyoide quod integrum fere ex sex ossiculis per syncondrosim vnitis conformatur, ex sesaminis ducenta ex quadraginta sex putauerim sequentis tabellæ disticho comprehensa.

IV.

PLATE 13

14 Female flap-anatomy (with a flap over the left trunk kept open by a white card) from J. Remmelin, *Catoptrum microcosmicum* ..., 1619. Woodcut (Wellcome Institute Library). 42.0 × 30.4 cm.

The main figure possesses folding pieces which can be pulled back so as progressively to expose more of the abdominal and thoracic contents. It must be said that the anatomy that is revealed underneath the flaps is not particularly distinguished, and in many cases is extremely difficult to make out. When the two flaps covering the external genitalia are lifted the labia majora are found to be very crudely drawn.

Many of the small diagrams surrounding the main figure are Vesalian. The second figure, the base of the skull, has three folding parts: it features a snake issuing through the foramen magnum, perhaps figuratively representing the spinal cord, and, at the same time, the serpent at the Fall of Man. On the page opposite the drawing a list is given to help identify the parts in the illustration.

Figures 5, 6, and 7 all demonstrate a lack of comprehension of the anatomy of the female external genitalia. Any aspiring obstetrician of the time would have experienced great difficulty in learning very much from them. This is largely due to the lack of artistic ability, because the identification of the parts and their descriptions in the text are quite excellent for the early part of the seventeenth century.

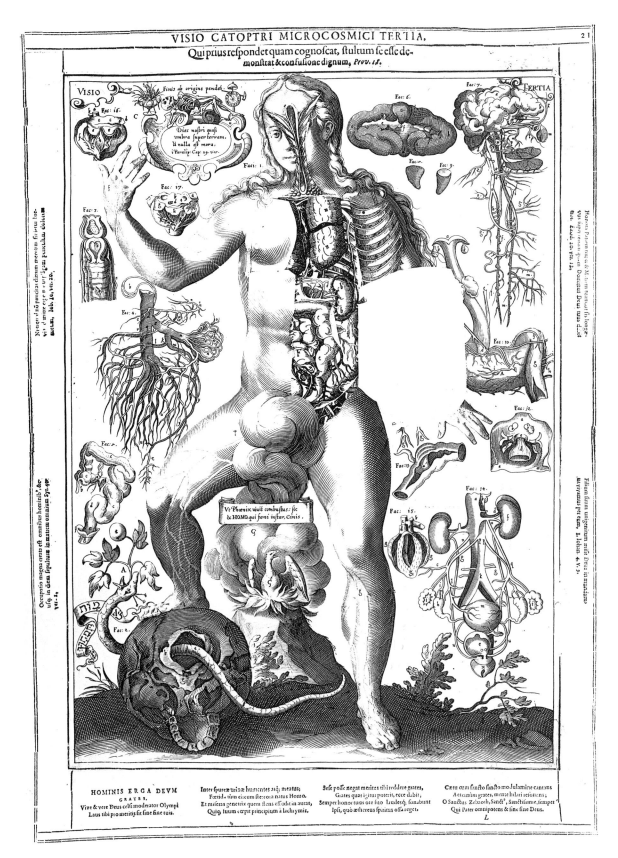

PLATE 14

Chapter 2: Selected reading

Arber, A. (1940). The colouring of sixteenth-century herbals. *Nature,* **145,** 803.

Blunt, W. and Raphael, S. (1979). *The illustrated herbal.* Thames and Hudson, New York.

Boase, T. S. R. (1972). *Death in the middle ages . . . .* Thames & Hudson, London.

Blackman, J. (1977). *Popular theories of generation* . . . in Woodward, J. and Richards, D. *Health care and popular medicine* . . . Croom Helm, London.

Bullough, V. L. (1972). Magnus Hundt. *Dict. sci. Biog.,* **6,** 562–3.

Crummer, L. R. (1923 and 1925). Early anatomical fugitive sheets. *Ann. med. Hist.* **5,** 189–209; **7,** 1–5.

Cushing, H. (1962). *A bio-bibliography of Andreas Vesalius.* Schuman, New York.

Garrison, F. H. (1926). *The principles of anatomic illustration before Vesalius: an inquiry into the rationale of artistic anatomy.* Hoeber, New York.

Herrlinger, R. (1970). *History of medical illustration from antiquity to A.D. 1600.* Pitman, London.

Holbein, H. the younger (1971). *The dance of death.* (Facsimile of the original 1538 edition.) Dover, New York.

Jones, P. M. (1984). *Medieval medical miniatures.* The British Library, London.

de Lint, J. G. (1924). Fugitive anatomical sheets, *Janus* **28,** 78–91.

MacKinney, L. (1965). *Medical illustrations in medieval manuscripts.* Wellcome Historical Medical Library, London.

Mende, M. (1978). *Hans Baldung Grien: Das graphische Werk* . . . Dr Alfonns Uhl, Unterschneidheim.

Morris, A. G. and Keen, E. N. (1982). Lawrence Herbert Wells and the history of anatomical illustration [pre-Vesalian]. *S. African med. J.,* **61,** 40–3.

Saunders, J. B. de C. and O'Malley, C. D. (1950). *The illustrations from the works of Andreas Vesalius of Brussels.* World Publishing, Cleveland.

Sigerist, H. E. (1960). *The foundation of human anatomy in the renaissance.* In *On the history of medicine* (ed. F. Marti-Ibañez). M. D. Publications, New York.

Singer, C. (1925). *The Fasciculo di medicina, Venice 1493.* R. Lier, Florence.

Singer, C. (1955). A study in early renaissance anatomy. In *Studies in the history and method of science* (ed. C. Singer). Dawson, London. (Reprint of 1917 edn.)

Singer, C. and Rabin, C. (1946). *A prelude to modern science. . . .* Cambridge University Press.

Streeter, E. C. and Singer, C., Fifteenth century miniatures of extramural dissections in *Essays on the history of medicine presented to Karl Sudhoff* . . . edited by C. Singer and H. E. Sigerist (Reprint of 1925 edn.). Books for Libraries Press, Freepost NY.

Sudhoff, K. (1964). *Ein Beitrag zur Geschichte der Anatomie in Mittelalter. . . .* (Reprint of 1908 edn.) Georg Olms, Hildesheim.

Sudhoff, K. (1910). Die Bauchmuskelzeichnung von 1496. *Archiv. f. Gesch. Med.,* **3,** 131–4.

Sudhoff, K. (1924). *The Fasciculus medicinae of Johannes de Ketham Alemanus. Facsimile of the first (Venetian) edition of 1491* . . ., (ed. C. Singer). R. Lier, Milan.

Vesalius, A. (1965). *Andreas Vesalius Bruxellensis: Tabulae anatomicae.* Culture et Civilisation, Brussels.

Weitzmann, K. (1977). *Late antique and early Christian book illumination.* George Braziller, New York.

Wells, L. H. (1966). The 'Sabio' and 'Sylvester' families of anatomical fugitive sheets. . . . *Bull. Hist. Med.,* **40,** 467–75.

Wells, L. H. (1968). Anatomical fugitive sheets with superimposed flaps 1538–1540. *Med. Hist.,* **12,** 403–7.

Wickersheimer, E. (1913). L'Anatomie de Guido de Vigevano, médecin de la reine Jeanne de Bourgogne (1345). *Sudhoff's Arch.,* **7,** 1–25.

Wickersheimer, E. (1926). *Anatomies de Mondino dei Luzzi et de Guido de Vigevano.* E. Droz, Paris.

Wirth, J. (1979). *La jeune fille et la mort . . .* Droz, Geneva.

3

The beginnings of factual
anatomical illustration

*W*ITH THE spread of printing across Europe in the second half of the fifteenth century the production of multiple, satisfactory copies of illustrated books, including anatomy books, became possible. However, it was not for a full hundred years after printing presses were established at Mainz that Vesalius' works were issued from Basle in 1543—books that were the most comprehensive solutions to the problem that Renaissance anatomists set themselves: how to present synthetically and coherently ancient anatomy, recovered by the humanists, along with the newer and more accurate knowledge obtained by dissection of human subjects. Before Vesalius, there were other attempts at a solution, ranging from the poorly printed tome of Gabriele Gerbi (de Zerbis) *Liber anathomie corporis humani* ..., Venice, 1502, to Alessandro Achillini's lecture notes on anatomy, *Anotomicae annotationes* ..., published in Bologna in 1520, but written earlier. These were not illustrated; one's heart sinks when turning the dense pages of Gerbi. The elegant volume of Ketham's works, produced in Venice in 1493, was no solution; it was not, compared with Gerbi, an academic anatomy text, and the figures relating to anatomy were medieval in concept, even if Renaissance in execution.

Anatomy was also included in volumes coming from German-speaking cities:

the illustrations were, with few exceptions, symbols rather than images of anatomy, and the texts often included a section of anatomy only within wider surveys of knowledge, as in Hundt's *Antropologium* (1501) and Reisch's *Margarita philosophica* (1503). Partial solutions to the problem, however, began to appear: the early work of Vesalius (1538) combined, as we have seen, words and pictures coherently. In this chapter we come to the anatomical work of Berengario da Carpi (1521 and 2), Dryander (1536 and 7), and Canano (?1542).

Having explored the remoter landscapes of pre-scientific illustration, we are now in more familiar country.

Giacomo (or Jacopo) Berengario da Carpi (Berengarius) c. 1460–1530

His family name was Barigazzi, but he adopted the name of Berengarius, perhaps after the Emperor of that name; he signed himself usually just Carpi. He was an anatomist, surgeon, and physician, and, from 1502–1527, a teacher in the medical school at Bologna.

The illustrated anatomical works by Berengario that concern us are: *Commentaria ... super anatomia Mundini*, Bologna, 1521 and *Isagogae breves ...*, Bologna, 1522. The first book, of more than a thousand pages, was a detailed anatomy reference text, giving, and then discussing, Mondino's fourteenth-century dissecting manual (Fig. 3.1). The printer set the original text by Mondino and the commentary by Carpi in different typefaces. This work was in the same style as that of Gabriele Gerbi, who was Berengario's teacher, and to whom he repeatedly refers. The *Isagogae* was a digest or précis of the larger book in about a hundred and fifty pages, again written more or less to accompany an actual dissection. It was described by the author as a 'little book than which no other on this subject was ever shorter or clearer'. 'It represents', he wrote, 'our present state of knowledge; its use will save the reader long hours of study.' However, in this same introduction, no mention was made of the illustrations. The shorter work was the one that was reprinted a number of times, (including a translation into English in 1660). In the *Isagogae* Berengario frequently suggests that the reader refer to his larger *Commentaria* for more information.

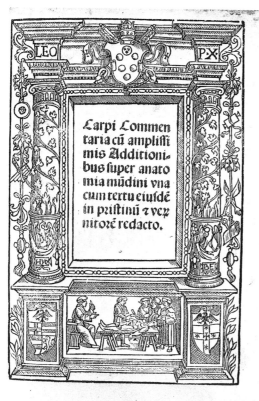

3.1 Title-page of Berengario, *Commentaria*, 1521.

The two works contain essentially the same type of illustration; they obviously have greater impact in the shorter work. Only some of the regions or systems of the body are illustrated, namely: the muscles of the trunk; the uterus and other parts of the female reproductive tract; the veins, but only those of the extremities; the muscles beneath the skin, shown in flayed men (*écorchés*); and the skeleton. In the 1523 edition of the *Isagogae* new figures of the brain, and the heart were added.

There are six dramatic woodcuts of men standing four-square with their legs apart. These show the muscles of the anterior abdominal wall (*Plate 15*). The muscles are indicated by lines representing in a diagrammatic way the direction of the muscle fibres. In all but one the figures show us their own dissected parts by holding skin and muscle flaps away. All stand in a sketched-in landscape, with a few hillocks and a few grass tufts or weeds. The second plate is the most dramatic: behind the gesturing man are bold rays of light in a dark sky—technically and aesthetically a fine woodcut (Fig. 3.2).

Berengario and his artist must have seen an illustration that appeared in various printed Venetian editions (including 1496, 1504 and 1521) of the *Conciliator . . .* by the fourteenth-century physician and philosopher, Pietro d'Abano. This illustration represented two male figures standing side by side, each with his near arm on the other's shoulder (Fig. 3.3). The muscles of the anterior trunk wall were shown in a similar diagrammatic way to that in the Berengario illustrations—but even more inaccurately. The criss-crossing muscles shown on the left-hand figure's right side in the *Conciliator* illustration are changed in Carpi's figures. It is possible that they were drawn somewhat arbitrarily in both cases, but the Carpi representation is the less inaccurate.

In Berengario's *Isogogae* three figures of women showing their reproductive organs are strongly drawn, and bold. The women either sit on a plinth in the *Fasciculo* (1493) tradition, or stand beside it. They have drapery behind them—in one case hanging from a curtain-rail suspended incongruously in a landscape (Fig. 3.4), in the other two, held high above their heads. The anatomical content of these figures

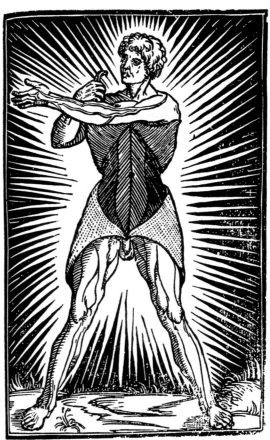

3.2 'Sunburst' muscle-man
from Berengario,
Commentaria, 1521.

I

H

K

O

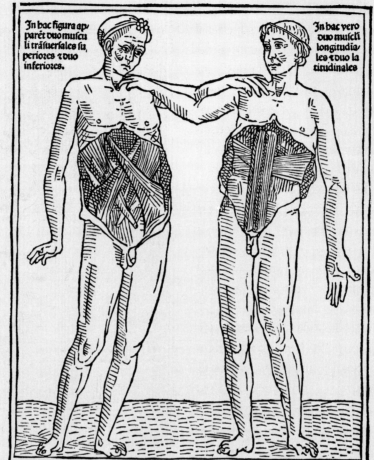

In hac figura apparét duo musculi trásuersales superiores τ duo inferiozes.

In hac vero duo muscli longitudinales τ duo latitudinales.

L

P

M

Consideras vo denuo anothomiã sensibili huius visione pcepi ordinez musculoz tactũ zᵉ. Uidetur eni intrã aliqñ pfundi vt nequeãt sensu discerni: τ iõ diuersimode ipsozuz pruntiatur situs: si tñ aliud apparebit subiungeï in bis ñ deinceps. ℂ Partes vo vétris ad interius ipsius procedeti occurrétes primitus vt cutis insenties: deinde spermatica sensitiua: postea pãniculus seu mẽbzana sub ipsa exté sa: deide lacertus myrach dict°: deinceps vo tunica tunicaq lacerti ventris: τ demũ pãniculus q fm veritate syphac existit quod periteneum siue circum extensum appellatur sub quo zirbus continetur τ intestina. Est autem bozum musculozum cum bis que ipsozum triplex iuuamé tum. vnum quidem vt eozum constructione intestina vesicam τ matricem quod in eis continetur: cogat expellere suo tempoze. secundũ vt sustentent τ robozét diapbzagma quando pectus exufflatione constringitur τ vocis adiuuét tumitionem. Reliquum vt ventris augmentent calozez in

alimenti digestionem. Qui autem continuantur vtilitatez pzebent ab instrumentis subleuando cibi soliditatem augendo ipsius nequãdo extenditur ei contigerit scissura vel quando ventri acciderit inflatio. ℂ Pzopter quartum bu iusmodi sciendum ɋ euacuatio aque vel saniei fm cauterium debet fieri paulatine fm ɋ virtus poterit tolerare. Nam fm veterez Quicũqꝫ empici aut hydropici vrñtur vel inciduntur: bis effluente sanie vel aqua multa τ repente omnino pereunt: cum omne subitum nature sit pzeliatiuum. Afoi. z. Modus autem incisionis: quoniam ascliticus existat rectus aut super sedem eleuatam vt tendantur ventralia: tuncꝗ ministri latera ventris deozsum compzimant τ consideretur an hydropisis sit ab itestinis vel renibus: epate vel splene. Cũ siquidem ab intestinis per tres digitos fm latũ sub vmbilico directe facienda est incisio. Si vo sit ab epate i latere fiat leuo. ɋ fi a splene tafr a dextro vt eductio accidat p ɜriũ: deiñ pellis cleueï ad supe

Afoi.6°
afoi. iȝ.

Afoi. τ
cõ. ȝi.

Q

3.3   Muscle-men from Pietro d'Abano, *Conciliator*, 1496.

is not great, but their influence may be seen in similar illustrations in Charles Estienne's *De dissectione . . .*, published 1545.

The next three figures are of the superficial veins of the extremities 'that are usually phlebotomized [that is, used in blood-letting] . . .'. In these printed books of Berengario, there were illustrations that were indeed useful for that purpose (Fig. 3.5). Previous blood-letting manuscript illustrations were practically useless. In the early printed venesection figures, such as the beautiful one in the *Fasciculo*, 1493, the artists did not seriously address the task of usefully representing the course of the superficial veins. In Berengario, a correctable venesection anatomy was distributed in identical copies to a wide readership of medical men.

The *écorchés* were included to assist physicians 'in recognizing the heads and middle parts of the muscles so that they may both prognosticate wounds . . . and know how to make incisions . . . without lesions of the tendons'. But, Berengario notes, the figures 'also assist painters . . .'. The *écorchés* were drawn as if they were living men, in a landscape sket-

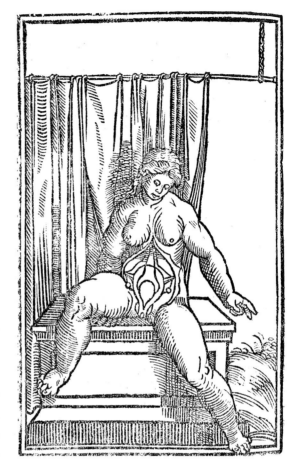

3.4 Female reproductive organs from Berengario, *Commentaria*, 1521.

ched in with greater detail than that to be seen in the figures of muscle-men. One, showing the superficial back muscles, stands with an axe; another, drawn from the side, holds a long staff; the frontal figure shows a man with a heavy rope, one end tied into a noose, with a single tree in the landscape behind— is this a figure of Judas? (Fig. 3.6). A fourth figure in Berengario's *Commentaria* is a woodcut showing a crucified man, perhaps Christ (Fig. 3.7). This possible lack of propriety was sometimes repeated by other Renaissance anatomists.

The two complete skeletons are again shown in the foreground against a landscape—trees, hills, buildings. . . One presents a front view, another a rear view (*Plate 16*) in which the skeleton holds a skull in either hand—potentially useful to show its various aspects, but in execution drawn in such an uninformed way that little information is conveyed; the drawings are as unsatisfactory as an anatomical image as some cuts done to illustrate 'Dance of Death' sequences.

Each of these woodcuts has a descriptive paragraph accompanying it; it is not always easy

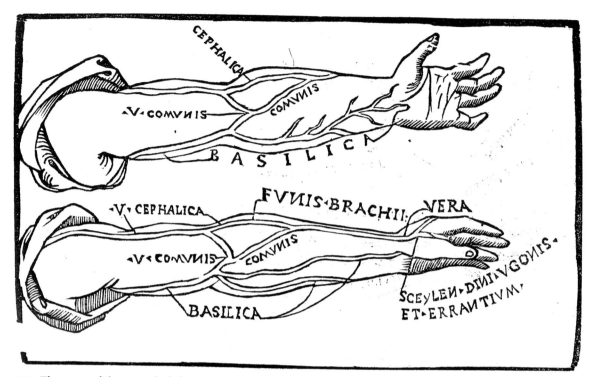

3.5 The veins of the upper limb from Berengario, *Commentaria*, 1521.

to connect the description and the figure. The body of the text and the illustrations are hardly related at all. Moreover, Berengario showed an uncertainty in attitude to illustration: 'the testicles [that is, the ovaries] in this picture are in the place where they belong'; in another picture: 'the testicles are not in their natural place ... so that the seminal vessels may be better seen'; again, 'in these pictures and in other pictures are shown some small branches ... [but] the vein shown in these pictures does not have them, this makes no difference'. The figures of the bones of the foot and of the hand have to be turned upside-down to read half the lettering (*Plate 17*). (The lettering is more easy to read in the 1522 *Isagogae*.) Some of these early sixteenth-century figures are however recognizably in the same manner as figures in the texts of our own time; it is not surprising that these early attempts lack some sophistication.

In Berengario's writing one can see a respect for Mondino and the authority of the works of Galen, but he also expresses independent opinions: 'one must not believe other authorities when experience and perception run counter to them'. This may have been a conventional statement, echoing Galen himself; nevertheless, Berengario did criticize these writings, and was regarded by his contemporaries as a bold, independent man having insufficient respect for authority. Indeed he challenged the traditional Galenic canon; his description of anatomical structures was based not only on the classical authorities, but also on direct observation. His familiarity with anatomy came, he says, from the dissection of hundreds of cadavers. His close and critical reading in Latin and Greek of classical, Arabic, and western medieval sources put him in touch with humanistic scholarship, with medieval and Arabic anatomy, and with scientific independent inquiry based on actual observation.

What natural abilities and background enabled Berengario to initiate this enterprise, the forerunner of Vesalius' anatomy and thence many subsequent texts? He received training from his father, a surgeon at Carpi, a town near Modena in north Italy. He studied under Aldo Manuzio (Aldus Manutius, *c.* 1450–1515), the humanist who became a great Venetian printer and publisher. The dedication of the *Isagogae* ... was to 'Alberto Pio, Count and Most Meritorious Master of Carpi ...', who, it later states, shared schooling 'under our Roman teacher, Aldus Manutius ... We both enjoyed it when we had to dissect a pig. The task fell to me, since I had practised the surgeon's art under my father's direction ever since childhood. From that time onward I was so fond of anatomy that I spent all my time at it.' Berengario obtained his medical degree in 1489 in Bologna, where Gerbi was a teacher. Early in the century, during a

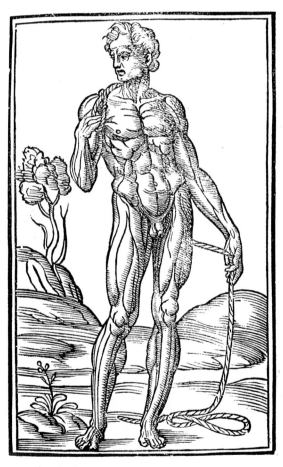

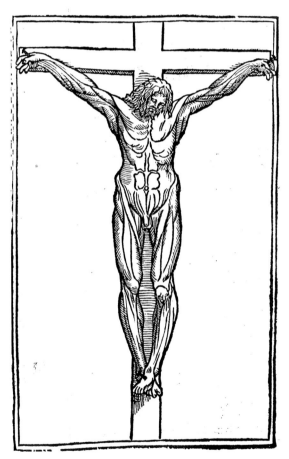

3.6 *Écorché* from Berengario, *Commentaria*, 1521.

3.7 Crucifixion figure as an *écorché* from Berengario, *Commentaria*, 1521.

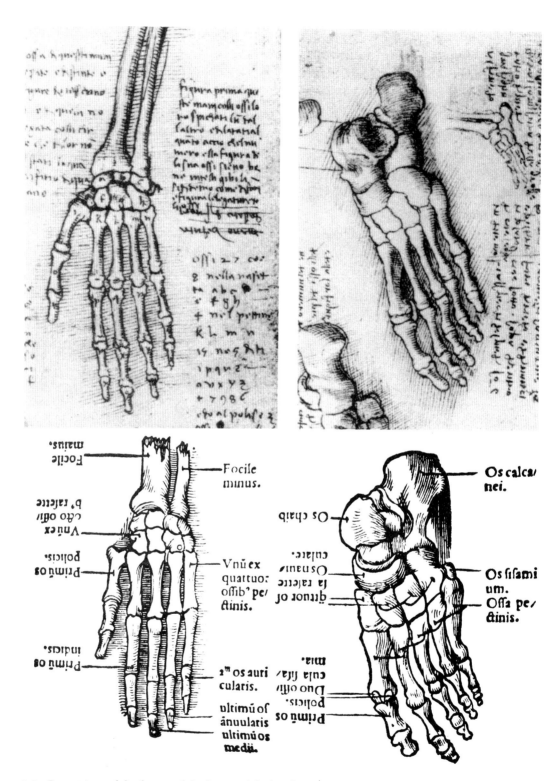

3.8 Comparison of the figures of the bones of the hand and foot, from Leonardo *Notebooks*, and Berengario, *Commentaria*, 1521.

plague epidemic, he was involved in public health in Bologna; but his reputation rested primarily on his skill as a surgeon and physician, being consulted by many of the more prominent families, including that of Pope Leo X. He cared for Lorenzo dé Medici, a nephew of the Pope, when he was recovering from a head wound received in battle in 1517. A year later Berengario published *Tractatus de fractura calve sive cranei*, Bologna, which was reprinted many times. With his eye firmly on the main chance, Berengario made a fortune in Rome treating the new disease, syphilis, with mercury. A riotous man, he has been described as rapacious, greedy, and worthless; certainly he was involved in a number of affrays. Yet for all that his illustrated anatomical books are surprisingly uncontentious by the standards of sixteenth-century academic argument.

With his education in humanist learning, Berengario had comprehended Greek, and, through translation, Arabic anatomy; by attending and carrying out many dissections, and by intensive study of the work of Mondino and his successors at Bologna, he completed his knowledge of contemporary anatomy and advanced beyond it. He, his illustrator(s), and his publisher realized some of the potentialities of the printing press and of illustrated books. Certainly he continued to respect Aldo, the greatest printer of the period; he was writing, in 1522, of Aldo 'of happy memory'. Ugo da Carpi, writing master, chiaroscuro artist, and maker of woodcuts, may have been the artist for Berengario's anatomical illustrations. Berengario was himself an art collector and patron—apparently not too generous a patron. He accepted a Raphael painting of St John in the Desert as a fee for medical attendance; the story is told by Vasari. Benvenuto Cellini, who made him two silver vases, also wrote about him.

There was behind some of the Berengario illustrations the tradition of an anatomical series, with dissected figures portrayed as if standing alive in a landscape. As we have seen, his sources also included a figure altered from the *Conciliator*. It is possible that Berengario, or more likely his artist, was influenced from another source: in at least one instance a drawing by Leonardo da Vinci and a Berengario illustration have close correspondences. The background shading in the drawing of the bones of the hand was possibly copied in the woodcut; moreover the Leonardo drawing of the bones of the foot and hand and the Berengario woodcut may be seen to be closely similar (Fig. 3.8, where the Leonardo drawing of the hand has been reversed for easier comparison.) Leonardo's anatomical drawings are the subject of the next chapter; his notebook sketches could have been seen by a few artists, even fewer anatomists. Other correspondences noted by some authorities seem to us to be less convincing.

During the first half of the sixteenth century Berengario's illustrated *Isagogae* was widely distributed, and many, including Vesalius, noted his findings. The mid-century publications of Vesalius, Estienne, and Eustachio all show directly or indirectly, in various ways, the influence of this work. Falloppio, looking back to a supposed Greek golden age of anatomy, wrote about him that he was, beyond all doubt, 'the first restorer of that anatomical science which Vesalius afterwards perfected'.

15 Standing figure showing the anterior abdominal muscles on fo. 80ᵛ Berengario da Carpi, *Commentaria ... super Anatomia Mundini ...*, Bologna, Hieronymus de Benedictis, 1521. Woodcut (Wellcome Institute Library). 15.4 × 9.9 cm.

This is a frontal view of a male with the abdominal skin and superficial fascia cut transversely, at about the level of the umbilicus, and also sagitally in the mid-line. The upper two flaps are held up by the hands, the lower two hang down over the antero-lateral thigh. It is the first of six illustrations of muscle dissections, each progressively deeper.

The rectus abdominis muscles are represented on each side of the mid-line. In two of the subsequent drawings the recti are shown detached from the chest and hanging downwards, with, interestingly, two horizontal tendinous intersections depicted on the posterior aspect; a then presumed posterior rectus sheath is shown. As the shading of the muscle in those plates is different to that of this plate it is most probable that, in this drawing, the anterior rectus sheath is represented. Indeed the text refers to 'two small skins ... underneath and above' the recti. On either side the external oblique muscles are represented by downward and medially directed shading.

Thigh muscles can be made out through the skin, and one can identify the rectus femoris anteriorly, flanked on either side by vastus medialis and lateralis. In the left thigh a rather wide sartorius muscle can be seen passing obliquely downwards and medially, with the adductor muscles lying medial to it.

In hac fi/
gura hés du
os musculos
obliquos de
scédétes, un
um a dextris
aliũ a siniſtris
q̃ sunt supra
oẽs muscu/
los eoᵱ pars
carnea appa
ret a laterib'
& in medio
uẽtris: supra
musculos lũ
gos ſũt eorũ
cordæ.ſ.una
adextris/alia
a siniſtris pel
liculares : &
latæ q̃ termi
nant̃ i linea:
q̃ eſt in me/
dio uẽtris:ut
uides/ & cor
dæ iſtæ ſunt
duarum pel
licularũ .ſ. ſe
cũdum ſub:
& ſupra.

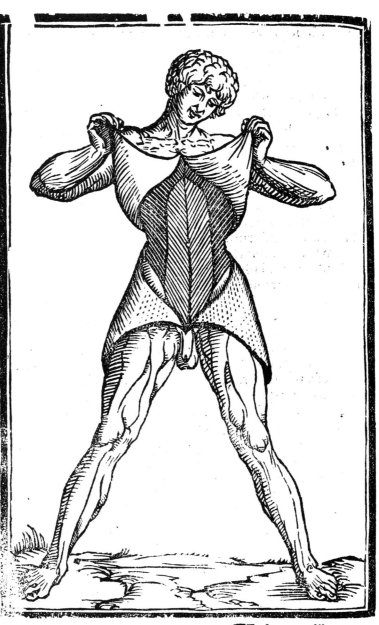

Et ita quælibet

PLATE 15

16 Skeletal figure, back view, holding skulls on fo. 521ᵛ in Berengario da Carpi, *Commentaria ... super Anatomia Mundini ...*, Bologna, Hieronymus de Benedictis, 1521. Woodcut (Wellcome Institute Library). 15.3 × 9.2 cm.

This is a rear view of a skeleton holding two skulls in uplifted hands, the one on the left showing the vertex, the other the right side.

Seven ribs are featured, and, below them, five sharp crescents. Possibly the rib cartilages were missing; but even so they are much too short. The scapula exhibits no real spine, and the upper limb bones are crudely drawn; all that can be determined is that there are two in the forearm and one in the upper arm. The pelvic bones are the most poorly drawn of all, and the superior tibio-fibular joint was obviously considered to be situated anteriorly. The upper part of the femur is enormous, and the thumb appears to have only one phalanx.

¶In ista si,
gura uidenť
ossa ptis po,
sterioris hois
uiděť ēt due
calue : in q̃rū
dextra uī co,
ronalis ꝓmis,
sura,q̃ ē i pte
supiori: uī &
sagittalis: q̃ ē
i medio:uī ēt
laude cōmis,
sura: q̃ ē i pte
iseriori:a late
rib' ēt uiděť
due cōmissu
re a me supra
noiate in ana
tomia cranei
q̃ sunt supra
ꝓmissuras sq̃
mosas exñtes
ꝓpe'aures:sƺ
iste sunt sere
isensibiles : a
sinistris ē alia
calua: in q̃ ui
děť mādibu,
le:& pars cō,
missure coro
nalis : &'due
cōmissure in
fra sagittalē
ad unū latus
existentes: &
uī unū os de
duob' ossib'

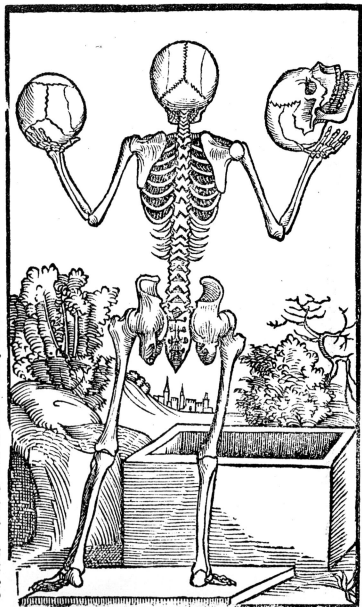

paris:qď est a regiōe oculi sen ab osse dictū pomū faciei tēdens p latū ca,
pitis uersus aurem.

PLATE 16

17 Bones of the hand and foot, on fo. 522$^\text{v}$ in Berengario da Carpi, *Commentaria ... super Anatomia Mundini ...*, Bologna, Hieronymus de Benedictis, 1521. Woodcut (Wellcome Institute Library). 16.0 × 9.4 cm.

This features the skeleton of the anterior aspect of the right hand and also that of the left foot viewed obliquely from above. Latin names are placed alongside, those on the left of the drawings (when viewed from the side of the book) being for some reason upside-down.

In the upper drawing the thumb correctly possesses one metacarpal bone and two phalanges, but the metacarpal does not articulate with any of the carpal bones! The latter in general, albeit inaccurate by later standards, are very good when compared with other printed early sixteenth-century illustrations. The bone proximal to the fourth metacarpal has a circle placed on it which probably represents the hook of the hamate.

The skeleton of the foot shows the second toe as being much longer than the big toe (as it is in the drawing of the foot skeleton, with similar perspective, by Leonardo, see *Fig. 3.8, p. 76*). The tarsal bones are better drawn than are the carpal bones; all are present and more or less correct. It is interesting that, at the base of the fifth metatarsal, there is a sesamoid bone ('os sisamium'), which was thus illustrated prior to Vesalius.

Also seen, stretching distally from the calcaneum, is either what is meant to be the plantar aponeurosis or, less likely, the long plantar ligament.

The illustrations in Berengario, of which these plates are but a very small sample, are anatomically quite the best that had been *published* up to this date.

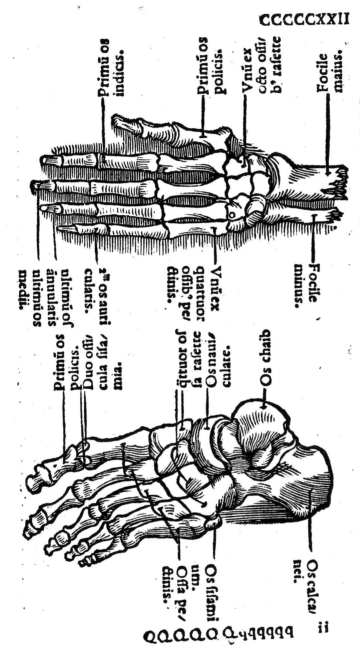

Primū os indicis.

Primū os policis.

Vnū ex octo offi/ b² rafette.

Focile maius.

2ᵐ os auri cularis.

vltimū of annularis vltimū os medii.

Primū so policis. Duo offi/ cula fifa/ mia.

qttuor of fa rafette Os nauicu lare.

Vnū ex quattuor offib² pe/ ctinis.

Os chaib

Focile minus.

Os fifami um. Offa pe/ ctinis.

Os calca nei.

ii

❡Habes in hac figura numerū: for mā:& fitū of/ fiū manus & pedis. In ma nu funt extre mitates duo/ rū fociliū bra chii: & octo offa rafette: & quattuor pectinis:& quindecim digitorum.

❡In pede habes os cal/ canei:& os chaib:& os nauiculare: & quattuor offa rafette: & quinq os/ fa pectinis:& offa qttuor/ decim digito rum.

PLATE 17

Johannes Eichmann or Dryander 1500–1560

Dryander's first illustrated work was a short monograph of 14 leaves: *Anatomia capitis humani* ..., Marburg, Eucharius Cervicornus, 1536. Berengario had also written on the head, but his book, unillustrated except for a single woodcut of a man's head being attacked by all manner of weapons, was about injuries. Dryander's anatomy of the head had eleven numbered full-page woodcuts. The artist who made the woodcuts has identified himself on some by a monogram of a pair of compasses with various initials: G. VB, GVB ... This is probably Georg Thomas of Basle, the compasses being a symbol of St Thomas the Apostle. His work is central to the whole enterprise; the workmanship is straightforward, with shading well used to give solidarity to the structures pictured. The same publisher issued the following year the first volume of what was to have been a complete illustrated anatomy by Dryander: *Anatomiae, hoc est, corporis humani dissectionis. . . .* This includes, among other figures, the dissection series of the head and ten other woodcuts. (Further volumes did not appear.) Dryander's illustrations in this book formed a dissection sequence starting with removing the scalp and skull-cap, and then continued to expose the meninges and the cerebral hemispheres (*Plate 18*), then the cerebellum, and finally the base of the skull. There was also, in the 1537 volume, a diagram illustrating physiological concepts of the integration of the various senses in relation to the 'cells', that is the stylized ventricles, of the brain (*Fig. 3.9a*). The purely diagrammatic nature of this figure, inserted to convey ideas as to how the brain works, is in sharp contrast to the images of the appearance of the actual cerebral ventricles in the other figures. The diagram was derived from concepts of the localization of *imagination*, *common sense*, and *memory* within these three ventricles. Similar diagrams had appeared in many manuscripts for at least two hundred years—for example in Guido da Vigevano, 1345. They also appeared in early printed work, as in Hundt's *Antropologium*, 1501 (*Fig. 3.9b*), which was the basis of Dryander's figure. In Dryander's figure the organs of vision, hearing, olfaction, and taste are labelled. 'Feeling is diffused throughout the entire body by means of nerves and muscles.' Each sense is connected to one or more 'cells'. The figure in this respect was intended as a physiological diagram to explain function; it is intermediate between the medieval figures and the much-admired, but equally unscientifically speculative, reflex figure in Descartes' *De homine. . . .* In Dryander, the physiological diagram is incongruously placed on a realistic representation of the head. The figure also shows the *rete mirabile*, which does not exist in the human being.

Dryander's woodcuts of brain dissection followed the pattern used first in the accessory woodcuts to the Schott–Fries visceral figure (1517), which we have shown and discussed (see *Fig. 2.16*, p. 46). The drawing in Dryander's dissections, undoubtedly taken from actual specimens, is more realistic and precise.

The illustrations added to the *Anatomiae* of 1537 were made by the same artist, and include skulls (*Plate 19*), which the neurosurgeon Harvey Cushing described as 'excellent', and visceral figures (*Plate 20*), which are much less convincing to us than those of the head.

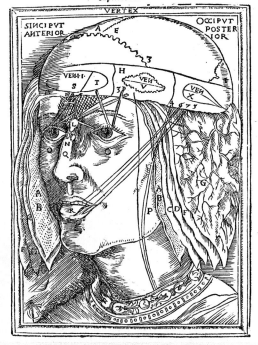

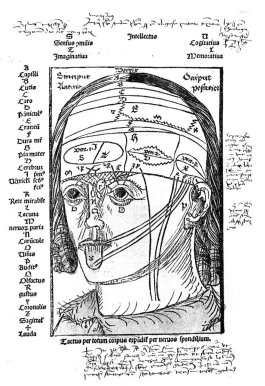

3.9a Diagram of brain 'cells' or ventricles from Dryander, *Anatomiae*, 1537.

3.9b A similar diagram from Hundt's *Antropologium*, 1501.

Dryander was a prolific writer: his books included works on astronomy (he was a professor of both mathematics and medicine), as well as various aspects of medicine. A work of his that shows well the transitional state of medicine, including anatomy, at this period is *Der gantzen Artzenei . . .*, Frankfurt, 1542, which was reissued, enlarged as *Artzenei Spiegel . . .*, in 1547. These books were directed primarily at laymen. There were more than two hundred illustrations in about three hundred pages; some blocks were used more than once. Some of these illustrations were symbolic diagrams, such as had been characteristic of medieval anatomy; other images were of newer, more realistic anatomy: not only traditional pictures of fetuses *in utero* and zodiacal, blood-letting figures, but also his own realistic brain figures, and others equally modern taken from Fries and Berengario and from Vesalius' *Tabulae*, 1538. Some of the images, in turn, anticipate both Estienne's *De dissectione, 1545* and Vesalius' *Fabrica, 1543*. Dryander, like Berengario, wrote a commentary on Mondino's fourteenth-century anatomy. The early sixteenth-century anatomists, whether in Italy or in Germany, tried very hard to reconcile traditional authorities with what they saw during their own dissections.

Dryander was born near Marburg. He studied for five years in Paris, where he overlapped in time with Vesalius. His doctorate was from Mainz. At the age of thirty-five years, he was appointed to the Protestant University of Marburg, founded only eight years previously. Dryander's anatomical work was encouraged by the Landgrave of Hesse and by the university authorities. With their support, he conducted four public anatomies in the period from 1534 to 1558. The phrase *inevitable fatum* (or *vatum*) appeared on the title-page of Dryander's monograph on the anatomy of the head, and was cut into the wood-blocks for his anatomy book issued the next year. This call for the reader to remember the end of life was appropriate to a professor in a Protestant university in the middle of Europe during the years of Reformation and Counter-Reformation. Public dissections became not uncommon in German-speaking cities in the later sixteenth and the seventeenth centuries, and some municipal authorities appointed surgeons as city anatomists.

In 1543, Vesalius, in his letter to Oporinus, accused Dryander of pirating figures from his *Tabulae*, 1538. A figure in Dryander's 1541 edition of Mondino and in his 1542 volume, *Der gantzen Artzenei ...*, was certainly modified from the Vesalian plates. Dryander had possibly taken it from a not-yet-published Estienne woodcut, itself derived from the Vesalian 1538 figures (see later, Chapter 5). Without actually naming him, Vesalius calls Dryander the 'slave of the sordid printer at Marburg and Frankfurt'—the slave being Dryander and the printer, who moved from the one city to the other, Christian Egenolff. His accusations seem intemperate, especially since he himself, in his *Fabrica*, 1543, modified Dryander's figures showing dissections of the head. This situation seems rather more the give and take of scholarship and science than criminal plagiarism. Dryander followed the Schott–Fries sequence, and Vesalius incorporated some ideas from Dryander. Was there, however, a sense in which some German writers on anatomy became 'wage-slaves', attached to printer-publishers who demanded a high level of output and were willing to pay for it? Certainly W. H. Ryff appears to have been in that position, with dozens of books issued on many subjects. The more scholarly monograph and the incomplete anatomy that Dryander produced for Cervicornus contrast with the more popular, extensively illustrated books that he wrote for Egenolff. Vesalius, the son of an Imperial official, and soon to be one himself, had a quite different, and a much more aristocratic, relationship with his publisher, a fellow academic.

18 Dissection showing cerebral hemispheres. *Figura tertia*, on Bii recto in Dryander, *Anatomia capitis humani ...*, Marburg, E. Cervicornus, 1536. Woodcut (Wellcome Institute Library). Height 13.9 cm.

The skull-cap has been removed and is placed upside-down, partly underneath the chin. The inner aspect of it reveals the lambdoid, sagittal, and coronal sutures, together with some blood-vessels, or their grooves, on the right parietal bone. From the level of the horizontal cut through

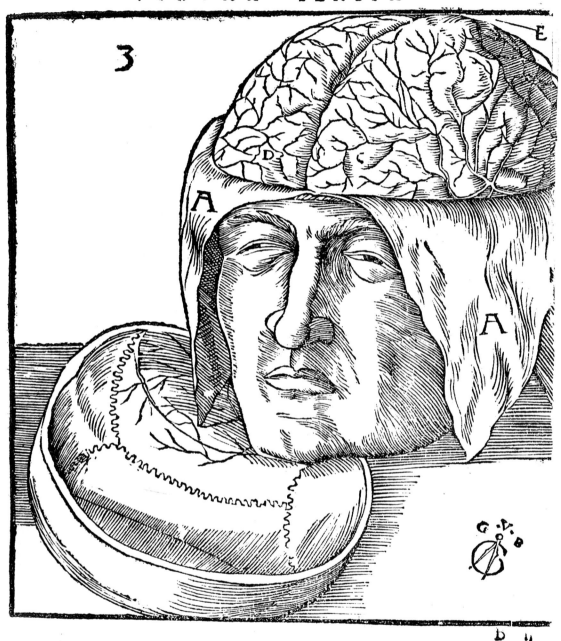

PLATE 18

the skull one would have expected it to have passed through the frontal sinus, but there is no sign of this on the cut surface.

The dura mater (A) has been cut and folded down on each side. There is no evidence that the superior sagittal sinus and the falx cerebri were left *in situ*, neither are they seen attached to the cut portions of the dura; and, indeed, no mention of the sinus is found in the accompanying text. The gyri and sulci of the exposed cerebral hemispheres have been drawn more or less at random, but at least the surface of the brain presents a more lifelike appearance than any previous drawing: in addition there is an attempt to show some blood-vessels on the surface. It is interesting that certain of these appear to emerge from the median longitudinal fissure, that is, they are representing branches of the anterior cerebral artery.

19 Skull resting on hour-glass. *Figura undecima* on gi. recto in Dryander, *Anatomiae ... corporis humani dissectionis ...*, Marburg, E. Cervicornus, 1537. Woodcut (Wellcome Institute Library). 13.6 × 12.0 cm.

The skull is shown balanced both on a sundial surmounting an hour-glass and also vertebrae. All are placed on a plinth bearing the date 1536 and the inscription 'Inevitabile Fatum'.

The coronoid process of the mandible is deformed, and the horizontal ramus has a very wavy outline and contains (as does the upper jaw) uniform teeth.

A metopic suture is seen dividing the two parts of the frontal bone (this suture seems to have been unusually prevalent in the sixteenth and seventeenth centuries; however, in other Dryander figures it is absent). The coronal and squamosal sutures are also seen, but the latter has rather too small an arc. This results in the antero-inferior part of the parietal bone (C) having a long thin tongue. The fronto-zygomatic suture is very strange, and no suture is shown on the zygomatic arch; nor is there any differentiation between the zygomatic bone and the maxilla. The orbits are very small and the margins irregular.

It must be presumed that the supporting vertebrae were intended as cervical; but their transverse processes contain no foramina for the vertebral artery.

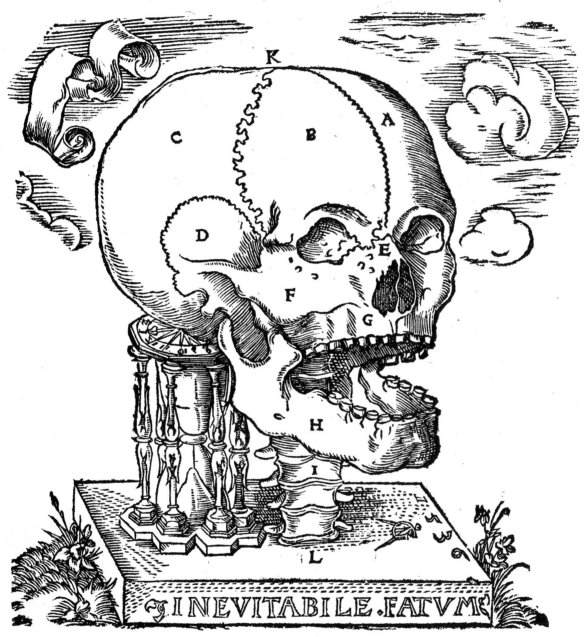

PLATE 19

g

20 Posterior view of lungs, etc. on iii verso in Dryander, *Anatomiae . . . corporis humani dissectionis . . .*, Marburg, E. Cervicornus, 1537. Woodcut (Wellcome Institute Library). 17.0 × 12.5 cm.

In this posterior view of the lungs, trachea, and oesophagus, the latter (L) is a very thin tube seen posterior to the trachea and lungs and piercing the diaphragm (K) inferiorly.

The trachea (A) is large, with regular rings, and is opened up as it enters the lungs, which seem not to be divided into right and left lobes. The bronchial branching, as well as that of the vessels, is quite fanciful, with the large bronchi passing to the most inferior parts of the lung and sending out smaller offshoots.

The lungs themselves are shown as being very globular, and can hardly be considered human. The large vessel (G) seen anteriorly on the right probably represents the aorta. The other smaller vessels on the left (M, N, O, reversed) are figments of the imagination.

Inferiorly (F) possibly represents the inferior portion of the heart, with part of the pericardium (H).

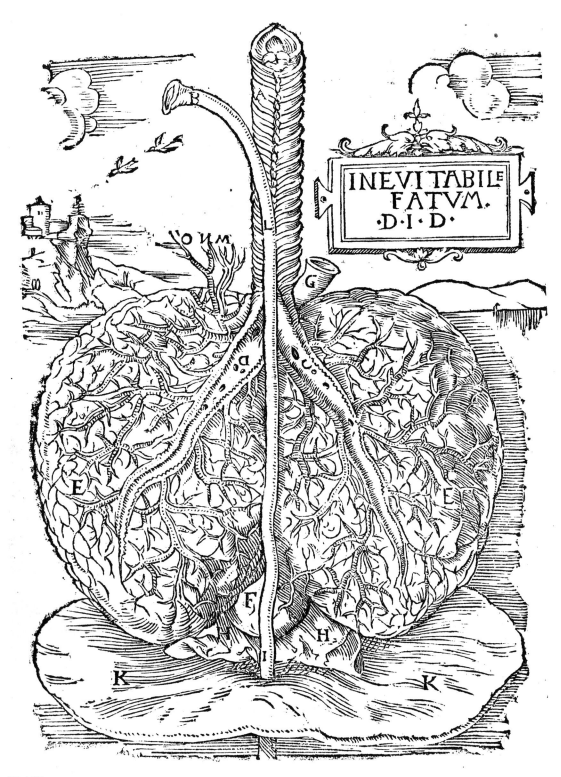

PLATE 20

Giovanni Battista Canano (Joannes Baptista Cananus) 1515–1579

In a sweeping statement, which need not be taken entirely at its face value, Falloppio wrote that, in the 1540s, besides Vesalius and Colombo, 'there was no one else capable of teaching anatomy skilfully, with the single exception of Joannes Baptista Cananus, a most celebrated physician and anatomist'. Canano was born in Ferrara, a city close to Bologna in north-eastern Italy. Many of his family, which was of Greek ancestry, were prominent physicians. At the age of twenty-six, Canano replaced his uncle as Professor of Anatomy at the *Studium*. Ferrara, already a prominent medical centre, under Canano became known to the scientific community for work in anatomy. John Caius, the English medical humanist who had lodged with Vesalius in Padua, made a visit to Canano to search for classical manuscripts, and praised his library.

At least two discoveries were made by Canano, the more significant of which is, in retrospect, the demonstration of valves in deep veins—a discovery to be, in the hands of Fabrici and Harvey, a spring board for the elucidation of the circulation of the blood. The other discovery was of a small muscle in the hand, the palmaris brevis. He was also the first to illustrate the interossei and lumbrical muscles.

Canano held the chair of anatomy for only four years or so, the succeeding professor being Falloppio. Canano's subsequent career took him to Rome in 1552 as physician to the Pope, and then back to Ferrara, where he was active in medical practice, and also in public health, on which he advised the Este family.

During his brief career as an anatomy professor, Canano prepared what may be regarded as the first satisfactory illustrated monograph on a detailed anatomical subject: *Musculorum humani corporis picturata dissectio*. Dryander's work on the head is, in comparison, much less rigorous. The date of publication, which was not given, has been variously estimated as 1541, 1542, or 1543. The publisher is also unknown. The volume is of modest size, only twenty-three leaves, and consists essentially of a short introduction and annotated figures of the muscles of the upper limb. The majority of the figures, all of which were carefully thought out, were designed to indicate the action of particular muscles. These images are both realistic representations and demonstrations of function. They represent a close collaboration between the anatomist and the illustrator, Girolamo da Carpi, whom Canano praised highly. The images are not to our eyes wholly satisfactory, since bone and muscle are not well differentiated.

The quantum jump taken by this modest man should be noted; the intent and execution of these small figures greatly surpass the achievement of Berengario's *Isagogae* .... (Berengario, it may be noted, found myology difficult. 'In order to expose these structures to view, extensive, long, and painstaking labour is required', and, therefore, 'I have made very little comment'.) A present-day anatomist, without historical interests, can recognize that Canano's figures would be appropriate to a text on functional anatomy.

The figures of Canano's book were impressions from engraved copperplates—the first time that this printing technique had been put to use in anatomical illustration. The delicate lines of intaglio engraving may be contrasted with the coarser, bolder statements of Berengario's relief woodcuts. Even the master craftsmen who cut Vesalius' wood-blocks could not achieve such fine lines as are possible with the burin. The engraving and the presswork did not do justice to Canano's innovations; the images, which by their shading give a roundness and depth, are somewhat blurred (*Plate 21*). But it should be noted that their quality in the original, which shows poor presswork, is nevertheless much better than that seen in facsimile and reproduction.

This little work was intended to be the first of a series of five volumes on the anatomy of all the muscles of the body, but the others were not published. It may be relevant that Vesalius in 1543, having sent off to his printer the manuscript, wood-blocks, and trial proofs of the *Fabrica* . . . and the *Epitome* . . ., made a journey to see his brother, who was studying at Ferrara. The two teachers of anatomy, at Padua and at Ferrara, may thus have had opportunity for discussion, and it has been suggested that Vesalius showed Canano proofs of his illustrations. Further speculation, for which there is no direct evidence, suggests that Canano, realizing the extent of Vesalius' achievement in illustration, abandoned his plans to issue the remaining instalments of his work on muscles.

Vesalius, of the renowned medical faculty at Padua, employed artists with a sense of the dramatic, used a publisher with wide international connections, and achieved and relished fame, even notoriety. Canano, whose temperament seems to have been much less pushing, prepared his work in the *Studium* at Ferrara, a medical school with a high reputation among professional anatomists, but without the fame of Padua. He chose to issue the first part of his work, in what must have been a small edition, from his own city, which was not a well-known centre for medical publishing, and the remaining parts—apparently ready for the press—were never issued. What we have today—there are only a dozen or so known copies of the book—may indeed be the remnant of a small proof edition that Canano distributed to a few friends and collaborators; one may originally have been in the hands of the engraver, Agostino de' Musi. As the *Liber primus* it would undoubtedly have had an appropriate title-page listing publisher and date, and, one presumes, would have been printed with more care on better paper-stock. We must regret, for whatever reasons, Canano's failure to complete the publication of his work; because of this, he has been denied significant influence on the subsequent development of anatomy.

21 a. Muscles of the forearm. The first figure, on Bii recto, of *Musculorum corporis picturata dissectio. Liber primus*. No place, publisher, or date. Engraving (Yale University Library). Size of the engraved figure 13.4 × 5.6 cm.
b. the same figure from a facsimile of that book published 1925, Florence, R. Lier, edited by H. Cushing and E. C. Streeter (Wellcome Institute Library).

The first drawing in Canano's book is of the flexor aspect of the left upper extremity, the forearm rather foreshortened. Identifiable muscles are the flexor carpi ulnaris (A), palmaris longus (B), flexor digitorum superficialis (C), flexor carpi radialis (D), pronator teres (E), and brachio-radialis (F). In the upper part of the arm the biceps and brachialis are drawn but not labelled.

It might be mentioned here that in Lind's *Studies in pre-Vesalian anatomy*, 1975, the mis-attribution of flexor digitorum profundus to muscle (E) and of extensor digitorum profundus [sic] to muscle (F) would seem to have arisen by considering 'bending' the hand to mean flexion and extension at the wrist, rather than 'turning' the hand, that is, pronation and supination.

A facsimile edition of Canano's publications was made from an original copy in the possession of Harvey Cushing. When a comparison is made between the 'facsimile' and the original, side by side, two interesting facts emerge with regard to this particular drawing. In the original there is an (F) placed on the muscle belly of brachio-radialis ('musculus manum supinam redens'), but this capital letter is absent in the 'facsimile'. Again, in the original, the tendon of muscle B (palmaris longus or 'musculus volae'), shown passing to the index finger, terminates on the base of the proximal phalanx, while in the 'facsimile' it reaches the distal part of this phalanx.

Canano's drawings are remarkable in that the muscles are so clearly delineated, whether drawn separately or together, and this makes it easier to understand their actions than do Vesalius' drawings in the *Fabrica*. It is a thousand pities if, as has been suggested, Canano was so overcome by a preview of the *Fabrica* woodcuts that he gave up his expressed intent to publish further anatomical drawings. From this one small book it is very clear that his understanding of muscles, and his ability to illustrate them, were far greater than those of any of his predecessors.

The poor quality of the paper used is shown by the fact that the printing on the following page comes through, as can be seen in the photograph from the original, *Plate 21a*.

Canano was also aware of the existence of valves in veins (as mentioned earlier in this book), and discussed these at a chance meeting with Vesalius at Regensburg three years after the *Fabrica* was published.

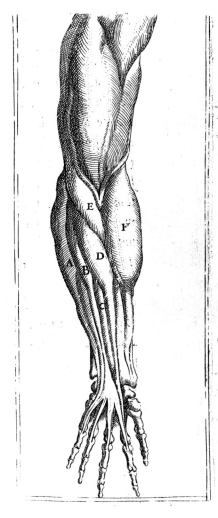

Hac in pictura hi nu
dantur musculi vide-
licet.
A. MVSCV-
LVS Flectens bra-
chiale ad minimum
digitum.
B. MVSCV-
LVS Volæ.
C. MVSCV-
LVS Tendonum
scissorum, sub quo est
musculus habens ten
dines non fissos am-
bo digitos flectunt.
D. MVSCV-
LVS Flectens bra
chiale prope magnū
digitum.
E. MVSCV-
LVS Manum pro
nam faciens.
F. MVSCV-
LVS. Manum su
pinam redens.

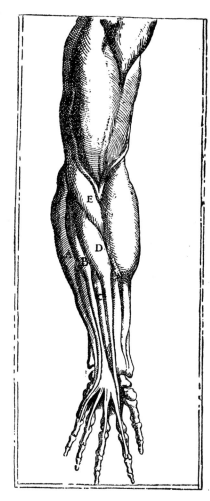

Hac in pictura hi nu
dantur musculi vide-
licet.
A. MVSCV-
LVS Flectens bra-
chiale ad minimum
digitum.
B. MVSCV-
LVS Volæ.
C. MVSCV-
LVS Tendonum
scissorum, sub quo est
musculus habens ten
dines non fissos am-
bo digitos flectunt.
D. MVSCV-
LVS Flectens bra
chiale prope magnū
digitum.
E. MVSCV-
LVS Manum pro
nam faciens.
F. MVSCV-
LVS. Manum su
pinam redens.

PLATE 21

(a)

(b)

Chapter 3: Selected Reading

Cushing, H. (1932). *A bio-bibliography of Andreas Vesalius*. Archon, Hamden, CT;

Cushing, H. and Streeter. E.C. (ed.) (1925). *Musculorum humani corporis picturata dissectio (Ferrara 1541?). Facsimile edn.* Lier, R. Florence.

Lind, L.R. (1959). *Jacopo Berengario da Carpi 'A short introduction to anatomy'* .... University of Chicago Press.

Lind, L.R. (1975). *Studies in pre-Vesalian anatomy* .... The American Philosophical Society, Philadelphia.

Lowry, M. (1979). *The world of Aldus Manutius* .... Blackwell, Oxford.

Muratori, G. (1971). Giovan Battista Canano. *Dict. sci. Biog.* **3**, 40–1.

O'Malley, C.D. (1970). Giacomo Berengario da Carpi. *Dict. sci. Biog.*, **1**, 617–21.

Putti, V. (1937). *Berengoria da Corpi: Saggio biografico e bibliografico* ... Cappelli, Bologna.

Sudhoff, K. (1910). Die Bauchmuskelzeichnung von 1496. *Archiv. f. Gesch. Med.*, **3**, 131–14.

Thorndike, L. (1941). *A history of magic and experimental science*, Vols V and VI: The sixteenth century [includes Berengario and Dryander]. Columbia University Press, New York.

Leonardo da Vinci

Leonardo was born in 1452 in a house near Vinci, a small town thirty kilometres from Florence. His mother was a young peasant woman called Caterina; she was not married to his father, Piero da Vinci, a lawyer. Leonardo stayed at first with his mother, but by the age of five was living with his father. His father had married another woman, who seems to have treated her stepson kindly. (Caterina also married shortly after Leonardo's birth.) When a separate household was established by his father in Florence in 1469, Leonardo, seventeen years old, moved there and was apprenticed to Andrea del Verrocchio (c.1435–88), whose workshop produced, on demand, sculpture, painting, goldsmith work.... Leonardo in 1472 was placed on the registry of the Company of St Luke's, the painters' guild; his apprenticeship was over when he reached twenty, but he continued to live in the Verrocchio household for at least four more years.

Leonardo's childhood and years of apprenticeship were in a society where books were in manuscript. Although undoubtedly Leonardo saw printed books in his youth, the first printing press in Florence was not established until about 1471. In this transition period books were produced both in the scriptorium and in the printing-house. In the years from 1461 onwards, a Florentine bookseller had, under commission from Cosimo de' Medici, employed forty-five scribes to produce books needed for a new library; although the work proceeded for at least five years, only a few hundred books were produced.

Leonardo cannot, however, have suffered from cultural deprivation in a city where the writings of Dante and Boccaccio were a common heritage, and where the architecture of Brunelleschi, the painting of Masaccio, and the sculpture of Donatello, Ghiberti, and the della Robbias were there for everyone to see. Perugino and Botticelli probably worked in Verrocchio's studio alongside Leonardo. Another successful establishment was that of the brothers Pollaiuolo; they and their pupils produced works in many media.

When he was thirty Leonardo left Florence for Milan, for a formal appointment to the Duke, Ludovico Sforza, nicknamed *il Moro*, 'the Moor'. Leonardo had recommended himself to Ludovico primarily as an engineer, in particular a designer of war machines: 'as the variety of circumstances shall necessitate, I can supply an infinite number of different engines of attack and defence'. But *il Moro* obtained also a courtier who was skilled in music, painting, sculpture, horsemanship, and the design of pageants and displays. Leonardo stayed with Ludovico until 1499, when the French forces began an occupation of Milan that lasted for thirteen years. For much of the period until 1506, Leonardo was again in Florence (the second Florentine period), with an appointment, 1502–3, as a military engineer to Cesare Borgia during the campaigns in the Romagna. From 1506 to 1513 he lived in Milan at the invitation of the French Governor (the second Milanese period), making several visits to Florence. From late 1513 he was in Rome, but in 1516 King Francis I invited him to join the cultural invasion into France of persons and ideas Italian. Generously, Francis gave him the use of a manor-house, the *Château de Cloux* on the Loire, near the royal residences and connected to them by an underground passage. Leonardo died in 1519, shortly after his sixty-seventh birthday; Vasari wrote mistakenly that he died in the arms of the king.

The notebooks of Leonardo

We have inherited from Leonardo but few paintings, many in poor condition, some unfinished; nevertheless these paintings have remained the object of great admiration to the present day. Leonardo's great sculptural project, an immense equestrian statue of Ludovico Sforza's father, was worked on during a period of fifteen years, but was never cast; the bronze set aside for it went to making cannon, while the clay model was used as target-practice and destroyed. It is not possible for us to appraise the ephemeral displays and ceremonies Leonardo designed and co-ordinated for ducal weddings and the like—the spectacles have passed; the music of his lute has been long silent. The hydraulic engineering projects, canals, and attempted diversions of rivers, often came to nothing, and plans for imaginative military and other machines remained ideas not put into practice. Leonardo published no books; a few of his illustrations were printed well after his death. He discussed with his friend, Luca da Pacioli, 'divine proportion' in architecture, the human body, and the design of letters; his contributions were used in the latter's book of that title (*Divina proportione*, Venice, 1509).

The work on which Leonardo spent most time is to be found in his notebooks. From an early date in Florence until his last years, Leonardo added to these pages, which eventually came to be a collection of many hundred sheets. These were willed to Leonardo's young pupil Francesco Melzi. They were subsequently dispersed, and what remains is to be found in various libraries of the world; but only a third or so of the original number have survived. These are distributed in libraries in Europe and America, including the following:

MILAN, in the *Biblioteca Ambrosiana* and at the Castello Sforzesco; PARIS, in the *Bibliothèque Nationale* and at the *Institut de France*; GENEVA, in the Frato Collection; NEW YORK, in the Morgan Library; LOS ANGELES, in the Dr Armand Hammer Collection; MADRID AND ENGLAND (see below).

In the eighteenth century the catalogues of the Royal Library in Madrid recorded two volumes of Leonardo's manuscripts concerned with mathematics and engineering, but they were mislaid, and only rediscovered in 1966, to be published in 1974.

The manuscripts in England are in London—the Arundel manuscripts in the British Library and the Forster Bequest manuscripts at the Victoria and Albert Museum—and in the Royal Library, Windsor.

The wide range and great depth of subjects annotated in these manuscripts have been a continual source of amazement. How could one man have investigated, often more imaginatively, carefully, and constructively than his contemporaries, the atmosphere and the flow of water; geology and geography; some aspects of mathematics and astronomy; many aspects of natural history; the physics of flight ... *and*, at the same time, be so mechanically inventive in the design of flying machines, submersibles, engines of war, and a hundred other devices? Nor was this all, for amongst trivial matters—jokes, collections of words, tales, records of household effects, and even what appear to be laundry lists, the notebooks include serious and interesting philosophical speculations, aphorisms, discussions on the theory and practice of the fine arts, architecture and music, and above all, pages devoted to human biology, human proportions, the senses (particularly eye and ear), physiology, and—not least—anatomy.

Not all the anatomical manuscripts have survived; there was at least one collection in small notebooks (*libricini*), which has disappeared; moreover, some pages were left at the Hospital of S. Maria Novella when he went to France in 1516. Nearly all the surviving notebook pages relating to anatomy are to be found among the Leonardo manuscripts in the Royal Library at Windsor. They comprise some 200 leaves, 400 pages. Much of the text of the notebooks is available in MacCurdy's 1938 translation. The Windsor anatomy pages have been reproduced with annotations by O'Malley and Saunders (1952).

The Windsor anatomical manuscripts

When he went to France towards the end of his life Leonardo took with him, among his other papers, his manuscript notes and drawings. They were seen there by the Cardinal of Aragon, as noted by his Secretary, Antonio de Beatis:

[Leonardo] has written of anatomy with such detail, showing by illustrations the limbs, muscles, nerves, veins, ligaments, intestines and whatever else there is to discuss in the bodies of men and women, in a way that has never yet been done by anyone else.

When Melzi inherited these manuscripts he kept them carefully, as noted by Giorgio Vasari when, in 1566, he visited Leonardo's pupil, now grown into a 'beautiful and gentle old man'. Many of the manuscripts came into the hands of a sculptor, Pompeo Leoni, who had them partly rearranged, and, about 1605, bound; one volume, with *Disegni di Leonardo da Vinci restaurati da Pompeo Leoni* on its front cover, is the basis of the Windsor notebooks, another the basis of the *Biblioteca Ambrosiana* collection in Milan. The exact route by which the volume travelled to the Royal Library is not known. Probably Thomas Howard, Earl of Arundel, bought it, some time before 1630, from a Spaniard who had acquired it after Pompeo's death in Madrid in 1608. Wenceslaus Hollar made etchings of some of the anatomical drawings about 1645; by 1690 they were certainly in the Royal Library, for that year Mary, who with William III ruled in England, showed them to a visitor from the Low Countries. Although the notebooks were listed as being in the Bureau at Kensington palace in 1735, they seem then to have been mislaid. In 1796, John Chamberlaine, Keeper of the King's Drawings and Medals, published seventeen plates reproducing some of the anatomical drawings—including a coitus figure. They were engraved by Bartolozzi; Chamberlaine described how they were 'discovered soon after his present Majesty's accession in the same cabinet where Queen Caroline found the five portraits of the court of Henry VIII by Hans Holbein...'.

The anatomical manuscripts were known to William Hunter, who had written enthusiastically about them in a letter to Haller dated 1773. However, it was not until 1916 that all the anatomical drawings of the Windsor collection were generally available in reproduction.

The Pompeo Leoni binding was disassembled in the nineteenth century, and the pages were rebound into three volumes. Recently these have again been dismembered for restoration, each leaf being carefully photographed in a laboratory set up in Windsor Castle, before being enclosed between protective sheets of acrylic. Facsimiles of the Windsor corpus were then published, along with translations and scholarly notes, by Keele and Pedretti (1979).

The Leonardo manuscripts cannot be reconstructed into a consecutive journal; nevertheless, there was originally a degree of chronological organization, disturbed during the notebooks' complex history. In 1508 Leonardo described his methods:

This will be a collection without order, made up of many sheets which I have copied here, hoping afterwards to arrange them in order in their proper places according to the subjects of which they treat; and I believe that before I am at the end of this I shall have to repeat the same thing several times; and therefore, O reader, blame me not, because the subjects are many, and the memory cannot retain them and say 'this I will not write because I have already written it'.

Leonardo often did turn back to older pages to add new thoughts; in an extreme case, nineteen years elapsed between the original and the last annotation. Almost all Leonardo's written notes in the manuscripts are in looking-glass writing, right to left on the page written with his left hand. In correspondence, of course, he wrote left to right. The purpose of the mirror-writing was, perhaps, to maintain a minimal degree of privacy. The language is Italian, in the Tuscan dialect.

Most pages have both text and illustration, but the latter has pride of place, with the writing usually glossing but not describing the figures. In general the drawings are anatomical, the writing physiological.

With what words O writer can you with a like perfection describe the whole arrangement of that of which the design is here?

For lack of due knowledge you describe it so confusedly as to convey but little perception of the true shapes of things, and deceiving yourself as to these you persuade yourself that you can completely satisfy the hearer when you speak of the representation of anything that possesses substance and is surrounded by surface.

I counsel you not to cumber yourself with words unless you are speaking to the blind ... do not busy yourself in making enter by the ears things which have to do with the eyes, for in this you will be far surpassed by the work of the painter.

How in words can you describe this heart without filling a whole book? Yet the more detail you write concerning it the more you will confuse the mind of the hearer. [This was put at the side of a drawing of the heart.]

And you who think to reveal the figure of man in words, with his limbs arranged in all their different attitudes, banish the idea from you, for the more minute your description the more you will confuse the mind of the reader and the more you will lead him away from the knowledge of the thing described. It is necessary therefore for you to represent and describe.

The words and sketches have been so well placed on the page that asymmetrical and often seemingly unrelated material is elegantly and informally composed into a unified structure.

Anatomy in the notebooks

Not all the anatomy is human. For example, one leaf illustrates the hind foot of a bear, to show how far it differs from that of the human being. Another pictures the structure of a bird's wing—Leonardo had studied the flight of birds, at first in relation to the possibility of human flight, and then for its own sake. On one leaf, in which the drawings explore the muscles and bones of the human lower extremity, the skeleton of the hind limb of a horse seen from the side is juxtaposed to the same parts of a human being (*Fig. 4.1*).

Some of the anatomical drawings are of human proportions, the most famous of these (not at Windsor) being an attempted resolution of the Vitruvian problem of containing the human form within a square and a circle.

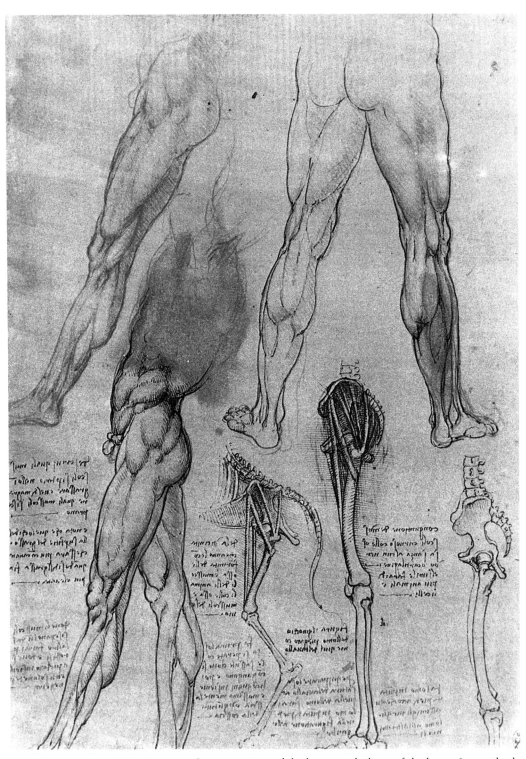

4.1 The lower limb in the human, with a comparison of the bones with those of the horse: Leonardo da Vinci.

Most remarkable of the anatomical illustrations are, however, the pages where human anatomy is shown. Some of the figures are merely diagrams illustrating received anatomical doctrine of the late fifteenth century. On one sheet for instance three brain ventricles are depicted in a manner not too different from many medieval and early printed diagrams of the brain—all related to the texts of ibn Sina (Avicenna) rather than to the results of observation. This diagram was drawn about 1490 (*Fig. 4.2*). Some fifteen or so years later Leonardo carried out experiments in which he injected molten wax into the brain ventricles of an ox; on another leaf of the Windsor notebooks, the solidified cast is drawn—still, however, with the medieval attribution of function to each ventricle: perception, common sense, and memory being associated with the present day lateral, third, and fourth ventricles (*Fig. 4.3*).

There are other anatomical drawings in which diagrams, derived from then-current doctrine, are superimposed on a realistically drawn human figure. This type calls to mind the illustration in the *Fasciculo ...* (1493) where diagrams of the female reproductive organs are shown superimposed on a Renaissance figure (see *Plate 8*, p. 43). Indeed Leonardo almost certainly consulted this particular book, in the Italian edition rather than the Latin, a language which he

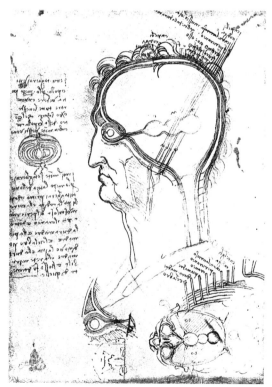

4.2 Diagram of the head showing, among other structures, the supposed brain 'cells': Leonardo da Vinci.

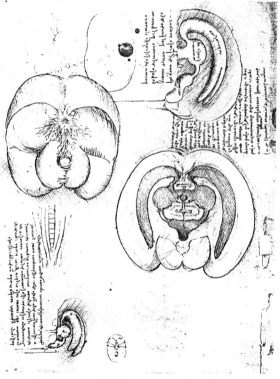

4.3 The structure of the brain ventricles of the ?ox revealed by Leonardo's wax casts.

never fully mastered. Leonardo's early illustration of the venous system (*Plate 24*) was based on a figure taken from the *Fasciculo*.

For most of his later anatomical studies, however, Leonardo did not rely on authority, for which indeed he had contempt:

I am fully aware that the fact of my not being a man of letters may cause certain arrogant persons to think that they may with reason censure me, alleging that I am a man ignorant of book-learning. Foolish folk! ... Do they not know that my subjects require for their exposition experience rather than the words of others? ... And if they despise me who am an inventor [innovator] how much more should blame be given to themselves, who are not inventors but trumpeters and reciters of the works of others?

Leonardo's more advanced work in anatomy was done during his second Milanese and his Roman periods. It was the result of painstaking dissections of the human cadaver, often supplemented by studies of animal anatomy.

Leonardo's anatomical methods

Leonardo stated for himself, and indeed for all anatomists at all times, the operational problems in achieving a successful image of any human anatomical structure:

This plan of mine of the human body will be unfolded to you just as though you had the natural man before you. The reason is that if you wish to know thoroughly the parts of a man after he has been dissected you must either turn him or your eye so that you are examining from different aspects, from below, from above and from the sides, turning him over and studying the origin of each limb; and in such a way the natural anatomy has satisfied your desire for knowledge. But you must understand that such knowledge as this will not continue to satisfy you, on account of the very great confusion which must arise from the mixture of membranes with veins, arteries, nerves, tendons, muscles, bones and the blood, which of itself tinges every part with the same colour, the veins through which this blood is discharged not being perceptible by reason of their minuteness. The completeness of the membranes is broken during the process of investigation of the parts which they enclose, and the fact that their transparent substance is stained with blood prevents the proper identification of the parts which these cover ... Therefore it becomes necessary to have several dissections ... [thus] by my plan you will become acquainted with every part and every whole by means of a demonstration of each part——And would that it might please our Creator that I were able to reveal the nature of man and his customs even as I describe his figure!

On another page, Leonardo writes:

And you who say that it is better to look at an anatomical demonstration than to see these drawings, you would be right, if it were possible to observe all the details shown in these drawings in a single figure, in which, with all your ability, you will not see nor acquire a knowledge of more than some few veins; while, in order to obtain an exact and complete knowledge of these, I have dissected more than ten human bodies ...

But though possessed of an interest in the subject you may perhaps be deterred by natural repugnance, or, if this does not restrain you, then perhaps by the fear of passing the night hours in the company of these corpses, quartered and flayed and horrible to behold; and if this does not deter you then perhaps you may lack the skill in drawing essential for such representation; and even if you possess this skill it may not be combined with a knowledge of perspective; while, if it is so combined, you may not be versed in the methods of geometrical demonstration or the method of estimating the forces and strength of muscles, or perhaps you may be found wanting in patience so that you will not be diligent.

It was not uncommon for Renaissance artists to study human anatomy by participation in dissection either as onlookers or as an actual operator. The influence of a direct anatomical study of at least the superficial muscles of the human body is evident in the nude figures of Antonio Pollaiuolo and Luca Signorelli, both contemporaries of Leonardo. Many drawings of skeletal and muscular anatomy were made by late-fifteenth and sixteenth century artists, for instance by Battista Franco (c.1510–1561). But, as so often, Leonardo carried his studies much further, and for different and less utilitarian, more scientific purposes. His context was to give a complete account of human biology:

This work should commence with the conception of man, and should describe the nature of the womb, and how the child inhabits it, and in what stage it dwells there, and the manner of its quickening and feeding, and its growth, and what interval there is between one stage of growth and another, and what thing drives it forth from the body of the mother, and for what reason it sometimes emerges from the belly of its mother before the due time.

Then you should describe which are the limbs that grow more than the others after the child is born; and give the measurements of a child of one year.

Then describe the man fully grown, and the woman, and their measurements, and the nature of their complexions' colour and physiognomy.

Afterwards describe how he is composed of veins, nerves, muscles and bones. This you should do at the end of the book.

Then represent in four histories, four universal conditions of mankind namely, joy, with various modes of laughing, and represent the cause of the laughter; weeping, the various ways with their cause; strife with various movements expressive of slaughterings, flights, fear, acts of ferocity, daring, homicide and all the things which connect with cases such as these.

Then make a figure to represent labour, in the art of dragging, pushing, carrying, restraining, supporting and conditions such as these.

Then describe the attitude and movement.

Then perspective through the office of the sight or the hearing. You should make mention of music and describe the other senses.

Afterwards describe the nature of the five senses.

The first period of Leonardo's investigation of human functional anatomy, beginning in Milan about 1485, involved dissections of at least some human material. These were private dissections, not made in association with any academic anatomist. Leonardo was especially concerned with the organs of the senses, particularly the eye—to a painter-philosopher, the noblest of them.

In Leonardo's second period of anatomical dissection (the second period in Milan) there was apparently the beginning of a collaboration with young Marcantonio della Torre, an anatomist who taught at the medical school in Pavia. It is possible that they contemplated preparing an illustrated anatomical text together, but the project was cut short by Marcantonio's death, of the plague, in 1511. In this second period of anatomical study, Leonardo paid much attention to the anatomical basis of movement—again relating to his artistic work:

This demonstration is as necessary for good draughtsmen as the derivation from Latin words is to good grammarians; for anyone must needs make the muscles of figures badly in their movements and actions unless he knows which are the muscles that are the cause of their movements.

The study of the muscles of the body was, until Canano and Vesalius in the 1540s, to remain a neglected science; Berengario agreed in the 1520s that he had little to contribute concerning myology.

Leonardo, with his anatomical drawings, wished to do two things; first to include in one series of drawings the results of a number of dissections, and secondly, to present each structure as seen from a number of viewpoints—at least from front, side and back, preferably from other points. *Plate 23* shows a series of views of the upper limb.

The true knowledge of the shape of any body will be arrived at by seeing it from different aspects. Consequently in order to convey a notion of the true shape of any limb ... I will observe the aforesaid rule, making four demonstrations for the four sides of each limb, and for the bones I will make five, cutting them in half and showing the hollow of each of them, one being full of marrow the other spongy or empty or solid.

Leonardo would have been delighted with the technical freedom of the movie camera and of video computer-simulation to achieve satisfactory flat images of a solid object.

It is not possible to be certain how many human cadavers Leonardo dissected. In his first stay in Milan, there is evidence that he had the opportunity of dissecting a head, possibly of an executed man; and there was also a dissection of a lower limb. Returning to Florence, in 1499, Leonardo appears to have had access to the Hospital of Santa Maria Nuova. There is a touching description of the death of an old man. Leonardo describes the event:

an old man, a few hours before his death, told me that he had lived a hundred years, and that he did not feel any bodily ailment other than weakness, and thus while sitting upon a bed in the hospital of Santa Maria Nuova at Florence, without any movement or sign of anything amiss, he passed away from this life. And I made an autopsy in order to ascertain the cause of so peaceful a death ...

Leonardo noted the structure of the blood-vessels of this old man, and the corpse provided material for studies on the musculature, which were completed by observations on living subjects. There is a note that a two-year-old child too was anatomized, and Leonardo undoubtedly had access to an unborn child of about seven months' gestation, although the drawing of this fetus is associated with a placenta obviously not of human origin (*Plate 27*). A note made by Leonardo about 1505 states that he had dissected at least ten bodies; but these were not necessarily complete cadavers.

In the final Italian period, in Rome in the years from late 1513 to 1516, Leonardo had access to the Hospital of the Santo Spirito, and studied anatomy there, paying particular attention to the human heart, until, on complaints from a rival artist, the Pope excluded him from the hospital. There is a sentence in Leonardo's notebooks that may refer to this: 'Make a discourse on the censure deserved by scholars who put obstacles in the way of those who practice anatomy . . .'.

Untrammelled by the precedents and procedures of academic anatomy, Leonardo developed his own methods of investigation and recording; the multi-viewpoint drawings and the wax casts of brain ventricles are evidence of this.

Make two air holes in the horns of the great ventricles and insert melted wax by means of a syringe, making a hole in the ventricle of the memoria, and through this hole fill the three ventricles of the brain; and afterwards when the wax has set, take away the brain and you will see the shape of the three ventricles exactly. But first insert thin tubes in the air holes in order that the air which is in these ventricles may escape and so make room for the wax which enters into the ventricles.

Other new methods used to investigate functional anatomy, and exploited by Leonardo, include the drawing of cross-sections of limbs (*Fig. 4.4*), the use of glass models of the heart valves, and the representation of muscles and muscle action by geometric diagrams. In some diagrams, otherwise realistic, he substituted cords and wires for muscles in order to indicate their function (*Fig. 4.5*).

Before you represent the muscles make, in place of these, threads which may serve to show the positions of these muscles, which should abut with their extremities in the centre of the attachment of the muscles above their bones. And this will supply a speedier conception when you wish to represent all the muscles one above the other. And if you make it in any other way your representation will be confused.

As may be seen from the notes already quoted, Leonardo writes as if this work were in preparation for the production of a textbook of functional anatomy. This didactic orientation of the notes appeared before he had any association with Marcantonio della Torre. Vasari's story that Leonardo and Marcantonio were to collaborate on such a text was obtained second-hand; he was born the year Marcantonio died, and was but eight years old at the time of Leonardo's death. Such instructive notes may be read two ways: either they can be regarded as preparation for the production of a textbook of human biology—anatomy, physiology, development, pathology and medicine placed in the context of human behaviour and emotions—*or* they can be seen as schemes for future investigation, schemes obviously so grand that even Leonardo must have vacillated, thinking along one line at one time, another at another.

On the one hand, Leonardo certainly had the vision and the ability to be able to prepare, from his notes, a book of illustrations of anatomy that would surpass by far works previously produced. On the other hand, Leonardo was notoriously unable to complete great projects; the horse for *il Moro* was just one such unfinished work. (There are those that would have that unhappy quality to be associated with left-handedness and uncertain cortical laterality. Others, with equally little evidence, would associate it with the separation from his natural mother in infancy.)

Parenthetically it may be wondered what might have been the consequences of a real collaborative association between Leonardo and a professional anatomist. First Leonardo would have had to define rather more rigidly the subject matter of his anatomy, probably in terms of Galenic anatomy. (A liberal-minded anatomical investigator might nowadays be more sympathetic to Leonardo's wide-ranging inquiry.) Secondly, Leonardo would have ben-efited from a somewhat more developed terminology, even though anatomical nomenclature was not systematized satisfactorily until centuries later. Thirdly, he would perhaps have been forced to study all anatomy and not only those parts that intrigued him. To balance out such possible benefits of association with an academic collaborator, Leonardo would have had to narrow his field of inquiry; no longer could we be certain that he would have been willing or allowed to look in an unprejudiced manner at any structural arrangement that took his fancy. The conclusion must be reached that Leonardo was not suitable academic material!

Are there other ways in which we can understand Leonardo's failure to make known his findings?

He spent his life as a courtier. He was proud of his professional abilities that had put him in this position, and he demanded respect, and received it, in the castles and mansions of his aristocratic patrons—the King of France, the Medicis, the Sforzas, the Borgias. His situation was later to be paralleled by many other painters in succeeding centuries. The view of the artist as artisan had been characteristic of an earlier, but still remembered, period. Leonardo maintained a lavish household in keeping with his position as courtier. (It is not known how he paid for this.) His attendance at the court of Ludovico Sforza included playing the lute, at which he was

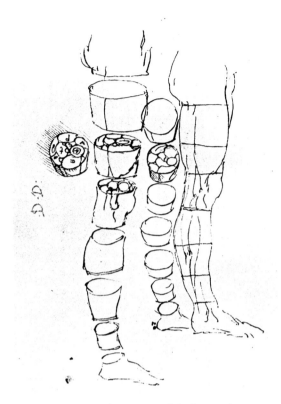

4.4   Cross-sectional anatomy of the human lower limb: Leonardo da Vinci.

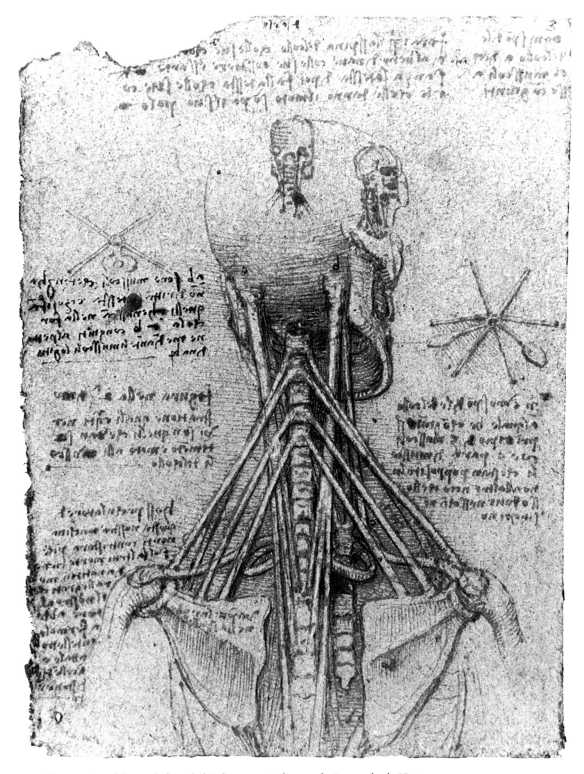

4.5   The muscles of the neck from behind represented as cords: Leonardo da Vinci.

proficient. Michelangelo spoke disparagingly, and rather bitchily, of him as 'the lute player from Milan'.

Contrast Leonardo with his younger contemporary, Albrecht Dürer (1471–1528) who was indeed influenced by Leonardo's work, which he saw on his second Italian journey, made 1505–7. In Dürer's *Dresden Sketchbook*, there is a copy, on folio 130 verso, of one of Leonardo's anatomical illustrations of the upper limb. Like Leonardo, Dürer worked with many techniques during his years of apprenticeship. But unlike Leonardo, Dürer was involved, in Michael Wolgemut's workshop, in the making of woodcut book illustrations. Even after he had been appointed court painter to Emperor Maximilian, he had begun to associate with scholars, and had started to explore the natural world objectively, Dürer continued to produce book illustrations and to make single prints for sale and on commission; his patrons for these wonderful works of art included not only the Emperor, but also humanists, merchants, and the more general public. For example, in the series of 15 woodcuts illustrating the Apocalypse, published first in 1498 and republished in 1511, Dürer was his own printer and publisher, as well as drawing and possibly cutting the illustrations. (Leonardo had none of these particular distractions.) Of equal stature to his artistic contemporaries in Italy, Dürer was also a business-man, jealous of his reputation as a print-maker; as was customary among northern wood-cutters and engravers, he usually signed and, after 1505 or so, dated his work.

It was perhaps a courtier's indifference to multiple publication that explains Leonardo's neglect of the printing press for reproduction of his works and drawings. Leonardo did consult illustrated books: his knowledge of the *Fasciculo*, the Italian version of Ketham, has already been noted; he also read Roberto Valturio's *De re militari*, Verona, 1472. But Leonardo would not have been inspired by publications such as the Savonarola sermons, printed soon after delivery, with accompanying popular woodcuts, 1489–98. References to printing, while not exactly disparaging, are very few in number—which surprises us knowing Leonardo's intense interest in all machines. He seems to have remained indifferent to the potentialities of even the finest products of the northern Italian book trade.

Another reason that separated Leonardo from publishing was his lack of facility in Latin, and his ignorance of Greek. Leonardo thus placed himself far from humanistic scholars. Undoubtedly he considered them the 'trumpeters and reciters of the works of others'. He was by training and inclination a very different man from the scholarly printer-publisher Aldo Manuzio, whose printing press, established in Venice at the end of the fifteenth century, produced Latin and Greek classics widely read by the learned public.

Leonardo thus came to ignore what was to become the principal transforming factor in the development of anatomical science. His notes were certainly not designed with their immediate publication in mind. How can these pages, with mutually interdependent text and illustration, be reproduced except in facsimile? The drawings lose much when separated from text, and the text by itself is often incomprehensible. The pages are structured in a non-linear manner; they are decidedly pre-Gutenberg in intent, and execution. It was not until photographic techniques enabled them to be accurately and easily reproduced in facsimile that these wonderful drawings could become known—much too late, however, to be anatomically influential. And by this time academic anatomy had in general long outstripped the knowledge acquired by Leonardo. Consequently, the Leonardo anatomical corpus, existing precariously in single form, remained essentially unknown. Leonardo's investigations in anatomy, so profound and so well illustrated, were perforce ignored. They have played, until this century, no historical part in the development of the subject. It is ironic that the proud Leonardo made little or no mention either of history or of persons in any of his notebooks.

22 Details of articulated skeletons from Leonardo da Vinci, *Anatomical notebooks* (Keele and Pedretti, 1979, 142 recto). Pen, with brown ink (Windsor Castle, Royal Library. © 1990. H.M. Queen Elizabeth II.). 28.8 × 20.0 cm.

Though it may seem remarkable it is nevertheless very probable that Leonardo never possessed a single complete individual skeleton. Had he done so he would surely have illustrated it *in toto*. Of course, it may be that such a drawing or drawings were among those that have been lost. Of his extant work this plate, probably drawn about 1510, is the closest approach.

The combination of a most gifted and experienced artist, one possessed of an insatiable curiosity, and with access, albeit limited, to human material—all this might well be expected to produce something out of the ordinary in skeletal illustrations. One only has to realize that these drawings fall in time between Hundt and Berengario (see *Plates 7 and 14, 15, and 16*) to appreciate how far ahead Leonardo was in anatomical artistry; not least, the bones *look* human! These drawings are far and away the most faithful arrangement and portrayal of human bones that existed up to that time—and indeed long after.

Among many excellent anatomical features are the curvatures of the vertebral column, the positioning (tilt) of the pelvic girdle, the slope of the ribs (*pace* the lateral view), the sterno-clavicular joint (lower left), the bowing of the femur, and the posterior positioning of the superior tibio-fibular joint. Leonardo also demonstrates his knowledge of the sesamoid character of the patella.

There are, as might be expected, some short-comings. The scapulae are much too long (in the posterior view reaching to the tenth rib). One also notes the too-long clavicles, the knob-like thoracic spines, the massive cervical vertebrae, a long and drooping coracoid process, too-long first, eleventh, and twelfth ribs, proportionately too broad a sacrum (central figure), and poor greater trochanters. A seven-piece sternum (inclusive of the manubrium and xiphisternum) is erroneously shown, in accordance with the teachings of Galen and Mondino. In addition, the eighth costal cartilage, although fused with the seventh, attaches separately directly to the lower part of the sternum.

In the lower left drawing there is an additional bone situated at the lateral end of the clavicle. This could possibly represent an ununited acromial epiphysis, though this is very rare. The head of the humerus ('the pole of the arm') is not very well portrayed in any of the three drawings where it is present.

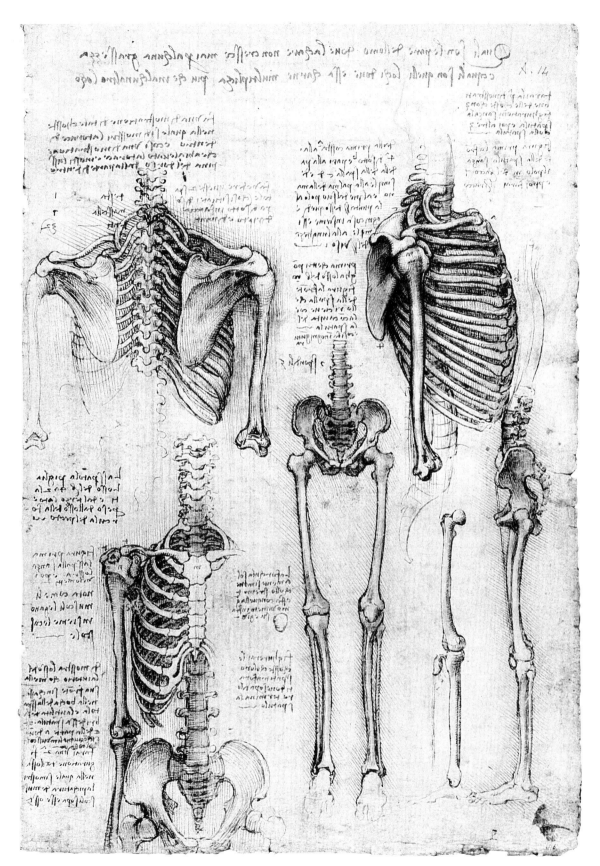

PLATE 22

23 The muscles of the upper limb from Leonardo da Vinci, *Anatomical notebooks* (Keele and Pedretti, 1979, 140 verso). Pen with brown ink and some chalking (Windsor Castle, Royal Library. © 1990. H.M. Queen Elizabeth II.). 28.6 × 20.1 cm.

The three upper drawings are vignettes of muscles attached to the vertebral spines; from left to right, semispinalis cervicis; splenius capitis; and, on the right, the upper portion of trapezius (with perhaps the rhomboid muscles, though the slope of the latter is too vertical).

The lower four drawings, essentially of the more superficial muscles of the arm, are superb, though one may regret that the two on the right were not shown with the forearm rather more supinated.

The origins of sternomastoid and trapezius, the reversed insertion of the two parts of pectoralis major, the two heads of the biceps, and the depiction of the deltoid, brachialis, brachioradialis, pronator teres muscles, etc. are most accurate and felicitous.

With regard to functional considerations, O'Malley and Saunders (1952) translate part of the accompanying notes: 'And the muscle o [biceps brachii] is appointed to rotate the arm from the elbow downwards, and it rotates it whether the arm is extended or flexed; and if the hand presents its dorsal surface [that is, is pronated] this muscle then assists the power of the muscle m [brachialis].' Thus Leonardo was aware that the biceps was a supinator of the forearm as well as a flexor of the elbow joint—although, in fact, when the elbow is extended this muscle is at a mechanical disadvantage as an elbow flexor when the forearm is supinated rather than pronated.

The eight-pointed star (lower right) indicates that Leonardo, properly to illustrate the anatomy of the upper limb, considered eight viewpoints (three lateral, three medial, one from the front, and one from the back) to be necessary.

These drawings present what one would see in an actual superficial dissection, and in this respect remind one of the drawings of John and Charles Bell, made in the dissection rooms in Edinburgh (see *Plates 104* and *105*, pp. 495 and 497) three hundred years later.

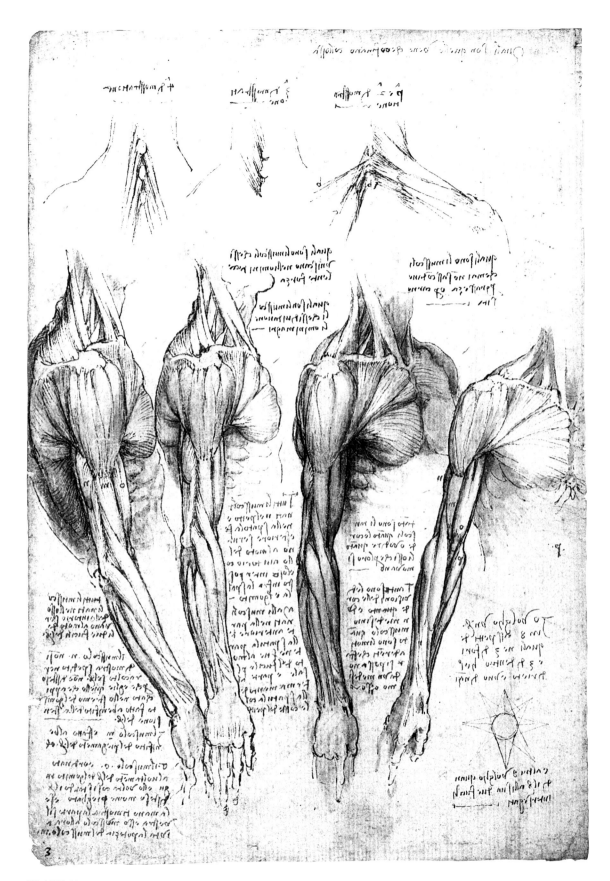

3

PLATE 23

24 The venous figure, from Leonardo da Vinci, *Anatomical notebooks* (Keele and Pedretti, 1979, 36 recto). Pen with brown ink and washes over black chalk (Windsor Castle, Royal Library. © 1990. H.M. Queen Elizabeth II.). 28.0 × 19.8 cm.

One can safely say that Leonardo's fame as an anatomist does not rest on this drawing, which must have been an early attempt, probably *c.*1494, before he had access to human dissection. An effort, so to speak, to put written anatomy into a human figure, quite in line with anatomical practice up to this time. Its purpose was to present the 'tree of the vessels' juxtaposed with the 'spiritual parts', the liver and heart. The stance of the body owes much to a blood-letting figure in the *Fasciculo* ... (1493).

Though the cephalic vein of the arm, the long saphenous vein in the leg, and the spleen are not too far-fetched, most of the rest of the anatomy follows earlier anatomical beliefs and teaching.

One notes the caval system (which was considered to convey the natural spirits to the rest of the body) springing like a bean-shoot from the liver, which latter seems to disappear behind the inferior vena cava and aorta; the heart appearing rather as an appendage; and the arterio-venous anastomotic arrangement of the blood-vessels near the heart.

The urinary bladder is shown with an open urethra but no prostate: the kidneys are oddly shaped, with the right positioned higher than the left: perhaps the hatched structure atop the left kidney represents a suprarenal gland.

The ureters seem to enter the urethra rather than the bladder. Someone (not Leonardo) has incorrectly labelled the right one 'vena cilis', the hollow vein, the term by which Leonardo referred to the vena cava. The right spermatic artery and vein, though large, are reasonable, although their relationship to the renal vein is not usual. No left spermatic vein is shown entering the left renal vein, though there is a stub of a left spermatic artery, just visible, arising from the aorta.

Perhaps the most pleasing feature of this drawing is the portrayal of the somewhat sad face.

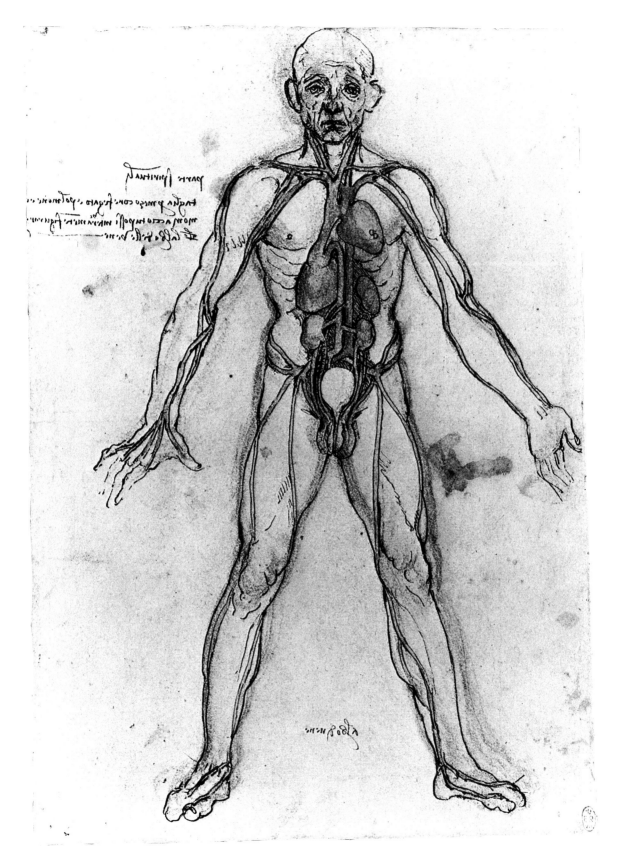

PLATE 24

25 The nerves of the human body from Leonardo da Vinci, *Anatomical notebooks* (Keele and Pedretti, 1979, 76 verso). Pen with brown ink (Windsor Castle, Royal Library. © 1990. H.M. Queen Elizabeth II.). 18.9 × 13.3 cm.

It is difficult to be sure when these sketches were drawn, though they most likely date before 1500. Over the years Leonardo's illustrations of the nervous system demonstrate increasing accuracy and understanding of this complex subject. For example, later drawings illustrating the distribution of the median and ulnar nerves in the hand, *circa* 1510, are beautiful and extremely accurate.

Thus these two drawings should more properly be regarded as *aides-mémoires* or sketches of ideas than as a serious attempt to illustrate the nervous system. Here Leonardo was essentially making the point that the spinal cord was continuous with the brain, the two being of the same 'substance', and also that the nerves originated (mainly) from the cord.

Thus too much should not be made of obvious anatomical crudities, such as the configuration of the brain, and that, in the left figure (evocative of a tiptoeing sleep-walker), the left leg possesses but one nerve below the knee. It is interesting that in this lateral view nerves to the back are shown, and two large nerves, almost certainly meant to represent the vagi, descend directly from the brain. By 1505 or thereabouts Leonardo knew that at least the right vagus reached to the stomach.

The right-hand figure serves the purpose of demonstrating the symmetry of the spinal nerves. In both figures the spinal cord is over-long.

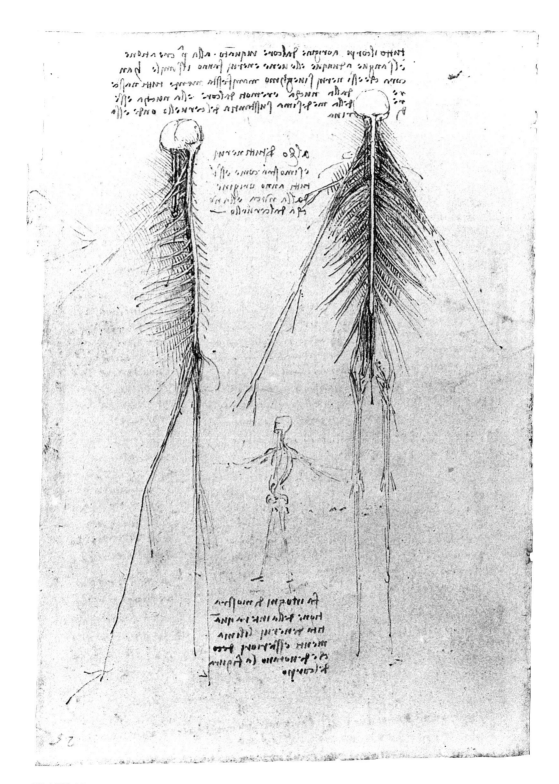

PLATE 25

26 The viscera of a pregnant woman from Leonardo da Vinci, *Anatomical notebooks* (Keele and Pedretti, 1979, 122 recto). Pen with brown ink and washes and chalks (Windsor Castle, Royal Library. © 1990. H.M. Queen Elizabeth II.). 47.6 × 33.2 cm.

This large, somewhat faint, drawing is one of Leonardo's most arresting anatomical illustrations. Alas, in spite of its immediate visual impact, from the point of view of human anatomy there is much in it that is erroneous.

It is almost as though, after drawing and describing various portions of human anatomy as he saw and understood them over a period of years Leonardo now become seduced by early writings, particularly of Galen and Mondino, which treat more of animal anatomy than human, and that he then included many of these precepts in this illustration.

It is quite impossible that Leonardo could have drawn this illustration at the time of making or viewing a dissection, or even from memory. Much of the anatomy is fanciful, and some is certainly derived from that of animals, such as the tributaries of the superior vena cava, the relative positioning and shape of the kidneys, the banding in the heart ventricles, and the arrangement of the branches of the aortic arch. With regard to the latter Leonardo, in a sketch entitled 'artery of the old man', was probably the first person accurately to draw the three main branches of the human aortic arch. Although the chronology of Leonardo's drawings remains in doubt it seems not impossible that the artery sketch preceded this visceral drawing.

The liver, suggestive of being multilobular, lies totally on the right side, with a blunt left extremity; it drains into the inferior vena cava by a single long hepatic vein seemingly formed from a venous plexus on the surface of the organ. The fundus of the gall-bladder (and perhaps the cystic duct) can be seen at the mid-point of the liver.

The trachea is depicted as dividing into two equally inclined main bronchi, each of which divides symmetrically. That Leonardo believed this to be true is evidenced by a number of his other drawings.

The heart consists of but two chambers, the ventricles, as had been the traditional view for some thirteen hundred years, the present-day atria being considered part of the venous system, as illustrated here. Elsewhere in his notebooks Leonardo in a small sketch very clearly shows two atria, separated from each other, lying atop the ventricles and leading into these via 'gateways'. He then rather spoils things by stating that they (the atria) are outside the heart substance, even though the drawing strongly suggests otherwise.

The urinary bladder is represented by a faint circle over the lower part of the (presumably) pregnant uterus and the vagina. Into it enter the two ureters. The two oval ovaries are each connected by a short thick tube to the inferior portion of the uterus in its cervical region. The ovarian vessels are difficult to make out in this drawing, but Leonardo was certainly aware that the left vein was connected to the left renal vein and the right one to the inferior vena cava.

Two vessels—not at all easy to follow in their entirety, but, in their mid-portion, in line with

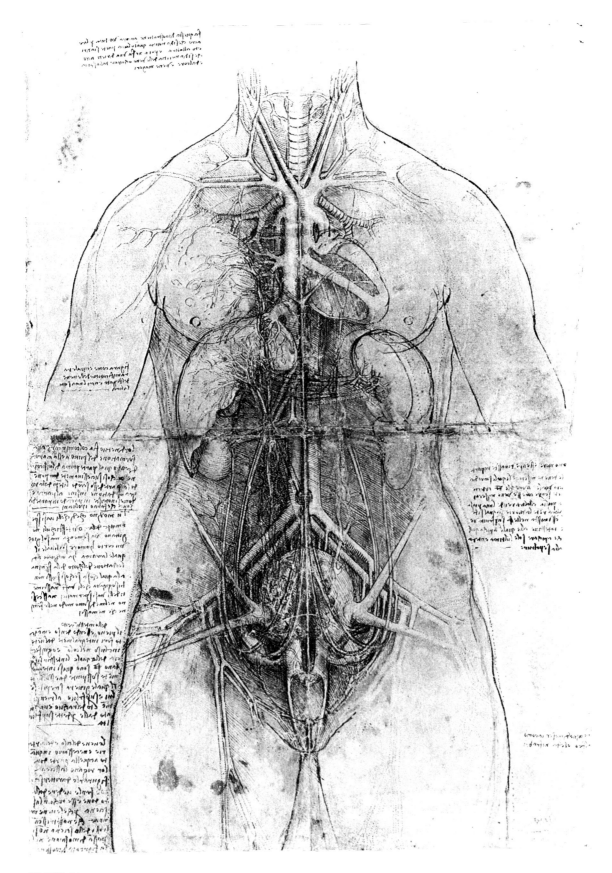

PLATE 26

where the epigastric veins would lie—lead from a plexus on the uterus to the breasts; that on the right breast ends in a vascular plexus. The physiological thinking of the day was that, in pregnancy, these vessels conveyed the retained menstrual blood to the breasts, where it was then changed into milk. This concept of these imaginary vessels is well exemplified in one of Leonardo's coition drawings.

The iliac vessels are poorly portrayed, being scarcely human. Umbilical arteries, presumably obliterated cords in fact, can be seen leading from the iliac arteries to the umbilicus; but, alas, they are accompanied by veins!

Perhaps what strikes one as the most puzzling part of this illustration are the two clearly delineated structures originating from a common attachment either side of the uterus. These are a triumph of the imagination, or perhaps dogmatic belief, over reality. They are too prominent to be round ligaments, which in any case are not bifid. It may be that the lower is representative of the ligament, the upper, despite its placement, being the Fallopian tube. Mondino earlier described such 'horns of the uterus', stating them to be two thick strong ligaments. It is also interesting to compare the portrayal here with that of the *Fasciculo ... 1493* (see *Plate 8*, p. 43). It is obvious that neither was taken from 'life', but rather they represent an adding-on, to conform with contemporary written anatomy and beliefs.

Two other points might be mentioned. The first is that this drawing seems to have been folded into four—the horizontal fold passing through the kidneys, the vertical one being in the mid-line. This latter passes through the vagina, and is largely responsible for the seeming division of this organ into two halves. The second point concerns the pin-pricks (seen best around the outline of the body) by which the drawing could be reproduced. One such reproduction, admittedly omitting certain structures such as the heart and liver, is extant. Whether or not this was made by Leonardo is in doubt—in the original the umbilicus is accurately positioned at the bifurcation of the aorta, but in the tracing it is placed just above the uterus, a mistake Leonardo himself would surely not have made.

27 Fetus *in utero*, etc. from Leonardo da Vinci, *Anatomical notebooks* (Keele and Pedretti, 1979, 198 recto). Pen with brown ink and wash and red chalk (Windsor Castle, Royal Library. © 1990. H.M. Queen Elizabeth II.). 30.4 × 22.0 cm

Considering the bizarre portrayals of fetuses *in utero* that had appeared prior to Leonardo's time (for an example see *Plate 1*) the fetus in the main drawing is revolutionary in its realism, even though, sadly, Leonardo believed that 'the heart of this child does not beat ...'. This portrayal of the form, proportions, and attitude of the fetus was unsurpassed until the illustrations of Smellie in the early eighteenth century.

To the left of the uterus one notes an ovoid ovary, with its short, thick tubular connection

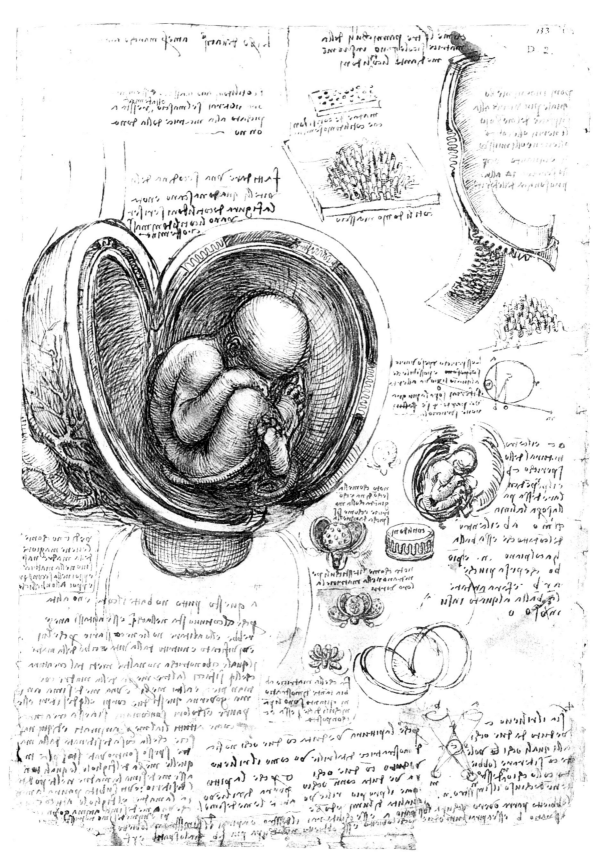

PLATE 27

to the lower part of the uterus. This is repeated in the small sketches to the immediate right of the uterus. In the main drawing the form of the cervix, projecting into the (outlined) vagina shows Leonardo's grasp of this part of human anatomy, which until then had been poorly and sparsely illustrated. Even Vesalius could have learned from it.

It seems strange to us that Leonardo appears to have been ignorant of the appearance of a shed human discoidal placenta. This may explain the non-illustration of the attachment of the umbilical cord in his drawing. The fetal membranes are shown attaching to the uterine wall in distinct and separate areas—the placentomes of the cotyledonary placentae of goats, cows, and deer. This concept of the placenta is emphasized in the more detailed smaller drawings, where 'male' and 'female' cotyledons are featured. One of Leonardo's notes refers to obtaining calves' placentae to determine which of these cotyledons they retain after parturition. The stripping apart of these is illustrated in the upper right-hand drawing.

The faint diagram in the lower right corner is unrelated to the other drawings, being concerned with Leonardo's views on binocular vision.

Chapter 4: Selected reading

Aaron, P. G. and Clouse, R. G. (1982). Freud's psychohistory of Leonardo da Vinci: a matter of being right or left. *J. interdisc. Hist.*, **13**, 1–16.

Barlow, T. D. (1948). *Woodcuts of Albrecht Dürer.* Penguin, Harmondsworth.

Clark, K. (1969). *The drawings of Leonardo da Vinci in the collection of Her Majesty the Queen ... Volume 3.* Phaidon, London.

Clarke, E. and Dewhurst, K. (1972). *An illustrated history of brain function.* Sandford, Oxford.

Keele, K. D. (1964) Leonardo da Vinci's influence on renaissance anatomy. *Med. Hist.*, **8**, 360–70.

Keele, K. D. (1983). *Leonardo da Vinci's elements of the science of man.* Academic Press, New York.

Keele, K. D. and Pedretti, C. (1977). *Leonardo da Vinci: anatomical drawings from the Royal Collection.* Royal Academy of Arts, London.

Keele, K. D. and Pedretti, C. (1979). Leonardo da Vinci. Corpus of the anatomical studies in the collection of Her Majesty the Queen at Windsor Castle. Johnson Reprint Company, London.

Kemp, M. (1976). Dr. William Hunter on the Windsor Leonardos and his volume of drawings attributed to Pietro da Cortona. *Burlington Mag.*, **118**, no. 876.

Kornell, M. (1989). Anatomical drawings by Battista Franco *Bull. Cleveland Mus. Art*, **76**, 302–25.

Linscott, R. N. (ed.) (1957). *The notebooks of Leonardo da Vinci*, trans. E. MacCurdy. Random House, New York.

MacCurdy, E. (1938). *The notebooks of Leonardo da Vinci.* Cape, London.

O'Malley, C. D. and Saunders, J. B. de C. M. (1952). *Leonardo da Vinci on the human body.* Henry Schuman, New York.

Popham, A. E. (1946). *The drawings of Leonardo da Vinci.* Cape, London.

Steinitz, K. T. (1958). *Leonardo da Vinci's Trattato della Pittura ... a bibliography of the printed editions 1651–1956.* Munksgaard, Copenhagen.

5

The great leap forward

T HE CHANGE in the attitude of scholars towards the natural world that occurred during the sixteenth and seventeenth centuries may be as well exemplified in their studies of anatomy as of other disciplines. This different attitude, which was to be the basis of the seventeenth-century scientific academies, occurred as early in anatomy as in any other subject: the study of the structure of the body rests quintessentially on ocular demonstration of natural phenomena. The scientific revolution in anatomy was in part a renaissance, a rebirth of classical enquiry, quite in accord with Galenic ideals—but not necessarily thereby acceptable to all Galenists, for the new anatomists rejected Galen's mistakes, at first hesitantly, then stridently. As confidence increased through their own discoveries, later anatomists of the seventeenth century rarely troubled themselves with references to the ancient authorities. Printed illustrations of structures revealed by dissection, rather than texts, became central to the transmission of anatomical knowledge.

In the first decades of the sixteenth century the potential of printed illustrations was beginning to be realized; the anatomy shown can be seen to be more observational, less schematic. From this springboard—a construction of Berengario and others—there occurred a great leap forward in anatomy and in anatomical illustration. The texts in these new anatomy books were at first not substantially different from those previously available, but the illustrations were. It was not the text of the *Fabrica*, 1543, that was widely copied, but the illustrations accompanying it.

Three sets of illustrations of human anatomy of great originality were made in the 1530s, 1540s, and 1550s—they were prepared under the direction of Vesalius, of Estienne, and of Eustachio, each an academic anatomist.

Andreas Vesalius, 1514–1564 (Andreas van Wesel; André Vésale)

Vesalius' family name was Witing (or Wijtinck—there were other spellings); they came from Wesel, a Westphalian town on the Rhine. The family had had, for at least three generations before Vesalius, connections with the royal courts. His great-grandfather was a professor in the medical school at Louvain, founded in 1426; he took as a family heraldic device the emblem of the town of Wesel—three weasels, which Vesalius was later to incorporate into the title-page of the *Fabrica*. Andreas' father was an apothecary in the service of Emperor Charles V. He married Isabel Crabbe and made his home in Brussels, where Andreas, the second child, was born. Although his mother's maiden name has long been thought to indicate an English background, there is apparently no evidence for this assumption.

At the age of fifteen years, Andreas Vesalius enrolled at Louvain and studied, for three and a half years, the liberal arts. A significant event for the Wesel family during this period was the successful petition to the Emperor by Vesalius' father asking that the 'blemish upon his birth' (he had been born outside marriage) should be removed. The Emperor's reply noted the medical and other services of the Wesel family to the Imperial House.

Vesalius travelled to Paris in August 1533 to study medicine. For foreign students the course in the faculty of medicine lasted a minimum of four years. The backbone of the course was separate morning and afternoon series of lectures given by professors-in-ordinary; during Vesalius' stay they were Jean Fernel, Johann Günther (Guenther or Winter) of Andernach, and Jacques Froment, or Fourment. These lectured on *natural subjects*, which included anatomy, physiology, and botany; *non-natural subjects*, hygiene and the regimen of health; and *subjects contra-nature*, pathology and therapeutics. The teaching relied heavily on the authority of the standard works by classical, Arabic, and medieval authors; but Mondino's anatomy, so influential in Italy and Germany, was less highly regarded in Paris. Important investigative work was carried out in establishing the textual accuracy of classical works: Günther brought out twenty-two translations, all issued by the Parisian publisher Simon de Colines. Günther's guide to Galen's anatomy, issued first in Paris in 1536, was later to be revised by Vesalius and republished in Venice in 1538. The library of the medical faculty contained many Arabic and medieval texts, but also such works as the Aldine edition of Galen in Greek, published in 1525.

Vesalius was later to write 'I have studied without the aid of a teacher'; but Günther was more gracious, and, in his 1536 textbook on Galen's anatomy, commended Vesalius as a student of great promise, with an extraordinary knowledge of medicine, and very skilled in dissecting bodies. Since Günther was known as a scholar and a translator, and had no reputation as a dissector himself, it is probable that Vesalius was given independent responsibilities in human dissection while still a student, duties in which he demonstrated his competence. The young man assisted Günther on one known occasion by dissecting the corpse of a hanged woman in a public anatomy. Another of Vesalius' teachers of anatomy was Jacobus Sylvius (Jacques Dubois). This physician was a forceful and popular lecturer on anatomy; he was known as a Galenist, but one who verified the texts by dissection of animals and human cadavers. It is possible that Vesalius did not attend any human anatomies carried out by Sylvius.

In 1536 Vesalius was obliged to leave Paris, his course not yet completed, because of an incipient war between the armies of France and the forces of the Emperor. Vesalius, with his close family ties to Charles V, sensibly returned to the Low Countries, and re-entered the University of Louvain. A man of enterprise, at Louvain he pursued particularly his anatomical studies; in one episode he reconstructed a skeleton from the corpse of an executed man. The body had been left to be picked by the birds at the side of a country road. Vesalius smuggled the skeleton through the gates of the city of Louvain, portion by portion. While still a medical student, he created excitement at Louvain by conducting an authorized anatomical demonstration in front of the medical and other faculties. Dissection had been a rare event. Before graduating in 1537 he also published, in both Louvain and Basle, a paraphrase of some of the writings of Muhammad ar-Razi (Rhazes)—*Regem Almansorem*.

Vesalius decided to complete his medical degree at Padua, where, after the prescribed series of examinations, in December 1537 he was appointed as teacher in surgery and anatomy. He had obtained clinical experience by work in the hospitals of Venice, only thirty-five kilometres distant. In order to help his students, and at their request, Vesalius published in 1538 a series of six large illustrations based on his first dissection at Padua as a professional anatomist. These were the *Tabulae anatomicae*, known also as *Tabulae sex* (see *Plates 12 and 13*, pp. 61 and 63). Three of these drawings were made to Vesalius' directions by Joannes Stephanus of Calcar. The book was printed in Venice at the expense of Calcar, who possibly received the profits. Pirated copies of the plates were published in a number of European cities: they were obviously popular. In 1539, Vesalius' salary was increased on account of his success as an anatomy teacher who not only lectured but who himself dissected and encouraged students to dissect.

In Padua, Vesalius became steadily more independent in his views and severe in his criticism of Galen's supposed infallibility. He realized fully that Galen's anatomy was substantially derived from that of animals, and that this had often created errors. As he writes in the dedication to the *Epitome*, 1543: '[Galen] although easily chief of the masters, nevertheless did not dissect the human body, and the fact is now evident that he described, not to say imposed on us, the fabric of the ape's [monkey's] body, although it differs in many respects'.

By 1543, Vesalius was a most experienced anatomist; and the confidence he had in himself was not only great but justified. His self-confident portrait appears in the *Fabrica*. It may be compared with a portrait of his Emperor (*Figs 5.1a and b*). Moreover he was capable of hard work, in teaching and research at the dissecting table and also in the preparation of the extensive manuscript for his great book: Andreae Vesalii Bruxellensis, Scholae medicorum Patauinae professoris, *de humani corporis fabrica libri septem*. Basileae: ex officina Ioannis Oporini …, MDXLIII Mense Iunio [Andreas Vesalius of Brussels, Professor in the medical school at Padua, *Seven books* [that is, a work in seven sections] *on the structure of the human body*. Basle, Oporinus, June 1543]. The word *fabrica* may be translated as *structure* or framework, but, as used by Vesalius, it has greater functional overtones. It could also mean a place where a thing is made, as well as the thing made. Obviously the word *fabric*, most commonly referring to material or cloth, can also be used as a metaphor for the intricacies of the tissues and organs of human anatomy.

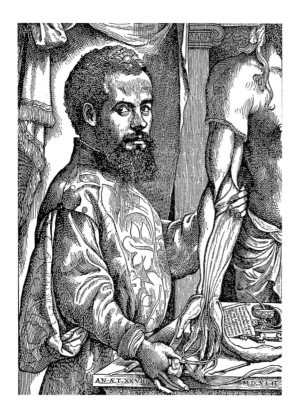

5.1a Portrait of Vesalius, aged twenty-eight, from the *Fabrica*, 1543.

The manuscript of the book was completed, and woodcuts were made in Venice under Vesalius' close supervision. The blocks and the text were sent to Basle, to the printer and scholar, Johannes Oporinus (1507–68), a man who had some medical training of a very different kind from that of Vesalius: he was for a time the pupil of Paracelsus. Vesalius himself travelled to Basle to see his book through the press. When it was published in 1543, he was twenty-eight years of age. While in Basle, he prepared an articulated skeleton from the corpse of a bigamist who had been beheaded for attempting to murder his first wife; much of this skeleton still remains in Basle. Vesalius wrote and Oporinus published, also in the summer of 1543, a less expensive companion book to the *Fabrica*; this was *De humani corporis fabrica librorum epitome* (*Plates 37 and 38*, pp. 163 and 165). The *Epitome* had nine anatomical illustrations, three of them similar to plates in the *Fabrica*. The unbound sheets of the *Epitome* may be compared with a set of 'fugitive sheets' (see Chapter 2, p. 44). The additional two woodcuts of a naked man and a naked woman, ostensibly to show surface anatomy or 'exhibit the Canon of Proportion', are perhaps the most beautiful figures to have been prepared for an anatomy text (*Figs 5.2a and b*). Like his earlier *Tabulae*, the *Fabrica* and the *Epitome* were copied or plagiarized in many centres; an authorized German translation of the *Epitome* was published in 1543 by Oporinus, the translator being the Rector of Basle University, Albanus Torinus.

Vesalius' former teacher in Paris, Sylvius, reacted most unfavourably and aggressively to the *Fabrica*; but only such diehard Galenists could fail to be influenced by this new science that Vesalius and other anatomists were creating in the Italian schools. While still on leave from Padua, Vesalius set out for Speyer on the Rhine, where the court of the Emperor Charles V was residing; he obtained a position as one of Charles's physicians at the Imperial Court, and remained there for the rest of his professional life, publishing little further— a few works which, though interesting, were comparatively insignificant in the history of medicine. He did however revise the *Fabrica*; Oporinus published the new edition in 1555. A year later Vesalius was, by Imperial charter, ennobled and made a count palatine. He died at the age of fifty years, returning from a pilgrimage to Jerusalem. He had possibly decided to take up academic life again, expecting to reoccupy his old anatomy chair in Padua, which had become vacant by the death of Falloppio. The reasons for his pilgrimage remain obscure.

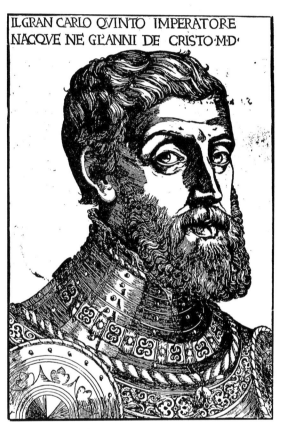

5.1b Portrait of Charles V.

Vesalius' methods

In January, 1540, when he was twenty-five years old, he was invited to Bologna to conduct an anatomy before the students. His ability in dissection was attested to by friends and enemies alike; his fame had spread. As the formal lecturer, rather than as the lecturer-demonstrator, was Matteo Corte or Corti (Matthaeus Curtius), a man of about sixty-five years who had moved a number of times from one medical school in north Italy to another, with successive increments to his salary. As a lecturer at Padua in 1524 he had received a salary of 800 gold ducats, which was 'a considerable sum in those days for a person who was not a lawyer' (Eriksson 1959).

By bringing these two popular anatomists together Bologna hoped perhaps to reaffirm its pre-eminence as a medical school; Padua had grown the more famous. The contrast between the two men, in age, attitude, and opinion was considerable; this must have been known to the authorities at Bologna when they invited Vesalius, apparently at the students' suggestion. They got their money's worth, for in their courses Curtius and Vesalius disagreed so emphati-

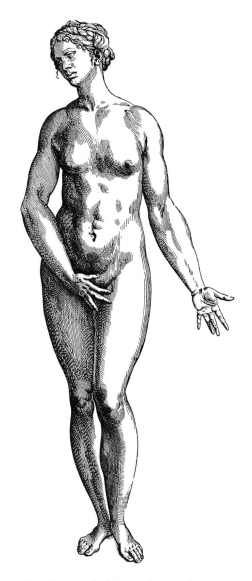

5.2a and b   The so-called Eve and Adam figures from Vesalius' *Epitome*, 1543 (as reproduced from the original wood-blocks in the *Icones*, 1934).

cally that the Rector had to intervene on more than one occasion. We know this much and much else about these courses because one of the students at the lectures and the demonstrations kept detailed notes, which were preserved, and are now in the Royal Library in Stockholm. Ruben Eriksson (1959) has, in an excellent work, transcribed these notes, with a translation and perceptive comments. The diarist was from Silesia, Baldasar Heseler by name; he was older than Vesalius, being a senior student who had read theology at Wittenburg under Martin Luther. He described vividly the excitement at the start of the first of Vesalius' demonstrations:

In the middle of Curtius' lecture our beadle, by name of Pelegrinus, presented himself, and by order of the anatomists informed us that the anatomy on our subject was now prepared. And they asked us ... that after the lecture we should go to the anatomy in good order and without disturbance: for we should all be well able to see wonderful things which we had not seen before ... And yet after the lecture we proceeded to the demonstration in great disorder, as the mad Italians do. The anatomy of our subject was arranged in the place [a church] where they use to elect the Rector medicorum; a table on which the subject was laid, was conveniently and well installed with four steps of benches in a circle, so that nearly 200 persons could see the anatomy. However, nobody was allowed to enter before the anatomists, and after them, those who had paid 20 *sol*. More than 150 students were present and D. Curtius, Erigus, and many other doctors, followers of Curtius. At last, D. Andreas Vesalius arrived, and many candles were lighted, so that all should see, etc ... And there was the body cut up and prepared beforehand, already shaved, washed and cleaned. He began with the outer skin, to which the inner one adhered, that is rightly called the skin, cutis, the outer one being better named hide.

Later Vesalius replies to one of Curtius' interruptions:

Here Curtius remarked that this, however, was not Galen's opinion. Vesalius answered: No, Dominus, he said, even if that is not Galen's opinion, we shall however demonstrate here, that in fact is it so. But now, he said, we do not want to fight with many words. Then the Rector interposed, rather clumsily: D. Doctor Andreas, do not be afraid of telling your opinion on these questions, do not fear those venerable masters.

The following extract from the notebooks indicates Vesalius' methods, and also his discovery that the source of Galen's errors was his reliance on non-human anatomy. Nevertheless both methodologically and scientifically Vesalius recognized his indebtedness to, and showed his respect for, Galen.

Please observe, he said, that all muscles issue from bones and beginning at their heads with sinews and ending in sinews or cordae they are again fastened to bones, in order to effectuate their natural voluntary movement in the body. The rest, he said, we shall demonstrate after dinner, when those muscles have been removed. And they had killed a dog upon which he showed that the muscles in dogs as also in other animals were fastened in quite another way than in man, so that they should be able to run faster. He promised to show us after dinner the anatomy of the muscles of an arm. In the meantime we ought to read about

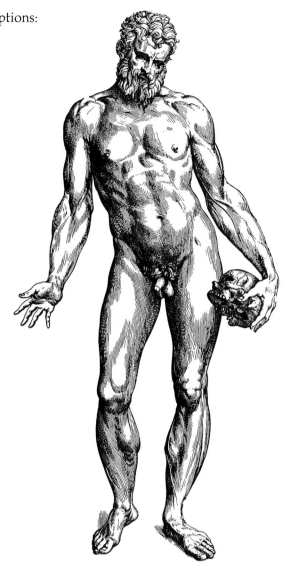

these matters in Galen, *De usu partium, I and II*, and *De anatomicis administrationibus, I*. However, he had on the dissection table put his anatomy of the bones [the skeleton] from which he on every occasion all the better demonstrated to us the position of the parts of the body.

The Fabrica

From the title-page onwards, it is apparent that Vesalius knew what he was about (*Fig. 5.3*). In that title-page, one of the most remarkable in the history of books, we can see that the old order of anatomy as textual explication is over; what now needs to be done is to find with

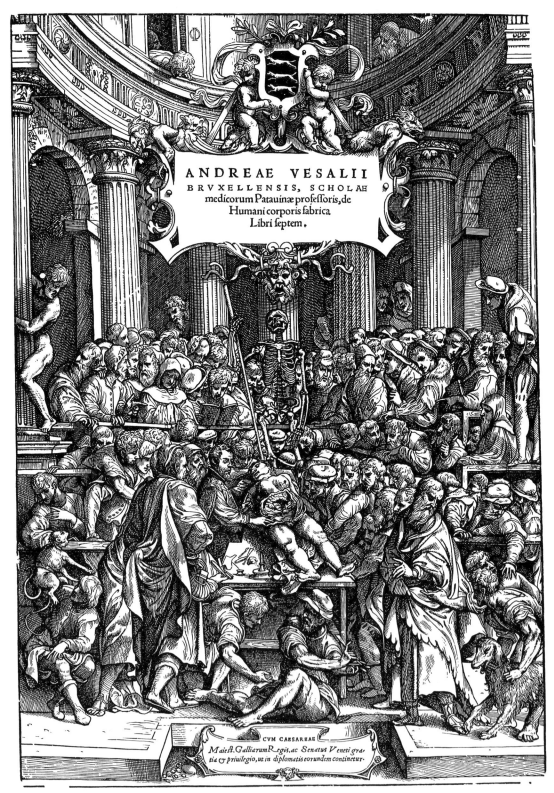

ANDREAE VESALII
BRVXELLENSIS, SCHOLAE
medicorum Patauinæ professoris, de
Humani corporis fabrica
Libri septem.

CVM CAESAREAE
Maiest. Galliarum Regis, ac Senatus Veneti gratia & priuilegio, ut in diplomatis eorundem continetur.

BASILEAE·

5.3   The title-page of Vesalius' *Fabrica*, 1543.

one's own hands and see with one's own eyes the real structures that exist in the human body, dissecting it apart not to show what was written on the pages of books but to demonstrate what almighty God had formed in his own image. In the crowds shown in the title-page dissection scene, there is only one onlooker with a book. The Professor of Anatomy, Vesalius himself—there is no doubt about it—is the centre of the crowd, dissecting and demonstrating. Behind and above, in the position occupied in some older anatomy scenes by a reader seated in his chair, there stands, supporting itself on a staff, an articulated skeleton—the structure to be understood first on learning anatomy. The assistants, who formerly had sometimes done much of the actual dissection, are shown preparing instruments under the table on which the cadaver lies. Animals are symbolically relegated to the wings, for, as we have seen, Vesalius was determined to base his anatomy primarily on the human, not on dissections of dogs or of primates other than man.

When we move from the title-page to the dedicatory preface addressed to the Emperor Charles V, in whose service Vesalius was to spend the remainder of his working life, there are further statements indicating that the old authority of Galen is under attack:

I am aware that by reason of my age—I am at present twenty-eight years old—my efforts will have little authority, and that, because of my frequent indication of the falsity of Galen's teachings, they [the books of the *Fabrica*] will find little shelter from the attacks of those who were not present at my anatomical demonstrations or have not themselves studied the subject sedulously; various schemes in defence of Galen will be boldly invented unless these books appear with the auspicious commendation and great patronage of some divine power [Charles V, of course!].

In the preface also he deplores:

that detestable procedure by which usually some conduct the dissection of the human body and others present the account of its parts, the latter like jackdaws aloft in their high chair, with egregious arrogance croaking things they have never investigated but merely committed to memory from the book of others, or reading what has already been described. The former are so ignorant of languages that they are unable to explain their dissections to the spectators and muddle what ought to be displayed according to the instructions of the physician who, since he has never applied his hand to the dissection of the body, haughtily governs the ship from a manual. Thus everything is wrongly taught in the schools, and days are wasted in ridiculous questions so that in such confusion less is presented to the spectators than a butcher in his stall could teach a physician.

That Vesalius developed an increasing confidence in his own ability and judgement may be seen by turning from the *Tabulae* (1538) to the first edition of the *Fabrica* (1543), and then to its revised edition (1555). Two examples may be given: one plate in the *Tabulae* includes a gross mistake taken over from the classical teaching recorded in Galen; a five-lobed liver is illustrated. This is corrected in the *Fabrica*. The text describing the interventricular septum of the heart in the 1543 *Fabrica* has:

The septum of the ventricles of the heart is very dense. It abounds with pits on both sides. Of these pits none, so far as the senses can perceive, penetrate from the right to the left ventricle. We are thus forced to wonder at the art of the Creator, by which the blood passes from the right to left ventricles through pores which elude the sight.

This may be taken in a straightforward manner, but was possibly meant ironically. In the 1555 edition, the doubts are brought into the open:

Although sometimes these pits are conspicuous, yet none, so far as the senses can perceive, passes from right to the left ventricle. I have not come across even the most hidden channels by which the septum of the ventricles is pierced, yet such channels are described by teachers of anatomy, who have absolutely decided that the blood is taken from the right to the left ventricle. I, however, am in great doubt as to the action of the heart in this part.

Vesalius' successor to the chair at Padua, Realdo Colombo (Realdus Columbus), and his pupil Valverde, were later to state that blood passed from right to left ventricle through the lungs, and not through the septum as Galen had it. This eventually led to the proof of the pulmonary circuit by William Harvey, a graduate of Padua, decades later. Vesalius' fellow student in Paris, Michael Servetus (Servet), had earlier, in 1540, made a statement about the pulmonary circuit in a book largely unread by anatomists; and, even earlier, ibn an-Nafis had described this circuit in work written in the thirteenth century, a fact that possibly only became known generally in the west in the 1920s.

The pages of the *Fabrica*, with their integral illustrations, form a text of modern anatomy; this can be said of no previous book. Other anatomists of Vesalius' time, and before, made summaries of the structure of the human body, many including original observations; some of these books were illustrated by instructive figures. Berengario's work published twenty-two years previously comes nearest in intent and achievement to Vesalius; he, like Vesalius, even issued an epitome, the *Isagogae . . .*, of his larger textbook. It is possible that German anatomical woodcuts made in the early 1500s suggested the potentialities of an illustrated textbook of human anatomy to Berengario. The resultant books he authored, and had illustrated, were innovative, but remained only a partial success, their simple illustrations in no way exploiting the possibilities of union between text and illustration. With Vesalius further strides were taken:

First the text, which covered the whole of anatomy, was based—to a greater extent than in any equivalent previous work—on the best information obtained from a critical re-examination of the manuscripts of classical authors, particularly Galen. Vesalius' work showed the beneficial results of his thorough education, his contact with humanist medical scholarship, in Paris with such men as Günther, in Padua with Caius, and in Basle with his publisher, Oporinus. That he was a competent scholar is shown by the part he played in editing Galen's work for the Giunta edition, Venice, 1541. (He contributed three short sections, including *Anatomical procedures* to this immense endeavour; in one copy the book has been bound in seven folio volumes weighing together some eighteen kilograms.) Vesalius' Latin prose has been described as having a 'complicated sentence structure heavily decorated with classic and late classic Latin nuances with metrical clauses and the like...', said by Singer to be much like spoken Latin. This was admired by some of his contemporaries, but deters all but a dedicated classical scholar today. The *Fabrica* has not yet been translated *in toto* into the English language.

Secondly, Vesalius cut through the tedious and sterile controversies concerning Galen's accuracy by demonstrating unequivocally that the classical author had derived much of his human anatomy from animal sources. This allowed Vesalius to benefit from Galen's inheritance, and yet made it possible to trust his own eyes and the findings of patient dissection of the human cadaver.

Thirdly, Vesalius incorporated in his book a *sufficient* number of illustrations, each one carefully considered in relation to the accompanying text, so that there could be consultation back and forth between words and pictures.

It is obvious that Vesalius was indebted to his predecessors, especially Galen; considerable errors taken over from Galen were indeed still included. However, in the *Fabrica*, Vesalius emphasized that the reference point for anatomy was the body on the dissecting table, and not the words of any authority, even such a great one as Galen. The book and its companion, the *Epitome*, were widely distributed, argued about, copied, and plagiarized, and no one at all involved in medicine could remain indifferent: Vesalius had either to be condemned as a dangerous heretic and destroyer of authority (a position taken by his Parisian teacher, Sylvius) or, alternatively, his attitudes and methods had to be adopted wholeheartedly. As William Osler wrote: 'Imagine the surprise and consternation of the easy-going professors who held the chairs of anatomy to have a huge volume thrust into their hands filled from cover to cover with descriptions and figures with which they were unfamiliar. And written by a young man of 28 ...'. Sylvius asked Charles V to *punish* Vesalius for his importunities. It is therefore justifiable to give to the *Fabrica* a considerable importance in the development of the scientific attitude. Few books of the sixteenth century can claim this; one other was *De revolutionibus orbium coelestium ...*, Nuremberg [*On the revolutions of the celestial spheres*], which also appeared in 1543. This latter book was the work of Nicolaus Copernicus, another medical doctor, published posthumously after many years of preparation. The *Fabrica* was the work of a man of twenty-eight years, published at the end of only five years of mature professional life, though five years of continuous investigation, writing, and teaching.

The printer and publisher of the Fabrica

The publisher of the *Fabrica*, and its companion book, the *Epitome*, was Johannes Oporinus (Oporin). His family name was Herbst or Herbster, referring to autumn, but when nineteen years of age he had adopted the name Oporin from the Greek word also signifying autumn; this was thought to be more appropriate to a dedicated humanist. In Oporinus's catalogue of 1567, only 27 of the 706 books listed related to medicine, yet Vesalius' *Fabrica* of 1543, and its edition of 1555, were Oporinus' master works. He put into the production of this book all the care he could, using fine type, including a beautiful italic, making sure that each page was well designed, and placing each illustration in an appropriate manner. He and Vesalius together saw the final work of production through the presses; there were probably six presses in the printing house, and printers must have worked at full speed to produce such a large work, in what was probably for that time a large edition, within a few months.

The question will be asked: Why did Vesalius choose to have these two books printed and published in Basle, when Venice, famous for its book production, was so close at hand? One factor, certainly, was Vesalius' previous association with and respect for the Basle publishers. Oporinus' brother-in-law, Ruprecht or Robert Winter, who had published editions of Vesalius' *Paraphrasis . . .* (1537) and *Venesection Letter* (1539), was one of the partners in Oporinus' first printing-house. When that venture failed in 1541, Winter remained with Oporinus for a time, but they were probably not associated at the time of printing the *Fabrica*. Nearly one hundred years after the first books were printed in Europe, Basle shared for a time with Venice the first place for scholarly printing. Basle, on the route between north and central Europe and Italy, was a centre of humanism. Erasmus (*c.*1466–1536) had chosen to live there, and in Basle Oporinus was considered second in scholarship only to him. It was a place for Catholics and Protestants alike; Oporinus went so far as to publish the Koran, which, even in tolerant Basle, put him in trouble with the law. What better place to publish an independent-minded work of anatomical research, which the author knew was going to upset many medical, and even some religious, authorities? The risks of publishing in those passionate times are seen in the fate of Servetus, Vesalius' fellow-student under Günther in Paris. The importunate Servetus was burnt at the stake by Calvin in nearby Geneva. In Lyons, the Catholics, unable to apprehend the man, burnt the book he had published along with his effigy.

The *Fabrica* and the *Epitome* were probably issued, as was customary, as unbound sheets. Copies were sometimes packed for distribution, carefully wrapped, into barrels. The works were on sale at the Frankfurt book fair.

The wood-blocks

The wood-blocks for the illustrations were cut for Vesalius in Venice. They represent some of the finest examples ever produced in this medium: in particular the portrait of the author, the title-page, the muscle-men and skeletons, and, in the *Epitome*, the male and female nudes, are rightly admired. The blocks were *cut* along the grain on the plane surface of the wood, probably pear-wood. (It was not until the end of the eighteenth century that Thomas Bewick in England perfected the technique of *engraving* with a burin on the end-grain of boxwood.) Vesalius complained of the expense of employing the Venetian artisans to cut the blocks. These blocks, more than two hundred of them, some as large as 35 × 24 cm, were sent over the mountains to Basle in the care of merchants. They were used in the production of the 1543 edition and again, with some careful re-cutting, in the 1555 edition; they then started on a journey which was to end centuries later in Munich, where all but a few were discovered in the University library. In 1934, as a co-operative venture between the New York Academy of Medicine, the University of Munich, and a printer, Dr Willy Wiegand, impressions of the blocks of the *Fabrica* and *Epitome* were again taken, using modern paper and the most careful techniques. These were published as *Icones anatomicae* (*Fig. 5.4*). After four hundred years the blocks showed little deterioration, and produced finer impressions than even those of Oporinus. Some of our plates are taken from this publication rather than the *Fabrica* itself. The wood had probably been soaked originally in hot linseed oil before being used, and this allowed fine cuts to be made and also preserved them through the centuries. The history of the blocks has a sad ending, for they were destroyed during the bombing of Munich in the Second World War.

ANDREAE
VESALII
BRUXELLENSIS
ICONES
ANATOMICAE
—
EDIDERUNT ACADEMIA
MEDICINAE NOVA-EBORA·
CENSIS ET BIBLIOTHECA
UNIVERSITATIS MONACENSIS
MCMXXXIV

5.4   The title-page of the *Icones anatomicae*, 1934.

In addition to the anatomical illustrations in the *Fabrica* there are woodcut pictorial initial letters to the various books and sections of the work, four larger initial (7.5 cm square) and seventeen smaller (3.25 cm square). The subjects are mostly connected with anatomy or surgery. The anatomists and surgeons, preparing skeletons, removing a corpse from a gibbet or grave-robbing, dissecting a pig and so on, are not men but cherubs or *putti*—plump male infants who go about their gruesome tasks with glee, and so lend elements of macabre humour and pathos to the inevitably heavy text (*Fig. 5.5a and b*).

The artists of the Fabrica

An obvious question concerns the identity of the artist or artists who drew the illustrations that were copied so well by the cutters. (The actual illustration was often pasted on the block, which was then cut with a knife through the paper.) The question has been discussed frequently through the centuries, but without resolution. What is probable is that they show the influence of Tiziano Vecelli (*c*.1485–1576), called Titian. This might be expected, since Titian and his school were the dominant influence in Venice at the time Vesalius was living in Padua. The

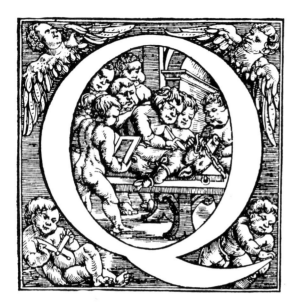

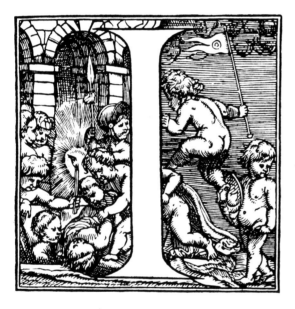

5.5a and b   Two initial letters from the 1543 *Fabrica*. The letter Q shows a dissection of a pig in progress: one *putto* is reading, most probably, the works of 'Copho'. The letter I shows a recently interred corpse being 'resurrected' at night by candlelight; a soldier-*putto* stands by, wearing a helmet and carrying a spear.

fine quality of some illustrations makes it not improbable that Titian himself actually drew some of them. Or did Titian's influence show through his pupil, Joannes Stephanus of Calcar, who as we have seen drew three of the six illustrations of the *Tabulae*? Vesalius had written of a possible collaboration with his fellow-countryman on a major work of anatomy. Calcar was said by his friend Vasari to have so absorbed Titian's vision that his paintings showed no trace of his Flemish origins. Moreover, the technique of shading of the title-page of the *Fabrica* is similar to that of the skeletal pictures of the *Tabulae*, undoubtedly by Calcar. However the draughtsmanship of the 1543 skeletons may be seen to be so much better than that of the 1538 figures that there must have been a most remarkable improvement in Calcar's technique if he had been responsible for both.

Did more than one artist contribute to the illustrations? That is likely, since inconsistent competence can be seen, especially in smaller illustrations. Possibly even Vesalius himself contributed some figures; John Caius, who knew him well when at Padua, said that Vesalius wrote *and* illustrated the *Fabrica*. What is certain is that in these two books there are a series of remarkable anatomical illustrations from the sixteenth-century Venetian school. We cannot, however, in respect to any plate, identify the artist with certainty.

The cultural influences shaping the illustrations in the *Fabrica* and the *Epitome* are complex. Many are in a contemporary mannerist style, in that they call attention to themselves by exaggerated poses and dramatic drawing (*Plate 33*). Others relate to the study of classical sculpture in Florence, Rome, and elsewhere in Italy—directly, as in the nudes of the *Epitome* (*Figs 5.2a and b*) and in the torso figures (*Fig. 5.6*), and less directly, as derived from naturalistic representation in the round of the human figure first seen in late-fifteenth-century sculpture, and later shown by academic models of flayed men—the *écorchés* (*Plate 31*). The Vesalian woodcuts were made in the 1540s in Venice, where, by this time, the work of northern European artists in this medium was known and assimilated.

An interesting secondary matter concerns the background to the muscle-men. When reverse prints of these plates are assembled in the order the muscle-men appear in the book, the landscapes form two continuous panoramas, one for the frontal views another for the series illustrating the muscles of the back. The landscape drawings were divided into fourteen parts, and the designs incorporated on to the wood-blocks after the figures of the muscle-men had been cut. The landscape drawing is in the style of Domenico Campagnola, another pupil of Titian; the treatment of the foliage of the trees, for example, is quite similar to that in signed woodcuts by Campagnola.

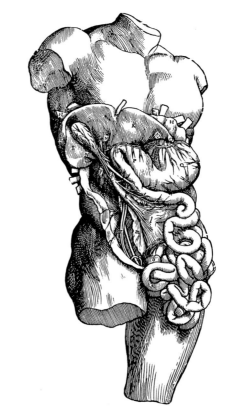

5.6 The viscera of the body shown within a classical torso, from the woodcut in Vesalius' *Fabrica*, 1555.

In the series of fourteen large plates of the muscles, the standing figures are on rocky ground some way out of a small city; there are also farmyards and ruins, and a quiet river winds through the town and the serene countryside. It is as if the men have removed themselves from society to be alone in their personal tragedies. The logical absurdity, even to the point of embarrassed laughter, of dissected men standing in such situations is diminished by the intense personal drama of the drawing and of the attitude of the figures, and, often, by the agony of expression. The theatricality of these plates calls to mind the characters of the most terrifying of the ancient Greek plays—these men are mutilated, maybe even self-mutilated, by events in the same way as Oedipus. Or, to look forward in time a further generation, one thinks of the tragedies of Shakespeare, and not only because of the plate where a skeleton contemplates, Hamlet-like, a skull taken from its burial place (*Plate 29*).

For four hundred years, people shown these plates for the first time have been immediately conscious of the drama, either turning away or looking more intently, as a spectator may at a violent, climactic moment in a play. It is not possible, even for anatomically-knowledgeable people, to stay indifferent; even they are caught in the tragedy, and, before reason reasserts itself, have identified themselves with the characters. This is a great achievement, for these drawings are not 'fine art', but useful, applied art. What seem at first glance to be drawings of feeling alone are instead instructional pieces, carefully arranged to show as much of the human anatomy to the scholar and the student.

Geminus' copies of the Vesalian illustrations

In the introduction to his brother's *Epistola ... radicis Chynae ...*, Basle, [Oporinus], 1546 ('China root letter', that is, 'Letter on Ginseng'), Franciscus Vesalius had written:

Would that the books of the *Fabrica* with its *Epitome* had not been so shamefully and wholly spoiled by a certain Englishman—who had even, I believe, at one time lived with my brother. He added to the *Epitome* certain parts borrowed from [the Fabrica] and so completely spoiled that which had first caused it to be so much admired.

The culprit was thought to be the Englishman, John Caius, who indeed had shared lodgings with Andreas Vesalius in Padua; but Franciscus was mistaken. The guilty publication was Thomas Geminus' *Compendiosa totius anatomie delineatio ...*, London, [John Herford], 1545. It contained most of the illustrations in the *Fabrica*, together with the Adam and Eve figures of the *Epitome*, the smaller figures assembled in groups—the larger occupying, as in the *Fabrica*, a whole page. Only two figures, of nerves and of vessels, had been copied at significantly reduced sizes; they were on folding sheets in the *Fabrica*. Thomas Geminus engraved the figures on copper ('brass'), and they were accompanied by some of the relevant explanations from the *Fabrica* and by the text, slightly modified, of the *Epitome*.

Andreas Vesalius, in the body of the same *China root letter*, repeated his brother's complaint:

Just now in England ... the illustrations of my *Epitome* have been copied so poorly and without artistic skill—although not without expense for whoever must bear it—that I should be ashamed if anyone were to believe me responsible for them.

... everything has been shamefully reduced—although figures of this sort can never be exhibited large enough. [Translations from O'Malley 1964].

The two brothers had, it is plain, not actually seen Geminus' work, for the illustrations, from the *Fabrica*, are remarkably fine copies of those of Vesalius. The background landscapes have been simplified into a few rocks and tufts of grass, and a few figures have been reversed; but these anatomical figures have been engraved with accuracy and clarity, the lettering particularly standing out well in this finer medium.

Thomas Geminus was a 'stranger', a foreigner, perhaps a religious refugee, from the country north of Liège in Flanders. In his will, he names himself 'Thomas Lambrit, alias Geminy', the latter indicating that he was a twin; a brother, possibly his twin brother, Jasper, was his executor. (Both Lambert and Geminus had many alternative spellings in those days of uncertain orthography.) The quality of Geminus' engraving far outstripped previous print-work done in England. Perhaps from the experience of working on the Vesalian figures, he set himself up in medical practice. Two years after the *Compendiosa* was published, Geminus is referred to as a surgeon; he worked as such until about 1555, when the College of Physicians 'examined and penalized' him for practising without a licence from them. But he had other work: as an engraver, as we have seen; as a maker of astrolabes and other scientific instruments; and as a printer and publisher.

Five years before the *Compendiosa* was first printed, anatomy had become an important subject in plans supported by the Crown to further good surgical practice. Henry VIII had, in 1540, given assent to an Act uniting Barbers and Surgeons into one Company, and in this same year another Act authorized the supply of four corpses of executed felons to be available to them for dissection (*Fig. 5.7*). The *Compendiosa* was a text for such studies. It was dedicated to the king, who was said to have suggested that the Vesalian plates should be made available to English surgeons. There is a fine portrait of Henry in the book. The work sold well, being 'notably well accepted and hath dooen muche good in Italye, Fraunce, Spayne, Germaine, and other foren parties'. It was soon realized that it would be even more useful, and profitable, if it were translated into English: the work 'set foorth in the Englishe tounge might greatly avail to ye knowlage of the unlatined surgeons ... [and] bee muche more beneficiall, then in latin ...'. An excellent translation was prepared by Nicholas Udall, Headmaster of Eton and author of the pioneer comic drama, *Ralph Roister Doister*. In his prefatory remarks, Udall addresses the surgeons of England 'for whose ease and profitable instruccion this present weorke is sette foorth'. The publication, also called *Compendiosa . . .*, London, Nicholas Hyll for Thomas Geminus, 1553, was again dedicated to the monarch, now Edward VI. The text was modified, and included a *Treatyse* on anatomy, taken from a number of sources, principally Thomas Vicary's *Anatomie of mans bodie*, which itself was partly based on a late-fourteenth-century manuscript. The copperplates were reprinted for this edition and for the next one, 1559, dedicated to Queen Elizabeth. (This latter has a fine portrait of the Queen, newly ascended to the throne.) The same plates were acquired by a French medical humanist, Jacques Grévin, in 1560, and taken to Paris by him to be used in his *Anatomes totius . . .*, Paris, André Wechel, 1564 and again 1565. In 1569, this book also was issued in the vernacular: *Les portraicts anatomiques . . .*, but by now the plates were well-worn—copper engravings take far fewer impressions than woodcuts before deteriorating. Grévin's books contain no acknowledgement to Geminus, and neither do re-engravings of these figures published at various places—Nuremberg, Cologne, Amsterdam—during the next hundred years.

In the first Latin edition of Geminus' book, he acknowledges his debt to Andreas Vesalius, but in the English version this has disappeared. Vesalius could not understand or forgive Geminus' plagiarism of a book for which he had worked so hard and for which he had obtained 'privileges'. Even if this form of copyright did not extend to England, had he not said in the

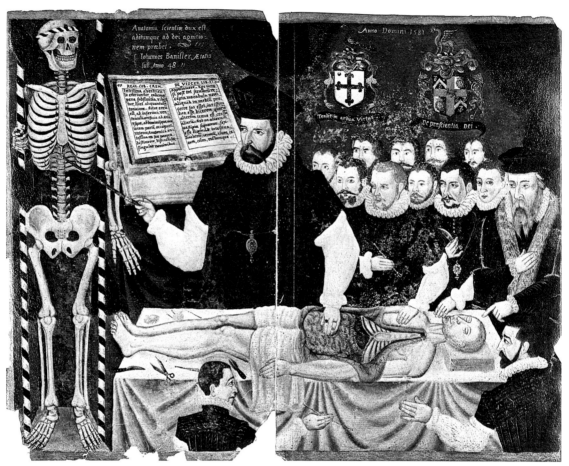

5.7 Dissection scene commemorating lectures by John Banister, 1581, to the *Mystery and Communality of Barbers and Surgeons of London* (Hunterian MS 364, Glasgow University Library).

Fabrica that he would 'provide printers with the illustrations [that is, the blocks themselves] rather than have them copied unskilfully'? One can indeed appreciate Vesalius' viewpoint. These copper engravings were however at least well copied from Vesalius, and served in turn, and again without acknowledgement, to spread anatomical knowledge in England and on the Continent.

Our *Plates 29, 33, and 36* are not taken from the original Vesalian woodcuts, but from Geminus' engraved copies.

Plates 28–38: the Vesalian figures

It is fascinating to imagine the reactions of the 'professors of dissection' if one morning in the late summer of 1543 they arrived to find, out of the blue, a complimentary copy of the *Fabrica* lying on their desks. Would they first tut-tut over the title-page, showing the professor down in the thick of things, or turn to the preface for enlightenment as to the young author's intent? If the latter, what would they make of 'jackdaws', 'everything wrongly taught', 'off-hand and superficial display', 'schools with hardly a thought of dissecting a human body', 'detestable practices', 'purblind old men', and so forth?

Most likely they would thumb through the vast book and perhaps goggle at the unaccustomed illustrations. Some would be excited and stimulated by these, some awed; some would reach for denigratory pens; but none, surely, would remain unmoved. What a revelation they must have been to those accustomed to the illustrations of Fries, Berengario, or Dryander! Canano might sigh for his pre-empted ambitions; Estienne gnash his teeth in frustration at the long hold-up in publication of his own book; Sylvius denounce his former pupil's apostasy; while plagiarists and copyists would probably rub their hands in joyful anticipation.

28 The first skeletal figure from A. Vesalius, *De humani corporis fabrica . . .* [the *Fabrica*], Basle, J. Oporinus, 1543. Woodcut (Cambridge University Library). 35.0 × 20.5 cm.

When viewed from the front an articulated human skeleton usually presents a very 'static' appearance; but the whole-skeleton drawings in the *Fabrica* are dynamic. This one could almost be an X-ray of a weary grave-digger resting on his implement, his weight mainly on the left leg, head tilted argumentatively and left arm thrown expressively outwards. One can almost hear him asking 'Is that deep enough?'—and, from the positioning of the handle of his implement in respect to its blade, one can imagine him fervently hoping to receive an affirmative answer!

So arresting is the immediate visual impact that one is reluctant to cavil at certain anatomical short-comings. These include a too wide and short chest, leaving an over-large gap between the costal margin and the pelvic crest; too long a radius and ulna relative to the humerus (the radius also being rather sinuous), and an unanatomical backward tilt of the pelvis on the vertebral column. A student of anatomy might presume that the breastbone consists of seven portions; in the text, however, Vesalius makes it clear that usually only three are present.

It was the view of Vesalius, as quoted by Saunders and O'Malley (1950), that in the adult the articulated skeleton 'to speak the truth, contributes more to display than to instruction': this plate well epitomizes this sentiment.

HVMANI COR-
SIMVL COMPACTO-
EX FACIE EXPRES.

PORIS OSSIVM
RVM ANTERIORI
SIO.

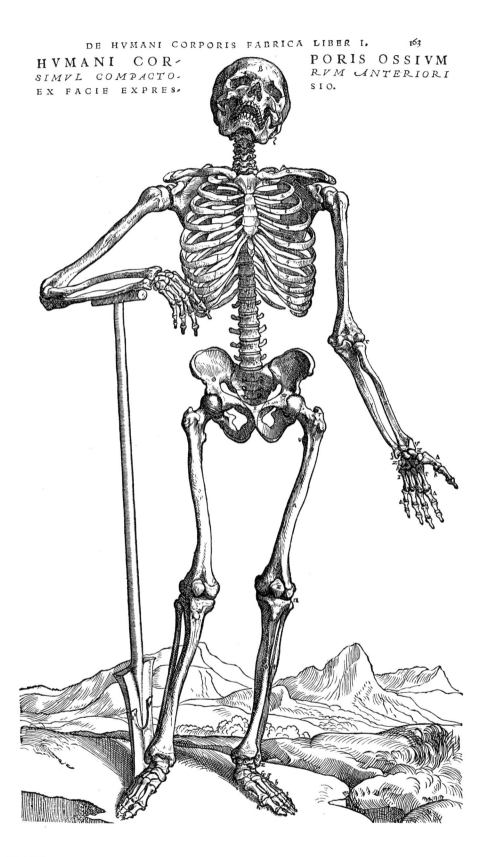

PLATE 28

29 The second skeletal figure (after Vesalius, *Fabrica*, 1543) from T. Geminus, *Compendiosa totius anatomie delineatio ...*, London, J. Herford, 1545. Engraving (Wellcome Institute Library). 39.0 × 26.8 cm.

In this plate Geminus omitted Vesalius' original motto on the front of the plinth—*Vivitur ingenio caetera mortis erunt*. This has been rendered 'genius lives on, all else is mortal'; or, more extravagantly, 'Man's spirit lives; all else Death's hand shall claim'; or even 'It is his genius that yet walks the earth; all else of him may go down into silence'.

This is probably the most reproduced and most famous of all the *Fabrica* drawings.

The cross-legged, contemplative, and Yorick-evocative pose is superb in both concept and draughtsmanship. The side view does, however, reveal the normal anteriorly convex lumbar curve to be non-existent; and the similar cervical curvature is also suspect. Oddly, Vesalius never seemed to appreciate the correct curvatures of the vertebral column, and used a rigid iron bar to support it for the drawings.

The thick, strong spine of the second cervical vertebra is evident, although the spine of the seventh is little different from the other cervical spines, hardly a 'vertebra prominens'. The hip-bones are tilted too far backwards, the pubic symphysis being on the same level as the junction of the third and fourth parts of the sacrum, instead of at the level of the tip of the coccyx. The hyoid bone (H) on the plinth is certainly not human; but it is a tribute to Vesalius' industry that two of the three very small bones of the middle ear, the malleus and incus (the latter name coined by him) appear to the right of the skull. At the time of the *Fabrica* the third and smallest bone, the stapes, was unknown: it has been claimed that it was discovered a few years later by Ingrassia, but he did not publish this fact until 1603. Meantime Gimeno, 1549, and Collardo, 1555, had both described the stapes; the latter it was who gave it its name, from a resemblance to a horse's stirrup.

Vesalius was somewhat of an authority on sesamoid bones, and the two carpal pisiforms are clearly shown, particularly the left. Purists may perhaps consider that the right patella is placed too low, and that on the left too high.

At the distal end of, in particular, the left tibia there is a wavy line presumably demarcating the lower epiphysis of this bone (designated 'malleoli' in the text). This would suggest the age of the skeletal material to be approximately eighteen years. The presence of an upper epiphysis of the right humerus would tend to confirm this age; but there is no evidence of an epiphyseal line at the distal end of the femur, although one such is present at the lower extremity of the right fibula; this latter usually unites with the shaft of the bone a little earlier than do these previously mentioned.

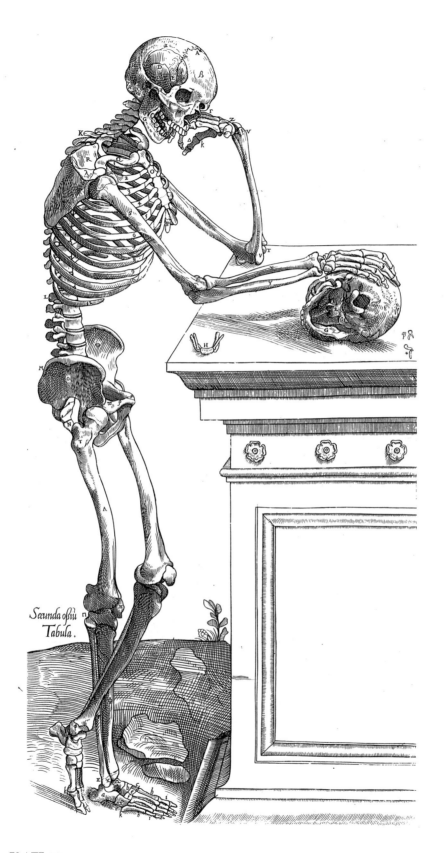

Secunda ossiu
Tabula.

PLATE 29

30 The third skeletal figure from A. Vesalius, *De humani corporis fabrica ...*, Basle, J. Oporinus, 1543. Woodcut (Cambridge University Library). 33.5 × 20.8 cm.

In this bent-over skeleton the sacrum is far from ideal. For illustrations elsewhere in the book, Vesalius used a six-piece rather than a five-piece sacrum. In his text (*Fabrica*, p. 83) he states 'six [bones] constitute the sacral bone', but on the following page 'sometimes it consists of only five bones'. Some five years earlier he had illustrated a five-piece sacrum in the *Tabulae Sex*. In fact, a five-piece sacrum occurs in 80 per cent of skeletons, a six-piece one in only approximately 20 per cent. Some twenty years later, in response to criticism by Falloppio, he correctly pointed out that, although he had previously stated the sacrum to be composed of five pieces, as he had had available a 'beautifully constructed' six-piece sacrum of a middle-aged man, he used this, as being more easily adaptable to Galenic description.

Returning to the figure, the spiral groove of the left humerus, the angulation (though not the actual positioning) of the ribs, and, again, the strength of the spine of the axis are well portrayed. The delineation of the lambdoid suture of the skull indicates that the presence of sutural or Wormian bones was recognized. The scapular spines are poorly drawn; but it is interesting to note the epiphyses of the inferior angles of the scapulae, which again suggest a skeletal age of eighteen years. As this was the same skeleton used for the previous plates it is interesting that the epiphyses noted in those are no longer clearly shown here, though there is a suspicion of epiphyseal lines on the left fibula. There is an awkwardness about the angulation of the neck of the left femur and the articulation of its head with the hip-bone. No Vesalian bone can be seen in the skeleton of the left foot, where it might have been featured.

For a number of reasons, not least the uniform curve of the vertebral column, this is the least felicitous of the three skeletal drawings in the *Fabrica*.

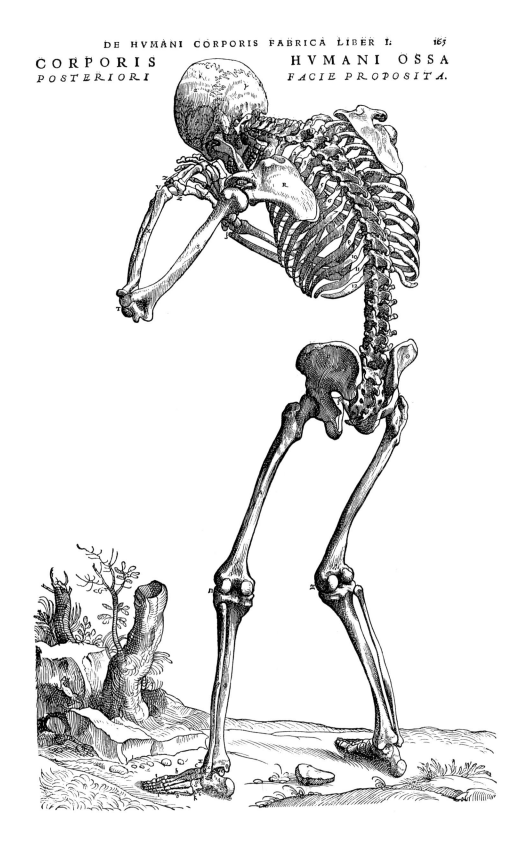

CORPORIS   HVMANI OSSA
POSTERIORI   *FACIE PROPOSITA.*

PLATE 30

31 The first muscle figure from A. Vesalius, *De humani corporis fabrica . . .*, Basle, J. Oporinus, 1543. Woodcut (Cambridge University Library). 35.0 × 21.0 cm.

The *Fabrica* drawings of the muscular system, long referred to as 'muscle-men', are equally esteemed with those of the skeleton, and represent progressively deeper dissections, illustrated first from the front, then from the back. Vesalius emphasized this progressiveness, and exhorted students always to refer to other plates so as to gain a proper appreciation of any particular muscle or muscle group.

Throughout his text Vesalius employs a rather confusing terminology for the muscles, referring to them in terms of their general functional activity: for example, the first, second, third, fourth . . . muscles 'moving the arm' (pectoralis major, deltoid, teres major, latissimus dorsi . . .) or ditto 'moving the thigh' (gluteus maximus, gluteus medius, gluteus minimus, piriformis).

In this plate, the first muscle-man, the skin, superficial blood-vessels, and fascia have been removed, the left inguinal lymph nodes being left intact. The platysma muscle has also been removed with the fascia; but Vesalius illustrates this elsewhere.

Allowing for some anatomical licence, such as the size of the forearm and calf muscles, the general muscle morphology is excellent and accurate. Such muscles as sterno-mastoid (F), sterno-hyoid (C), pectoralis major (L), brachio-radialis (a), tibialis anterior (Z), etc. are easily recognized, although it does appear that the extensor pollicis longus has a shorter tendon on the left thumb than does the brevis!

As Vesalius himself commented, this drawing, showing many muscles which can be identified in the living person, could have been designed as well for the use of artists as for anatomists and physicians. Indeed the oversized limb musculature would seem to lead one almost inevitably to this conclusion.

Errors are conspicuous by their absence, and, quite apart from the remarkably lifelike pose, much else is admirable. The folding of the sternal portion of pectoralis major under its clavicular head is particularly well portrayed, as are the extensor retinaculae (4, 5, and 6) and the crossing of the radial wrist extensors (b) by abductor pollicis longus and extensor pollicis brevis (c). The two extensor tendons to the index finger are clearly seen, as are also the tendons of extensor digitorum brevis (rather more faintly) in the left foot.

The tendinous intersections of the rectus abdominis are more marked, thicker, and more numerous than is usual. The issuance of the spermatic cord (k) through the aponeurosis of the external oblique is placed rather too lateral.

PRIMA
MVSCVLO,
RVM TA-
BVLA.

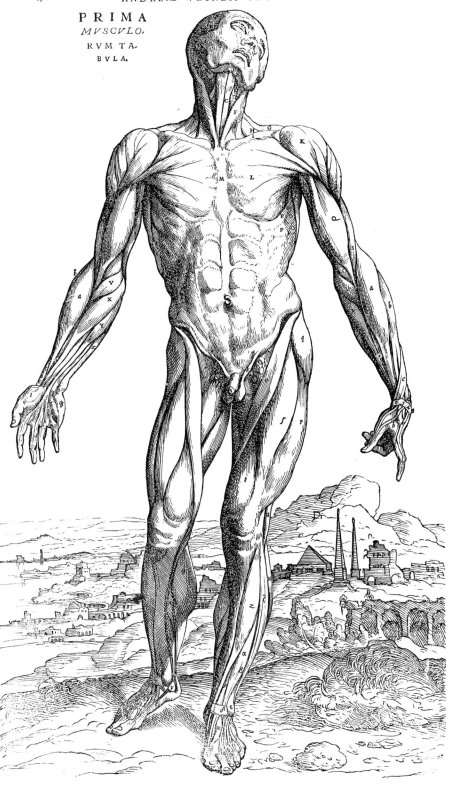

PLATE 31

32 The fifth muscle figure from *Andreae Vesalii Bruxellensis Icones anatomicae,* Munich, University of Munich (Bremer Press) 1934. This was printed from the original wood-blocks used in the 1555 edition of the *Fabrica.* (Private collection.) 33.0 × 20.1 cm.

In this figure, the dissection has progressed so that many previously described muscles are now either removed or turned down from their attachments.

Modern anatomists have been amazed, not to say dismayed, to observe the upward extension of the rectus abdominis muscles almost to the clavicle, and also puzzled by the muscle (X) descending on to the chest wall, deep to the clavicle. Cushing (1962) stated 'it is curious that Vesalius' opponents did not point out the two glaring faults in his own figures where the scaleni muscles run over [*sic*] the clavicle on the chest (p. 184) and the rectus abdominalis reaches to the clavicular level; the description is evidently drawn from the pig'. This seems at first sight a valid criticism, but Vesalius' text makes it clear that, with regard to the rectus muscle, it was illustrated as such to indicate the appearance in lower animals, and in fact the upper limitation of the muscle in man is indicated by a line marked by the letter r. The text also clearly states that the recti are 'inserted wide and fleshy into the cartilage connected to the pectoral [sternum] bone at the side of the xiphoid process'. In any case reference to the preceding drawing shows the recti to be inserted correctly. For an explanation of the peculiar scalene muscles, see comments, *Plate 33*.

The long head of the left biceps appears as if it arises from the head of the humerus. The more superficial forearm muscles of the right arm have been removed, and flexor carpi ulnaris ('ulnae exporrectus') hangs down; flexor digitorum superficialis is well shown, with its tendons on the fingers dividing to allow the deep flexor tendons to pass through them. In the right leg the rectus femoris has been detached from its origin and hangs downwards, together with sartorius ('the second muscle moving the tibia'), similarly treated, just lateral to it. The extensor digitorum longus has also been detached from its origin, and lies on the ground, revealing the small extensor digitorum brevis. The extensor hallucis longus is intact (joined by the brevis tendon), but is better seen in the left leg. Lateral to the rectus abdominis is the transversus abdominis muscle (Y), with the cut spermatic cord 'piercing' it. The 'sheet' over the right loin and buttock is the internal oblique cut away and allowed to fall downwards and outwards.

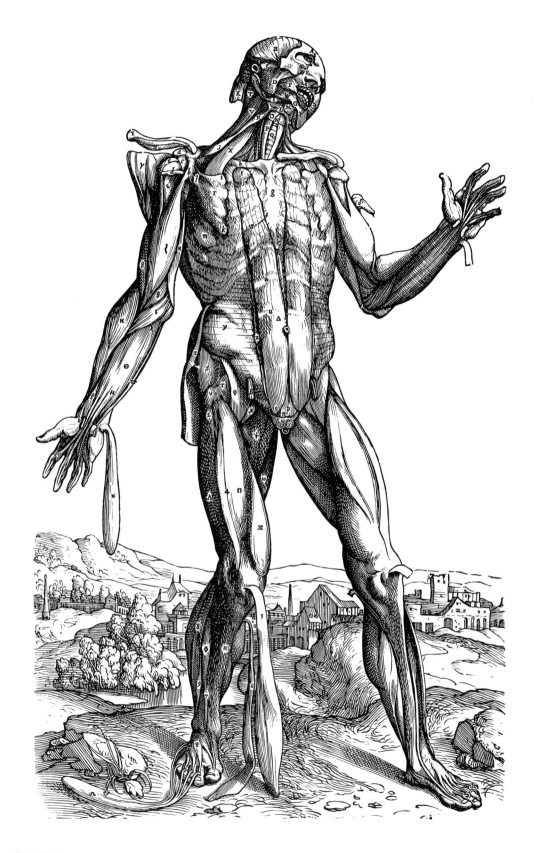

PLATE 32

33 The sixth muscle figure (after Vesalius, *Fabrica*, 1543) from T. Geminus, *Compendiosa totius anatomie delineatio ...*, London, J. Herford, 1545. Engraving (Wellcome Institute Library). 33.6 × 20.5 cm.

In this sixth muscle-man, the mandible is divided in the mid-line and turned to either side to reveal the two medial pterygoid muscles, together with the tongue and tonsils (F). On the left side the anterior belly of the digastric (I) has been detached from the mandible and left dependent.

The puzzling scalene muscles are here shown even more blatantly than in the previous plate. It is perplexing why they were included—they do not figure, for instance, in any of the muscle drawings in the *Epitome*. When one considers the time and effort spent in preparing the material, the artistry of the illustrators and blockmakers, and the skill and care of the printer of such a work as the *Fabrica* (and, in this instance, of the *Compendiosa ...*) one is led inescapably to the conclusion that Vesalius intended his book to be a lasting monument of his work. Yet he states, in the explanation to this plate, that, on consideration, he thought it a good opportunity 'to show this muscle of a dog, of which Galen speaks, arising from the transverse processes of the cervical vertebrae, marked O, having a fleshy belly extending to the fourth rib, where it is marked P, ending rather lower on certain ribs by a thin membranous tendon'. To go to the trouble of so portraying these muscles just to make a point of Galenic animal anatomy seems extremely odd, not to say inexplicable.

Apart from the 'bagginess' of the calf musculature and the extremely miserable gluteus minimus (V) the rest are pleasingly drawn. Although the lumbrical muscles of the hand were known to and described by Vesalius in the text they are not shown here, even though the deep flexor tendons, from which they arise, can clearly be seen.

Although the intersections in the down-turned rectus abdominis muscle are once again more prominent than one would expect to see on its posterior aspect, it is interesting to find the superior and inferior epigastric vessels depicted. These are almost the only blood-vessels shown in the muscle-men illustrations, save for the inferior phrenic shown in the next plate (*Plate 34*).

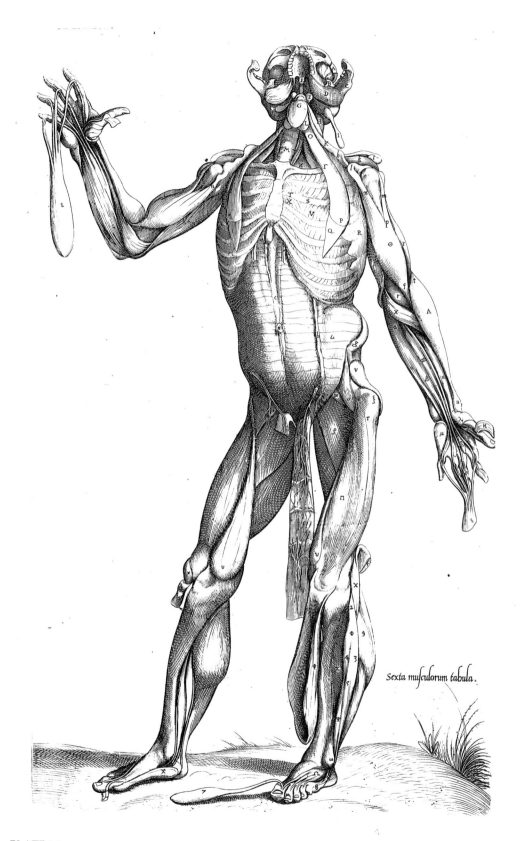

Sexta musculorum tabula.

PLATE 33

34 The seventh muscle figure from *Andreae Vesalii Bruxellensis Icones anatomicae,* Munich, University of Munich (Bremer Press), 1934. This was printed from the original wood-blocks used in the 1555 edition of the *Fabrica.* (Private collection). 33.3 × 20.0 cm.

Here the cadaver has been eviscerated and suspended in a rather grotesque manner. The diaphragm, together with its poorly portrayed crura, central tendon,. and apertures for the inferior vena cava and oesophagus, is shown separately. In the main figure the inferior phrenic arteries arising from the cut aorta, together with the veins entering the inferior vena cava, are seen.

The posterior abdominal wall muscles psoas major and quadratus lumborum are shown, together with, rather poorly, the iliacus.

The thigh musculature has pectineus ('the eighth muscle moving the femurs') appearing much too large.

The pronator teres (Q) and quadratus muscles are the only two forearm muscles left in place; it must be said that the small muscles of the thumb are confusing, probably because their attachments and functions were poorly understood by Vesalius.

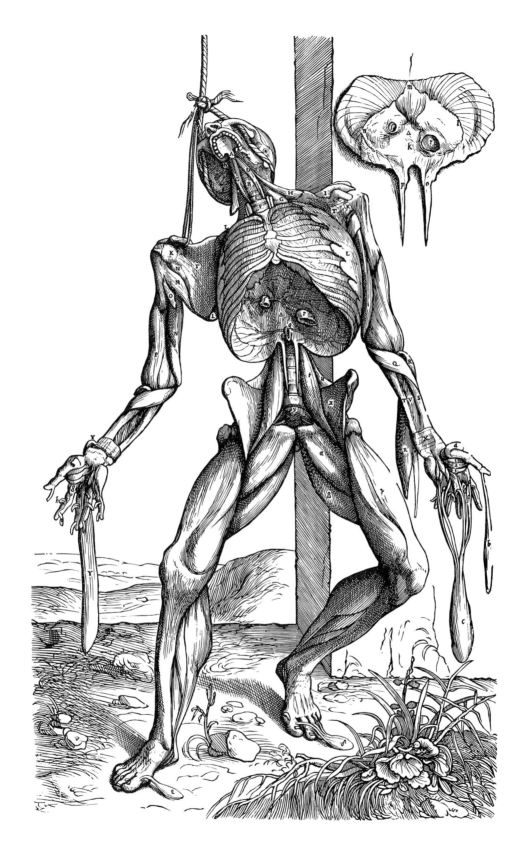

PLATE 34

35 The vein figure from A. Vesalius, *De humani corporis fabrica ...*, Basle, J. Oporinus, 1543. Woodcut (Cambridge University Library). 35.0 × 19.5 cm.

This is the vein-plate from Book III of the *Fabrica*. Because of the then prevalent practice of blood-letting as a therapeutic tool it is not surprising that this drawing of the venous system is so much more detailed than that of the arterial system, which appears twenty-seven pages later. It also possesses twice as many pages of annotations.

As mentioned earlier, a number of errors have been carried over from the *Tabulae Sex* into this illustration. The superior and inferior venae cavae are again shown as a single trunk; this because the right atrium was considered a part of the caval system, and not a heart chamber in its own right. The oval opening seen to the left of (E) thus represents the right atrio-ventricular orifice. The vein indicated at (E) ('like a crown embracing the root of the heart') passes to the left to become continuous with a 'hatched' vein which appears to enter the caval trunk posterior to the atrio-ventricular orifice. The latter portion, at least, represents the coronary sinus; in the explanatory text the reader is referred to a later drawing of the heart (Book VI, Figure 7) where the opening of what is certainly the coronary sinus is seen. The anterior portion of vein (E) is probably an anterior cardiac vein.

The upper limb veins are basically accurate, but those of the root of the neck are not. The cephalic vein (a) joins the external jugular (T) (drawn larger than the internal jugular) instead of the axillary vein (m); and the configuration of the brachiocephalic veins is that obtaining in lower animals. Significantly, (H) is described in the text as the place where butchers stick their knives when slaughtering cows and pigs.

Although unlabelled, the superior sagittal, lateral, and sigmoid cranial sinuses are recognizable, as are the vertebral veins, though the actual arrangement of these vessels is somewhat erroneous, to say the least.

In the lower limb the short saphenous vein (15) is displaced laterally, and the tibial veins and tributaries are very large. The long saphenous vein is correctly shown entering the femoral vein, and the profunda femoris vein is well portrayed.

The right renal vein enters the inferior vena cava slightly superior to that of the left. The right and left testicular veins correctly drain into the inferior vena cava and left renal vein respectively. The internal iliac veins are mainly formed by an unduly prominent gluteal vein, and what, from the description ('passing through the foramen of the pubic bone'), would seem to represent a very large obturator vein. The veins draining the pelvic structures are very inconspicuous. The azygos (F, 'vein lacking a mate') is far too large; but the inferior and superior epigastric veins, and the continuance of the latter as the internal thoracic, are particularly well portrayed.

This plate, when compared with that from the earlier *Tabulae Sex*, well exemplifies the quantum leap from diagrammatic stylization of the venous system to a more factual topographical presentation.

INTEGRA ET   A B OMNIBVS
PARTIBVS   *LIBERA AC*
nuda uenæ   *cauæ delineatio.*

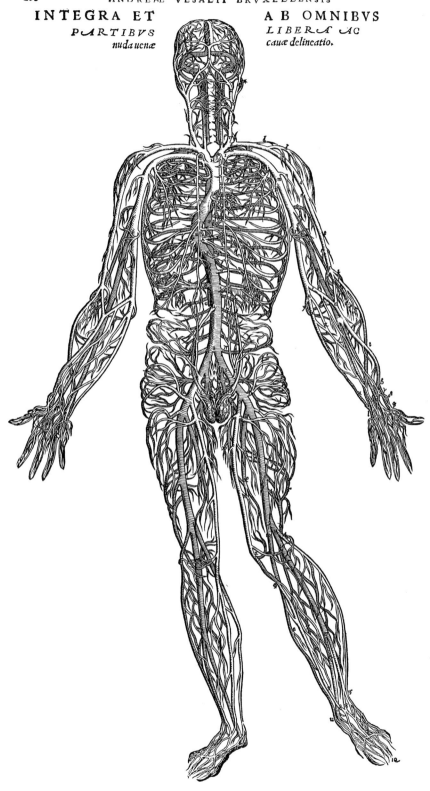

PLATE 35

36 Dissection of the brain on the second page of figures of the head (after A. Vesalius, *Fabrica*, 1543) from T. Geminus, *Compendiosa totius anatomie delineatio . . .*, London, J. Herford, 1545. Engraving (Wellcome Institute Library). 33.0 × 22.5 cm.

This brings together, in a single plate, four illustrations from Book VII of Vesalius' *Fabrica*, namely figures three, four, thirteen, and fourteen (the small centre drawing originally formed part of the fourth figure). They retain their *Fabrica* numbering, though Geminus chose to employ Roman numerals for the lower two drawings, which were labelled 'decima tertia' and 'decima quarta' in the *Fabrica*.

In the upper left drawing the arachnoid and dura (O and P) are shown turned down. The falx cerebri (D) lies over the retracted left hemisphere, but the superior sagittal sinus is not seen: (F) identifies the inferior sagittal sinus. The corpus callosum (L) is visible at the bottom of the cleft between the two hemispheres, with, posteriorly, the great cerebral vein of Galen.

The upper right drawing contains the choroid plexus ('plexus reteformis, O'), the caudate nucleus (indicated by the lower (L,M), though in the annotation these letters denote the lateral brain ventricles themselves), and a somewhat crudely portrayed corpus callosum (I), described in the English edition of Geminus as the 'harde bodye of the brayne'.

The lower left figure (XIII) shows the frontal lobes pulled backwards, together with the olfactory tracts (L). Also seen are branches of the internal carotid arteries and the optic nerves (O,N—'the sinowes of sight'). Anterior to the optic chiasm is a structure labelled (S)—'a portion of the basyne whiche receaveth the flegme from the brayn'—which in spite of its indicated position must be presumed to represent the pituitary fossa. This is also seen (CC) in XIIII, with (D) being the infundibulum, 'whiche bryngeth downe the flegmatyke humoure of the brayne'.

The middle meningeal vessels (K) are seen to advantage on the left in XIII, though the identity of the structure labelled (I)—'whiche vessell runneth furth into the thynne pannicle [arachnoid] of the brayne'—remains in doubt.

In Figure XIIII (G) presumably denotes the oculomotor nerve, but the other nerves featured really cannot be correlated with present-day cranial nerves, even when Vesalius' numeration, or pairing, of these is taken into account.

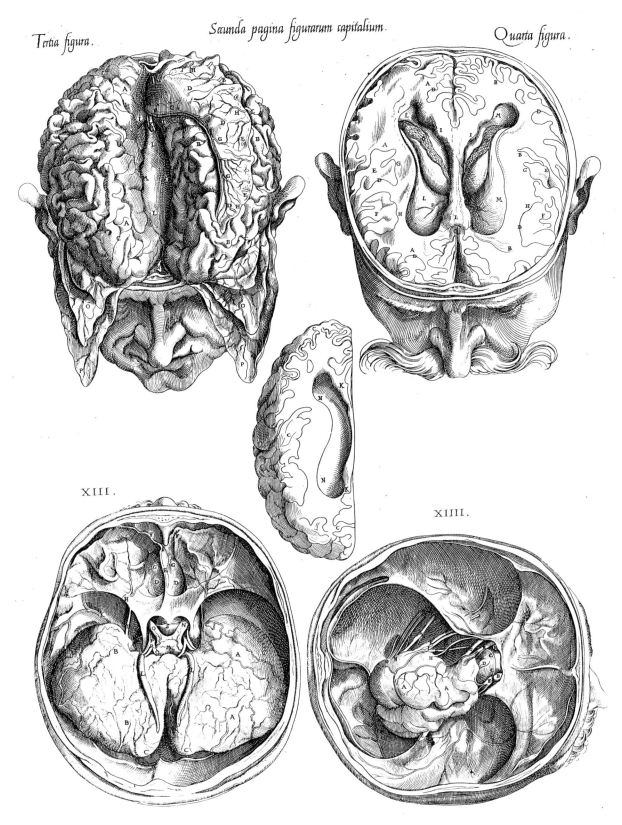

Tertia figura.

Quarta figura.

XIII.

XIIII.

PLATE 36

37 The fourth muscle figure from A. Vesalius, *De humani corporis fabrica librorum epitome* [the *Epitome*], Basle, J. Oporinus, 1543. Woodcut (Yale University Library). 41.4 × 21.5 cm.

To paraphrase Vesalius' introductory description, this fourth muscle figure, from the *Epitome*, illustrates those muscles of the back of the body that were hidden on the left side of the second muscle figure: here the muscles of the right side are superficial to the few shown on the left, which include those of the calf and foot, seen lying on the ground.

The horizontal sections show the brain in progressive dissections; they are derived from drawings in the *Fabrica*, but have different lettering.

The muscles of the right back include ilio-costalis (R), longissimus (S and P), probably semispinalis capitis (M), and cervicis (N), and levator scapulae (V). What the muscle (O) is meant to represent is obscure; it is annotated as part of what is now the semispinalis, but, if so, is situated too lateral.

The triceps (l, m, n, o) and supinator (r) are the only muscles of the upper limb.

Gluteus minimus and obturator internus with its gemelli can be seen in the right buttock region, as also quadratus femoris, part of adductor magnus, semi-membranosus, and vastus lateralis (biceps femoris has been removed) in the thigh.

The 'bag' of muscles hanging down from the left greater trochanter are the obturator internus and gemelli. In the left leg are seen tibialis posterior (r) and the peronei, together with flexor hallucis longus (z), flexor digitorum longus (y), and flexor digitorum brevis (x), reflected from their origins; also portrayed is what may best be described as a *mélange* of small muscles of the sole of the foot. In the (separate) right sole are seen the tendons of flexor hallucis longus, flexor digitorum longus, and, cut short, flexor digitorum brevis.

QVARTA MVSCVLOS COMMONSTRANTIVM FIGVRA, OMNES IN POSTERIO

RI CORPORIS SEDE SVB ILLIS QVI SECVNDAE FIGVRAE SINISTRO LATERE EXPRIMVNTVR
reconditos proponit musculos, dextro quidē latere eos qui primū occur
pes & caput humi collocata pariter iuuant. Tres uerò in hac figura
sequuntur, ac harum prima in integri hominis consistens capite, sinistro
dextra manu hic cōtinetur: illa quae sinistra complectitur, ultimū locum

runt, sinistro autē qui sub ipsis adhuc cōduntur, quibus ostendendis
conspicuae cerebri partium imagines inuicē sectionis ordine sub
lateri secundae figurae capitis succedit, primam autem excipit quae
sibi uendicante.

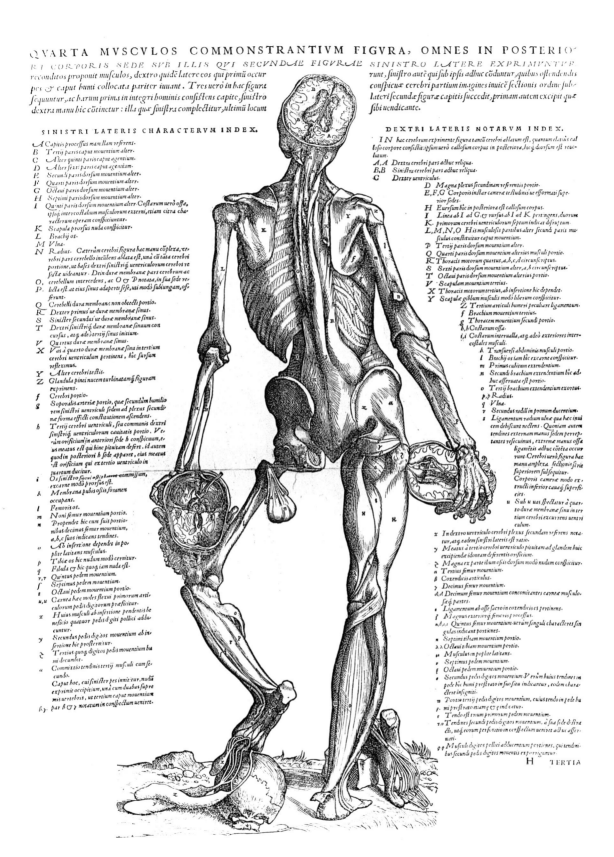

SINISTRI LATERIS CHARACTERVM INDEX.

A Capitis processus mamillam referens.
B Tertij paris caput mouentium alter.
C Alter quinti paris caput agentium.
D Alter sexti paris caput agentium.
E Secundi paris dorsum mouentium alter.
F Quarti paris dorsum mouentium alter.
G Octaui paris dorsum mouentium alter.
H Septimi paris dorsum mouentium alter.
I Quinti paris dorsum mouentium alter. Costarum uerò ossa,
ipsiq́ intercostalium musculorum externi, etiam citra cha
racterum operam conspiciuntur.
K Scapula prorsus nuda conspicitur.
L Brachij os.
M Vlna.
N Radius. Caeterum cerebri figura hac manu cōplexa, ce
rebri pars cerebello incūbens ablata est, una cū tata cerebri
portione, ut bases dextri sinistriq́ uentriculorum cerebri re
sectae uideantur. Dein durae membranae pars cerebrum ac
O, cerebellum intercedens, ac O & P notata, in sua sede re
P. lella est. at eius sinus adaperti sese, uti modò subiungam, of
ferunt.
Q Cerebelli durae membranae non obiecti portio.
R Dexter primus ue durae membranae sinus.
S Sinister secundus ue durae membranae sinus.
T Dextri sinistriq́ durae membranae sinuum con
cursus, atq́ adeò tertij sinus initium.
V Quartus durae membranae sinus.
X Vas à quarto durae membranae sinu in tertium
cerebri uentriculum pertinens, hic sursum
reflexium.
Y Alter cerebri testis.
Z Glandula pinei nucem turbinatamq́ figuram
exprimens.
f Cerebri portio.
g Soporalis arteriae portio, quae secundum humilio
rem sinistri uentriculi sedem ad plexum secundi
nae forma effecti constitutionem ascendens.
h Tertij cerebri uentriculi, seu communis dextri
sinistriq́ uentriculorum cauitatis portio. Ve
rùm orificium in anteriori sede conspicuum, e
ius meatus est qui hinc pituitam deferit. id unum
quod in posteriori hac sede apparet, eius meatus
est orificium qui ex tertio uentriculo in
quartum ducitur.
i Os sinistro sacri ossis latere commissum,
excarne modò prorsus est.
k Membrana pubis ossis foramen
occupans.
l Femoris os.
m Noni femur mouentium portio.
n Propendet hic cum suis portio
nibus decimus femur mouentium,
a, b, c suos indicans tendines.
o Ab insertione dependet in po
plite latitans musculus.
p Tibiae os hic nudum modò cernitur.
q Fibula & hic quoq́ iam nuda est.
r,r Quintus pedem mouentium.
s Septimus pedem mouentium.
t Octaui pedem mouentium portio.
u,u Carnea haec moles flexui primorum arti
culorum pedis digitorum praeficitur.
x Huius musculi ad insertione pendentis be
neficio quatuor pedis digiti pollici adducuntur.
y Secundus pedis digitos mouentium ab in
sertione hic proferuntur.
ʒ Tertius quoq́ digitos pedis mouentium hu
mi decumbet.
a Commixtio tendinis tertij musculi cum secundo.
Caput hoc, cui sinister pes innititur, nudū
exprimit occipitium, una cum duabus supre
mis uertebris, ut tertium caput mouentium
ß.γ par ß & γ notatum in conspectum ueniret.

DEXTRI LATERIS NOTARVM INDEX.

IN hac cerebrum exprimente figura tantù cerebri ablatum est, quantum elatius cal
loso corpore consistit: ipsum uerò callosum corpus in posteriora, hicq́ deorsum est reuc
luum.
A,A Dextra cerebri pars adhuc reliqua.
B,B Sinistra cerebri pars adhuc reliqua.
C Dexter uentriculus.
D Magna plexus secundam referentis portio.
E,F,G Corporis instar camerae testudinis ue efformati supe
rior sedes.
H Euersum hic in posteriora est callosum corpus.
I Linea ab I ad G, rursus ab I ad K pertingens, duorum
K primorum cerebri uentriculorum septum indicat disiunctum.
L,M,N,O H is musculosis partibus alter secundi paris mu
sculi constituitur caput mouentium.
P Tertij paris dorsum mouentium alter.
Q Quarti paris dorsum mouentium alterius musculi portio.
R Thoracis motorum quartus, a,b,c,d circunscriptus.
S Sexti paris dorsum mouentium alter, a,b circunscriptus.
T Octaui paris dorsum mouentium alterius portio.
V Scapulam mouentium tertius.
X Thoracis motorum tertius, ab insertione hic dependet.
Y Scapulae gibbum musculis modò liberum conspicitur.
Z Tertium articuli humeri peculiare ligamentum.
f Brachium mouentium tertius.
g Thoracem mouentium secundi portio.
h,h Costarum ossa.
i,i Costarum interualla, atq́ adeò exteriores inter
costales musculi.
k Transuersi abdominis musculi portio.
l Brachij os iam hic excarne conspicitur.
m Primus cubitum extendentium.
n Secundus brachium extendentium hic adhuc asseruata est portio.
o Tertij brachium extendentium exortus.
p,p Radius.
q Vlna.
r Secundus radij in pronum ducentium.
s Ligamentum radium ulnae qua haec inui
cem dehiscunt nectens. Quoniam autem
tendines externam manus sedem percep
tantes resecuimus, extremae manus ossa
ligametis adhuc cōtēta occur
runt. Cerebri uerò figura hac
manu amplexa, sectionis serie
superiorem subsequitur.
Corporis camerae modo ex
tructi inferior cauaq́ superfi
cies.
u Sub u uas spectatur à quar
to durae membranae sinu in ter
tium excurrens uentri
culum.
x In dextro uentriculo cerebri plexus secundam referens nota
tur, atq́ eadem sinistri lateris est ratio.
y Meatus à tertio cerebri uentriculo pituitam ad glandem huic
excipiendae idoneam deferentis orificium.
ʒ Magna ex parte ilium ossis dorsum modò nudum conspicitur.
α Tertius femur mouentium.
β Coxendicis articulus.
γ Decimum femur mouentium.
d,d Decimum femur mouentium concomitantes carneae musculo
saeq́ partes.
ε Ligamentum ab osse sacro in coxendicis es pertinens.
ζ Magnus exterioris femoris processus.
η,θ,ι Quintus femur mouentium ut eum singuli characteres sin
gulas indicant portiones.
λ Septimi tibiam mouentium portio.
λ,λ Octaui tibiam mouentium portio.
μ Musculus in poplite latitans.
ν Septimus pedem mouentium.
ξ Octaui pedem mouentium portio.
ο Secundus pedis digitos mouentium. Verùm huius tendines in
pede hic humi prostrato in suo situ indicantur, eodem chara
ctere insigniti.
π Portio tertij pedis digitos mouentium, cuius tendo in pede hu
ρ mi prostrato etiam σ & indicatur.
σ Tendo est trium primorum pedem mouentium.
τ,υ Tendines secundi pedis digitos mouentium, à sua sede distra
cti, utq́ eorum perforatio in conspectum ueniret adhuc asser
uati.
φ,φ Musculi digitos pollici adducentium portiones, qui tendini
bus secundi pedis digitos mouentis exporriguntur.

H TERTIA

PLATE 37

38 Composite male visceral figure from A. Vesalius, *De humani corporis fabrica librorum epitome* [the *Epitome*], Basle, J. Oporinus, 1543. Woodcut (Yale University Library). 44.0 × 23.7 cm.

This plate has a special interest in that the smaller drawings were intended to be cut out and pasted on to the central figure; detailed instructions as to how to proceed were given in the marginal notes. The resulting 'flap-anatomy' sheet was then to be attached to a whole-figure plate of the brain and nervous system, which in the book preceded this particular folio.

There was also another illustration, with the same central figure, but where the male organs were replaced by female ones.

If one follows the instructions (using photocopies from facsimiles, *not* the originals!), it must be admitted that the results are really not very informative. Presumably Vesalius utilized this idea in an endeavour to get as much morphological anatomy as possible into a minimum of plates, quite in keeping with the textual format of the *Epitome*—a masterpiece of condensation of information.

While Vesalius was not the first to employ an overlay or flap technique, his method of setting one up was certainly detailed and complex.

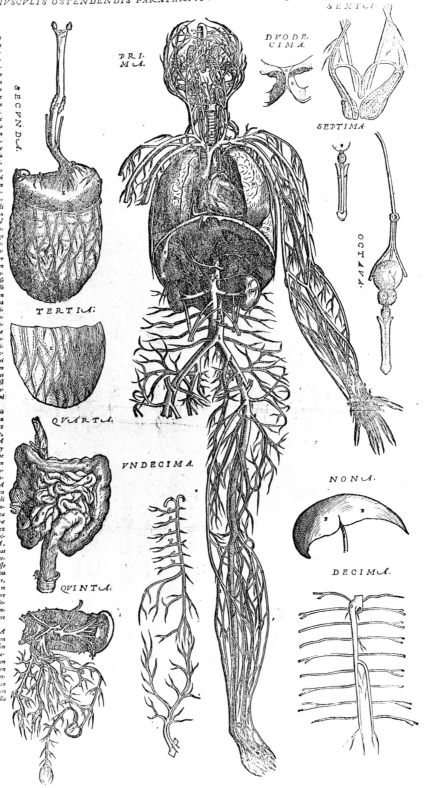

PLATE 38

Printers in Paris: the Estienne family

The earliest printers in Paris were from German-speaking cities and from the Low Countries. Their books were usually printed from Gothic (black-letter) type. Among these printers was Johannes Hygman, who was issuing mathematical and science books in 1492 and, in company with Wolfgang Hopyl, in 1496. The firm continued under a new partner, a French scholar Henri Estienne, whose family name was Latinized as Stephanus. His position was assured by his marriage to Guyone Viart, Hygman's widow. From 1502 to 1520, Estienne published about seven books a year—mathematical, humanist, liturgical, and medical works. When he died in 1520, Guyone Hygman married a third printer, the type-cutter Simon de Colines. It was an honorable custom for widows of printers to marry the partner or foreman of their lately deceased husbands so as to ensure the continuation of the craft. (There is a history yet to be written on women publishers of the first two centuries of printing.) Colines combined another press with that of Estienne, and issued books under his own imprint. After 1525, Robert and François, sons of Henri Estienne, started publishing themselves. Robert married the daughter of a printer of Flemish origins, Josse Bade, one of the early generation of Parisian scholar printers, and so inherited the Bade press. It was a third son, Charles (*c*.1505–64), who wrote a book containing a major series of illustrations to anatomy. This was *De dissectione partium corporis humani ...*, 1545; a translation appeared the next year, *La dissection des parties du corps humain*. The publisher was Simon de Colines: the Estiennes were apparently on good terms with their stepfather, which is seen also by the issue in 1543 of another book by Charles under the joint imprint of Simon de Colines and François Estienne.

The period from Henri Estienne through to the publication of *De dissectione ...* overlaps the reign of François (Francis) I, King of France 1515–47. There has not been a monarch more supportive of printing than Francis. He appreciated the role of the printing presses in their scholarly endeavours, and he brought this appreciation into public policy. Geoffrey Tory, the bookseller, poet, translator, artist, and designer, who had worked with Simon de Colines and Estienne, was appointed the first royal printer; Robert Estienne was the second, publishing material coming from the court and *Parlement*. Francis, as in other things, encouraged his printers to follow Italian models. At his palace at Fontainebleau, his architects grafted Renaissance ideas on Gothic structures; Italian artists, including Leonardo da Vinci and Andrea del Sarto, were brought to France. Domenico del Barbiere, at Fontainebleau after *c*.1537, produced an anatomical copper engraving in a mannerist style, possibly as a model for French painters and sculptors (*Fig. 5.8*). And the models for the printers were equally Italian: the Gothic typeface was for the most part rapidly abandoned—quite unlike the situation in Germany or in England, where Gothic and Roman continued to exist side by side. Particularly remarkable were the roman typefaces by Charles Garamond—faces that determined the direction of much of subsequent printing history. An early model of such founts was that used by Robert Estienne in printing Sylvius' *Isagogae ...* 1531, a Latin–French dictionary that would probably have been known to

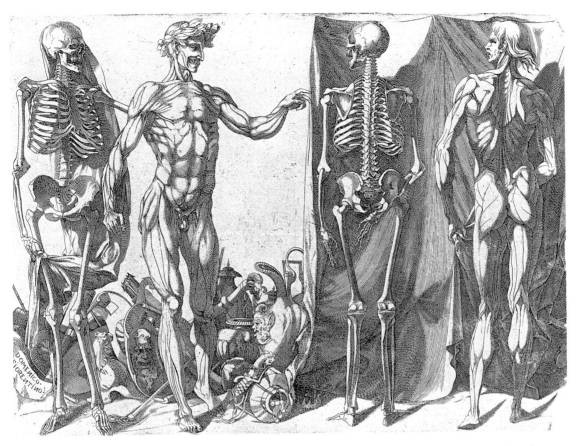

5.8 Two *écorchés* and their skeletons; copper engraving by Domenico del Barbiere. The laurel garland and discarded trophies indicate the vanity of pride.

Vesalius, for he was in Paris shortly thereafter. Simon de Colines followed particularly the example of Aldo Manuzio in printing smaller-format classics, in printing Greek texts, and in the use of italic. (Francis in 1538 ordered that a copy of every work issued in Greek by Estienne should be placed in the royal library; this was a forerunner of the national copyright libraries of the world.) The printers in France of this period, particularly the ones mentioned, were responsible for the form of present-day French orthography through their adoption of the use of accents—though the text of Charles Estienne's *La dissection . . .*, 1546, does not always follow the modern usage in this respect.

During the twenty years or so of his business life Simon de Colines published, on average, more than a book a year of importance in science and technology: many works by Galen; the work of Soranus (the classical writer on obstetrics), and of the thirteenth-century Englishman Roger Bacon; and books by contemporaries on clinical medicine, blood-letting, pharmacy, physiology, veterinary medicine . . . His authors included two of Vesalius' teachers—Jean Fernel and Günther of Andernach; and also a work by Vesalius' tragic fellow student, Michael Servetus.

Illustration in the books of this golden age of French printing also followed Italian models. Simon de Colines in 1526 published for Geoffrey Tory a fine Book of Hours, a devotional work in the tradition of heavily-ornamented manuscript texts, such as that produced for the Duke of Berry. Tory's illustrations to his *Horae* were very much in the style of the *Fasciculo* published in Venice in 1493, or of the Aldine *Hypnerotomachia*, Venice, 1499. (The elaborate borders for Tory's book were derived from manuscript sources; the forms were Italianate.) The ability of the French cutters to produce the delicate lines of these illustrations was such that it has been suggested that some were cut in metal, rather than wood, relief.

Charles Estienne (Carolus Stephanus, c. 1505–1564)

Charles was the third son of Henri and Guyone Estienne. He continued his education in Italy, 1530–4, studying classics at Padua, and becoming interested in botany and medicine. Later in Paris he was a pupil of Sylvius, whose work his brother was publishing. Fellow-students were Vesalius and Servetus. Charles was eventually awarded his medical doctorate in 1542. He was a lecturer in anatomy at the Faculty of Medicine in Paris from 1544 to 1547, and it was during this period that his anatomy book was published. But his literary output was not confined to this subject, for starting in 1535 he had written a series of books, mostly published by his brothers, on agriculture and horticulture—the French version of these, collected together, was *L'agriculture et maison rustique . . .;* he also wrote a glossary of Latin and Greek words for plants, fish, and birds.

In 1546, the date of publication of Estienne's anatomy in French, Martin Luther's final edition of the German-language New Testament was published. And Protestantism was a force not only in the German states but also in France. Robert Estienne, printer to Francis I, considered it wise to leave for Geneva in the period following the death of his Royal patron. The family publishing house was now split in two, with one centre at Geneva under Robert, and another in Paris under Charles, who had to give up medical practice. (François Estienne died in 1550.) The firm continued as printer to the King, and books were issued on a wide range of subjects— for instance, a fine Cicero, 1555, and a guide to the routes of France, a prototype Michelin guide. One book was wisely dedicated to an Inquisitor. But the business fell into debt, and the last years of Charles Estienne's life were spent in prison.

De dissectione . . ., 1545 was translated into French and published as *La dissection des parties du corps humain . . .,* 1546. (It is the latter to which reference is made in the following.)

This folio volume has over four hundred pages, with nearly sixty full-page woodcut illustrations, some repeated; at the end of the volume there are smaller figures of individual muscles, shown, not very helpfully, detached from their origins and insertions. The text was set in a beautiful italic (*Fig. 5.9*), and the volume is as much an exemplar of fine Parisian sixteenth-century printing as was Vesalius' *Fabrica* of the printing at Basle in the same period.

The origins of the book and its illustrations date back at least to 1530, when Estienne was

Le premier liure de Lanatomie,

& diſſection des parties du corps humain.

Proeſme contenant largument de tout loeuure.

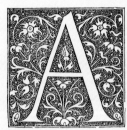

NAXAGORAS, interrogué pour quelle cauſe principalement il penſoit les hommes auoir eſte formez:adonc leuant les yeulx en hault, & monſtrant le ciel au doit, pour cela (dit il) ie croy les hommes eſtre nez en ce monde. Par ceſte parole/a bon droit dung chaſcun priſee/& grandement eſtimee/comme digne de vray Philoſophe: ſembloit attribuer toute excellence & nobleſſe au ciel/auquel ne ſe trouue riens pareil ou ſemblable. Par ce dire/nous eſtimoit auoir eſte eſueillez de la terre/haultz & droitz eſleuez/ a ce que regardans & contemplans ceſte ſi excellente couuerture/peuſſions auoir congnoiſſance de noſtre Dieu:de qui tenons origine / lequel cöme ſouuerain prince de ce monde/tient la hault ſon ſiege:A la cötemplation duquel ont eſte faictz les hommes:non point comme habitas ou heritiers de la terre:mais cöme ſpectateurs des choſes ſuperieures & celeſtes:que nulle aultre choſe animee/ſans luſaige de rayſon peult cöcepuoir ou cöprëdre. Au ciel/eſtimoit Anaxagoras reſider ceſte haulte & diuine nature/embraſſant & cötenant toutes choſes.Du ciel croyoit eſtre produictz les hommes/ & a lutilite diceulx les fruictz & aultres biens de la terre: les ſayſons & changemens de temps:deſquelles toutes choſes produictes/ ont croyſſance/ & paruiennent a maturite. De ce pouuons inferer,noſtre meilleure vacation & ſolicitude/debuoir eſtre/ſoy principalement employer/a linueſtigation des diuins ouuraiges de nature: & aduertir ſongneuſemët/comment du ciel(duquel eſt Dieu le grand prince & gouuerneur)ſont entretenues les choſes terriennes/auſquelles luy ſeul donne nourriture & accroiſſement/& par conſequent defenſe/& tutelle:& ce tout pour lhomme & a la cömodite diceluy. Car tout ainſy(diſoit Chryſippus)que leſtuy eſt faict pour le bouclier/& le fourreau a cauſe de leſpee: auſſy toutes les choſes de ce monde fault eſtimer auoir eſte faictes pour lhomme : les fruictz / pour la vie diceluy:les cheuaulx/pour le porter:les beufz/ pour luy labourer la terre: les chiens/pour le garder/& luy chercher proye: les porcz & poyſſons/ pour ſon manger : les ouailles/ affin que de leur lene taincte & accouſtree/ il ſen puiſſe veſtir & couurir. Mais luy,ſans doubte, a eſte faict pour la contemplation de ſon formateur:& pour imiter Dieu en tout:duquel pour ceſte cauſe principalement a receu la conſtante rayſon.

Trop long & prolixe ſeroit le propos/ par lequel on pourroit demonſtrer les hommes auoir eſte faictz pour la cötëplation des grandes & incredibles oeuures de Dieu:lequel ignorans aulcuns des anciens/ont appelle Prouidence:les aultres/diſoient que ceſtoit le monde/qui toutes choſes cötenoit & embraſſoit:Zeno lappelloit Nature/maiſtreſſe/nourriſſe/& prouidëte a toutes vtilitez & opportunitez.Aulcuns(cöme ceſtuy Anaxagoras)ont pëſe que le ciel feuſt le Dieu eternel:duquel toute conſeruation de toutes choſes procedaſt/auquel riens ne feuſt plus perfaict ou conſummé/riens plus noble/ſaige ou excellent. Ainſy de toutes partz & toutes rayſons/pouuons cöclure:que cöme il ſoit vray/ que par le conſeil & prouidence de Dieu / les choſes de ce monde ayent eſte admirablement produictes pour la ſanté & conſeruation dung chaſcun:ſans doubte nous ſommes auſſy nez,& produictz pour icelles contempler & conſyderer.Mais par ce que les choſes qui ont eſte a noſtre vſaige faictes par ce grand architecteur/ſont infinies:trop ſeroit difficile que chaſcun de nous les peuſt toutes bien congnoiſtre/& perfaictement contempler: tant pour la varieté dicelles/comme pour lim-

A. j.

side notes: Les hömes auoireſté faictz pour contempler louuraige diuin. — En cötëplant le ciel, no⁹ admirons Dieu. — Lhomme. — Nature. — La principale vacation de lhomme. — Toutes choſes auoir eſté faictes pour lhomme. — Queſt ce que les anciës philoſophes ont eſtime eſtre Dieu. — La diuerſite des choſesque lhomme peult contempler.

5.9 The first page of the first book in Estienne's French-language edition of *La dissection*, 1546.

in his twenties—to a period eight years before Vesalius' *Tabulae*, and only ten years after Berengario. The book as a whole, and more particularly its illustrations, must therefore not be compared with the *Fabrica*, to which it perforce owed nothing; it should instead be thought of as another early attempt to resolve the problem of using figures to illustrate anatomical text. That Estienne's attempts were not as successful as that of Vesalius does not alter the fact that Estienne's book was the fourth fully illustrated text of the whole body to be issued in Europe, preceded only by Berengario's two works and the *Fabrica*; Dryander's text was never completed; others, such as Hundt's, were not texts of anatomy.

The sequence of events in the printing and publishing of Estienne's book may be listed:

1526: decorated initial letters, to be used in *De dissectione* . . . and other books, designed by Tory (see *Fig. 5.9*).

1530–2 dates on four of the full-page woodcuts.

1532–9 most of the other full-page cuts made.

1536 *Anatomica* by Charles Estienne advertised in a list of Robert Estienne's publications; no copy of this *Anatomica* is known—possibly it was not published.

1539 *De dissectione* . . . printed, up to the middle of the final book.

1539 Estienne de la Rivière complains to *Parlement*.

1541 completed sections of *De dissectione* . . . submitted to Faculty of Medicine.

1545 Latin edition, published by Simon de Colines.

1546 French edition, same publisher.

Estienne de la Rivière (Stephanus Riverius) was a surgeon who was associated with Charles Estienne at the beginning of the project (the similarity of the names is confusing). He made the dissections and assisted with the illustrations; the first of the plates had the initials S.R., which probably refer to him (see *Plate 39*). Estienne de la Rivière's legal case, submitted in 1539, but not resolved for some years, was that his efforts should get due recognition in the final work— and indeed his name did appear on the title-page, and his contributions were acknowledged. How the actual credits should be distributed is not now certain. The book—relying on the authentic corpus of Galen's work then being published—nevertheless does contain a long list of original anatomical discoveries showing familiarity with the appearance of dissected human bodies. That Charles Estienne based his text on Galen is not surprising considering the environment in which he was brought up and educated: his father was a classical scholar; his stepfather, for a decade, produced volume after volume of Galen's works, with a major work on anatomy, *De usu partium corporis humani* . . ., published in 1528; his teachers in Padua and Paris provided advanced humanist education. Estienne de la Rivière's contribution may have been to carry out dissections from which material not in Galen was added to a text written by Charles Estienne. Rivière's role in producing the woodcuts is unknown.

The illustrations themselves present a formidable challenge of classification and attribution, for they are in such varied styles. Even when signed by Jollat, as artist or cutter or both, the woodcuts are uneven in quality, some very much in an earlier popular or vernacular style, others recalling Italianate, mannerist work, not unlike that of the Fontainebleau artists, Primaticcio and Rosso (see *Fig. 5.8*, p. 167). Jollat's work may be identified through the monogram he used—the alchemical sign for mercury; in some cases his name is written in full, with the J replaced by the mercury sign. Another monogram present is a Lorraine cross, which was used during much of the sixteenth century by Geoffrey Tory and others associated with him.

In Book I, there are standing skeletons, a vessel-man, *écorchés*, surface anatomies ... These have landscape backgrounds of varying complexity: some have a few flowering plants, others classical views; while some have entire scenes of large buildings, towns, and so on. It is certainly frustrating to attempt to follow the indicator lines in many of the figures from legend, number, or letter to the part intended; they cross each other and they disappear (see, for example, *Plate 40*).

In Book II there are included a series of dramatic figures purporting to show the anatomy of the brain. These are arranged in landscapes in which there are numerous conceits and elaborations quite unconnected with any didactic purpose. The actual anatomical parts may occupy one-thirtieth or less of the printed area of the illustration; the rest includes the naked figures of muscular men placed in extravagant poses, holding tablets on which are cut lists of features identified by letters. These small figures of brain dissection follow the examples of Fries (1517) and Dryander (1536) in showing successive dissections of the brain after removal of the skull-cap—in one picture this hangs on a branch of a nearby tree. Because of the smallness of the brain figures and their indistinctness, the features can only be interpreted, and that only partially, by the use of prior knowledge; no one could learn brain anatomy from them. Other illustrations in Book II constitute a series in which the anatomy of the abdomen is shown in successive layers dissected from the front. The same criticisms apply to this series and to a series of three illustrations of neck dissections: the picture of the intestines is particularly unrealistic, resembling very much the diagrams in Fries or even those in Hundt, and in no way as satisfactory as those in the series of torso figures in Vesalius' *Fabrica*, inaccurate though these are in some respects.

Book III deals, among other structures, with the reproductive organs, and includes matters of obstetrical interest. The dispositions of the women in the illustrations of female organs were taken from earlier examples, and some resemble the equivalent figures in Berengario (see *Fig. 3.4*, p. 73). But the same criticisms, both of small size and unclear drawing, again hold. On one illustration, for instance, a woman on a three-legged stool has her thighs apart to show the pudenda; but the drawing is so bad that it is impossible to make out any structures. This illustration includes a syringe placed on the floor, a vicious-looking mechanical dilator, and a curved probe.

These obstetrical illustrations owe much to a mildly erotic series of figures by Perino del Vaga, a pupil of Raphael. Some figures are luxuriously spread out on a bed with excessive pillows and bedding. Later French voluptuous and erotic pictures—by Watteau for example—use, naturally enough, similar positions within similar settings. The areas in these abdominal and gynaecological woodcuts that show anatomical structures amount to no more than one-fiftieth of the printed area. The work ends with a manual of practical anatomical procedures; in the French edition this is entitled: *Ladministration & dissection de chascune partie du corps humain . . . .*

In many of the figures, but not all, the appropriate anatomical areas, with their associated numbering and lettering, may be seen to have been mortised into the original woodblocks with more, or with less, technical expertise (see, for example, *Plate 45*). Why was this done? Was an original anatomical wood-block of the early 1530s modified later in the light of new anatomical knowledge, by having the relevant portion cut away and a new woodcut mortised in as a replacement? This seems unlikely, for the anatomy is to say the least hesitant, and surely no one would go to the trouble involved to put in such poor modifications. It seems more likely that these blocks were cut originally for another purpose, perhaps for the Estienne or the Simon de Colines printing-houses; not being used, they were modified for anatomical use, by replacing central areas and by recutting the surrounds. This coming together of disparate parts conse-quently exaggerates to us, and perhaps exaggerated to contemporary readers, the already mannered, even surrealistic, impression discernible at first glance.

Estienne's anatomy text was Galenic, clearly expressed and well organized. The illustrations, while often astounding and sometimes elegant, are remarkably varied, and often unclear and inconsistent in quality and usefulness. Estienne and de la Rivière were attempting to marry text and figures; they put forward a number of solutions, some less, some more satisfactory. These considerations serve to underline the success of Vesalius' more sure and consistent resolution of the same problems; but the Parisian authors' achievement may be seen when the book is compared with those of Ketham, 1491 and 1493; Berengario, 1521 and 1522; and Dryander, 1536 and 1537.

Two bibliographic postscripts may be added. The first concerns the figure that shows the venous and the arterial systems in one drawing of a standing man (*Plate 41*). At his left side there is some decorated masonry, with a frame within which the letterpress refers to the numbering and lettering given on the figure; the perspective of the plinth, frame, and lettering is awry. A similar vascular man may also be seen, re-cut, in Dryander's book: *Der gantzen Artzenei . . .*, Frankfurt, Egenolff, 1542. From the dates of publication one would suspect that Estienne's artists copied from Dryander; but the reverse is the case. In the introductory matter to the reader Estienne discusses how, by 1539, the work

was in print up the middle of the third book, when because of a controversy brewing, it became necessary to suppress the whole work ... But the typographers could not, long enough, guard the portion of the work already in type ... and some of it was secretly carried away ... to Germany, where copies of it, more especially of the pictures of the nerves, veins, and arteries, were later procured here by our Paris friends who apprised us of the theft thus committed, to which however we paid no attention [quoted from Cushing 1962].

It seems probable that Estienne used the two vascular figures published by Vesalius in 1538 as the starting point for this figure (see *Plate 12*, p. 61), combining the venous diagram with the one of the arteries to put them in the context of a human figure (*Plate 41*). We are here, of course, pre-Harveian, so there are no interconnections shown between the two vascular systems. Vesalius commented, in his letter of complaint to Oporinus, 1542: 'At Paris they have copied the first three plates very well, but the others they have omitted, perhaps because they were difficult to engrave, though it was these first three which students could have best dispensed with'—it was Vesalius himself who drew the first three figures, and Calcar the three skeletal figures, so was Vesalius referring to the first figures cut, viz. Calcar's skeletons? But Estienne's book, in the Latin and French editions, has no skeletal pictures that could be said to be derived from the *Tabulae Sex*.[1]

From all this one may surmise, first, that Estienne used the Vesalian 1538 diagrams to supervise the drawing and cutting of the venous–arterial wood-block some time between 1538 and 1542, probably either in 1538 or 1539. Secondly we may deduce that Vesalius, as well as Dryander, saw prints taken from some blocks prepared for Estienne's work, even though the completed book had not yet been published.

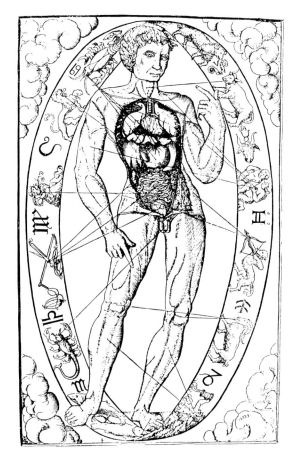

5.10 A dissected astrological figure showing the viscera in relation to the signs of the Zodiac, dated 1533, and signed with a Lorraine cross. This figure was probably intended to be used in Estienne's *De dissectione*, 1545, but was not included. It was printed in Kerver's *Les figures*, Paris, 1557.

The second postscript is short and straightforward: the Estienne wood-blocks came into the possession of Jacques Kerver, and were publised by him in book form: *Les figures et portraicts des parties du corps humain*, 1557. This book included as well five extra full-page woodcuts, obviously prepared for Estienne and his collaborator, but not chosen for the final version published in 1545. These were produced in the Jollat–Tory workshop, four with Jollat's mark and the other unsigned, but with the cross of Lorraine. All but one were dated 1532 or 1533.

[1] A publication dated 1543—Jean Tagault *De chirurgica institutione*, Paris, Chrestien Wechel—contains the Calcar skeletal figures reduced in size. These may have been obtained by Vesalius before his letter to Oporinus was written (1542).

Three of these additional illustrations have an astrological basis dated 1533, and this may have seemed to Estienne outdated by 1545 (*Fig. 5.10*). Nowhere are Estienne or Rivière acknowledged.

39 Skeletal figure seen from the front, on page 39 of Charles Estienne, *De dissectione partium corporis humani ...*, Paris, Simon de Colines, 1545. Woodcut (Cambridge University Library). 27.7 × 17.7 cm.

This is a hideous portrayal of a human skeleton. The proportions of the foot to the leg and the leg to thigh are all wrong—the foreshortened foot is half the length of the femur! The greater trochanter of the femur, particularly the right one, is truncated, and the lesser trochanter is an enormous wedge. The radius and ulna are grossly curved and the shaft of the humerus is much too thick; it does, however, show both the bicipital groove and the nutrient foramen or 'feeding hole'. It is interesting that the little sesamoid bones of the thumb are depicted and named.

The ribs are thin and rounded, and spaced much too far apart; the costal cartilages are indicated, but the proportions of the manubrium relative to the too-thin sternum are much too great, though the depiction of manubrium, sternum, and xiphisternum as three entities is good. Those vertebral bodies that are visible are squashed supero-inferiorly, and skull details are very difficult to make out, other than that an egregious metopic suture is present.

Between the two tibia can be seen the hyoid bone (1), the cartilaginous patella (5), tracheal cartilaginous rings (4), thyroid cartilage (3), and, presumably, cricoid cartilage (2). This illustration, probably drawn about 1538, but not published until 1545, is very poor anatomically—comparable to the similar figure in Vesalius' *Tabulae Sex* (see *Plate 13*, p. 63). Perhaps the best that can be said for it is that it seems to have been intended more to place the bones together than to serve as an anatomical portrayal of their actual appearance.

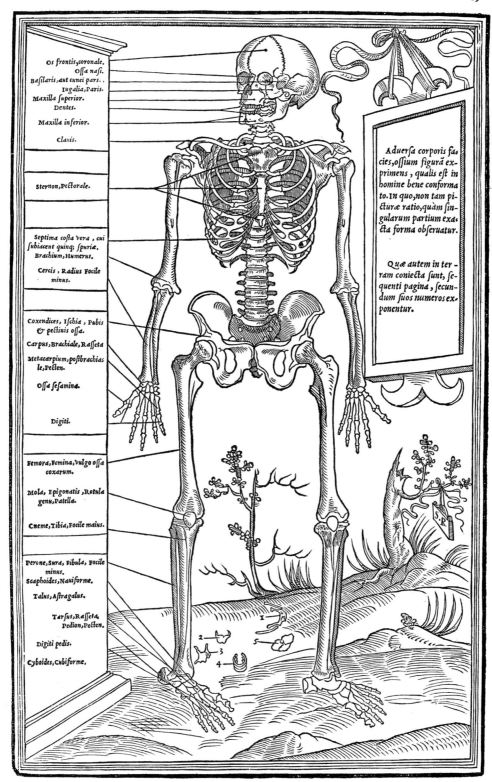

Os frontis, coronale.
Ossa nasi.
Basilaris, aut cunei pars.
Iugalia, Paris.
Maxilla superior.
Dentes.

Maxilla inferior.

Clauis.

Sternon, Pectorale.

Septima costa vera, cui
subiacent quinq; spuriæ.
Brachium, Humerus.

Cercis, Radius Focile
minus.

Coxendices, Ischia, Pubis
& pectinis ossa.
Carpus, Brachiale, Rasseta
Metacarpium, postbrachia=
le, Pecten.

Ossa sesamina.

Digiti.

Femora, Femina, vulgo ossa
coxarum.

Mola, Epigonatis, Rotula
genu, Patella.

Cneme, Tibia, Focile maius.

Perone, Sura, Fibula, Focile
minus.
Scaphoides, Nauiforme.

Talus, Astragalus.

Tarsus, Rasseta
Pedion, Pecten.

Digiti pedis.

Cyboides, Cubiforme.

Aduersa corporis fa=
cies, ossium figurã ex=
primens, qualis est in
homine bene conforma
to. In quo, non tam pi=
cturæ ratio, quàm sin=
gularum partium exa=
cta forma obseruatur.

Quæ autem in ter=
ram coniecta sunt, se=
quenti pagina, secun=
dum suos numeros ex=
ponentur.

PLATE 39

40 A figure of the nerves of the body on page 59 of Charles Estienne, *De dissectione partium corporis humani . . .*, Paris, Simon de Colines, 1545. Woodcut (Cambridge University Library). 27.7 × 17.7 cm.

This very odd figure shows the nerves of the body from the front, entwined around a skeleton whose right hand holds up the mandible. The distal portions of the nerves are flourishingly curled, and resemble spaghetti more than nerves.

The inferior alveolar nerve in the mandible and its mental branch are well drawn. Both the origin and pattern of the brachial plexus, quite apart from being different on the two sides, are obscure and certainly inaccurate, though once the ulnar nerve (A) has become an entity its course and distribution are reasonably correct, as is true of both the median (E), and, to a lesser extent, the radial (C). The less attention paid to the nerves of the neck and thorax the better; the recurrent laryngeal nerves arising from the vagi are perhaps the most accurate.

The sciatic nerves are rather disappointing—reasonable as far as their origin is concerned, but their distribution is certainly not a strong point. For example, one has to believe that the branch appearing from behind the knee, passing medially around the tibia and extending on to the dorsum of the foot, was considered to be a sciatic branch. This is certainly an error; and nowhere can one see the common peroneal (a big nerve indeed)—one would expect it to be shown at the lateral side of the neck of the left fibula.

The origin of the femoral nerve is acceptable, but its saphenous branch is non-existent; no obturator nerve appears anywhere.

The nerves of the head are largely imaginary and meaningless squiggles, save only the supra- and infra-orbital.

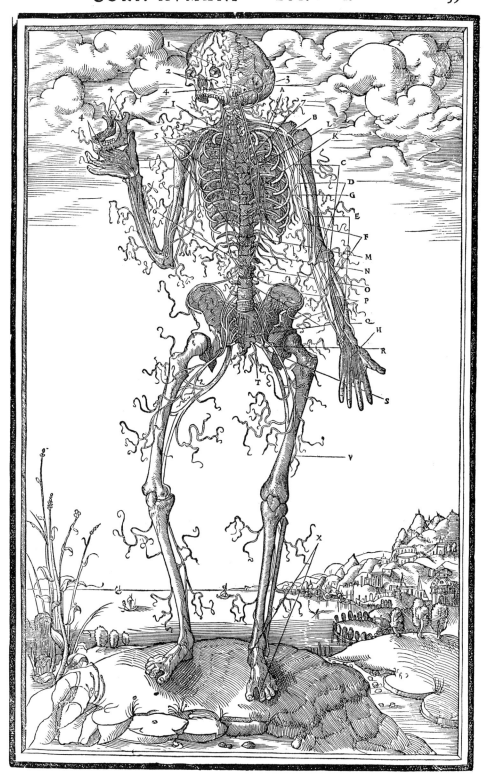

PLATE 40

41 A figure of the veins and the arteries, on page 134 of Charles Estienne, *De dissectione partium corporis humani ...*, Paris, Simon de Colines, 1545. Woodcut (Cambridge University Library). 27.7 × 17.5 cm.

Turning to the aorta in this woodcut it is obvious that, just after it leaves the heart, its form is certainly not human. The heart itself is very small, perhaps partly because it has been deprived of its right atrium! It was obviously considered unnecessary to know the branches of the aorta, and, from what little this drawing shows of them, in Estienne's view they certainly were not of very much importance.

There is a small four-lobed liver; a kinked inferior vena cava has seemingly no obvious connection with the heart, both the upper and lower parts 'draining' into the liver. The azygos vein is correctly pictured draining into the superior vena cava.

The pelvic veins are extremely fanciful; they were considered of little importance in those days. The femoral artery was obviously considered to parallel the enormously large great (long) saphenous vein. It is perhaps odd that the obliterated umbilical arteries are so well shown— virtually the only recognizable branches of the internal iliac arteries. The straight ligamentum teres is shown passing from the umbilicus to the liver. The course of the cephalic vein above the shoulder is totally inaccurate, and causes one to wonder where the left one might drain; the right one joins with the superficial temporal vein! Though large, the representations of the basilic, axillary, and subclavian veins are much better, and their merging with the jugulars and formation of the superior vena cava are not too inaccurate, though the axillary receives a prodigious tributary from the lateral thoracic wall.

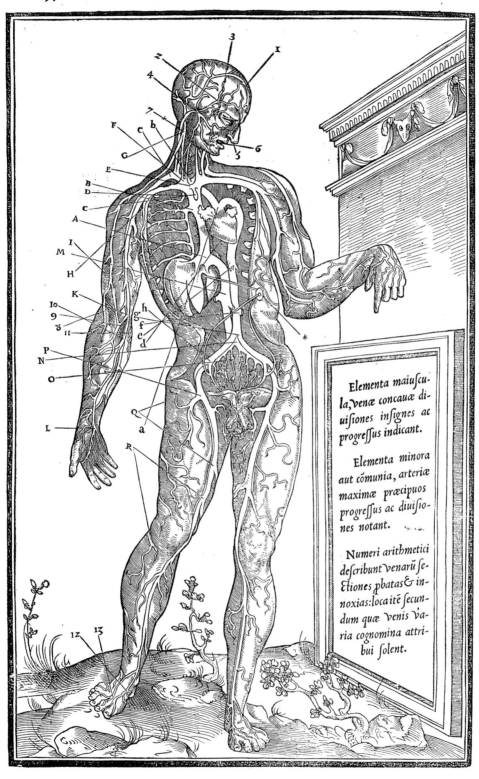

Elementa maiuscu-
la, venæ concauæ di-
uisiones insignes ac
progressus indicant.

Elementa minora
aut cómunia, arteriæ
maximæ præcipuos
progressus ac diuisio-
nes notant.

Numeri arithmetici
describunt venarū se-
ctiones pbatas& in-
noxias: loca itē secun-
dum quæ venis varia
cognomina attri-
bui solent.

PLATE 41

42 Male visceral figure, on page 180 of Charles Estienne, *De dissectione partium corporis humani ...*, Paris, Simon de Colines, 1545. Woodcut (Cambridge University Library). 28.0 × 18.0 cm.

This figure, supported by tree branches in each axilla, possesses a face very reminiscent of the Friesian plate, (see *Plate 9*, p. 54). His abdomen is shown widely opened, with the guts removed: the stomach is shown lying on a tree stump (lower right) with a very thin duodenum issuing from it.

There is a very reasonable representation of the spleen (N), though it is too far separated from the left kidney (which is shown lower than that on the right).

The liver has been turned upwards to show the entry of the hepatic portal vein into it and the gall-bladder, though no real common bile-duct is seen. The liver is shown 'slung' from the diaphragm by the triangular ligament (A).

The inferior vena cava and aorta are felicitous, but the common iliac arteries do not divide into internal and external iliacs, nor are internal and external iliac veins differentiated. The ureters (K) are seen descending anterior to the iliac vessels to enter, much too low, the bladder (L). Oddly, neither testicular arteries nor veins are featured. The hepatic portal vein (C) is correctly shown as being formed by the rather thin splenic and the two mesenteric veins (though the text describes the portal vein as dividing into them, in accordance with the physiological beliefs of that period).

The diaphragm and its central tendon (M) can be seen, with the inferior vena cava piercing the latter. The cut oesophagus, alas, is shown doing likewise: the aorta can be seen entering the abdominal cavity just posterior to the oesophagus.

The representation of the viscera here is once again a woodcut inserted into the figure—the lower extent of this is just below the scrotum; the upper can be seen cutting across the neck. All in all this is one of the more informative, accurate, and pleasing illustrations in Estienne's book—certainly one of the least grotesque.

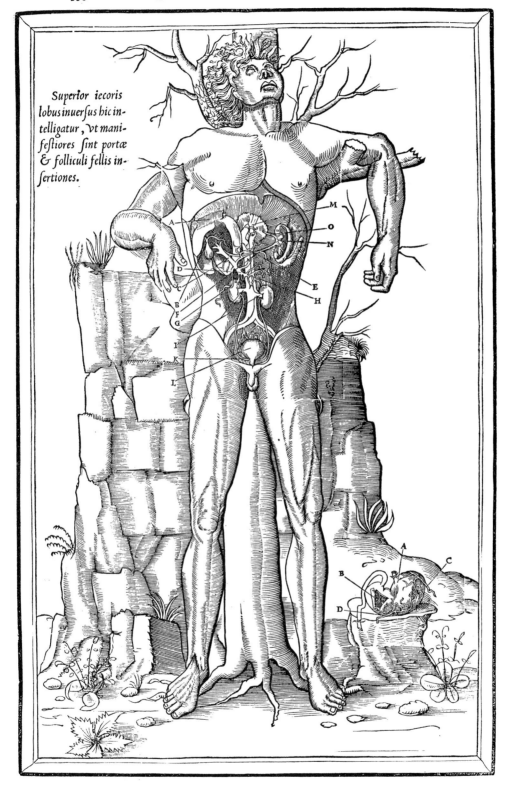

Superior iecoris
lobus inuerfus hic in-
telligatur, vt mani-
feftiores fint portæ
& folliculi fellis in-
fertiones.

PLATE 42

43 Figure showing a dissection of the thorax, on page 224 of Charles Estienne, *De dissectione partium corporis humani . . .*, Paris, Simon de Colines, 1545. Woodcut (Cambridge University Library). 28.0 × 18.0 cm.

This illustration portrays a man lolling in a massive chair, with his thorax open, with his head twisted grotesquely upwards to the left, and virtually devoid of a neck.

There is here certainly a lot of plate for very little anatomy. The heart and lungs have been removed, and the aorta has been cut across. Again, the arterial pattern is certainly non-human. The left recurrent laryngeal nerve once again is nicely shown arising from the left vagus (this had been described by Galen), but then the vagus goes on to end by supplying the diaphragm! An unworthy thought that perhaps this nerve was meant to be the phrenic is disposed of in the French-language edition, where it is described as the *nerf de la sixiesme conjugaison*, which was then the description of the vagus (so where is the phrenic?).

A small oesophagus and trachea are visible, and the 'frill' is seemingly a poorly separated composite of pleura and pericardium.

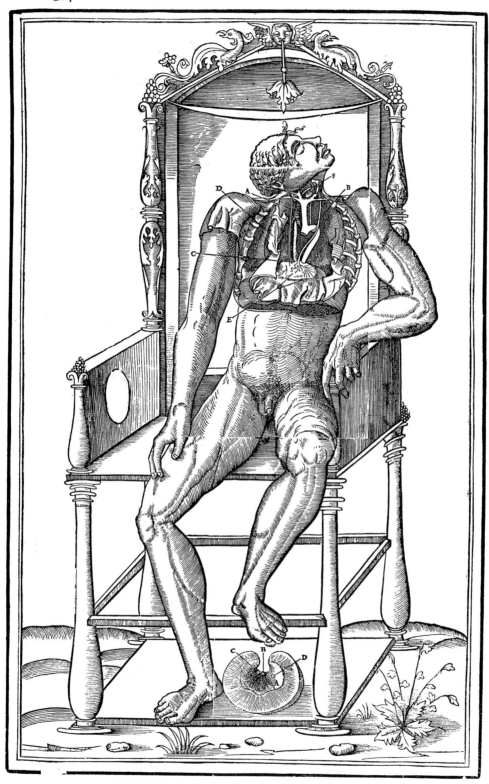

PLATE 43

44 Figure showing a brain dissection, on page 242 of Charles Estienne, *De dissectione partium corporis humani ...*, Paris, Simon de Colines, 1545. Woodcut (Cambridge University Library). 27.8 × 17.9 cm.

This shows a man bending over a table, presenting the top of his head cut off in a horizontal plane. It is a pointless illustration if what the author presumably wished to convey was the structure of the brain; it is very difficult to follow the markers, as the brain area is so small and indistinct. The cerebellum and the opened ventricular system are recognizable, but very little else. In fact it is a better representation of the surface anatomy of muscles than of the brain!

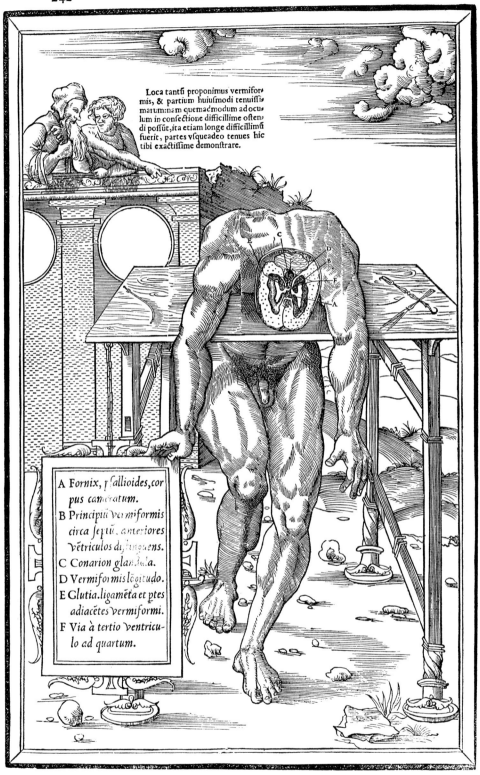

Loca tantū proponimus vermifor/
mis, & partium huiuſmodi tenuiſſi/
matum:nam quemadmodum ad ocu/
lum in confectione difficillime often/
di poſſūt,ita etiam longe difficillimū
fuerit, partes vſqueadeo tenues hic
tibi exactiſſime demonſtrare.

A Fornix, pſallioides,cor
  pus cameratum.
B Principiū vermiformis
  circa ſeptū, anteriores
  Vētriculos diſtinguens.
C Conarion glandula.
D Vermiformis lōgitudo.
E Glutia.ligamēta et ptes
  adiacētes Vermiformi.
F Via à tertio Ventricu/
  lo ad quartum.

PLATE 44

45 Figure showing the female reproductive system, on page 291 of Charles Estienne, *De dissectione partium corporis humani . . .*, Paris, Simon de Colines, 1545. Woodcut (Cambridge University Library). 27.9 × 17.8 cm.

In this drawing of a seated woman with her abdomen opened it is obvious that the central area is yet another separate wood-block insert.

Posteriorly can be seen the inferior vena cava, with the aorta dividing into iliac vessels, while anterior to these is the cut and tied rectum. The uterus has rather exaggerated vessels, and is pulled up by strings held in the beak of a parrot, which latter is the end of an arm-rest. The bladder (F) is very small, and the vagina and vulva are not drawn, though there is something that looks like a folded scroll of parchment, perhaps representing cut skin, obfuscating this area. Indeed all of Estienne's illustrations that could inform students on the anatomy of the female genitalia are poor in both detail and accuracy.

In general it may be considered that Estienne's illustrations represent not so much the dissection of cadavers, as rather posed human beings, in which, almost incidentally, a modicum of anatomy is revealed. Most of them sadly betray the numerous excellent and original observations contained in the text.

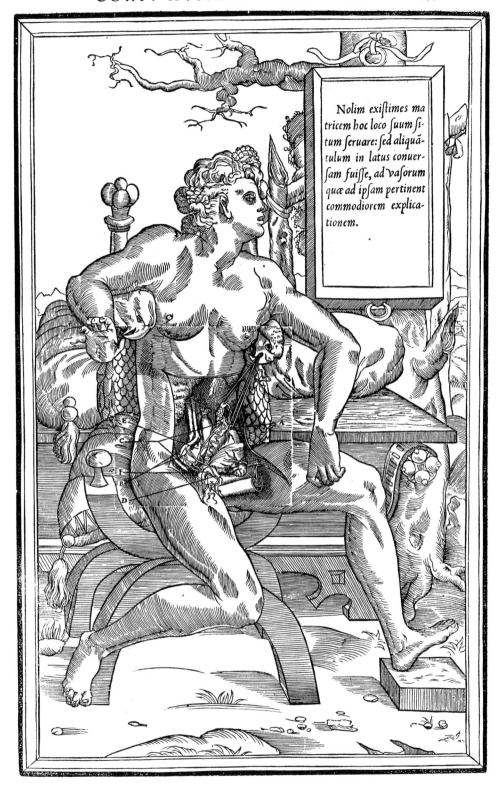

Nolim exiſtimes ma
tricem hoc loco ſuum ſi-
tum ſeruare: ſed aliquã-
tulum in latus conuer-
ſam fuiſſe, ad vaſorum
quæ ad ipſam pertinent
commodiorem explica-
tionem.

PLATE 45

Eustachio and his anatomical plates

Bartolomeo Eustachio, or, in the Latinized form, Bartholomaeus Eustachius, was born in the first years of the sixteenth century (the actual date is unknown) at San Severino, near Ancona in north-eastern Italy. He spent much of his professional life in Rome. Although life in this city was far from placid—in 1527 soldiers occupied and sacked Rome—it was a quiet medical centre when compared with the excitements of Padua at that time, the time of Vesalius. Before his move to Rome, Eustachio was physician to the Duke of Urbino, and then to that Duke's brother, Cardinal Guilio della Rovere, in whose service he remained; indeed Eustachio died—in 1574— on a journey from Rome when summoned to attend the Cardinal. He was a teacher of anatomy in the medical faculty of the *Sapienza* at Rome, where he himself was probably trained. He carried out autopsies at some of the Roman hospitals, and was allowed subjects for dissection. While his published writings were influential during his lifetime, his fame as an anatomical illustrator rests principally on a series of copper engravings of the skeleton and muscles that sadly were not published until a hundred and forty years after his death. These plates were

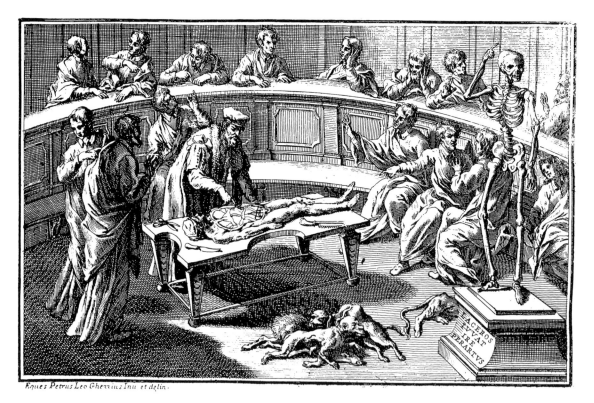

5.11 The dissection scene from Lancisi's edition of the Eustachian plates, 1714, drawn and engraved by Petrus Leo Ghezzius.

prepared by Giulio de' Musi, a Roman artist, under the direction of Eustachio and his assistant Pier Matteo Pini of Urbino. The majority of them were not published while Eustachio was alive; why, has not been satisfactorily explained. They were obviously treasured by Eustachio, for he bequeathed them to the family of Pini; but they were then lost to view, even though Marcello Malpighi searched for them. They were later acquired by Pope Clement XI through the efforts of his physician, Giovanni Maria Lancisi (1665–1720). Lancisi published them for the first time in 1714: *Tabulae anatomicae ... quas e tenebris tandem vindicatas ... Jo. Maria Lancisius*, Rome, Francis Gonzaga (*Plates 46–50*). The title illustration (*Fig. 5.11*), to this book was drawn by Petrus Leo Ghezzius, but it seems to represent the spirit of anatomical science in the Rome of Eustachio, in the mid sixteenth century: only a few of those present are seen to be actually looking at the anatomist, who is demonstrating a partially dissected cadaver; the remainder of the students are politely disputing with each other, in a scene that resembles a late-medieval anatomy. This is most unlike the dissection taking place on the title-page of Vesalius' *Fabrica*, but it was perhaps more conducive to the discovery of the *minutiae* of anatomy.

Eustachio's text to the plates was either never completed or was lost, and Lancisi and subsequent editors had to supply an anatomical commentary. In 1972 Luigi Bellini identified a manuscript written by Eustachio and his pupil Pier Matteo Pini in the city library at Sienna. This was in the form of a dialogue, a *syngramma* and an *antigramma*, arranged under 150 headings of the parts of the body: bones, muscles and ligaments, veins, arteries, nerves, viscera, reproductive organs, heart, lungs, and brain. The relevance of this to the proposed text of Eustachio's anatomy is not clear. Certainly he intended to publish an illustrated volume entitled *Liber de dissensionibus ac controversiis anatomicis*, for such was announced in his *Opuscula anatomica*, 1564.

Other eighteenth-century editions were printed from the original copperplates, or from re-engravings. The best of the latter are those of B. S. Albinus, Leiden, 1744. The figure of the nervous system, and in particular the sympathetic nervous system, (see *Plate 46*) was considered so useful that it was included in the 1817 edition of *Encyclopaedia Britannica*, about two hundred and fifty years after it was first engraved.

Eustachio suffered cruelly from an arthritis, perhaps gout. He was a sarcastic and ungracious man in controversy, particularly in his earlier writings, with special scorn for Vesalius and Falloppio. '[Vesalius] today is considered by everyone as the discoverer and almost the architect of the art of anatomy ...' 'Although no honest person ought to disparage the general benefit which that man brought to the art of medicine ... yet I believe that his misleading errors ought to be revealed so that they may be carefully shunned'; and Eustachio proceeded to do so, demolishing Vesalius' faulty account of the innervation and structure of the auditory apparatus, stating for example that 'there is no truth either in his text or his illustration' concerning the cavities of the ear. The monograph on the ear, *De auditus organis*, included in *Opuscula anatomica ... 1564*, has been translated by O'Malley, 1971, and it is from him that the above quotations have been taken. Eustachio gives such an accurate description of the auditory tube—the Eustachian tube—that the eponym is justified, though the tube had been known to some ancient writers, including Aristotle.[2]

The diligence of Eustachio as a dissector is shown in this same work by his discovery and description of the tensor tympani muscle. The accuracy of the engravings may be seen in the depiction of the anomalous remnant of the thyroglossal duct, as noted by Morgagni (1764). There is also correspondence between the engraving and the actual appearance of this structure; Eustachio probably considered it to be a thin muscle. Wilhelm His described, in 1885, its embryological significance.

Eustachio criticized specifically the Vesalian illustrations. Anatomy may be seen to be in process of maturing as an observational science; illustrations, correctable illustrations, were major factors in achieving this maturity. Illustrations that were made in one city, printed in another, and distributed in identical copies, became available throughout Europe. Non-correspondences between actual anatomy and illustration could be noted and corrected. The integrity and honesty of anatomist and illustrator may be seen when detail, previously unrecognized or meaningless to them, was shown in illustrations.

Eustachio's plates are remarkable not only for the advanced anatomical knowledge shown, but also for the original method of identification of structures drawn on the plates, and for their strange artistic qualities. Each of the illustrations is provided with a graduated border on both sides and at the top of the plate; the smaller illustrations have a further rule at the bottom. To identify a structure it is only necessary to give the reference number for a horizontal or east–west latitude and for a vertical or north–south longitude. In order to assist the student, there were provided in Lancisi's edition two printed rules; each rule, or geometrical *gnomon*, is a scale suitable for moving in a parallel across the plate. One rule was intended for the smaller, and another, with a different scale, for the larger plates. With a little practice, it is both quick and easy to pin-point structures using grid references, which apparently were to be indicated in an accompanying text. The divisions of the scale of the plates and the rules are only approximately the same; it is difficult to understand why they were not more accurately drawn. As in geographical maps, the figures often intrude into the margins where the numbered references for latitude and longitude are engraved. This method of grid referencing allowed Eustachio to present his figures without superimposed lettering or numbering; the figures therefore can be clearer; moreover, structures can with practice be very easily identified from a text reference.

Students of Vesalius' *Fabrica* must often have wasted time searching for an obscurely-placed

---

[2] The extraordinary method by which Hamlet's father was murdered—emptying a vial of poison into his ear while he slept—may have occurred to Shakespeare because of common knowledge of Eustachio's findings. If the drum were perforated by otitis media, poison could pass from the external meatus to the pharynx, and so be swallowed. This theory was put forward, perhaps in the spirit of Sherlockian argument, by Eden and Opland (1982).

letter; indeed some of the wood-blocks were recut for the 1555 edition precisely in order to make the letters more easily identifiable.

A third method of identification, the one that many modern textbooks employ, is that of a marginal letter or number, or a descriptive word or phrase, with a line from there to the structure in question: this was used in the sixteenth century by Estienne, for example, and has a long history traceable to medieval cautery figures.

A fourth method is to redraw and present an entire figure at the same size but in outline only, and on this to place easily-seen letters or numerals; cross references can then be made between the outline and the lifelike main illustration. This was Albinus' technique in his edition of Eustachio, and for his own works (*Fig. 5.12*); it was a method that was used extensively in the days of the great eighteenth- and early-nineteenth-century atlases of anatomy.

Eustachio was concerned with measurement in more ways than are indicated by his use of these marginal rulers. He left, in his will, many items to his pupil Pier Matteo Pini—his books in Latin, Greek, and Hebrew, for instance; but also included were scientific and measuring instruments of many kinds. It is to be noted that the eight smaller plates appearing in Lancisi's 1714 publication, with

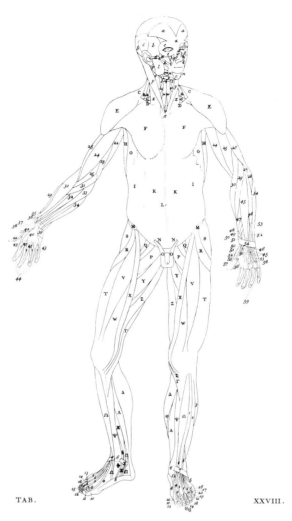

5.12 Outline diagram to accompany Eustachio's Tabula XXVIII (see *Plate 49*), as reproduced in Albinus' edition, 1761.

graduated borders, were included with other works in Eustachio's *Opuscula anatomica . . .*, Venice, 1564, a work dedicated to Pini. In this book there are to be found instructions on how to use the rulers described above when looking at the plates (*de usu tabularum*). This method of identifying structures in an illustration has thus been known since 1564, yet has rarely been used since—Arent Cant used it in a folio anatomical atlas issued in Leiden in 1721.

Eustachio's *Opuscula . . .*, published ten years before his death, collected together some of his monographs, including not only those on the organs of hearing, 1562, but also a treatise on

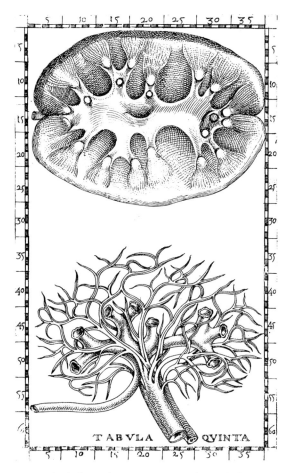

5.13 The kidney shown in section, above; below, the relationships of the vascular and urinary elements of the kidney from Eustachio's *Opuscula anatomica*, 1564.

teeth, 1563, and, what is perhaps his published masterpiece, the small book on the kidney, 1563. In this latter book anatomy, draughtsmanship and engraving contribute to the excellence of the plates, the technique of copper engraving being well suited to such detailed and precise work. These figures may be taken to represent the culmination of an extraordinary development that had taken place during a period of forty years: the figures of anatomy in Berengario's pioneering *Commentaria ...*, 1521 are at the beginning of scientific anatomy (see *Plate 15*, p. 79, for instance); the figures of the kidney published in Eustachio's lifetime (*Fig. 5.13*) already show all the elements of a developing observational science. Indeed many of these figures, with their concern for measurement and for the study of variation, look forward to analytical biology.

Eustachio's illustrations make no attempt to represent cadavers as they would appear when lying dissected on an anatomy table. Even when illustrating anomalous structures—a subject of great interest to Eustachio, there are no details that make the viewer think of the specific dissection that must have been made to demonstrate that particular anomaly. The figures of Vesalius attempt to copy the natural appearance of anatomical structures; Eustachio's figures are *maps* of human anatomy, not representations from a single viewpoint. They demand careful study, and not a quick all-embracing glance. Nevertheless, the appearances of the figures are easily reconciled in the imagination to actual slender men, gesturing in an unexcited, stylized manner. They are elegant, classical figures, not at all mannered, romantic, or dramatic; the precise soft line of copper engraving is entirely appropriate to the unhurried drawing. And yet, where faces can be seen, there is in them depth of expression.

It has been said that the figures are not lifelike but to us, in the latter part of the twentieth century, they appear as living characters in a formal play or in a classical ballet. That they gesture in front of, and sometimes partly obscure, measuring rulers reinforces the formality.

There are no backgrounds, only the baseboard, drawn with uncertain perspective. Such attention to measurement in quiet, intense men, variously anatomized and precisely and clearly drawn, disturbs the viewer's equanimity, in the same way that the memory of figures clearly seen in dreams disturbs a waking state.

46 Figure showing the base of the brain and associated nerves, Tab. XVIII, from G. M. Lancisi's edition of B. Eustachio's *Tabulae anatomicae . . .*, Rome, F. Gonzaga, 1714. Engravings made *c.*1555 (private collection). 28.2 × 18.6 cm.

If one ignores the imaginary convolutions of the cerebral hemispheres there is much to admire in this portrayal of the base of the brain—the olfactory bulbs and tracts; the optic chiasm; the infundibular opening to the third ventricle; and the (rather small) mammillary bodies behind the chiasm, together with the oculomotor nerves (rather large) issuing from the interpenduncular fossa. The pons is foreshortened, but shows the origin of the trigeminal and abducent nerves. These latter are depicted as giving rise to the cranial portion of the sympathetic trunk, which has a prominent superior cervical ganglion giving communications to the spinal nerves.

From the ponto-medullary junction spring somewhat artificial facial and stato-acoustic nerves, while cranial nerves nine, ten, and eleven are conjoined as the vagus. The hypoglossal nerve (cut on the left-hand side) gives off a descending branch, which is joined by a slender (presumed) contribution from a cervical nerve.

The most lateral branch of the right vagus, seen crossing the brachial plexus, possibly represents a rather large cardiac branch. Medial to it is seen the phrenic nerve, of accurate origin.

It is interesting that the right and left brachial plexus show quite different patterns. That of the right side is quite excellent, with the shaded posterior cord forming the radial and giving off the axillary nerve. The origins of the musculo-cutaneous, median, and ulnar nerves are very accurate, conforming to the most usual configuration.

The vagal trunks do not give rise to recurrent laryngeal branches, which is curious, as these nerves are quite large, and were certainly known when this drawing was being produced.

Below the level of the diaphragm the nerves become rather stylized. Only one long sympathetic ganglion is present in this region, although the concept of the branches descending anterior to the sacrum is felicitous, as are the rami from the spinal nerves to the sympathetic trunk (though these are continued too far caudally).

The four smaller drawings do not greatly add to the lustre of the central figure, which is a more superior rendering of the nerves concerned than any to be found in the *Fabrica*.

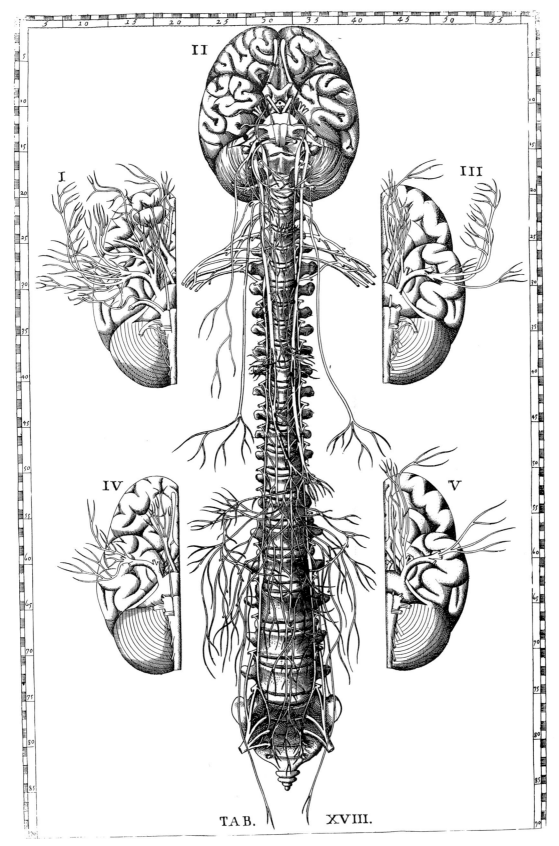

II

I

III

IV

V

TAB. XVIII.

PLATE 46

47 Figure showing dissection of the nerves of the body seen from the back, Tab. XX, in G. M. Lancisi's edition of B. Eustachio's *Tabulae anatomicae ...*, Rome, F. Gonzaga, 1714. Engravings made *c.* 1555 (private collection). 28.2 × 18.3 cm.

This shows the distribution of the spinal nerves viewed from the back. The uplifted right arm shows the radial nerve distribution, with its deep branch seen entering the forearm by piercing the supinator muscle. The termination of the suprascapular nerve is seen on the dorsum of the scapula, as is the left axillary entering the deltoid. The nerve medial to the scapula can only represent the spinal accessory, but it is not well-drawn.

The sciatic nerve in the buttock is inaccurately portrayed as giving rise to the superior and inferior gluteal nerves and also the pudendal nerve. However, knowing how difficult it is accurately to determine exactly where the sciatic nerve as such originates from the sacral plexus, too much should not be made of this error.

The hamstrings have been pulled apart (biceps femoris cut across and retracted laterally) to show the sciatic supplying them, before it divides into tibial and common peroneal in the popliteal fossa.

The cross-legged pose enables the medial and lateral plantar branches of the tibial nerve to be displayed in the right sole—the latter crossing superficial to flexor accessorius.

It is difficult to identify the two white lines seen disappearing into the left sole: the anterior one may be meant to represent a rather crude peroneus longus tendon, but the other, seemingly winding round the lower leg from the front, is a mystery. It certainly is not a misplaced superficial peroneal nerve, as the distribution of the peroneal nerves was very accurately shown in the succeeding illustration. The two identical structures also appear in Tabula XXIV, but there on the medial side of the leg; so presumably here they are an artistic error.

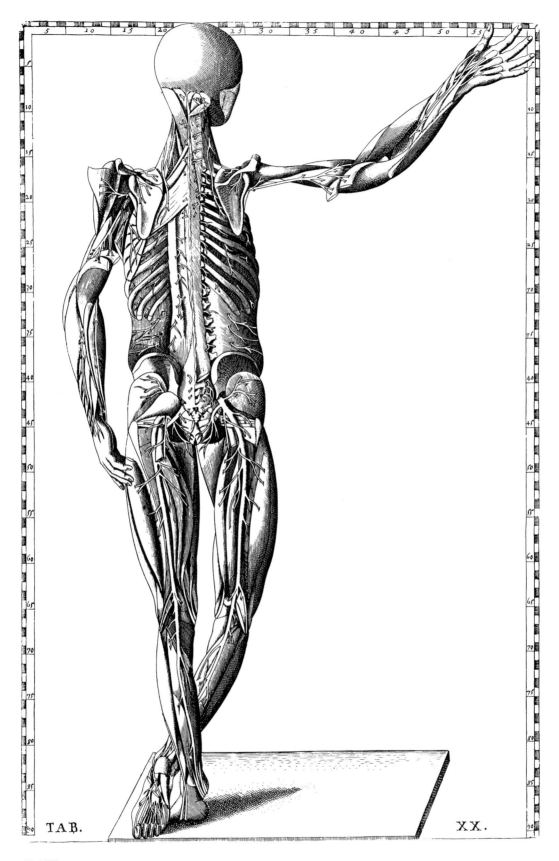

TAB.   XX.

PLATE 47

48 The vein figure, Tab. XXV, from G. M. Lancisi's edition of B. Eustachio's *Tabulae anatomicae . . .* Rome, F. Gonzaga, 1714. Engravings made *c.* 1555 (private collection). 29.1 × 18.9 cm.

It seems not unlikely that this pose inspired the plate by Haller reproduced later in this book (see *Plate 80*, p. 353). It is concerned primarily with the deep veins, as the superficial ones, for example, the saphenous, are covered in earlier drawings.

It would be difficult to determine the origin of the basilic and cephalic from this drawing, but their terminations are accurate; and it is gratifying to see that the jugular veins, brachiocephalic veins, and superior vena cava are certainly human (cf. the *Fabrica*), though it is strange that no glimpse of the azygos arch is vouchsafed.

The clinically important communication between the facial vein and the orbital veins is clearly suggested.

The heart is rather puzzling. At first sight it appears that the right portion of it is the right atrium, with the right coronary vessels in the groove on its left side and the great cardiac vein tributaries appearing around the left border. However, the venae cavae seem separated from the presumed atrium, and indeed, in an earlier figure of the heart from the back, the cavae are clearly shown as being continuous with each other. No matter how many human hearts one examines it is difficult to understand how this belief, common as it was in the sixteenth century, could have been sustained.

Turning to the inferior vena cava, the numerous small 'stubs' would appear to represent a multiplicity of hepatic veins. The positioning of the kidneys (the right correctly lower than the left) and renal veins is good, but the veins on the surface of the kidney are not. As Eustachio was well acquainted with the suprarenal glands it is a pity that they are not featured in this plate, though their veins can be seen.

The cut-short testicular vessels are accurate, spoiled only by having arterio-venous anastomoses. Emphasis is given to the external iliac vessels; the internal iliacs are sorry vessels indeed. The deep dorsal vein of the penis is shown draining into a pelvic venous plexus, but no prostate is identifiable.

The veins of the thigh are somewhat stylized, but the cut-off upper end of the long saphenous can clearly be seen. The lower leg vessels are presumably the anterior tibial artery and veins; the venous pattern on the dorsum of the foot is different on the two sides. The arcuate artery and its communicating branch with the sole is excellent, particularly in the right foot.

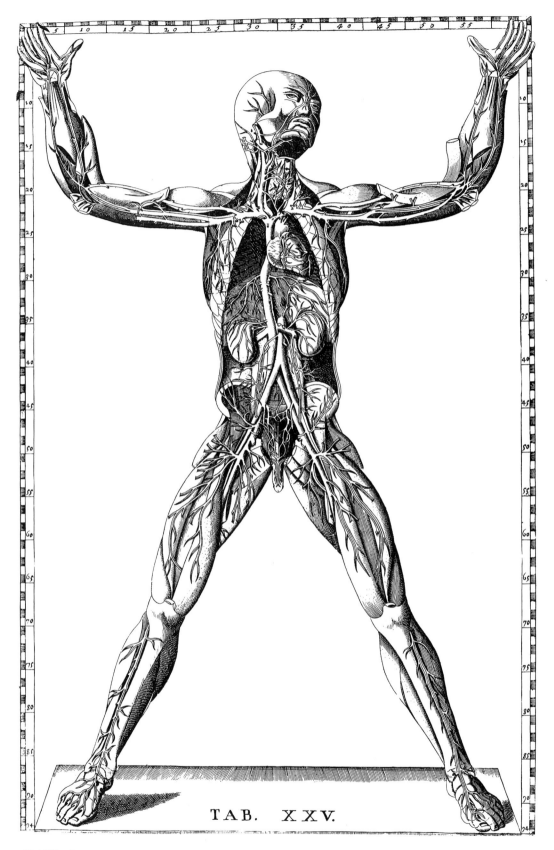

TAB. XXV.

PLATE 48

49 A muscle figure, an *écorché*, Tab. XXVIII, from G. M. Lancisi's edition of B. Eustachio's *Tabulae anatomicae . . .*, Rome, F. Gonzaga, 1722. Engravings made *c.*1555 (private collection). 29.0 × 18.7 cm.

This figure is posed very similarly to the first muscle-man in the *Fabrica* (see *Plate 31*, p. 151), even to the left-facing head, pronated left forearm, outflung right arm, and bent and laterally rotated right leg: but what a difference there is in presentation of the same musculture!

It is a fine example of how Eustachio formalized the structure of the human body. The muscles are extremely clearly delineated, for example the right sartorius, gracilis, and semitendinosus, with their conjoint insertion. It is true that there is no ilio-tibial tract into which to insert tensor fasciae latae, and the depiction of the muscle itself is rather poor.

The ankle and wrist retinacula are crude yet sharply defined, and the digitations of serratus anterior and the external oblique muscles are stylized, but certainly interdigitate!

One might perhaps quibble over the insertion of the tibialis anterior tendon, and certainly the relationship of pectoralis major and the deltoid is not at all clear.

Considering such illustrations as this one must bemoan the fact that Eustachio did not publish them in his lifetime. They might well have been more helpful to students of anatomy than those of Vesalius and his imitators.

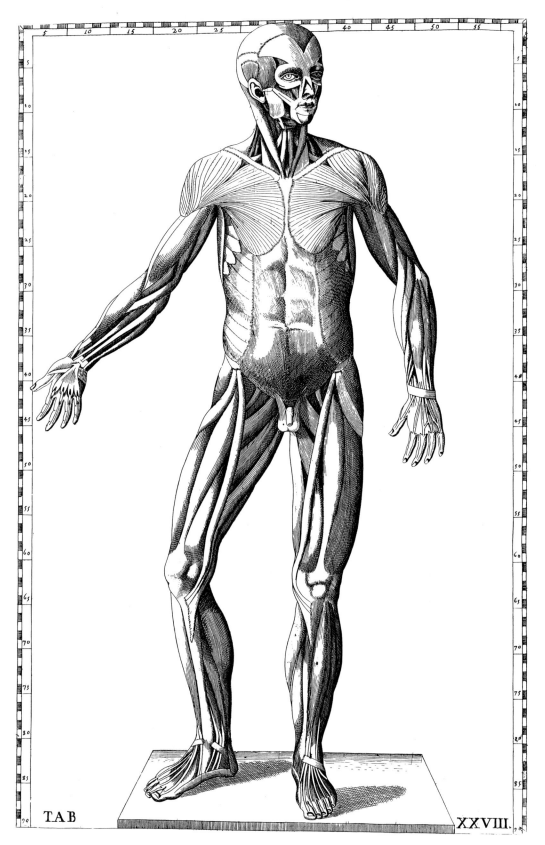

T.A.B   XXVIII.

PLATE 49

50 A skeletal figure, Tab. XXXXV, from G. B. Lancisi's edition of B. Eustachio's *Tabulae anatomicae . . .*, Rome, F. Gonzaga, 1714. Engravings made *c.* 1555 (private collection). 28.1 × 18.3 cm.

It must be stated that this is far and away the best of the three Eustachian whole-skeleton plates, and this not least because of its policeman-like pose. There is the typically clear, no-frills portrayal, and, in addition, proper vertebral curvatures are present. The neck is long—the cervical vertebrae being too massive—but then some people do have longer necks than others.

Minor blemishes include the unduly sinuous spine of the scapula; and the too-weighty left ulna, the rather-too-wide mandibular ramus, and the incorrect relative lengths of the femur and tibia.

The small drawing, lower right, is a section through the temporal bone, and shows the opened bony cochlea and semicircular canals.

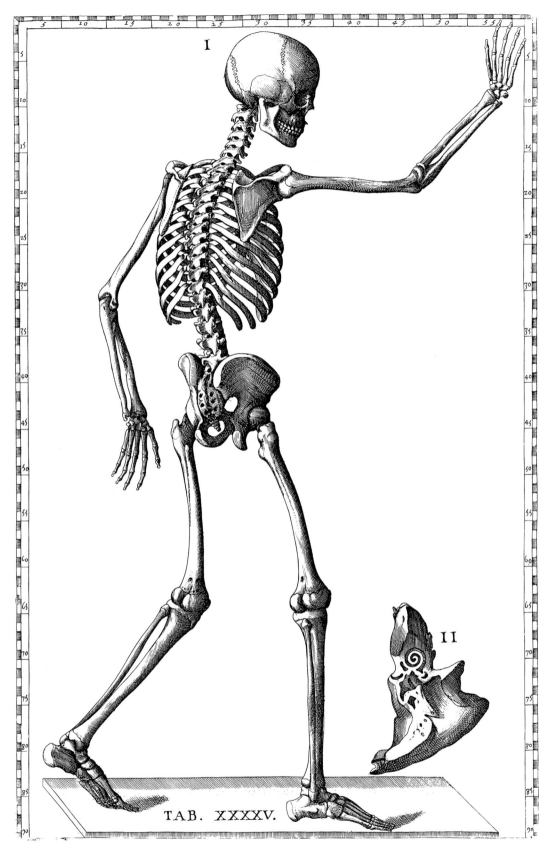

I

II

TAB. XXXXV.

PLATE 50

Chapter 5: Selected reading

Andreas Vesalius

Anson, B. J. (1949). Anatomic tabulae and initial letters in Vesalius' Fabrica and in imitative works. *Surg. Gyn. Obstet.*, **89**, 97–120.

Cavanagh, G. S. T. (1983). A new view of the Vesalian landscape. *Med. Hist.*, **27**, 77–79.

Clark, H. (1981). Why did Vesalius take his Fabrica to Basel to have it printed? *Library Quart.*, **51**, 301–11.

Copeman, W. S. C. (1963). The evolution of anatomy and surgery under the Tudors. *Ann. roy. Coll. Surg. Eng.* **32**, 1–21.

Cushing, H. W. (1962). *A bio-bibliography of Andreas Vesalius.* Archon, Hamden CT.

Eriksson, R. (1959). *Andreas Vesalius' first public anatomy at Bologna 1540 ...* Almqvist and Wiksells, Uppsala.

Farrington, B. (1932). The preface of Andreas Vesalius to De Fabrica Corporis Humani, 1543. *Proc. roy. Soc. Med.*, **25**, 1357–66.

Fulton, J. F. *et al.* (1944). [Symposium on Vesalius' De humani corporis fabrica]. *Yale J. Biol. Med.*, **16**, 106–48.

Grendler, P. F. (1977). *The Roman inquisition and the Venetian press: 1540–1605.* Princeton University Press.

Guerra, F. (1969). The identity of the artists involved in Vesalius' Fabrica, 1543. *Med. Hist.*, **13**, 37–50.

Kemp, M. (1970). A drawing for the Fabrica; and some thoughts upon the Vesalius muscle men. *Med. Hist.*, **14**, 277–88.

Lambert, S. W., Wiegand, W., and Ivins, W. M. (1952). *Three Vesalian essays.* Macmillan, New York.

Levey, M. (1975). *High renaissance.* Penguin, Harmondsworth.

Lind, L. R. (1969). *The Epitome of Andreas Vesalius ...* The M. I. T. Press, Cambridge, MA.

Lindberg, S. G. (1953). Chrestien Wechel and Vesalius. *Lychnos*, 50–74.

Lindeboom, G. A. (1964). *Andreas Vesalius 1514–64. ...* Erven F. Bohn, Haarlem.

Moes, R. J. (1976). Andreas Vesalius and the anatomy of the upper extremity. *J. Hand Surg.*, **1**, 23–8.

O'Malley, C. D. (ed.) (1959). *Thomas Geminus Compendiosa totius anatomie delineatio: A facsimile...* Dawson, London.

O'Malley, C. D. (1964). *Andreas Vesalius of Brussels 1514–1564.* University of California Press, Berkeley.

O'Malley, C. D. (1964). Andreas Vesalius 1514–1564: *In memoriam. Med. Hist.*, **8**, 299–308.

O'Malley, C. D. (1965). *English medical humanists: Thomas Linacre and John Caius.* University of Kansas Press, Lawrence.

Rosand, D. and Muraro, M. (1976). *Titian and the Venetian woodcut.* International Exhibitions Foundation, Washington.

Saunders, J. B. de C. M. and O'Malley, C. D. (1950). *The illustrations from the works of Andreas Vesalius of Brussels.* World Publishing, Cleveland.

Sigerist, H. E. *et al.* (1943). [Symposium on Andreas Vesalius]. *Bull. Hist. Med.*, **14**, 541–717.

Singer, C. (1961). Eighteen years of Vesalian Studies. *Med. Hist.*, **5**, 210–20.

Singer, C. and Rabin, C. (1946). *A prelude to modern science ... the 'Tabulae anatomicae sex' of Vesalius.* The Wellcome Historical Medical Museum, London.

Oporinus

Bietenholz, P. G. (1971). *Basle and France in the sixteenth century.* . . . Droz, Geneva.

Rostenberg, L. (1944). Johann Oporin, printer, publisher, and scholar: 1507–68. *Library Quart.* **14**, 207–13.

Steinmann, M. (1967). *Johannes Oporinus.* . . . Helbing and Lichtenhahn, Basle.

Charles Estienne

Armstrong, E. (1954). *Robert Estienne: Royal printer* . . . . Cambridge University Press.

Herrlinger, R. (1967). Carolus Stephanus and Stephanus Riverius (1530–1545). *Clio Med.,* **2**, 275–87.

Huard, P. and Grmek, M. D. (1965). *L'Œuvre de Charles Estienne et l'école anatomique.* Au cercle du livre précieux, Paris.

Kellett, C. E. (1955). Perino del Vaga et les illustrations pour l'anatomie d'Estienne. *Aesculape,* **37**, 74–89.

Kellett, C. E. (1957). A note on Rosso and the illustrations to Charles Estienne's De dissectione. *J. Hist. Med.,* **12**, 325–36.

Kellett, C. E. (1964). Two anatomies. *Med. Hist.* **8**, 342–53.

National Gallery of Canada (1973). *Fontainebleau: L'art en France 1528–1610.* National Gallery, Ottawa.

Rath, G. (1964). Charles Estienne: contemporary of Vesalius. *Med. Hist.,* **8**, 354–9.

Bartolomeo Eustachio

Belloni, L. (1969). Testimonianze dell'anatomico Bartolomeo Eustachi . . .. *Physis,* **11**, 69–88.

Belloni, L. (1981). Ancora sul manoscritto 'De dissensionibus ac controversiis anatomicis' di Bartolomeo Eustachi. *Physis,* **23**, 581–7.

Eden, A. R. and Opland, J. (1982). Bartolommeo Eustachio's 'De auditus organis' and the unique murder plot in Shakespeare's 'Hamlet'. *New Eng. J. Med.,* **307**, 259–61.

O'Malley, C. D. (1971), Bartolomeo Eustachi: an epistle on the organs of hearing . . . *Clio. Med,* **6**, 49–62.

6

Consolidation

DURING THE years from 1522 to 1541 the printing and publishing house of the Giunta family of Venice produced a number of editions in Latin of Galen's complete works, the most carefully collated being the 1541 issue to which Vesalius contributed. This *Opera* included the *Usefulness of parts* and other of Galen's anatomical and physiological writings. The house of Froeben based their 1542 edition on this triumph of international humanist scholarship, initiated by Lucantonio Giunta. Certainly anatomists themselves on occasion, as well as printers, would initiate the publication of their own work: this may have been the case with Berengario and his *Commentaria*. Eustachio planned, and partly carried through, an illustrated work on the whole of anatomy; most of his plates, as we have seen, did not find a publisher until the eighteenth century, and his text was never completed or has been lost. Printer/publisher and scholar/scientist often had the same background, with the same sort of education: Oporinus was a humanist scholar, Froeben a specialist in Greek publication and a friend to the city's humanists, and the presses in Basle that they controlled published work by the scholars and scientists Andreas Vesalius and Felix Platter. The relationship of humanist printer and anatomical scholar was even closer with Simon de Colines and Charles Estienne in Paris. In a different context, some publishers—Schott and

Egenolff for instance in the German states—seemed to be able to exercise considerable control over their medical authors, such as Ryff, with direct commissions.

Books, newly printed, were distributed across Europe by agents of the publisher, with the book fair at Frankfurt as a major centre. They would be bought, then as now, if the potential customers' desire to own the book was matched by a willingness to part with the required sum. The print-run of a book in the sixteenth century would most likely be of the order of a thousand copies, sometimes as many as three thousand, rarely more. Twelve years after the *Fabrica* was issued, another edition was produced by the same printer/publisher with the text re-set and with the wood-blocks slightly modified to make the identification numbers and letters more clearly visible. (One presumes the first edition was sold out.) The book was widely distributed, and—for the most part—favourably received.

Over the first hundred years of its existence, the role of printing had been to disseminate texts, and, from about 1500, in addition to disseminate illustrated texts. From the time of Vesalius and Estienne, illustrated texts in anatomy became the predominant format, so that by 1650 anatomical knowledge was conveyed as much by illustration as by text. What was found useful and acceptable was naturally enough copied, as it would have been in earlier centuries when texts and illustrations were circulated in manuscript. Dissemination of illustrated anatomy books led to further demand, and this was met by copies and modifications. The illustrations in Vesalius' works were the ones most frequently copied and modified, for few other publications of this kind were as desirable and available. His predecessors' work was obviously less complete, and the figures of his contemporary, Estienne, were much less satisfactory and less effective. Most of Eustachio's plates were unpublished. Leonardo's work remained private and unprinted. Canano's work on the muscles was published only in part. Other anatomical texts were incomplete, or not illustrated, or both. Thus if any work was to be used as a basis of an illustrated anatomy it would be most likely to be that of Vesalius. Hence the centrality of his work in the hundred years following 1543. The alternative for an anatomist, or for a publisher, was to commission an entirely new series of illustrations—a lengthy, difficult, and costly business for which the printer/publisher, the author, and the illustrator might indeed be neither equipped nor prepared.

That Vesalius, his illustrators, and his printers had done such a good job of presenting a complete anatomy was due to a remarkable conjunction of diverse skills and imagination: from Vesalius, an education in Galenic and Renaissance medicine, especially in anatomy, and a dedication to dissection in pursuit of knowledge; from the artists, a sophistication in representing, on a plane surface, solid objects including the human figure; from the Venetian wood-cutters, a skill highly developed over the previous fifty years; and from the printer/publisher, ability and imagination in using every known device to make understandable the hundreds of cross references between illustration and text without diminishing the clarity of the one or the scholarship of the other.

But the *Fabrica*, and its companion volume, the *Epitome*, did not meet all needs: the *format*, the *cost*, and the *language* of these books were inappropriate for certain groups of customers and their particular requirements.

The Format: the *Fabrica* is a very big book. So extensive and so dense is its text that it has only once been translated *in toto* into another language (Oporinus' issue of a German translation—without illustrations—in 1543). The *Epitome*, although shorter, is an even larger folio. It should be remembered that many books in the sixteenth and seventeenth century were produced in sizes suitable for a pocket.

That there are still extant many copies of the *Fabrica* in good condition signifies that it was not often read to destruction. Fewer copies of the *Epitome* remain (was the print-run the same?); the others probably suffered that fate, especially if the unbound sheets of the *Epitome* were used as broadsides.

Cost: the extraordinary pains taken to produce fine woodcuts (Vesalius complained of their costliness) and to design and print to the highest standard the texts, references, and cuts, combined with the costs of the excellent paper used (which may have amounted to 40 per cent or so of the total costs of production)—all this would without doubt raise the price of the *Fabrica* and the *Epitome* beyond the means of many medical men and other potential purchasers, certainly beyond the means of the ordinary medical student.

Language: Vesalius was particularly mindful of the needs of surgeons. Training in surgery was provided in the universities of north Italy: indeed Vesalius was professor of both anatomy and surgery at Padua. In France, England, and other countries, however, a knowledge of surgery, even for those such as Paré or Banister whose practice brought them into the highest levels of society, was obtained outside universities. The trainees did not require a knowledge of Latin, yet their need to know anatomy was well recognized as being as great or greater than that of physicians. Moreover, the sale of medical works was, at that time, not confined to physicians and surgeons; there was a public, literate in their own language but not in Latin, who wished to keep abreast of the latest thought, and who could afford to buy books, including medical books.

Purpose and use: In spite of Sylvius' criticisms, Vesalius' books were used in two ways: first, when investigating anatomy in a scholarly manner (the marginal referencing to classical and contemporary work is extensive in the *Fabrica*), and secondly, when investigating anatomy at the dissection table. Many readers would not have had the library resources or the time and inclination to consult authorities. Moreover the book was less useful when subjects for dissection were not available, as must have been the case with general readers, or were only available from time to time, as was the case for medical students in many universities.

Particular requirements: The *Epitome* provided a survey of anatomy; for more details, the reader turned to the more complex illustrations and text of the *Fabrica*. As we have had cause to remark earlier, one of the consequences of printed anatomical illustrations is that they are 'correctable'. Mistakes were identified by Vesalius' contemporaries, and with this came, in some, an urge to produce figures that they considered more truthfully represented structures seen on dissection—not that the new figures were, in actual execution, always an overall improvement on those in the *Fabrica*. Where systems or regions of the body had been incompletely or inadequately dealt with, there was a desire to expand them by more detailed monographs.

When considering representative illustrations of anatomy in the hundred years following 1543, questions therefore arise concerning format, costs, language, use, and particular requirements. Few artists, anatomists, and their publishers attempted to produce, from scratch, totally new illustrations to a totally new text on the anatomy of the human body. The Casserian illustrations, along with the work of Berrettini and Martinez, remained either unpublished or incomplete at the time of the anatomists' deaths; their work is considered in Chapter 7. In this chapter we discuss some illustrated anatomical texts that owe much, directly or indirectly, to the work of Vesalius; in addition an example of an original work that focused on a particular aspect of functional anatomy is included.

It does not seem profitable to discuss plagiarism' at great length. Many of those authors that followed Vesalius acknowledged their debt to him, and, through him, to his illustrators, whose names Vesalius had not made known; they gave this acknowledgement more or less prominence. If an acknowledgement is given, then plagiarism—the passing off of another's work as one's own—is not present. Questions of *copyright* depend entirely on legal definitions and interpretations. These took time to develop, and evolved differently in different political regions. (There was no international copyright union until very recent times.) Vesalius had 'copyrighted' his work under authority from Emperor Charles V and the Pope, but the legal strictures seemed unenforceable, which left Vesalius testily complaining when others used work to which he had devoted such intense effort and dedication. Certainly he himself owed much to his predecessors; but equally certainly his books established his fame, if not his fortune. Imitation, in this case, was indeed a sincere form of flattery.

Juan de Valverde de Amusco (or Hamusco) (c. 1525–c. 1587)

In 1556, a year after the publication of the second complete edition of Vesalius' *Fabrica*, a book on human anatomy in the Spanish language was issued at Rome: *Historia de la composición del cuerpo humano* ... It was written by Valverde. In 1559 a decree by Philip II ordered Spanish students studying outside Spain to return home—they were too exposed to heresies. Such circumstances would not seem propitious to the success of this textbook. As it turned out, Valverde's anatomy became remarkably popular, appearing in many editions—Cushing lists fifteen up to 1647; it was printed in Rome, Venice, Antwerp, and Amsterdam by notable houses; and translated into Italian, Latin, and Dutch/Flemish. Jewish doctors at the court in Constantinople in the seventeenth century consulted their copies of Valverde. The success of the book owed much to the copperplate illustrations, nearly all of which were taken over from the woodcuts in the Vesalian books. As Valverde explains in the address to the reader:

Although it seemed to some of my friends that I should make new illustrations without using those of Vesalius, I did not do so, in order to avoid the confusion that could follow, not knowing clearly in what I agree or in what I disagree with him, and because his illustrations are so well done it would look like envy or malignity not to take advantage of them. [This, and the following translations, are taken from Guerra's most helpful account (1967).]

Valverde was thus no plagiarist, but nevertheless Vesalius was highly critical: '... Valverde, who never put his hand to a dissection and is ignorant of medicine as well as of the primary disciples, undertook to expound our art in the Spanish language only for the sake of shameful profit'. This comment is taken from Vesalius' 1564 publication on Falloppio's work. This was a sad return for the praise given by Valverde to his detractor: Vesalius 'has, without doubt, excelled everyone before [him] in this subject'. Valverde admired particularly Vesalius' ability to recognize the difference between the structure of monkeys, the basis of Galenic anatomy, and that of human beings: Vesalius 'began to open the eyes of many, showing that we are not to believe everything that is written [by Galen]'. Further praise came from Valverde, but this time somewhat tempered by a recognition that Vesalius did not get everything right; Valverde was not going to replace total reliance on Galen with total subservience to Vesalius:

[In certain things] he seems to have used less diligence than was required (perhaps tired of such arduous work), those things I will point out in the proper place, more with the intention of not missing a thing in this history than with the desire to reprimand him to whom we all owe so much.

To what can we attribute the success of Valverde's anatomy? First, its format, although folio, was significantly smaller than Vesalius' (approximately 29.0 × 19.5 cm compared with 43.0 × 28.0 cm). The text, entirely by Valverde though using Vesalius as a guide, was shorter, more direct, rearranged in a simpler manner, and less scholarly. Secondly, its cost was probably much less than that of the *Fabrica*, and more within the means of medical men and students. Thirdly, it was in a vernacular language, and would be available to Spaniards not fully at ease with Latin. Many of its later editions were also in living languages, but a Latin translation (by Michael Colombo, Venice, 1589, the son of Valverde's teacher Realdo Colombo), made the work available to scholars across Europe. Fourthly, Valverde's text was, as the author stated: 'a plain account in the manner of a commentary on what I have seen in corpses'. If readers wanted more, they were referred to Vesalius, who was, Valverde said, better read by experienced anatomists who have frequent access to dissections. He did not wish to injure Vesalius by 'exiling' his work from Spain—Vesalius' work could be read with greater understanding if the reader had first used Valverde's succinct account, the whole of anatomy in just over two hundred pages of text, as opposed to the *Fabrica's* more than eight hundred pages. Lastly, in Valverde's illustrations, that is in the re-drawn and engraved copies of selected illustrations from Vesalius (two-thirds of Vesalius' illustrations were used), many points were noted as being corrected or improved. Guerra (1967) has most helpfully given a careful description of these changes. However, Valverde, his artist, and his engraver, while perhaps improving some details, degraded others. As an example of this, comparison may be made between the woodcut of the fifth muscle-man of Vesalius—our *Plate 32*, p. 153—and the corresponding engraving from Valverde — our *Fig. 6.1*. It will be noticed straight away that the copperplate has been engraved from the printed Vesalian figure, and the subject is therefore facing in the other direction when the plate is printed. The stance of the dissected man has been changed so that one leg is now kneeling on the tree stump.

Improvements made by Valverde include shortening (though too much so) the upper extent of the rectus abdominis muscles, elimination of the scalene muscle passing anterior to the first rib, and clearer delineation of both the adductor muscles (though still inaccurate) and those of the antero-lateral compartments of the leg. Features that are better shown in the *Fabrica* woodcut include the tendons and small muscles on the dorsum of the feet and the ribs and intercostal musculature.

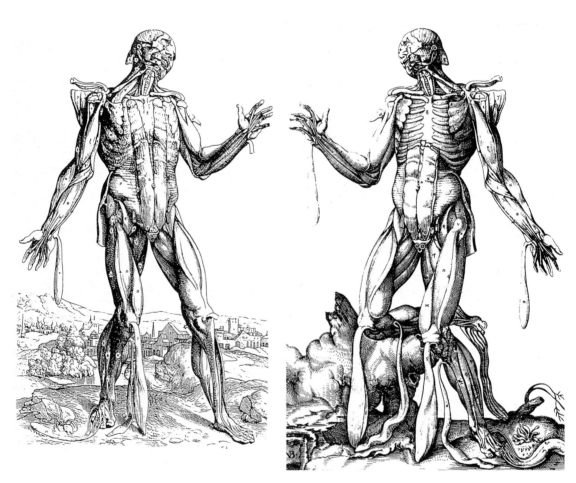

6.1 Comparison of Vesalius' fifth muscle figure with that reproduced by Valverde.

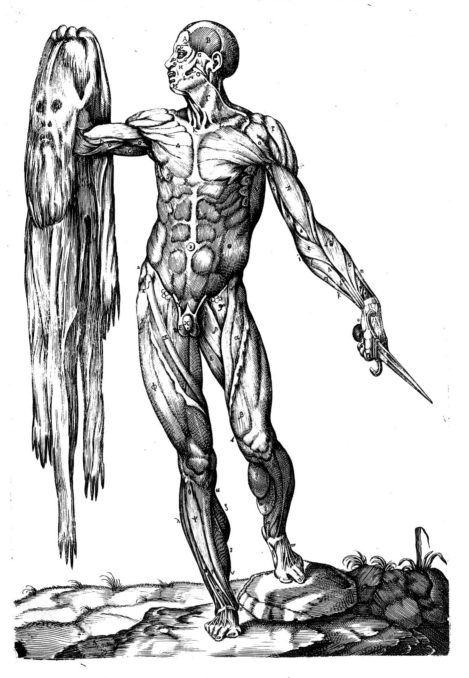

6.2 Flayed man with own skin, from Valverde, *Historia*, 1556.

It may also be noted that Valverde intentionally kept the Vesalian lettering, to facilitate reference to the text of the *Fabrica*. Valverde suggested that a student refer to the larger work for greater detail.

In Valverde's text there are to be seen fifteen apparently non-Vesalian illustrations, but, as we shall discover when we discuss the plate of the pregnant woman (*Plate 51*), some of these are composites derived mostly from originals in the *Fabrica*. However, the composite pictures are often quite striking to our eyes, notably these: an *écorché* figure from Book II—a flayed man holding not only a dagger (impossible to use as a skinning knife) but also the flayed skin of a bearded man (*Fig. 6.2*); the abdominal wall and abdominal contents from Book III, in which a man holds a dissected flap in his teeth (*Fig. 6.3*); and the figures showing the anatomy of the thorax from Book IV—a dissected man with his hands in the corpse of another, figures taken from two separate illustrations in the *Fabrica*(*Fig.6.4*). These are mannerist conceits. One of them — the flayed man—derives from classical times, from images of Hercules holding a lion's skin and of Apollo flaying Marsyas; the bearded face is taken more directly from a similar figure in the Last Judgement section of the Sistine paintings by Michelangelo, an ironic self-portrait by this artist. Valverde's artist was probably the Spaniard, Gaspar Becerra (1520–70), who had assisted Michelangelo in his work at the Vatican and was known as an anatomist. (The engraver was Nicolas Beatrizet, a Frenchman.) The Vesalian torsos, demonstrating the anatomy of the intestines, etc, were based on much-admired Grecian, and Greco-Roman, sculptures (see *Fig. 5.6, p. 139*); Valverde's artist used a different Roman conceit—the torsos showing the abdominal contents *in situ* are clothed with the breast- and belly-plates of a suit of Imperial armour (*Fig. 6.5*).

Juan de Valverde's academic life was tied up with that of Vesalius' successor in Padua, Realdo Colombo. Valverde went with Colombo from Padua to Pisa, and then, in 1548, to Rome. At Rome Valverde was personal physician to Cardinal Juan Alvarez de Toledo, the son of the Duke of Alba, Spanish governor of the Low Countries. He dedicated his anatomy text to this patron. The Roman ecclesiastical authorities did not disapprove of opening corpses: autopsies were performed in 1550 by Colombo on a cardinal—Valverde was present—and, in 1556, on Ignatius Loyola.

Before the move to Rome, Colombo wrote of Valverde: 'an uneducated man, a half-knower, who learned something from me about anatomy'. It was however in Valverde's text that the public first could read an argued account of the pulmonary circulation: ibn an-Nafis (1210-88) and Servetus (1511-53) stated, boldly, that the blood passed through the lungs as it travels from the right to the left side of the heart. Valverde gave reasons: the interventricular septum was impermeable; the pulmonary vein is indeed full of blood (some contemporary opinion thought that it contained air)—he and Realdo Colombo had many times experimented on living and dead animals and demonstrated this fact. Valverde may possibly have heard Colombo's views, but probably not Servetus', on the pulmonary circulation—views that Colombo did not put into print until 1559 in *De re anatomica . . .*, Venice, an unillustrated treatise.

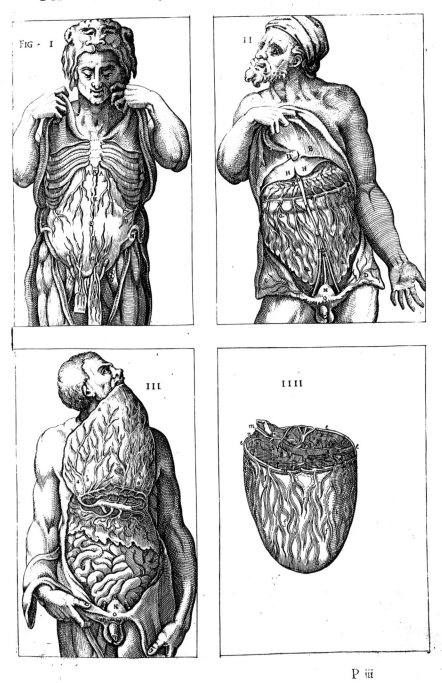

6.3   Abdominal wall and contents, from Valverde *Historia*, 1556.

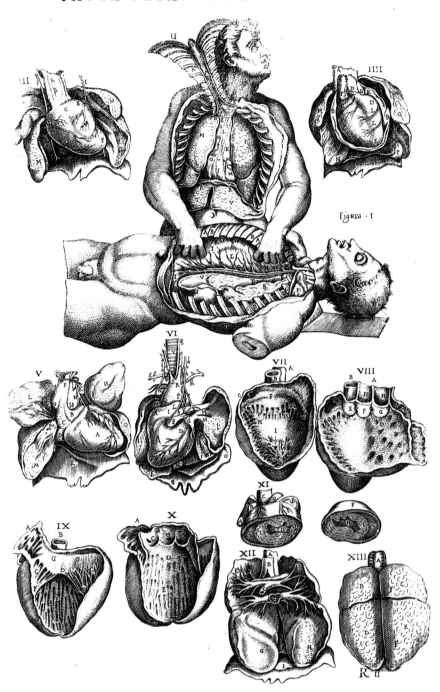

6.4   A dissected man dissects, from Valverde *Historia*, 1556.

As a young man, Valverde wrote a book of hygiene, including advice on diet and behaviour in relation to mental and physical health—a sort of 'advice to princes' on these matters. It was first issued in Paris by Charles Estienne, anatomist, printer, and publisher.

As a postscript it may be noted here that Valverde's anatomy had been preceded by another book in which the text was in Spanish and the illustrations were from Vesalius: *Libro de la anathomia del hombre*, Valladolid, S. Martinez, 1551. The figures were very crudely reproduced by an unskilled draughtsman; the head in many figures is tiny in comparison to the rest of the body.

Some books by Valverde

1. *De animi et corporis sanitate tuenda libellus . . .*, Paris, Charles Estienne, 1552. [Venetian edition 1553.]

2. *Historia de la composición del cuerpo humano . . .*, Rome, Antonio de Salamanca and Antonio Lafreri, 1556 [in Spanish].

3. *Anatomica del corpo humano . . .*, Rome, same publishers, 1560 [in Italian].

4. *Anatome corporis humani . . .*, Venice, Giunti, 1589 [in Latin: translated by Michael Colombo]. In a 1586 Giunti Italian edition four extraordinary mannerist muscle-men were added. These are not Vesalian figures, but are of little anatomical interest.

5. *Vivae imagines partium corporis humani . . .*, Antwerp, Christopher Plantin, 1566, in Latin. Flemish edition, same publishers, 1568.

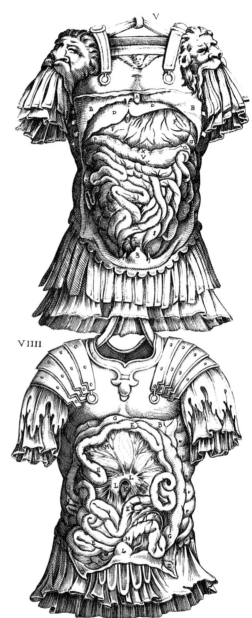

6.5 Dissected torso clothed in armour, from Valverde, *Historia*, 1556.

51 *Gravida.* Tabula sesta del libro tercero, from Valverde, *Historia . . .* , 1556. Engraving (Wellcome Institute Library). 24.0 × 15.6 cm.

The main figure is of a pregnant woman with the abdominal wall and peritoneum opened to show the gravid uterus (L), liver (E), stomach (F) with transverse mesocolon (G, H), and peritoneal folds [? broad ligament of the uterus] indicated by (OI) and (OK). The bladder (R) is hardly visible, but the median and the two lateral (nowadays confusingly termed 'medial') umbilical ligaments (the remains of the urachus and umbilical arteries) are shown hanging down over the right thigh. They come to a common point, representative of the umbilicus, and then a single cord, the ligamentum teres, continues onwards. This latter has been cut; the upper portion can be seen, entering the liver, between the two letters (E).

This is one of some fifteen illustrations of Valverde's not to be found as such in Vesalius' *Fabrica.* Valverde has surrounded it (figs xxxi–xxxiiii) with drawings of human placentae, which replace (and are a great improvement on) the non-human placentae that Vesalius featured. The amniotic fluid draining out in figures xxxii and xxxiii is an interesting touch, as also is the baby sitting on the floor with its umbilical cord around its neck.

Valverde has generally been considered—not least by Vesalius—to be a relatively ignorant plagiarist of Vesalius. True it is that over two hundred of Valverde's illlustrations are 'after' Vesalius, even to their actual lettering. But in his address to the reader Valverde gave full recognition to Vesalius' work, though saying that in certain cases he will correct or modify it; thus the charge of plagiarism must fail. However, the claims of such as Francisco Guerra (1967) that a goodly number of Valverde's illustrations 'improve' on those of Vesalius cannot always be validated when one examines the two authors' works side by side. For example, Valverde's frontal skeleton shows the coccyx well below the level of the ischial spines; the radius and ulna are very poor, and the fibula too thick; however, the pubic symphysis is an improvement on that of Vesalius. In Valverde's Book II, Tabula I the calf muscles are mainly imaginary, and the pectoralis major and deltoid most unanatomical. Certainly some of Valverde's illustrations do improve on those in the *Fabrica*—in Book II, Tabula VI he has eliminated those depressingly non-human scalene muscles, while in the same Book, Tabula XIII, the cut-off leg is much more clearly shown, as is also the case in Tabula XIIII. However only a few of his illustrations demonstrate innovative endeavour. *Plate 51* has been selected because it is one of them— certainly no real equivalent appears in Vesalius. Nevertheless it must have been inspired by a woodcut in the *Fabrica*, namely Book V, page 377. In this, the female figure is beheaded, the arms chopped off through the middle of the humerus, and the legs similarly through the mid- thigh. The Vesalian figure shows a normal non-pregnant uterus, the colon is differently arranged, and no liver is featured. In other words, Valverde modified the Vesalian drawing and placed the altered viscera in a whole female figure—same perspective but different content. Interestingly, Valverde includes in his Book III the above Vesalian drawing, but there is more neck, more leg, and the umbilical ligaments are draped to the right not the left. It must be said that the

TAB. SESTA DEL LIB. TERCERO

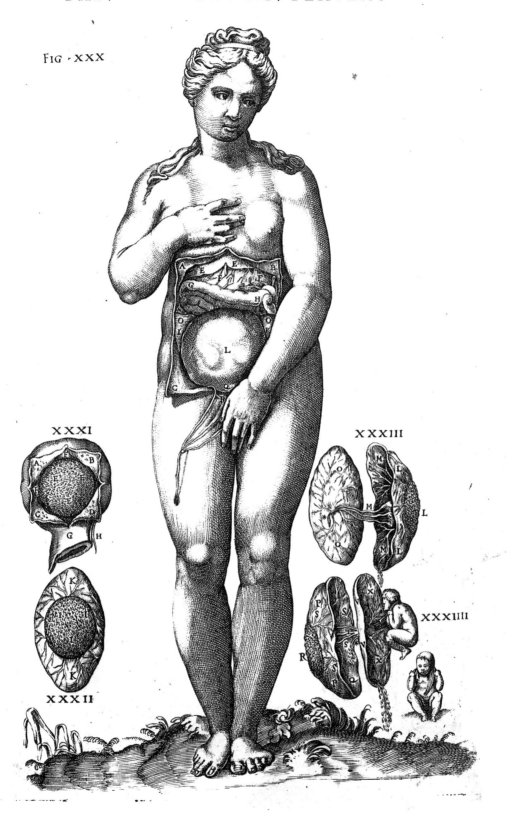

FIG · XXX

XXXI

XXXII

XXXIII

XXXIIII

PLATE 51

copperplate of Valverde is much clearer in detail and lettering than the woodcut of Vesalius.

There is no doubt that Valverde was much read and studied—the many editions of his work testify to this—so perhaps in some ways it is a pity that he felt constrained to copy the format and perspective of Vesalius' *Fabrica* illustrations so closely.

Coiter, Platter, and Bauhin

In the decade or two after Vesalius the science of anatomy must have seemed to some to have reached a perfection beyond which it would be difficult to make progress. Some subjects within anatomy, however, had not been exhaustively considered or illustrated in the *Fabrica*, and to these, particularly to developmental and to comparative anatomy, a number of investigators turned.

A fine series of studies by *Volcher Coiter (1534–76)* exemplified these new interests. In his book *Externarum et internarum principalium humani corporis* ..., Nuremberg, 1572 there are to be found large illustrations printed from copper engravings of skeletons of immature humans, as well as those of a range of animals — frog, tortoise, monkey, domestic fowl, mouse, bat. ... Coiter admired Vesalius greatly: *omnium in re anatomica princeps.*

Coiter, a Friesian from Groningen, had had an excellent medical and scientific education at Montpellier in France and in Italy, including work with Eustachio at Rome. His most influential teachers were Falloppio and Aldrovandi. His interests in development are said to have preceded that of Falloppio, and his work on the embryology of the hen to have been the first since Aristotle. Coiter also anticipated Harvey in embryology and by his studies on the living heart. He held academic posts at Bologna and Perugia, but his career in Italy was cut short when he was imprisoned by the Inquisition. The Counter-Reformation looked with suspicion on those anatomists and medical doctors who challenged received opinions. Heterodoxy in medicine could spill over into heresy in religious matters and *vice versa*; Servetus was a notorious example. Paracelsus too, in the decades after his death, was regarded as a dangerous influence by the zoologist and critic Konrad Gesner and others. Vesalius himself may have come under observation in this respect in his Paduan days. The humanist Günther von Andernach, who was Vesalius' anatomy teacher, adopted unorthodox religious views.

On his release from prison, Coiter left for Augsburg; he later went to Nuremberg, where he became the city's chief physician and anatomist. He bequeathed to this city an *écorché* statue, which is shown in a very fine portrait of Coiter in oils, painted in 1575 and owned by the city library.

Included in the illustrations to the 1572 text, published at Nuremberg, were modified Vesalian skeletons; in one, for example, a scythe replaced the non-functional spade in the original. More significantly, Coiter not only altered but actually improved the illustration of the weeping skeleton, repositioning the figure so that it showed the plantar aspects of the bones of the left foot. Other of the copperplates were quite original, owing nothing to Vesalius. Some were inscribed as having been drawn by Coiter himself. In these delicate figures one may see the potential of copper engraving for precise anatomical delineation brought to a sort of perfection. The skeletal figures of a child were particularly admired.

Some books by Coiter

1. *De ossibus et cartilaginibus humani corporis tabulae*, Bologna, J. Rossi, 1566.

2. *Externarum et internarum principalium humani corporis partium tabulae*, Nuremberg, Theodor Gerlach, 1572 (other copies 1573). (In this book *tabulae* refers to the text, not to the illustrations. There is a section of the book: *De foetus humani et infantum ossibus*.)

3. *Lectiones Gabrielis Fallopii de partibus similaribus humani corporis* ..., Nuremberg, Theodor Gerlach, 1575.

Felix Platter, sometimes Plater, Platerius, 1536–1614, was born in Basle, and after studies at Montpellier, where he and Coiter were friends, he returned there to become, aged twenty-four years, Professor of Medicine. In 1583 the publishing house of Froeben issued Platter's *De corporis humani structura et usu....* The text in the first two of the three sections of this is in the form of tables where the structures of the body are categorized and bracketed in a complex classification. It is the third book that is illustrated: *Corporis humani partium per icones delineatarum explicatio.* This has a separate title-page, and copies are noted dated 1581. The fifty single-page illustrations are each accompanied by a page of explanatory text; the reader is spared the searchings often needed when reading the *Fabrica*.

The illustrations were etched, rather than engraved, on the copperplate; this is a freer, less laborious and less expensive procedure, but one unsuitable for precise work, so important in representing anatomical detail. Some of the etchings, but probably not all, were done by Abel Stimmer, brother to the better-known Tobias. In his introductory remarks to the reader, Platter regrets the casual work of the artists, and suggests reference should be made to the *Fabrica* for doubtful points. Apparently Platter was offered the actual woodcuts, still in Basle, from Vesalius' 1555 publication, but the question of expense made him turn to reproduction by etching. One plate is taken from Coiter (none apparently from Valverde); most are direct copies of Vesalius— a few showing decided improvements. At least one appears to be an original illustration: our *Plate 54.* The skeletal figure is more a symbol than a useful anatomical drawing: the skeleton holds an hour-glass, a reminder of time passing and the approach of death. This emblem was, as we have seen, used by other anatomists at least as far back as Berengario in 1521. Much better in every way is an illustration of a skull (*Fig. 6.6b*), which, as Herrlinger (1970) demonstrated, is a copy, but an *improved* copy, of a woodcut in the *Fabrica* (*Fig. 6.6a*).

Platter's successor as chief physician to the city of Basle was *Gaspard*, or *Kaspar, Bauhin* (1560– 1624). He received a scientific and medical education in many parts of Europe, concentrating on

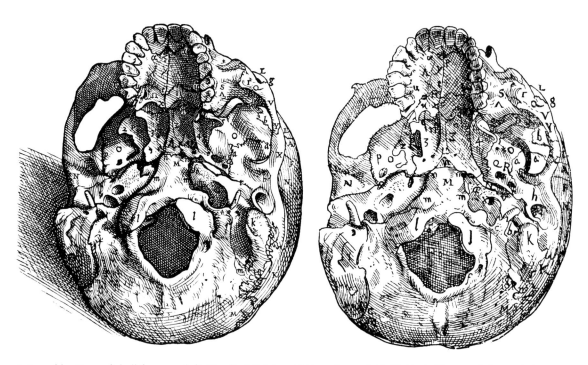

6.6a and b Base of skull from, on left, Vesalius' *Fabrica*, 1543, and, on right, Platter's *De corporis humani structura*, 1583.

two subjects: anatomy, which he pursued in winter; and botany, which took him into the countryside in summer. His first teacher was his father, a French physician, an Anabaptist, who had escaped religious persecution by fleeing to Basle. He studied under Platter, and spent a year and a half with Fabrici in Padua. Bauhin also anatomized at Bologna, Montpellier, Paris, and Tübingen. He returned to Basle aged twenty-one to receive his doctorate, and to be appointed to the faculty of medicine. A year later Bauhin was made Professor of Greek; later in his life, in 1615, he was appointed Professor of Medicine. He secured for the University, of which he was Rector four times, a permanent anatomy theatre, and, impartially, a botanic garden—one of the earliest in Europe.

Bauhin was responsible for introducing a more rational approach to anatomical nomenclature; it is quite appropriate that Basle was, in 1895, the site of an international conference to standardize anatomical names. The lists developed there became known as the B.N.A. (*Basle nomina anatomica*).

Bauhin's anatomical publications, originally issued in the years 1588 to 1620, were intended to make the new, revisionist, post-Vesalian anatomy more generally available. The format of his major anatomical collection *Theatrum anatomicum ...*, 1605, is a chunky quarto of more than thirteen hundred pages. It was written in Latin, probably with the needs of medical students and university-trained physicians in mind. In 1615 the text was used by Helkiah Crooke in an

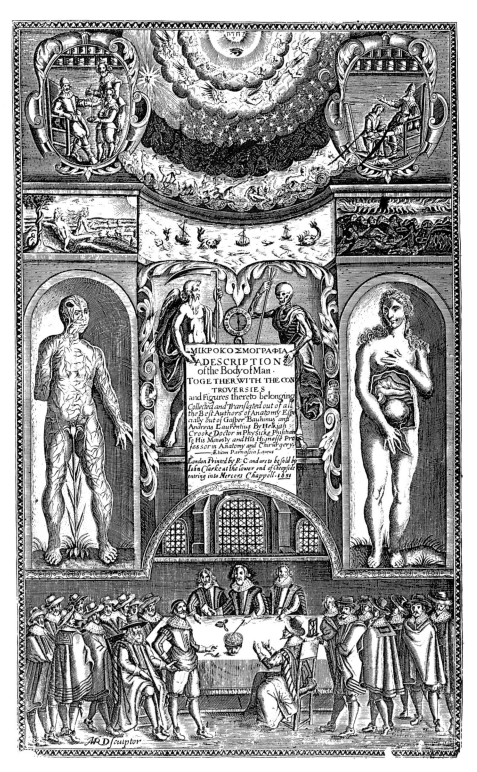

6.7 Title-page of H. Crooke's *Microcosmographia*, 1655.

English-language version *Microcosmographia. A description of the body of man* ... London (*Fig. 6.7*). It would have been a valuable adjunct to have by one when dissecting—a practical anatomy text in the tradition of much earlier texts, including that of Berengario.

Like Valverde, Coiter, and Platter before him Bauhin used Vesalius' illustrations. Pictures were also taken from the works of other anatomists; these he names in an appendix to the book. They are, in the order and with the dates he uses:

Carpus [Berengario da Carpi]   1522
Dryander   1537 and 1540
Stephanus [Charles Estienne]   1539[1], 1545
Vesalius   1543, 1555, and 1568
Paré   1561
Valverde   1559, 1566
Varolius   1573
Coiter   1575
Platter   1583
Salomon Albertus   1584
Valverde, in Latin   1589
Laurentius [du Laurens]   1600
Fabricus 1600
Casserius 1600[2]
Philippus Ingrassias 1603

Some books by Bauhin

1. *De corporis humani partibus externis tractatus*, Basle, S. Henricpetrus 1588.

2. *De corporis humani fabrica: libri IIII ...*, Basle, S. Henricpetrus [1590].

3. *Anatomes ... liber primus et secundus ...*, Basle, S. Henricpetrus [1591 and 1592]. This includes book 1 above.

4. *Theatrum anatomicum novis figuris aeneis illustratum ...*, Frankfurt, Matthew Becker 1605. Another edition, Frankfurt, J. T. de Bry, is dated 1621, but it is unillustrated; it is usually bound together with the illustrations under the title: *Vivae imagines partium corporis humani ...*, same publisher, but dated 1620. In this latter book, each of the plates faces its accompanying explanation, as in the anatomical

---

[1] There is no known publication in anatomy by Estienne dated 1539. Did Bauhin have the sheets of *De dissectione ...*, printed that year up to the middle of the last book, or was an *Anatomica* by C. Estienne issued before this date, as advertised in Robert Estienne's lists (see p. 170)?

[2] As we shall see, many of the copperplates of human anatomy prepared under Casserio's direction were not published until after his death in 1616. Bauhin could be referring to Casserio's work on the comparative anatomy of the larynx and the ear *De vocis auditusque ...* [1601].

text by Platter. The *Theatrum* ... is the book that Harvey used in his Linacre lectures on anatomy to the College of Physicians in London 1616.

5. *Appendix ad Theatrum anatomicum* ... was issued from Frankfurt: M. Becker with the title-page dated 1600. In the copies we have examined this *Appendix* ... was bound with the *Theatrum* ..., yet included a portrait of Bauhin dated 1605 and listings of references that continue beyond 1600.

52 Skeleton of six-month-old child, from V. Coiter, *Externarum et internarum principalium humani corporis . . . ,* 1572. Engraving (Wellcome Institute Library). 54.1 × 29.5 cm.

This drawing of the skeleton of a six-month-old child is probably the earliest attempt to illustrate such an immature skeleton. Not unnaturally it exhibits errors both of omission and commission: the facial skeleton, the sacrum, and the vertebral column generally leave something to be desired, and it must be noted that, oddly, the scapulae are absent in large part—the clavicles articulate with the acromial processes, and (g) denotes the coracoid processes (above the glenoid fossae), but of the rest of the scapulae there is no sign.

However, the illustration does show early cartilaginous epiphyses (stippled), crude though these may appear. The text describes the order of ossification of, for example, the pelvic girdle and the long limb bones. The letters (K) denote the epiphyses of the latter, (L) and (U) the compounded carpal and tarsal cartilaginous elements, (h) the costal cartilages and 1–5 the order of appearance of ossification centres in the sternum, 4 and 5 being bilateral.

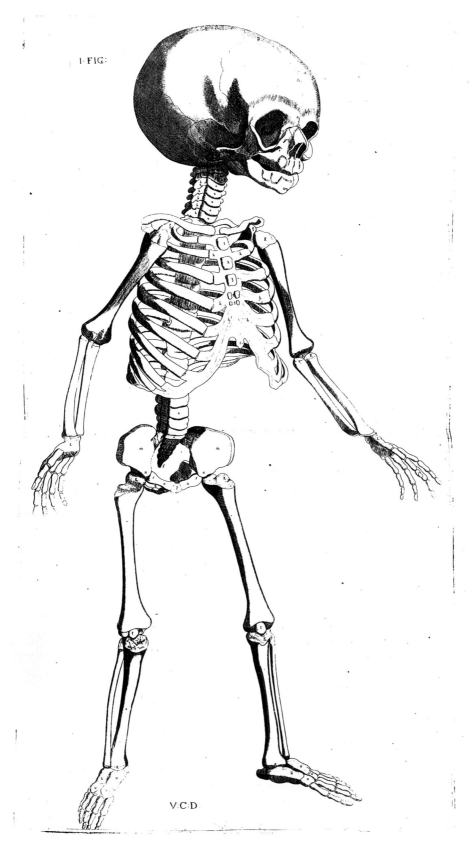

I·FIG:

V·C·D·

PLATE 52

53 Base of adult skull, from V. Coiter, *Externarum et internarum princialium humani corporis . . .*, 1573. Engraving (Cambridge University Library). 19.5 × 17.3 cm.

This is the first of two drawings of the adult skull—although it is not yet fully adult, as evidenced by the unfused suture between the sphenoid and occipital bones (nn).

Even taking into account Coiter's great interest in the skeleton, this plate of the skull base is truly excellent. Save perhaps for the portrayal of the teeth—little distinction between canines, premolars, and molars—it could almost be used without a blush in a modern text.

Especially to be commended are the curl of the lateral pterygoid plates (P3); the sutures, particularly the squamotympanic, occipitotemporal, and palato-maxillary, and those forming the pterion (P); the foramina in general (one notes the small lesser palatine); and the pleasing shading technique which brings out the texture of the skull bones so well.

Apart from the dentition, features one would like to be improved include the too-blunt pterygoid hamulus; the rounded spine of the sphenoid; the styloid processes (I), which incline too medially, and the rather peculiar insignificant mastoid processes (K), oddly different on the two sides. But really what most occupies one's thoughts is admiration at the skill and dedication of those responsible for producing this late-sixteenth-century plate. It is interesting to compare it with similar plates, such as those in Galen's *Opera Omnia*, 1538 (see *Fig. 2.17, p. 48*); Ryff, 1540 (*Plate 11, p. 59*); Vesalius' *Fabrica*, 1543, and Pauw, 1615 (*Plate 58, p. 245*); and, indeed, with those in present-day textbooks of anatomy.

With regard to the Vesalian woodcut (on page 22, repeated on pages 38 and 48 of the *Fabrica*, 1543) it is obvious that Coiter consulted this, because he employed exactly the same letters to identify certain portions of the skull. He did not, however, feature the small inconstant foramen—known eponymously as the 'foramen of Vesalius'—lying antero-medial to the foramen ovale, which is shown in the *Fabrica* drawing.

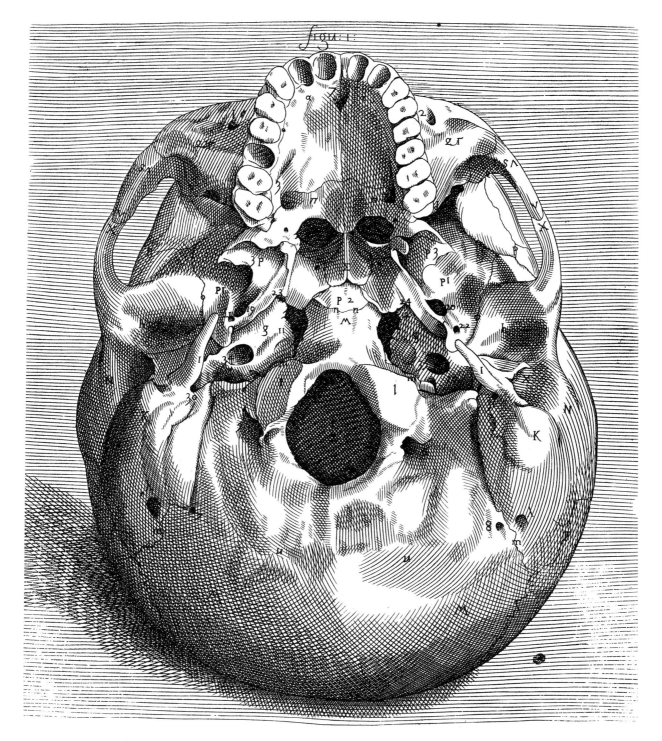

figu. 1.

PLATE 53

54 Female skeletal figure holding hour-glass, from Plate 2 in Book III of F. Platter, *De corporis humani structura* ..., 1583. Engraving (Wellcome Institute Library). 27.3 × 19.0 cm.

This illustration also appears, re-drawn, in Bauhin's *Theatrum*, 1605, though in the latter the figure is reversed, with the skeleton facing to its left; it also shows other differences—the feet point directly forwards, parallel to each other, the spine is quite straight, but with the sacrum tilted almost horizontally backwards; and the greater trochanter of the femur closely resembles a bony tumour. It must be said that both Platter and Bauhin portrayed the pelvic girdle very poorly—at first sight it would appear inadvertently to have been drawn back-to-front. The pubic symphyseal area is much better portrayed in this Platterian plate, although even so it is hardly felicitous. The lower limb bones are poorly drawn, very 'quavery' in outline; the lesser trochanters are virtually non-existent. Particularly in the dependent upper limb the ulna and radius are quite horrible, the ulna curved and the head and styloid process of the radius deformed and quite out of proportion. The tapering costal cartilages, the down-turned coracoid process, and the clavicles do not impress. Forty years after Vesalius, anatomically this is a poor skeletal figure.

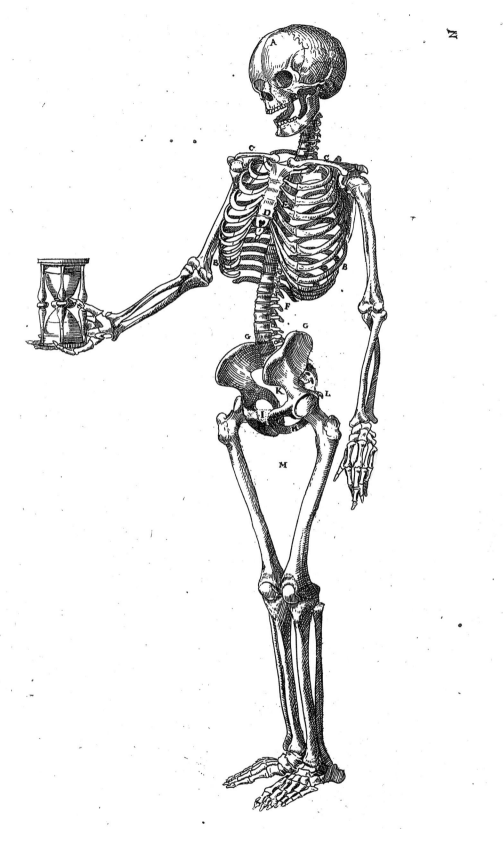

PLATE 54

55 Muscles of the torso seen from the back, from page 1047 of C. Bauhin, *Theatrum anatomicum...*, 1605. Engraving (Cambridge University Library). 15.0 × 8.6 cm.

This illustration is really a *mélange* based on the upper portions of two woodcuts in Vesalius' *Fabrica*, though in this plate the hair on the head is more curly and the indicator symbols are different. The portrayal of the superficial back muscles above the buttocks is after Vesalius' tenth muscle-man, whilst the gluteal musculature derives from the ninth.

The head is tilted and twisted to the right, and the muscles of the back are shown with trapezius removed. The splenius capitis is shown overlying semispinalis capitis; but, as represented here, it is too thick and has too constricted an origin. The deltoid (H, M), the rhomboid muscles (V), and latissimus (N) are fairly accurate, though the fascicle lines appear too horizontal in the lower portion of the latter; which in any case is aponeurotic, not muscular. A part of the external oblique can just be made out, lower right.

The positioning of supraspinatus is inaccurate, though infraspinatus (P) and teres major (O) are better; perhaps not surprisingly the teres minor is not differentiated from infraspinatus.

In the buttock the gluteus maximus and the gluteus medius are easily recognizable, but the posterior thigh muscles are different in configuration on the two sides. It is impossible to reconcile either pattern with the true state of affairs. In a later illustration in the book (Tab. XX), where the posterior thigh is shown more extensively dissected, the same musculature is depicted, and is once again markedly in error. Without doubt the *Fabrica* drawings are far more accurate than is this one from Bauhin.

LIB.IIII.   TAB.III.

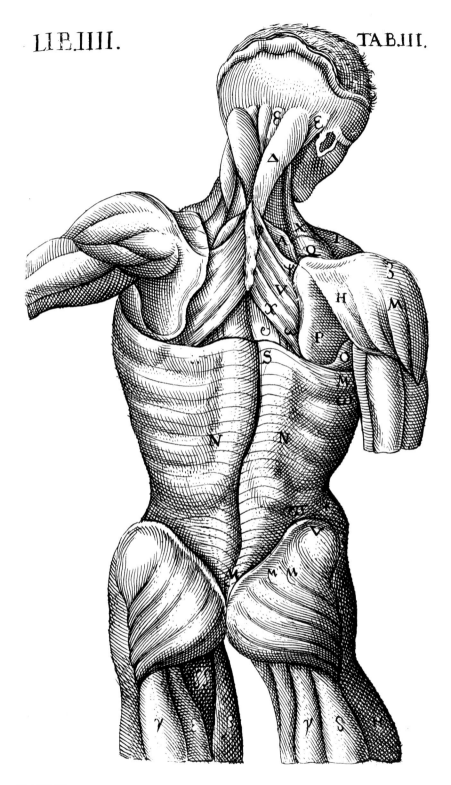

PLATE 55

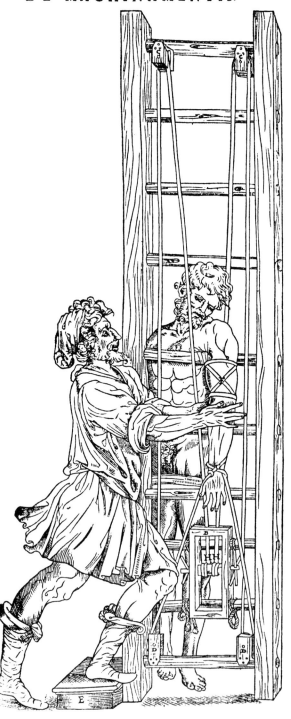

6.8 An illustration of reduction of a dislocation, from Guidi, *Chirurgia*, 1544.

Guidi, Pauw, and Vesling

Guido Guidi (in Latinized form, Vidus Vidius), c. 1508–69, is remembered chiefly for his *Chirurgia*, which contained translations into Latin of certain Greek manuscripts by Hippocrates, Galen, and Oribasius in the Library of Lorenzo de' Medici at Florence. This work by Guidi on surgery, published in 1544, stands alongside Vesalius' work on anatomy, 1543, and Fuch's on botany, 1542: all are humanist publications remarkable for the excellence of their woodcut illustrations. The *Chirurgia*, containing about two hundred woodcuts (*Fig. 6.8*), was a product of Italian–French co-operation of the time of Francis I. The Fontainebleau artist was possibly Primaticcio, more likely Salviati. The inspiration, however, was tenth-century Byzantine manuscript illustrations, derived themselves from earlier figures relating to the surgery of the Hippocratic collection. Some of the woodcuts in Guidi's book were signed with a Lorraine Cross (compare Estienne), and were from the workshop of Jollat.

Alas! Guidi published no book on anatomy, and what we have in printed work of the Fontainebleau school, in relation to anatomy, is only a single woodcut sheet of *écorchés* and skeletons by Domenico (see *Fig 5.8* on p. 162) and the illustrations, of variable quality, to be found in Estienne's *De dissectione . . .*, 1546 (see *Plates 39–45*, pp. 175–187). However, more than thirty years after Guidi's death, his namesake and relative collected together three volumes of his uncle's medical writings, the third volume being *De anatome corporis humani . . .*, 1611. This volume was illustrated by 78 copperplates, some taken from the *Fabrica*. It may be conjectured that others should be attributed to the elder Guidi (perhaps our *Plate 57*). Some—and these the weakest—were surely made for this posthumous publication (*Plate 56*). The title-page to this 1611 anatomy is a baroque extravaganza drawn and engraved by Franco Vallegio and Catarin Dollio (*Fig. 6.9*). On top of the architectural frame sits a skeleton holding an hour-glass in one hand, and in the other an apple indicating the fall from grace in Eden. Either side are the bones of the sacrum, each with two femora, making a sort of her-aldic shield. To the left and right of the title-stand two figures: one, a woman with a preg-nant uterus exposed, holding what may be a dissected uterus showing the placental site. This figure is a modification of Valverde's (see *Plate 51*, p. 219). The other figure is an *écorché* male figure holding in one hand a flaying knife and in the other his skin. The latter is again derived from one of Valverde's figures. Below there are two further skeletons, above which is a bull's skull with a floral wreath, and below them an assemblage of skulls and femora. The skeletons in this title-page are as equally far from reality as that in the first plate in the book (our *Plate 56*). The genre of all this resembles the title-page to the plates of Casserio, 1627 (see *Fig. 7.2, p. 260*); but the drawing and de-sign in the Guidi title-page is much less skilled.

Guido Guidi the elder was a Florentine, his mother a descendant of Domenico del Ghirlandaio. Guidi was a professor at the Collège Royale in Paris in the seven or so years preceding 1547, when he left to take up, at the invitation of Cosimo de' Medici, the

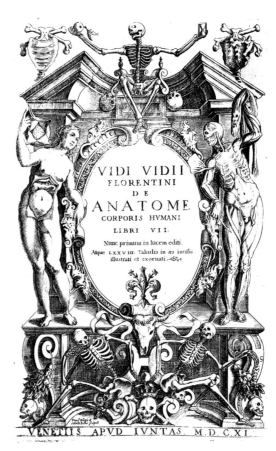

6.9   Title-page of Guidi, *De anatome*, 1611.

chair of philosophy and medicine at Pisa. (In Paris he had lived in the same house as Benvenuto Cellini.) Later in life, Guidi took holy orders.

Some books by Guido Guidi

1. *Chirurgia e graeco in latinum conversa . . .* , Paris, Petrus Galterius, 1544.

2. *Ars medicinalis* edited by Guido Guidi (nephew) in three volumes, in the third of which is *De anatome corporis humani libri VII*, Venice, Giunta, 1611.

3. *Opera omnia . . .* , another edition of 2 above. The third volume is *De anatome . . .* (without the engraved title-page). Frankfurt, Wechel, 1626.

Pieter Pauw (or Paaw) 1564–1617, was born in Amsterdam, and, like Platter, had studied with Fabrici at Padua. He was appointed Professor of Anatomy and Botany at Leiden, and was responsible for the building of its anatomy theatre (see Chapter 8). His special interest was in osteology. In his book *Primitiae . . .* we can see him using, and then extending, Vesalian anatomy of the bones. The title of the book is: *Primitiae anatomicae. De humani corporis ossibus* [that is, First fruits of anatomy. On the bones of the human body] Leiden, Justi à Colster, 1615. The title-page (*Fig. 6.10*) includes a picture of an orchestra of lemur-Deaths playing trumpets; a skeleton uses bones as drumsticks. One of the illustrations in the book is from the *Fabrica*— the skeleton with a spade—but others are original , with special emphasis on the skull, which is shown from all angles, and, as in Coiter and Platter, in fetuses (*Fig. 6.11*) and in animals. This interest is also seen in items 'kept in reserve' from the *Primitiae . . .* and published the next year as: *Succenturiatus anatomicus . . .*, Leiden, 1616. This contains a discussion on the treatment of depressed fractures of the skull, and shows Pauw's familiarity with the Greek and Latin literature on this subject. (A further volume issued the same year is on Celsus' *De re medica. . . .*) Pauw continued and refined the work of Dryander and Vesalius; his work leads on to that of Douglas, Monro–Sue, and Cheselden. Many of the illustrations of the skull and of other bones are common to Pauw's various books. They are thought to have been drawn and engraved by Jacob de Gheyn or his pupils.

Nearly three-quarters of a century after Vesalius had first written the *Epitome . . .* Pauw reissued that text with a commentary. *Andreae Vesalii Bruxellensis Epitome anatomica . . .*, Leiden, J. à Colster, 1616, small quarto. It was accompanied by thirteen Vesalian plates re-engraved in smaller format.

Again, in Pauw as in Valverde, Coiter, Platter, and Bauhin, we see the influence of Vesalius, and an attempt made to refine some of the original illustrations or, where these proved unsatisfactory, to add new ones.

Johannes Vesling, (1598–1649), born in Minden, became professor of anatomy at Padua in 1632. His anatomical studies are to be found in *Syntagma anatomicum . . .*, issued in an unillustrated quarto edition in 1641 and with twenty-four full-page copperplates in 1647, both books published by Paul Frambotti in Padua. The plates are formal representations of anatomy, tending towards the diagrammatic. Superficialities have been rejected; there are no landscape backgrounds. The figures have been thought through from the beginning, and owe little to Vesalius' figures or to any of his followers. Their formality may be seen, for example, in a plate of the muscles of the upper limb (*Fig. 6.12*), where one is reminded of the copper engravings of Canano; except for a certain amount of artistic licence shown, for example, in the disposition of the flexor muscles to the fingers, the diagrams are of the same character as those in many present-day manuals of anatomy. (The artist for the illustrations was Giovanni Georgi.) It will come as something of a relief to see at last, more than a hundred years after the *Fabrica*, figures in our book *not* based on those in Vesalius' work.

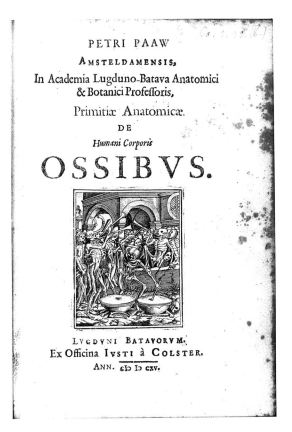

6.10 Title-page of Pauw, *Primitiae anatomicae*, 1615.

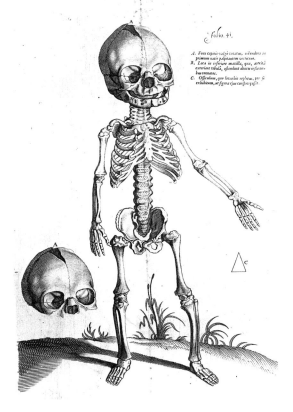

6.11 Fetal skeleton, from Pauw, *Primitae anatomicae*, 1615.

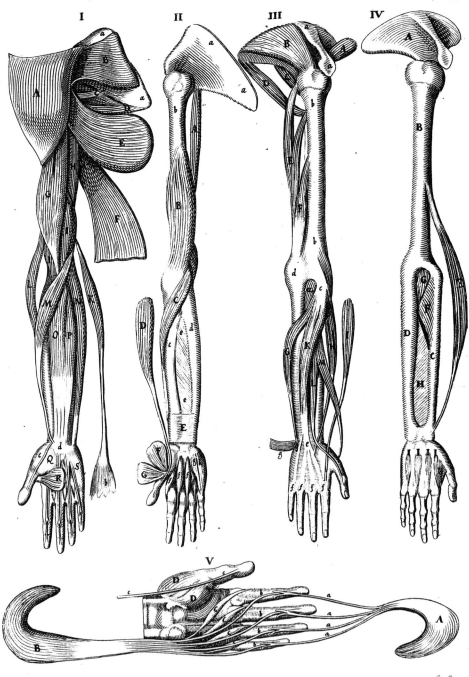

6.12   Arm musculature, from Vesling, *Syntagma*, 1647.

The work became popular, perhaps mainly because of the diagrammatic nature of the figures. It was republished a number of times, and was translated into German (1652), Dutch (1661), and Italian (1709). An English-language version was made by the herbalist and unauthorized physician Nicholas Culpeper: *The anatomy of the body of man* ..., London, Peter Cole, 1653. In an address 'To the Reader' he criticizes Vesling's text '... it is apparent that he drank too deep of Aristotle's spittle ...', but praises, we may think far too extravangantly, the engravings '... as for the brass cuts, they are performed very exactly, far exceeding any that ever were printed in the English tongue, inferior to none in the world'.

56 Skeleton holding scythe. Tab. I on page 15 of Book I, from G. Guidi, *De anatome ...*, 1626. Engraving (Cambridge University Library). 25.0 × 15.4 cm.

It must be admitted at the outset that other illustrations in this book display far greater accuracy and appeal than the one chosen for this plate. Several of the muscle illustrations, for instance, are somewhat reminiscent of Eustachio, though neither Guidi (nor the artist responsible for the drawings) could have seen his plates; many also are Vesalian in flavour.

The text makes mention of Vesalius, Valverde, and Realdo Colombo, and must therefore be presumed to have been written after 1543 and before Guidi's death in 1569. It is of a very much higher order of quality than some of the illustrations.

It is distressing to find, so long after Vesalius, a skeletal drawing such as this. The sinuous vertebral column and the sacrum are a disaster beyond comment; the clavicles curve over the first rib; the sternum is depicted as a broad shield; the delineation of the long bones of the limbs makes it doubtful that they could ever have been seen, let alone examined, and the carpal and tarsal bones are simply terrible (the right and left tarsal bones are shown as quite different!). Whoever caused (presumably Guidi Junior) or permitted the travesties of these illustrations of whole skeletons, of which this is an example, to be included with Guidi's text did no service to his name. They give a strong impression of being human skeletons designed by a committee; they must surely have made Guidi turn in his grave.

TABVLA. I.

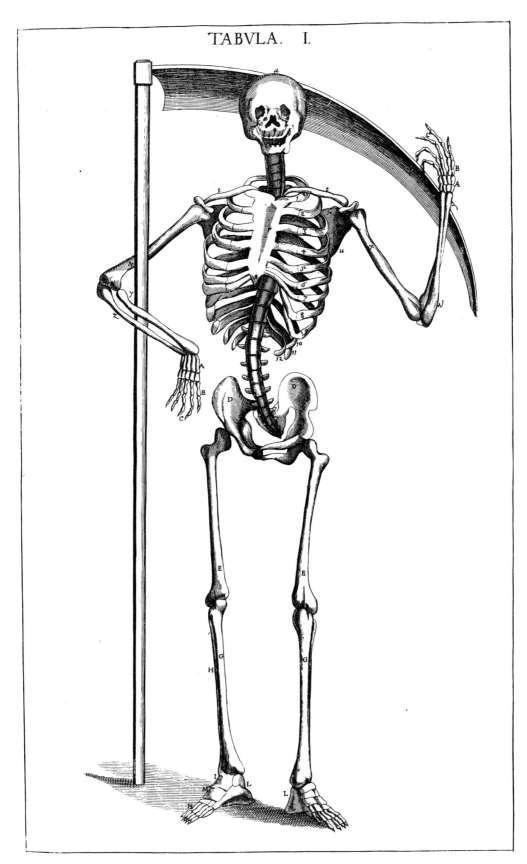

PLATE 56

57 Bones of the foot, Tabula XVII, on page 73 of Book II in G. Guidi, *De anatome* ..., 1626. Engraving (Cambridge University Library). 24.9 × 15.7 cm.

This plate, however, helps to restore one's balance, for here the bones of the foot (plus diverse cartilages, etc. from elsewhere in the body) certainly indicate that knowledge of anatomy and the illustrating thereof need not be totally divorced from one another. The bony skeletal elements (not least the sesamoid bones associated with the metatarsophalangeal joint of the big toe) are readily recognizable for what they are intended to be, and the thyroid, cricoid, and epiglottic cartilages are well depicted (agreed, figures XVIII and XIX *are* vile). True also it is that the portrayal, in the centre of the plate, of the temporo-mandibular cartilage (V, VI, and VII), the menisci of the knee (VIII and VIIII), the palpebral cartilage (X), a tracheal ring (XI), and the clavicular intra-articular discs (XII and XIII) leave something to be desired.

TABVLA. XVII.

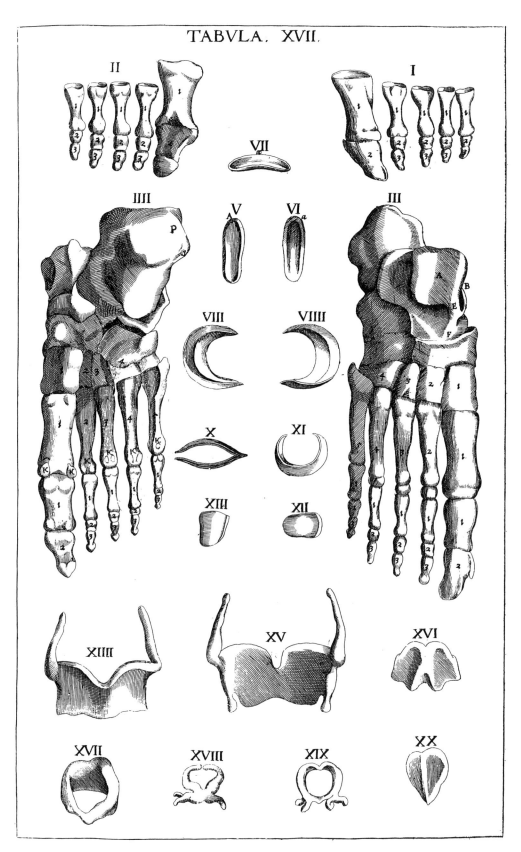

PLATE 57

58 Two skulls, on folded sheet, bound between pages 48 and 49 of P. Pauw, *Primitiae anatomicae*, 1615. Engraving (Glasgow University Library, Hunterian collection). The sheet measures 24.7 × 17.5 cm, and the two skulls virtually fill it.

The skulls that are featured here, Folio 48, are those of a young adult, probably male. The unerupted third molars, and, in the lower drawing, the unfused basi-occiput and basi-sphenoid (u) indicate an age of approximately twenty-one years.

The upper drawing shows a metopic or frontal suture between the frontal bones (a). The squamous part of the temporal bone (d) is too small: the lateral plate of the greater wing of the sphenoid, particularly its superior portion, extends too far backwards, thus vitiating the concept of a pterion. The mandibular notch is rather too wide and shallow, and the coronoid process conveys the impression of being a solid tuberosity rather than the pointed blade-like process that in fact it is.

The lower drawing suffers from very crinkled pterygoid plates, poor foramina ovalia, and a certain lack of right and left symmetry. However, the artist has captured the 'texture' of the bones most pleasingly, and, although both jaws lack a number of teeth, this fact has been faithfully rendered, and no attempt has been made to provide a full dentition. It would also seem likely that the styloid processes have been broken off, as they do not appear in either drawing.

One would have thought that the same skull would have been used for both drawings, yet the dentitions of the right upper jaws are different. The upper drawing shows the canine, second premolar, and first and second molars, while in the lower are featured the lateral incisor, the canine, and the first and second molars.

For the early seventeenth century the quality and clarity of the anatomy and the three-dimensional impact of this plate are impressive: but it should be compared with drawings of the skull base by Ryff (see *Plate 11*, p. 59) and Coiter (*Plate 53*).

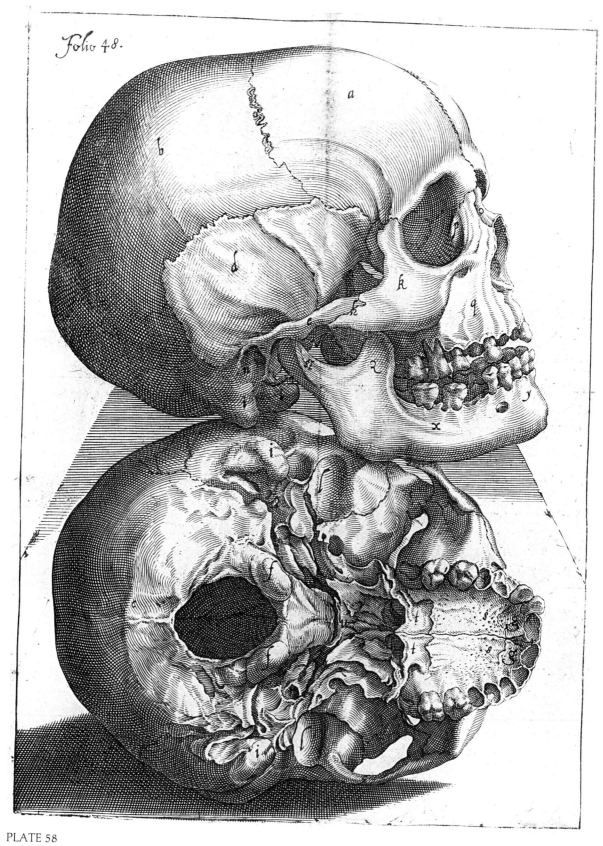

Folio 48.

PLATE 58

59 *In situ* visceral female and six other figures, Tabula Cap. VII, opposite page 80, of J. Vesling, *Syntagma anatomicum...*, 1647. Engraving (Cambridge University Library). 12.3 × 17.2 cm.

In the first figure the four abdominal wall flaps reveal the aorta and inferior vena cava, the kidneys with stylized suprarenals displaced from the upper poles of the kidneys, the rectum (c), the fundus of the uterus, and the urinary bladder.

In figure II, although in the text (L) and (K) are identified as arteries (M) and (I) as veins, they are seen to combine into a single tube (*pace* Harvey!), which descends to the ovaries (O). This was still common in anatomical drawings of this date, perhaps owing to the fact that the gonadal vein and artery are so closely wrapped together (see also *Plate 63*, p. 268).

The fundus of the uterus, its cervix, and a poorly drawn vagina (Y) are featured. The urinary bladder (Z), with its ureters entering it, seems almost to sprout out of the vagina. The uterine and vaginal vessels are largely imaginary in concept, but the area around the ovaries is interesting both in its portrayal and description, which followed the usual practice of that time. The structure labelled (d) is the ligament of the ovary, but is listed as the *ductus testium* or vas deferens. (Q) is the Fallopian tube (*tuba uteri*); but its function was obviously not known, and no ostium is shown. The structures labelled (S) are the round ligaments of the uterus.

Figure III is very typical of Vesling's formality of illustration, and shows the uterus and cervix, together with the round ligaments (F): the vagina is opened out to show transverse rugosities, although the lower margin is uninformative as to the vaginal opening. Figure IV is in part a repeat of figure II, and here the crura of the clitoris (I) and its glans (K) are portrayed, but shown arching over the (presumed) lower part of the vagina.

Figures V, VI, and VII all demonstrate a lack of comprehension of the anatomy of the female external genitalia. Any aspiring obstetrician of the time would have experienced great difficulty in learning very much from them. This is largely due to a lack of artistic capability, because the identification of the parts and their descriptions in the text are quite excellent for the mid-seventeenth century.

TABVLA CAP. VII.

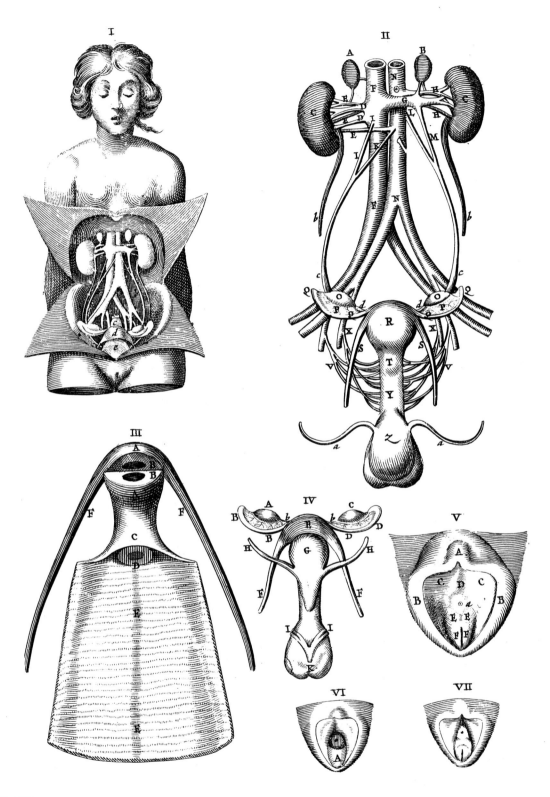

PLATE 59

Discoveries in anatomy 1550–1650

Naked-eye anatomy is a perfectible, descriptive science. From 1500 onwards, in association with printed illustrated texts, the structures of the most, and of many of the less, obvious parts of the human body were described and illustrated: the shape of the liver was no longer five-lobed; the heart had two, not three, ventricles; there was no *rete mirabile* to be seen at the base of the brain; the uterus was not bicornuate; there were three auditory ossicles not two ... The new anatomy was an improvement over the old; the idea of progress in anatomy is not a whiggish interpretative imposition on the history of that science, not an opinion, but a reality, demonstrable by comparison of illustrations with the actual structures to be seen in dissection, or at operation, or by computerized tomography, or by nuclear magnetic resonance scan. Some reservations, however, to this view must be made.

First, we must be careful not to confuse the image on the paper, put there for specific purposes (often for didactic, more rarely—after 1550—for symbolic purposes) with the knowledge and understanding of the anatomist who commissioned the woodcut or copper engraving. Berengario was not perturbed by altering the position of a part in an illustration to show other structures more conveniently; Vesalius described the rectus abdominis muscle correctly, but one of his muscle-men portrays it incorrectly; Leonardo's apparently realistic *gravida* figure is drawn not from dissection but from descriptions in a printed text.

Secondly, the question of variability of anatomical structures must be taken into account: that a particular anatomical arrangement is found in one dissection does not necessarily mean that other bodies will have precisely that same pattern.

Thirdly, theories of use can impose an interpretation on anatomical structures. How the structural relationships between the vessels of the liver and the heart and lung are seen depends on theories held by the anatomist of the time. The liver according to Galenic theory was the site of manufacture of the blood and the chief organ of the venous system: consequently the vein-man in the *Fabrica* shows no heart—Vesalius was a Galenist in this as in many things. Once Harvey's ideas on the circulation had been generally accepted, the venous system was pictured ending at the right side of the heart.

Fourthly, the more and the less precise organization of different structures may not be recognized. The structures may be illustrated, but the pattern of organization may not have been discernible to the anatomist or his artist. The appearance of the gyri and sulci of the cerebral hemispheres of the brain was compared with coils of intestines, and naturally enough, no fixed pattern of arrangement was illustrated. It was only in the latter half of the nineteenth century that the precise disposition of these was recognized and pictured correctly. An acute observer may however note and draw a structure even though neither he nor anyone else at the time had called attention to it. Scarpa, in the early nineteenth century, illustrates the carotid sinus, at the bifurcation of the common carotid artery, even though the significance of this structure was not realized until the present century.

Lastly, although facilitated enormously by the printing press and its ability to make multiple copies of illustrations, the dissemination of new knowledge was not completely efficient. Advances in anatomy would not necessarily be generally known—and therefore not incorporated into received, or normal, science—if they remained in manuscript or were printed in small editions, perhaps for local use; one thinks of Leonardo's notebooks and of Canano's work in this context.

In the hundred years from 1550 to 1650 a sheaf of knowledge was gathered that was considerably greater than that possessed by early-sixteenth-century anatomists. More accurate descriptions and illustrations of almost all the major organs of the body were available at the end of the period, though there was no one book that included all advances.

It is not our purpose here to list, illustrate, or acknowledge the major discoveries and insights of this century of anatomical consolidation. To unravel questions of priority, no matter how important to the protagonists, is often as tedious a business in this as in any other science, even though the possession of a discovery must be recognized as a major motivating force for scientific endeavour. During this hundred years, for instance, the third auditory ossicle was discovered and illustrated. To disentangle various claims for priority would be possible for this discovery, but at the end of the exercise we would still be left with the significant fact that from about 1550 on the stapes was known, and was illustrated in plates.

The interdependence of structure and function is an inevitable result of the evolutionary process. This relationship, interpreted as the wisdom of the Creator, was the stated basis of all biology and medical science. From Galen and his book, *The usefulness of parts*, to Platter and his *De corporis humani structura et usu* ... and beyond, anatomy was considered functionally. Of course, many functions were mistaken. Fabrici considered that the valves of the veins, which he described and illustrated, would merely discourage flow to the periphery. It needed the insights and experiments of Harvey to re-interpret the use of these valves in the economy of the body in terms of the circulation.

With these introductory remarks, an important set of illustrations will now be briefly discussed: Fabrici's illustrations of the valves of the veins.

Girolamo Fabrici

Girolamo Fabrici, (*c.* 1533–1619), or Fabrizio or in Latinized form, Hieronymus Fabricius ab Aquapendente, was named after the village near Orvieto where he was born.

Fabrici spent nearly fifty years teaching in the medical faculty at Padua, from which he had graduated. He both taught and practised surgery. He was also consulted as a physician on non-surgical problems, and counted important persons as his patients, Galileo among them. His chief involvement was in anatomy, both teaching and research, to which he dedicated the principal part of his life. It was due to him that a temporary anatomical theatre was constructed within the University buildings, and then, with money from Venice, in whose domains Padua lay, a permanent one (1594), which still can be viewed, with his name over the door.

Fabrici's pupils included men from many countries. His relations with German students were close, if often stormy. German-speaking students were grouped with those from Scandinavia, Bohemia, Hungary, and some other central European countries into a large German 'nation'. Poland was the second largest, and England and Scotland, at this time separately represented, were small 'nations' at Padua, in this ostensibly student-directed university. William Harvey, during his studies there, 1600–2, was one of the English 'nation's' *Councillors* to one of the Rectors. The University of Padua (*Universitas studiorum*) was split into two autonomous, but unequal parts, the larger for the study of law (*Universitas juristarum*), while the other comprised the schools of theology, philosophy, and medicine (*Universitas artisarum*). Bauhin, Pauw, Spieghel, and Caspar Bartholin all studied under Fabrici. His most famous pupil, William Harvey, regarded his teaching on the valves of the veins as one seminal factor in the idea of the blood-circulation. It is probable that Harvey was influenced by the ease with which Fabrici moved from work as a medical doctor to human dissection and to dissection and experiment on a variety of non-human species of animals, always showing himself to be a careful observer and precise note-taker.

Fabrici admired Andreas Vesalius, whose successor he was in the Chairs of Anatomy and Surgery, but he thought him preoccupied with structure, to the detriment of consideration of the 'uses of parts' dissected. Fabrici maintained the Galenic viewpoint that structure and function should not be considered separately. Fabrici's physiology was teleological rather than experimental; he arrived at concepts about the purposes of structures by imposing his, mainly Galenic, ideas as to their roles in the economy of the body. Vesalius was, Fabrici thought, engrossed with criticisms of Galen; moreover, the language of the *Fabrica* was too convoluted, and the descriptions sometimes too minute. A new illustrated text, incorporating advances made since the *Fabrica* by Colombo, Eustachio, and others, was needed. From the early days of his appointment at Padua until his death at the age of eighty-six or so, Fabrici laboured to prepare such a text of functional anatomy. It was not until 1600, when he was in his mid-sixties, that the first volume was published, a treatise on vision, speech, and hearing. The delay was due to scholarly caution—Fabrici wanted each part of the complete anatomy, to be called *Totius animalis fabricae theatrum*, to be exposed to the constructive criticisms of his colleagues. Some other manuscripts that had been accumulating over the years were published in succession, including monographs on the valves of the veins (1603), embryology (1604 and, posthumously, 1621), respiration (1615), and locomotion (1618). Many of these described and illustrated studies on an extensive range of other species besides the human. A Polish woman scholar, who discussed these matters with Fabrici, Hedwiga Mielecka, assisted him in obtaining rare animals. A study of the development of the hen's egg, and on the formation of the fetus in various species, was a time-consuming occupation not only of Fabrici but also of a number of late-sixteenth- and seventeenth-century scientists. Coiter, Platter, Bauhin, and Pauw all illustrated various aspects of the human fetus, as we have seen, and Spieghel, Needham, and Harvey wrote extensively on these subjects.

The embryological treatises of Fabrici are beautifully illustrated with detailed copperplates, drawn and engraved by unknown artists (*Fig. 6.13*). In *De formato foetu* not only are the uterus, placenta, membranes, and fetus of the human illustrated, but also those structures in many animals, in the sheep, ox, horse, pig, dog, rat and mouse, guinea-pig, shark, and snake. In the College of Physicians in Philadelphia there is a copy of *De formato foetu* in which there have

been bound thirty large original paintings on a black background. These reproduce in colour most of the engraved plates, plus an extra one. The paintings have printed explanatory pages text, not present in the ordinary copies. Another, but less complete example, of this 'de luxe' edition is apparently to be found in the *Biblioteca Marciana* in Venice.

Fabrici's treatise on the venous valves *De venarum ostiolis* discusses their role in slowing down the 'normal' flow of blood centrifugally in the limbs—a mistaken Galenic idea, that did not interfere, as we can see in *Plate 60*, with his showing in an accurate manner their structure in relation to the openings of side branches. The work was dedicated to 'The illustrious German Nation'.

Fabrici's project for a work on the whole of anatomy was only realized in part. However, more was prepared than was published. In his will Fabrici left to the Venetian state many large paintings of anatomy in oils; 167 of these are now in the *Biblioteca Marciana* in Venice. They have been bound in eight volumes, seven devoted to human and one to comparative anatomy. (We have not seen

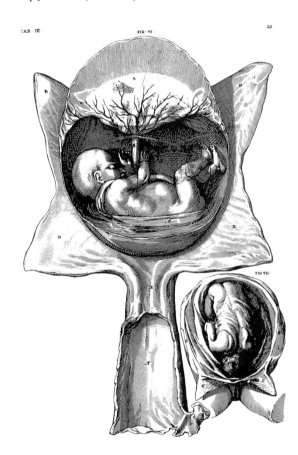

6.13 Opened uterus showing fetus and placenta, from Fabrici, *De formato foetu*, 1604.

these paintings, which are described in Sterzi, 1909.) The artists—there appear to have been a number—are unknown. The paintings are unlabelled. Engravings of some plates were apparently made; some have a note *intagliato* in Fabrici's hand, indicating that an engraving was made. They are mentioned in his will, but the present whereabouts of them or their impressions are not known. Thomas Bartholin may have had some of these large unpublished prints in his possession.

Some books by Fabrici

1. *Pentateuchos cheirurgicum . . .*, Frankfurt, 1592, edited by J. H. Beyer. Later, enlarged edition, *Operationes chirurgicae . . .*, Venice, 1619.

2. *De venarum ostiolis*, Padua, Lorenzo Pasquati, 1603.

3. *De formatu foetu*, Venice, Franciscus Bolzettam, 1604.

4. *De formatione ovi et pulli . . .* Padua, 1621 (a posthumous publication).

5. *Opera omnia anatomica et physiologica . . .*, edited by B. S. Albinus, Leiden, van Kerckhem, 1738 (an earlier edition was published in Leipzig, 1687).

60 The valves in the iliac, femoral, and saphenous veins, Tabula V, page. 17 of G. Fabrici, *De venarum ostiolis*, Padua, 1604. (This appears to be identical with the 1603 plate.) Engraving (Wellcome Institute Library). 34.7 × 23.6 cm.

In this plate the left external iliac vein and artery, together with their continuation as femoral vessels, and, in addition, the great or long saphenous vein, are all slit open along their length. Fabrici compared the presence of valves (*ostiola*) in the veins with their absence in the arteries. He did, however, consider the function of these valves to be that of delaying or impeding the flow of blood distally, that is, in this case, preventing it from pooling in the foot.

This beautiful illustration well demonstrates not only the form of the venous valves but also their positioning in the veins. In this regard it will be noticed, as is also shown in drawings of the saphenous vein in the leg and foot in Fabrici's Tabulae VI and VII, that the valves are placed just proximal to where smaller veins join the main veins.

The plates in *De venarum ostiolis* are the first portrayal of venous valves, except for rather crude woodcuts by Salomon Alberti in 1585.

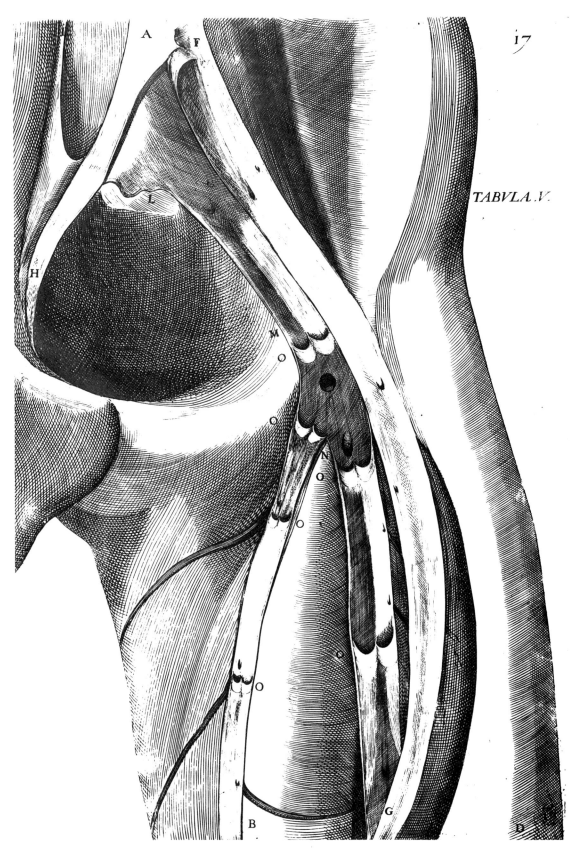

TABVLA. V.

PLATE 60

Chapter 6: Selected Reading

Adelmann, H. B. (1967). *The embryological treatises of Hieronymus Fabricius of Aquapendente* ... Cornell University Press, Ithaca, NY.

Bylebyl, J J. (1979). The School of Padua: humanistic medicine in the sixteenth century. In *Health, medicine and mortality in the sixteenth century*. Cambridge University Press.

Cole, F J. (1975). *A history of comparative anatomy* ... Dover, New York. (Reprint of 1949 edition.)

Cushing, H. (1943). *A bio-bibliography of Andreas Vesalius*. Schuman, New York.

Franklin, K. J. (1933). *De venarum ostiolis 1603 of Hieronymus Fabricius of Aquapendente (1533?–1619)*. Charles C. Thomas, Springfield, IL.

Grmek, M D. (1972). Guido Guidi. *Dict. sci. Biog.*, **5**, 580–1.

Guerra, F. (1967). Juan de Valverde de Amusco ..., *Clio Med.*, **2**, 339–62.

Herrlinger, R. (1952). *Volcher Coiter 1534–1576*. M. Edelmann, Nuremberg.

Herrlinger, R. (1970). *History of medical illustration from antiquity to A.D. 1600*. Pitman, London.

Jennett, S. (1961). *Beloved son Felix: The Journal of Felix Platter a medical student in Montpellier in the sixteenth century*. Frederick Muller, London.

López Piñero, J. M. (1979). The Vesalian movement in sixteenth-century Spain. *J. Hist. Biol.*, **12**, 45–81.

Schierbeek, A. and Nuyens, B. W. F. (1955) *Volcher Coiter* Opuscula sell. Neerland. Arte Med. **18**.

Schullian, D. M. (1971). Volcher Coiter. *Dict. sci. Biog.*, **3**, 342–3.

Sterzi, G. (1909). Le Tabulae anatomicae ed i codici Marciani con note autografe di Hieronymus Fabricius ab Aquapendente. *Anat. Anzeiger*, **35**.

Whitteridge, G. (1970). Gaspard Bauhin. *Dict. sci. Biog.*, **1**, 522–5.

Whitteridge, G. (1971). *William Harvey and the circulation of the blood*. Macdonald, London.

Zanobio, B. (1971). Girolamo Fabrici. *Dict. sci. Biog.*, **4**, 507–12.

7

Baroque anatomy

An extraordinary convention

ANATOMICAL dissections, until the technique of preservation was introduced, were carried out during the cool weather of the European winter. From the fourteenth century until the construction of anatomy theatres at the end of the sixteenth century some dissections were made in hospitals or churches, but they were also performed in the open air, sometimes under temporary shelter. These outdoor dissections may be one of a number of reasons why the skeletons or cadavers of anatomical texts were placed in the foreground against a landscape. This tradition persisted for more than two hundred years, from before Berengario to after Albinus. During these years, the landscape was indicated, sometimes by a rock or two and a few clumps of vegetation, but frequently by elaborate landscapes or townscapes. Behind Vesalius' muscle-men there can be seen confidently-drawn scenes, complex landscapes that extended from foreground shrubs and, perhaps, masonry, through midground trees, rivers, houses, and bridges, to hills and mountains in the background. Attention was called to the prominent foreground figure by placing it in such perspective views, giving an impression of solidity and roundness to the anatomical structures shown. Similar scenes are to be found behind a number of Estienne's figures, which were conceived independently of those of Vesalius.

Illustrations showing dissections of women were, as in the books of Berengario or Estienne, often but not always placed inside buildings, or at least shielded away by drapes and curtains— in one case incongruously hung up in the middle of a landscape.

Figures against landscapes were used to display anatomical structures discovered by dissection. But they were not shown as cadavers; they were shown as if, paradoxically, they were living human beings. A very early example of this convention was Guido de Vigevano's upright figure of a man being subjected to dissection. The abstract and diagrammatic frog-like stance of many manuscript figures was justified, and, as it were, brought to 'life' by picturing the individual sitting on a chair, or a simple three-legged stool, or maybe even an elaborate, decorated throne.

Of course, no one can submit to evisceration and the resection of many muscles and still remain upright and alive. To show a person so, leaning exhausted or anguished against a wall, is patently absurd; and yet a Vesalian muscle-man found himself in this situation. The results of a dissection, perhaps of a hanged person, carried out inevitably with a modicum of mess, were transformed to a scene in a pleasant landscape, where the anatomized person is shown apparently alive. This is indeed a strange convention to anyone unfamiliar with the traditions of anatomical illustration.

Dissected men and women, and skeletons as well, were set within a variety of circumstances. They could be provided with a spade, as in the first Vesalian skeletal illustration. They often conveyed moral instruction, as in hundreds of illustrations starting with Berengario and progressing through Dryander and Vesalius to Bidloo and beyond. And surprisingly these figures could express emotions: despair, pride, contemplation, and viciousness are called to mind by Vesalius' 'weeping' skeleton, Estienne's muscle-man, another Vesalian skeleton, and Valverde's *écorché* holding a flayed human skin—his own, seemingly; but that is too horrible a thought.

The convention whereby anatomized persons are shown as apparently alive comes also out of the macabre figures of the medieval *Totendanz*. Personifications of Death were shown as skeletons, or as partially decayed corpses—*lemures*, come from the underworld to claim the living. The grave is not however Death's final victory; the buried corpse, decayed to the bare bones, will rise up at the last trump as a 'living' skeleton, to be reclothed with flesh. In Orvieto cathedral, Signorelli's skeletons elbow their way out of the solid ground to stand upright on their former graves, waiting to become whole again and taken to judgement. The Bidloo–Lairesse skeleton of 1685 emerges from the tomb still with his winding-sheet (see *Plate 71*, p. 314). Even today the tradition is immediately understood; it is only when anatomy is emphasized at the expense of symbol that the picture becomes unacceptable to the lay person, and the convention becomes so extraordinary.

Relevant also to this convention is the association of art and anatomy, continuing from the days of Pollaiuolo, Michelangelo, and Raphael to the life studies of a thousand academies and art schools. Artists were indeed inspired by the sculptures of the ancient world; but it should be noted that, unlike their classical forerunners, some artists of the high Renaissance studied not only unclothed men and women but also dissections; they carried their analysis to deeper and formerly hidden levels, by actual dissection or by being present when anatomists dissected— Vesalius complained that artists crowded around him and interfered with his work.

The skeleton was regarded as the framework on which to build a drawing of a naked, classically inspired, figure: 'In painting the nude, begin with the bones, then add the muscles and then cover the figures with the flesh in such a way as to leave the position of the muscles visible.' Drawings by Michelangelo and other artists of the high Renaissance show attempts to follow Leon Battista Alberti's advice. The superficial muscles of the whole body, as shown in skinned cadavers, could be recognized and demonstrated also in living men—less easily in living women. Flayed standing figures (*écorchés*) were drawn, printed, or modelled for artists to study. It was for them, as much as for anatomists and surgeons, that so much attention was paid to the superficial musculature. *Écorchés* had a prominent place jn anatomy texts: Berengario, Eustachio, and Vesalius started a tradition that with Albinus reached some sort of culminating perfection. Whether this knowledge was, in practice, productive of exceptionally true-to-life figure drawing or sculpture is open to examination; classical sculptors, so much admired by critics in the sixteenth century, had not relied on dissection. Excessive emphasis on the 'anatomical' approach led (leaving behind the perfections of the late Renaissance) to exaggerations and distortions of musculature, seen for example in Goltzius' *Hercules* (Fig. 7.1), who would be more at home on a Californian 'muscle beach' than in any real world. Printed books of anatomy designed specifically for artists, of which there are examples from the seventeenth century onwards, often show nudes with identified muscles.

Some academic anatomy texts also included illustrations of naked men and women. These would have been useful if they had been well labelled to show structures that may be seen in the living person, such as the muscles beneath the skin, or even the details of the external genitalia; but they were not so labelled. Even though their purpose is not fully explained, we are grateful that Vesalius included such fine 'Adam and Eve' figures in the *Epitome* (see *Fig 5.2*, p. 130).

Anatomical figures in a landscape may resemble life drawings, but they are not: they are drawings of death. There is an outrage, suppressed maybe with familiarity, when a cut is made on the cadaver, and when the dissection is carried down to deeper layers. (Some anatomical artists have indeed exploited this horror of the dissecting room.) In order to exorcize this atavistic reaction, the dissected figure may instead, in the convention we have been discussing, be placed in the familiarity of a quiet landscape. In a third convention, seen in medieval manuscripts and in twentieth-century didactic texts, the anatomical structures were neutralized to a greater or lesser extent into diagrams, more or less remote from both the living and the dead.

The anatomical plates we are now to present were drawn within the convention of 'living' anatomies set against a landscape. They were made in the seventeenth century, after the high

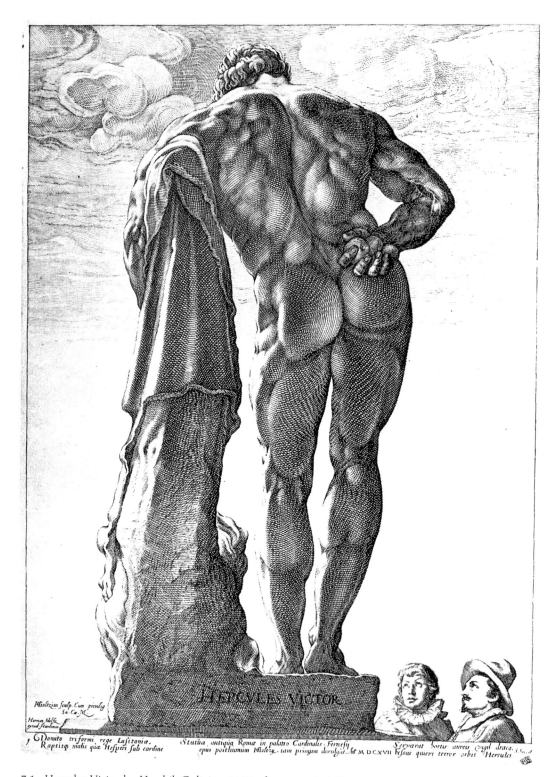

Domito triformi rege Lusitaniæ,
Raptisq; malis quæ Hesperi sub cardine

Statua antiqua Romæ in palatto Cardinalis. Fernesi
opus posthumum Goltzi. iam primum divulgat HG M D C XVII

Servarat hortus aureu vigil draco.
Iessus quieri terror orbis Hercules

7.1 Hercules Victor by Hendrik Goltzius, 1617, after an ancient Roman statue.

emotionalism of Vesalius' mannerist skeletons and muscle-men, but before the gentlemanly unperturbed neoclassical figures of Albinus. We have called such anatomy 'baroque anatomy'; the reader will decide whether this is an appropriate term. Whatever nomenclature seems right, the particular conventions shown by Casserian–Spieghelian plates, by Berrettini's work, and by that of Martinez seem to be foreshadowed by traditions of the Fontainebleau school that had influenced Estienne, as well as by Vesalius and his followers. In the work of the seventeenth-century anatomists and artists the extraordinary convention we have been talking of is taken to barely permissible limits.

In parenthesis, it would be of interest to examine the evolution of the title-pages of anatomy books. A series can be constructed: from the woodcut title to Vesalius' *Fabrica* (see *Fig. 5.3*, p. 132), through the symbol-laden engraved frontispieces of the work of Casserio (see *Fig. 7.2*), to the classical restrained elegance of the typographic title-pages of Albinus' and William Hunter's atlases (see *Figs 8.11 and 12.5*, pp. 323 and 469).

Casserio, Spieghel, and Bucretius

In *Plate 64* a beautiful woman is shown standing among rocks and trees with her Grecian hair blowing in the wind. But her abdominal and uterine walls are peeled back like so many leaves of a cabbage, to show a full-term infant and its placenta—all of which defies reason and gravity. Yet all is done in the most naturalistic manner. Other plates in this series are even more exaggeratedly strange, as in one showing a dissected cadaver, cut in half, ambling away from a river across an Italian landscape (*Plate 62*). We can think of the Vesalian muscle-men and skeletons as players in a highly-charged drama; but in these seventeenth-century plates it is impossible to imagine what action could precede or follow the scene shown. The irrational convention, not easy to accept for those previously unacquainted with it, has been excessively elaborated. The figures, though grotesque, are quite formal and even graceful, and certainly not so disturbing or emotionally charged as are those of Vesalius. So absurd in one way, they are nevertheless well disposed to show anatomical details. Moreover, unlike the engraved plates of Estienne, in most a significant portion of the illustration is taken up with anatomy, in spite of the richness of detail present in the background landscapes—a few, however, continue the extravagant tradition (*Fig. 7.3*).

These plates have been associated with the names of Casserio, Spieghel, and Bucretius.

Giulio Casserio (c. 1552–1616), the Latin form being Julius Casserius, was born at Piacenza (Placentia), a small mainland town not far from Venice. His training in anatomy was under Fabrici in Padua; he was successively his servant, assistant, and eventually deputy — perhaps even designated successor. Casserio however died before his long-lived master. Fabrici signed William Harvey's doctoral diploma from Padua, April 28, 1602, as Professor of Anatomy and Surgery; Casserio signed as teacher of anatomy, physic, and surgery.

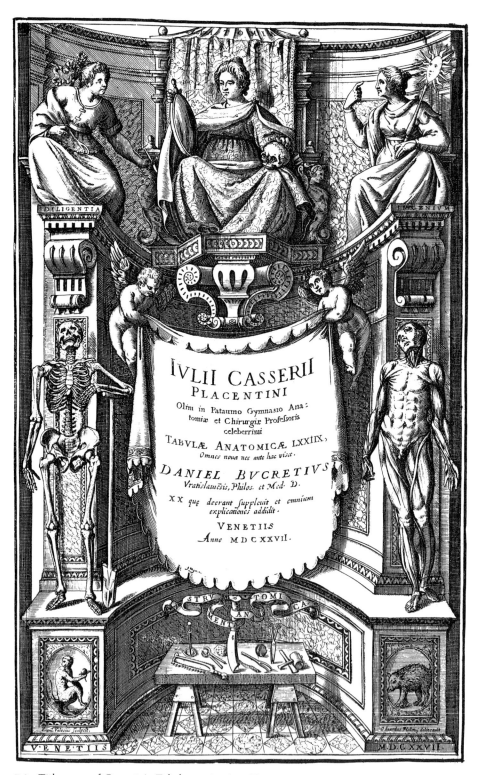

IVLII CASSERII
PLACENTINI
Olim in Pataumo Gymnasio Ana:
tomiæ et Chirurgiæ Professoris
celeberrimi
TABVLÆ ANATOMICÆ LXXIIX,
Omnes nouæ nec ante hac visæ.
DANIEL BVCRETIVS
Vratislauiensis, Philos. et Med. D.
XX que deerant suppleuit et omnium
explicationes addidit.
VENETIIS
Anne MDCXXVII.

7.2 Title page of Casserio's *Tabulae anatomicae*, Venice, 1627.

For more than two decades Casserio was involved in the production of illustrations of anatomy. Some of these were published in his lifetime; many were included in posthumous works, published with his, but also with other names attached.

His first publication was on vocalization and hearing: *De vocis auditusque organis* ..., Ferrara, V. Baldino, 1601, a beautifully-printed folio book with 34 large engraved anatomical plates. Casserio's approach in this monograph was that of a comparative anatomist. There are, for instance, a number of plates of the larynx of the cat. The artist, as draughtsman and engraver, of these plates was Joseph (or Josias) Maurer, perhaps a Swiss artist, pupil of Tobias Stimmer. Maurer, as described in this book, was resident in Casserio's house for this specific purpose. The wonderfully ornate baroque engraved title-page has been shown to be the work not of Maurer but of Jacopi Ligozzi. Cazort has cunningly unravelled its iconography. In this extravagant title-page there are two *putti* skeletons sporting wings!

Casserio's next work was *Pentaestheseion ... de quinque sensibus liber*, Venice, 1609. Twelve illustrations relating to hearing were taken from *De vocis auditusque* ... and twenty-one new illustrations were added concerning the other senses.

From before 1600 Casserio had been working towards a more ambitious project: to produces a fully-illustrated anatomy of all the parts of the human body. This he announced as a *Theatrum* of anatomy. He did not, however, live to complete it.

Adriaan van den Spieghel (c. 1578–1625), the Latin form being Adrianus Spigelius, came from Brussels, and took his doctorate at Padua.

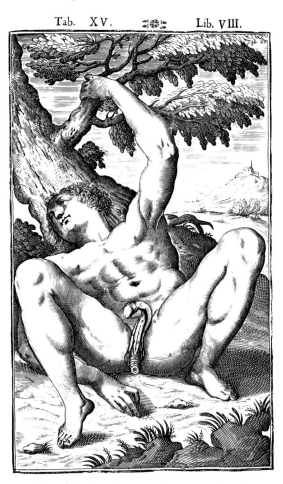

7.3 Casserio's plate showing the penis and anal musculature from Spieghel, *De humani corporis fabrica*, 1627.

He was appointed as successor to Casserio and taught at Padua, at first as a close associate of Fabrici, and then independently. He occupied a chair in anatomy and surgery which, nearly ninety years before, had been that of Vesalius, another citizen of Brussels. Spieghel was a practising surgeon; he wrote also on fevers and on botanical subjects. Spieghel's text on the whole of anatomy was not illustrated, and remained unpublished in his lifetime; in his will he asked Bucretius to see the work into print. Spieghel wrote a treatise on human development which was also published posthumously, having been given a similar title—*De formato foetu*—as Fabrici's work, 1600.

Danieles Bucretius (c. *1600–31*), the Latin name adopted by Daniel Rindfleisch, or Rindofleisch, was from Wrocław, Poland, formerly capital of German Lower Silesia. He had received his doctorate from Padua in 1626. Later in his short life, in 1629, he entered the Dominican order.

There are three books to be considered, published in 1627, or within a year of this date:

1. Julius Casserius, *Tabulae anatomicae ...*, Venice, 1627. (An edition from Frankfurt, 1632, contains these plates re-engraved and reduced in size.)
2. Adrianus Spigelius, *De humani corporis fabrica libri decem ...* Venice, 1627. (The title of this book is confusingly similar to Vesalius's *Fabrica*.)
3. Adrianus Spigelius, *De formato foetu ...*, Venice, [1626].

Bucretius was responsible for the first and second publications, both published by E. Deuchin. Liberalis Crema, who was married to Spieghel's daughter, put together the third book. The second and third have texts by Spieghel. (Casserio and Spieghel were both dead at the time of publication.)

Tab·VII

All these books contain plates originally made under Casserio's direction. Bucretius had acquired seventy seven from Casserio's heirs for works nos. 1 and 2 above, and Crema nine for work no. 3. These completed plates had been intended by Casserio to form part of his *Theatrum*. Some aspects of anatomy were not covered, so twenty more illustrations were made for number 2 above, under Bucretius' direction, by the same artists used by Casserio. In the complete series, the largest number of plates, forty three—and these perhaps the most memorable—are to be found in Liber IV, on the muscles. There are also interesting illustrations on the genito-urinary system in Liber VIII and on the brain in Liber X—one of these, showing the arterial circle at the base of the brain, predates the Willis–Wren illustration (*see Plate 91*, p. 403).

7.4 Full-term fetus, with partly dissected abdomen, and placenta from Spieghel, *De formato foetu*, [1626].

The third publication, Spieghel's work on fetal development (*Fig. 7.4* and *Plate 64*), was edited by Crema, who added his own commentary to that of his father-in-law.

The artists for most, but not necessarily for all, of the plates in these three books were identified in the Bucretius intoduction: Odoardo Fialetti, a pupil of Tintoretto and of Jacomo Robusti, drew the pictures. Francesco Valesio engraved them. In 1608 Fialetti had written a manual of artistic anatomy, illustrated with forty engravings emphasizing measurement and proportion. These men had been working with Casserio, and were employed by Bucretius in the production of the additional plates needed to complete the series for books nos. 1 and 2 above.

Except for those few plates which were derived from Vesalius, the anatomists—Casserio first and Bucretius later—had reconsidered ways of presenting human anatomy. In doing so they produced the first original series of illustrations of the anatomy of the human body since Vesalius, Estienne, and Eustachio. Casserio had, like Vesalius, realized the importance of a sufficient number of illustrations. In bringing his work to completion, Vesalius had taken at most five years; Casserio's work remained incomplete and unpublished after about twenty years. It does take longer to produce a copper engraving than a woodcut, but this cannot account for the delay. Casserio's series of illustrations were originally without text; Spieghel's manuscript was not originally written for that purpose. In Vesalius' *Fabrica* the full-page woodcuts and the text figures were fully integrated with the text—which is of course technically straightforward, the text and the woodcut being printed at one pull of the press. With copper-engraving, the price paid for increased subtlety of line is that the page has to be printed by two passages through the press, one for the intaglio copperplate and another for the relief printing of the text.

Spieghel's collected works were published in Amsterdam by J. Blaeu, 1645. This book, edited by J. A. van der Linden, contains among other writing the text of Spieghel's *De humani corporis fabrica* and all the illustrations, with impressions taken from the original copperplates. The book also incorporates editions of the classical work on lymphatics by Aselli and by van der Wale, and on the circulation of the blood by Harvey. The portrait of Harvey at the age of seventy-nine now in the Hunterian Collection at Glasgow shows him with a copy of this book.

61 The muscles of the scapular region. Tabula XVI, Book IV of A. Spieghel, *De humani corporis fabrica...*, Venice, 1627. Engraving originally made for Casserio (private collection). 33.7 × 21.7 cm.

In this plate, the figure, in a charming landscape, is posed so as to display to advantage the superficial musculature of the back, in particular that of the scapular region. Its execution is most impressive for so early in the seventeenth century—the shading well conveys the contours of the body, although the buttocks are somewhat exaggeratedly globular (see also Browne, *Plate 92*, p. 411).

Parts of the anatomy, however, leave something to be desired. The iliac crest (K) is malpositioned with regard to the buttock; the muscles labelled G ('which turn the humerus on the scapula'), viz. part of the deltoid, infraspinatus, and the teres muscles, are not too well portrayed. The unlabelled muscle appearing above teres major (lower G) is the long head of triceps, which here, erroneously, would appear to originate well back on the dorsum of the scapula, and not from below the glenoid fossa.

Latissimus dorsi and trapezius are reasonably accurate, and the obliquity of splenius capitis (Q) is well shown as it disappears beneath the cut skin border (R). The heavily shaded muscle partly detached from the upper ribs is the *quartus scapulae musculus*, that is, pectoralis minor.

Tab. XVI. ⁁⁁⁁ Lib. IV. 28

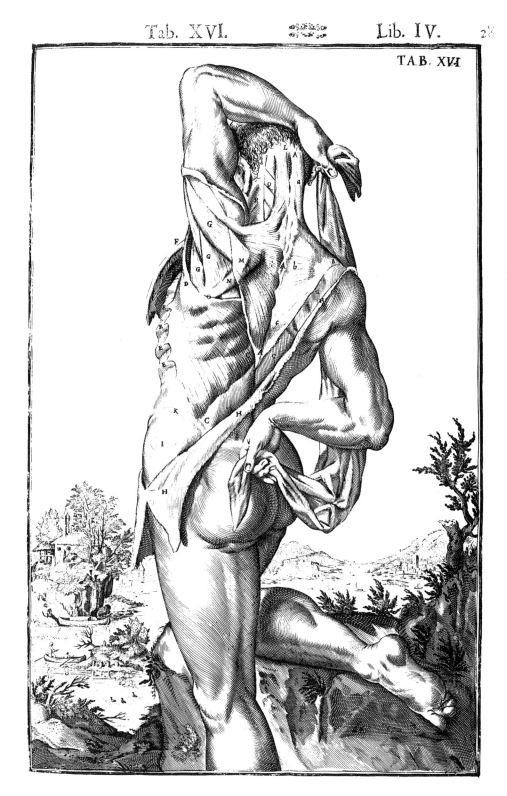

PLATE 61

62 Anterior thigh and pelvic muscles. Tabula XXXI, Book IV of A. Spieghel, *De humani corporis fabrica*..., Venice, 1627. Engraving originally made for Casserio (private collection). 33.2 × 20.8 cm.

This is an unusual presentation which displays some dubious anatomy. For example (AA) are described as thoracic vertebrae, but (B) (the twelfth rib) is seen to attach high up on the eleventh vertebra. Quadratus lumborum (a) is rightly shown stretching from the iliac crest to the twelfth rib.

Psoas major (G) and the (reflected) iliacus (L, M) are reasonably well depicted, but, because of the poor portrayal of the pubic bones, the origins of muscles attached to them are suspect: presumably they represent, from lateral to medial, pectineus, adductor longus, and gracilis, with adductor longus turned back in the left thigh to reveal adductor brevis and branches of the femoral nerve. On the right side there is poor delineation of the anterior superior iliac spine, which gives origin to sartorius (T)—the iliac crest seems to sweep without break to the inferior spine, from which part of rectus femoris (R) can be seen to arise.

The folded scroll-like structure (S) seen on the medial side of the right thigh is presumably meant to represent the fascia lata: the similarly-labelled structure on the lateral side of the thigh presumably represents the same, or perhaps the ilio-tibial tract.

Tab. XXXI.   Lib. IV.   43

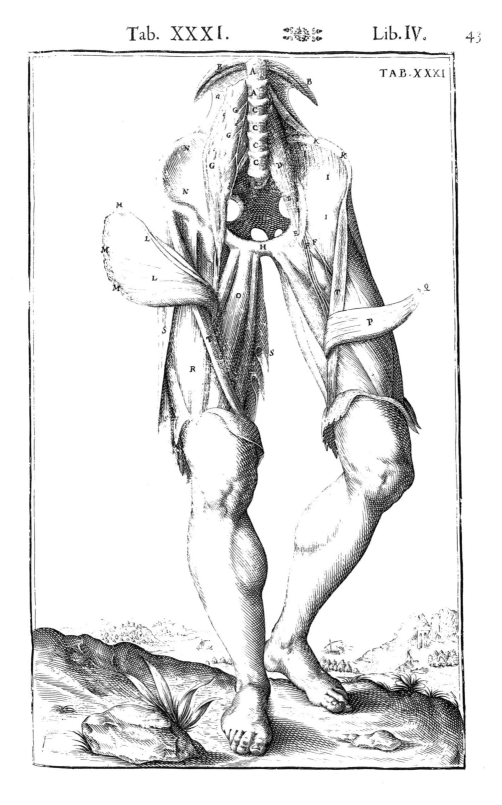

PLATE 62

63 Female figure: the genito-urinary tract, etc. Tabula XVIII, Book VIII of A. Spieghel, *De humani corporis fabrica . . .*, Venice, 1627. Engraving originally made for Casserio (private collection). 34.0 × 22.0 cm.

The essential anatomy of this is presented in an enlarged format later in the book. Here the liver (AB), bile-duct (H) attached to a portion of duodenum (G), spleen (D), pancreas (C), and suprarenal (N) are recognizable in the upper abdomen, while lower down are seen the kidneys (M) (the right correctly lower than the left), their veins and ureters, the rectum (S), the uterus (Z), the ovaries (a), and the bladder (Q) (with the attachment of the urachus, (R)), together with the inferior vena cava, aorta, and other structures. These include a vessel (T) that appears to be a *mélange* of artery and vein, part of which can clearly be seen, on the left side, to join the ureter (P). This is in fact curious, because in other plates this inaccuracy does not occur. There is another inaccuracy in the origin of the umbilical arteries (Y), the left of which is shown arising not from the internal iliac artery, but from the ovarian artery.

The state of knowledge of the relationships of the ovaries and their vessels, the uterine ligaments, and the oviducts revealed in this plate reflect the prevailing beliefs of the period, and need not be commented on further.

Tab. XVIII.   Lib. VIII.   81

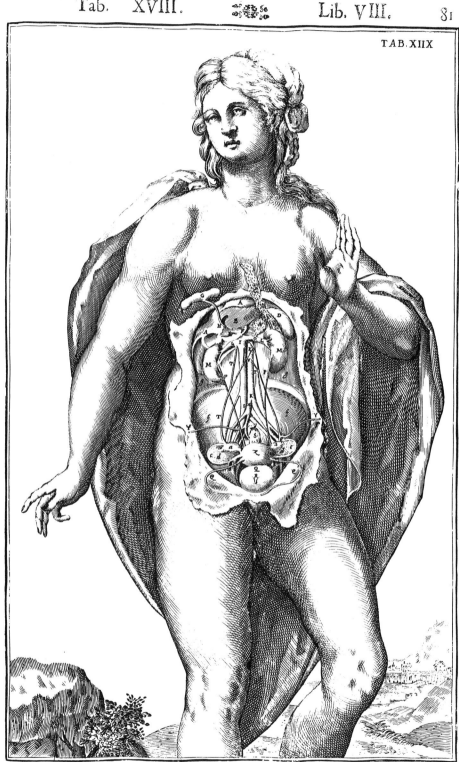

TAB. XIIX

PLATE 63

64 Pregnant woman with fetus and placenta displayed. Tabula I of A. Spieghel, *De formato foetu* ..., Venice, 1627 (private collection). 34.2 × 21.0 cm.

This is the last of a series of four stylized representations of the uterus, with membranes and fetus *in situ*: it could almost be entitled 'the flowering of the fetus'. Bearing in mind its date, this plate portrays the placenta, vessels, and umbilical cord ('vinculum') quite excellently. This is true also of the chubby, purportedly female, baby, with a good head of hair, although its lower limbs are rather awkwardly placed. The membranes, however,—(A) to (C)—are less good; they are too substantial and too numerous.

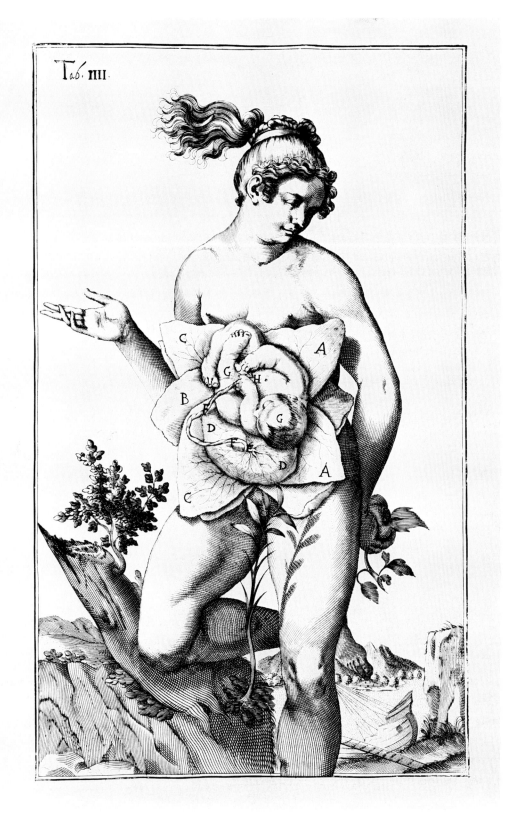

PLATE 64

Pietro Berrettini da Cortona, 1596–1669

The scholars and the artists of the Renaissance explored intensely the classical world, a world in which heroes and gods as well as philosophers were seen to play their parts. Each new artefact recovered and placed on show, privately and publicly, was studied and then copied. The Hellenistic sculpture of Laocoön and his two sons fatally struggling against sea serpents, made *c*.25 BC, was recovered and displayed in 1506. It became a model for many drawings, engravings, and sculptures. Titian drew it in a sardonic manner, as a group of three monkeys; it has been suggested that this was a comment on Vesalius' criticism of Galen's anatomy, that it was derived from the lower animals rather than from human beings.

This sixteenth-century attitude to the ancient world persisted into the following century, which was also permeated with an idea of a past in which the arguments of calm reason and the extravagant behaviour of mythical beings both played a part. The ancient city of Rome became a place of pilgrimage, with the Vatican—particularly when ruled by Urban VIII (Matteo Barberini)—leading the way in the serious attention it paid to ancient remains and collections of classical objects. Visitors to Rome could take away with them engravings of classical sites and sculptures, produced, as a lucrative enterprise, by artists, engravers, and printers.

The ancient world was looked on as a protracted golden age. When he drew plans of classical sites or of ruined buildings, the painter and architect Pietro da Cortona freely reconstructed the original structures, improvising where necessary. Artists like Cortona, in painting after painting, 'lionized heroes and dreamed of gods'. When Cortona painted the 'Rape of the Sabine women', or Ovid's 'Four ages of man', and when he produced complicated allegories, designed to show the glory of his patrons and divine providence, his settings were of the golden age. Yet this happy freedom of expression and interpretation came out of Cortona's sketchbook studies of actual objects. It is not surprising, then, that when, early in his career, Cortona made twenty anatomical drawings, the figures were noble and heroic, and positioned amidst archaeological ruins.

Pietro Berrettini was born in 1596 at Cortona, a town not far from Arezzo in Tuscany—Cortona was earlier the birthplace of the artist Luca Signorelli, also interested in human anatomy. Pietro's formative years as an artist were spent in Rome, where, after a relatively obscure beginning, he rapidly established himself in his twenties as one of the principal men in what has come to be known as the Roman High Baroque. His eventual patron was one of the nephews of Urban VIII, Cardinal Francesco Barberini; Cortona produced an allegorical picture glorifying another nephew, Cardinal Antonio Barberini. Some of the paintings done in his maturity were vast—for instance, his ceiling in the Barberini Palace, now the National Gallery in Rome, or the fresco painted for the Grand Duke of Tuscany in the Pitti Palace in Florence. Yet even in these, where so much is going on, the classically robed figures were graceful, well grouped and organized, and painted with remarkable freedom.

Pietro da Cortona's anatomical drawings were made in Rome, probably about 1618. They were apparently prepared from dissections made at the Santo Spirito Hospital. The anatomist is not known for certain, possibly Nicholas Larchée. The actual drawings have, surprisingly, been preserved, for they were acquired by Sir William Hamilton, FRS, British Ambassador to the King of Naples. He should be better known for his significant contributions to archaeology, or indeed to diplomacy; but it is his wife Emma's relationship with Horatio Nelson that comes first to mind. Cortona's drawings were presented by Hamilton to William Hunter, obstetrician, anatomist, and collector. The letter from Hamilton, dated 31 March 1772, sent with this gift is bound in with the drawings. It begins 'As I am truly sensible that these drawings of Pietro di Cortona could no where be placed to such advantage as in your Museum, allow me to present them to you ...' Hunter himself called attention to an accompanying seventeenth-century manuscript note that these studies were Cortona's original work. They were included in Hunter's bequest of his entire collection to the University of Glasgow, where they still are: Hunterian MS 653 is a bound folio volume containing the twenty drawings. In their present state they show signs of having been used to prepare engravings.

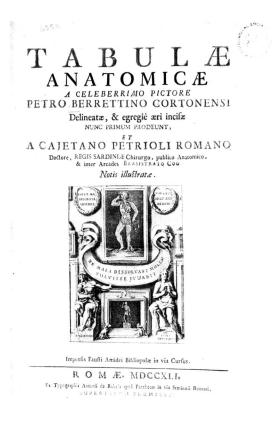

7.5 Title page of Petrioli's edition of Pietro Berrettini's anatomical plates, Rome, 1741.

These anatomical studies are highly finished, and are coloured in a subdued manner: the paper is greyish, the drawing is in brown ink and black chalk, washed with blue, sepia, and grey; certain structures, particularly nerves, are dramatically and effectively highlighted with white paint. The noble gestures of the figures can be seen to have been altered and corrected, in some cases more than once. Many of the dissected men hold oval or rectangular medallions—they look like framed mirrors—within which are drawn figures detailing the anatomy of various regions. Others have no accessory figures. The drawings are numbered, but for the most part have no text or lettering. The eleventh drawing was made in different colours, and may have been a replacement for one lost or damaged.

In 1741, that is some one hundred and twenty years after these drawings were made by Pietro da Cortona, the following book was published in Rome: *Tabulae anatomicae a celeberrimo pictore Petro Berrettino Cortonensi delineatae ...*, Antonio de Rubeis (*Fig. 7.5*). It was edited by

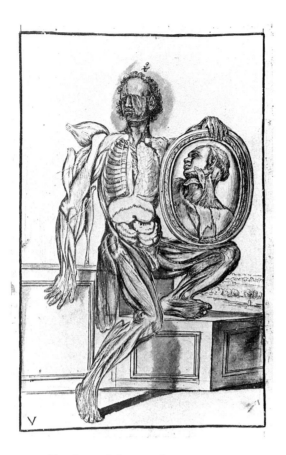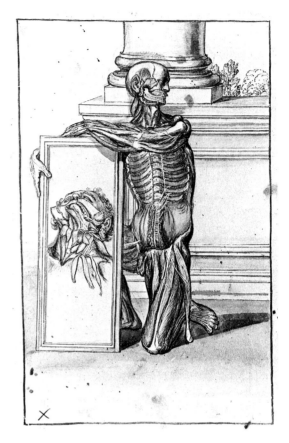

7.6a and b   Original drawings by Pietro Berrettini, presently in the Hunterian Collection of Glasgow University.

Gaetano Petrioli, surgeon to the King of Sardinia. Twenty of the 27 large engravings of this book, that is nos. 1 to 19 and no. 27, can be clearly seen to be closely, but not exactly, similar to the original drawings in the Hunterian Collection (*Plates 65 and 66*: compare *Figs 7.6 a and b*). The remaining seven are mostly copies of the figures in Vesalius' *Fabrica*, or taken from Vesling and others. Petrioli was making available, for the first time, engravings printed from copperplates that were prepared at about the same time as the original paintings, that is around 1618. For this first printed edition Petrioli added new, additional anatomical figures, engraved in an incongruous manner wherever there was sufficient space on the plate. The additional figures are from Vesalius, Valverde, and others.

It can be seen that the original engraver has admirably translated Cortona's drawings, full of life and grace in spite of the subject matter. The anatomical content has been clearly emphasized, but there is a decided falling off in the rendering of the faces (*Figs 7.7 a and b*). In some plates, the landscape background has been changed, but not for the better. Petrioli added a text and identification symbols. In some copies of the book that we have seen the presswork is remarkably fine.

Many of the engravings, following the drawings, emphasize the peripheral nerves. The first fourteen plates show successively deeper layers of dissection from the front; plates 15–19 show a similar progression from the back. The first engraving has 'Petr. Berret. Corton. delin.' at the foot of the impression. The twentieth plate is an inept portrayal from the back, reminding one of the absurd Guidi skeleton shown in our *Plate 56* (see p. 241). This portrayal, and those numbered 21 to 26, are not of the same quality; they are presumably *not* from drawings by Cortona. The last engraving, no. 27, is taken from an original drawing presently in the Hunterian Collection (our *Figs 7.7 a and b*).

Petrioli in 1741 is said to have been in possession not only of Berrettini's plates but also of Eustachio's plates, whose chequered history we have discussed in Chapter 5.

In 1788, another edition was produced. The plates were then a hundred and seventy years old: *Tabulae anatomicae ex archetypis egregii pictoris Petri Berrettini Cortonensis expressae . . .*, Rome, Venantio Monaldini. The editor this time was F. Petraglia. The intrusive figures added by

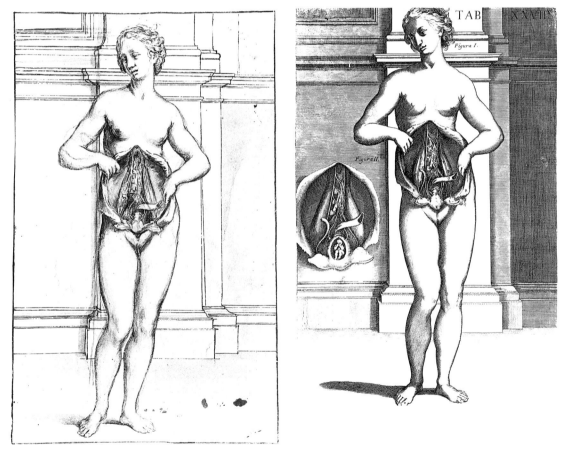

7.7a and b   Berrettini's drawing showing the reproductive organs of the female (Hunterian Collection, Glasgow University), compared with the engraving in Petrioli, 1741.

Petrioli for the first edition have now been erased, and the plates have been burnished and then re-engraved to effect repairs, in some cases clumsily. The accessory figures found in the original drawings have been retained. In an introduction, the history of the plates is described; in this an attribution of the original engraving to Luca Ciamberlano (born 1580, active 1640) is made. His monogram, C superimposed on an L, is to be seen on impressions of plates 1 and 4.

As a postscript, we may note that Pietro Berrettini da Cortona was referred to by his contemporaries, and is referred to by historians of art, as 'Pietro da Cortona' or as 'Pietro' or 'Cortona'. Because anatomists admire the published books of engravings from his drawings, and because they were issued with a title-page carrying his full name, they know him usually as Pietro Berrettini, or more simply, as Berrettini.

65 Seated, dissected male figure. Tab. V from P. Berrettini, *Tabulae anatomicae ...*, Rome, 1741. Engraving made *c.*1618 with two added figures (*Figures III and IIII*) by Petrioli, the editor for this edition (Wellcome Institute Library). 37.5 × 25.5 cm.

In the main figure, the thorax and abdomen have been widely opened and the legs and arms dissected. The left frontalis muscle has been detached and turned downwards, and what must be the supraorbital nerve is shown *deep* to it. (The frontalis muscle is, of course, supplied by a branch of the facial nerve.) The portrayal of the sternomastoid muscles is grossly inaccurate with regard to the positioning of their inferior portions.

There is a folded-down skin flap of the thigh (which more closely resembles thickened fascia lata) to which the lateral cutaneous nerve is distributed.

The superficial and deep peroneal nerves can be distinguished in the right leg, though the distribution of the superficial on to the dorsum of the foot is not portrayed; the deep peroneal is shown accurately terminating at the first cleft. In general the right leg muscular anatomy is accurate.

In the left leg the saphenous nerve is distributed to the medial part of the big toe, but there is a curving branch of the femoral, crossing the thigh medially, which is difficult to understand. The text identifies this as the 'short branch'; it could be the nerve to vastus medialis, displaced; but this nerve seems to be in its proper place anterior to the saphenous nerve.

In the abdomen the diaphragm (m) seems to be 'stitched' to an odd single-notched liver (n) (the 'stitching' may perhaps represent the cut edge of the diaphragm). Beneath the diaphragm is a haphazard and inaccurate grouping of the intestines.

In the thorax the right lung is turned over to the left side and the right vagus is nicely shown, with the recurrent laryngeal nerve hooking around the right subclavian artery; also a rather stylized sympathetic trunk, lying on the ribs. This trunk has rami associated with it, but the origin of these is obscure.

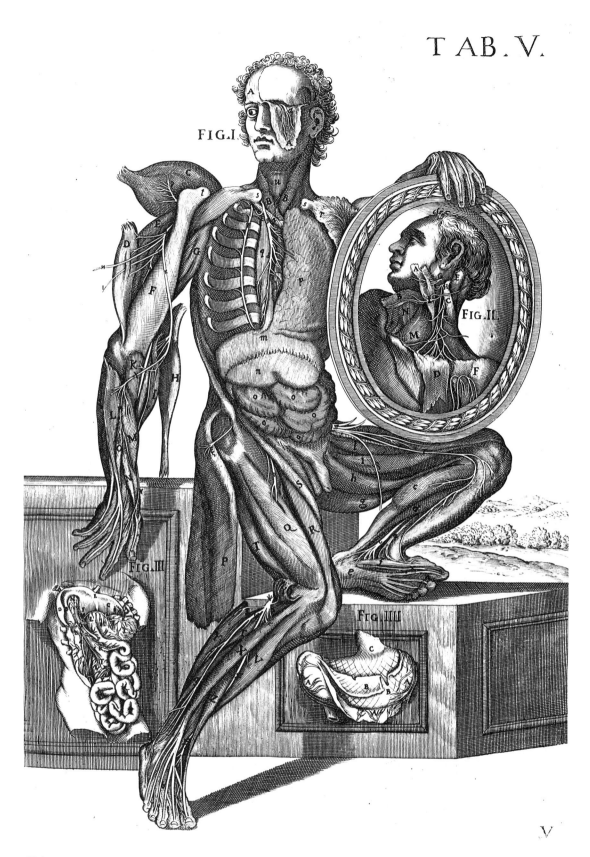

TAB. V.

FIG.I.

FIG.II

FIG.III

FIG.IIII

V

PLATE 65

Berrettini was much given to the twisting of limbs, and here medial rotation of the right arm at the shoulder joint, together with pronation of the forearm, makes the anatomy of this upper limb more difficult to determine than it otherwise would be. The radial nerve is seen winding around the humerus, and its deep and superficial branches are distributed in the forearm, the latter extending to the thumb and dorsum of the hand.

Figure II presents the cervical plexus of nerves and a mass of muscles that are difficult, indeed unnecessary, to identify. Figure III is a straight copy of Vesalius, from page 365 of the 1543 *Fabrica*. Figure IIII shows the oesophagus entering the stomach, which is covered by reflected peritoneum. The concept of the attachment of the greater omentum to the stomach seems poorly understood.

66 A kneeling dissected man showing muscles and nerves. Tab. X of P. Berrettini, *Tabulae anatomicae . . .*, Rome, 1741. Engraving made *c.*1618 with added figures (*Figures III–X*) by Petrioli, the editor for this edition (Wellcome Institute Library). 38.0 × 26.0 cm.

The sartorius muscle (S) of the left thigh has been displaced so as to show the femoral nerve. In the lower leg once again the superficial peroneal nerve is not shown supplying the dorsum of an awkwardly twisted foot. The way the left arm is draped over the board could, at first sight, lead one to think it ends in a right hand. The forearm muscles are very confused.

The thoracic and abdominal contents have been removed, revealing the sympathetic trunk in the thorax, its continuation in the abdomen, and also the splanchnic nerves.

The head shows the inferior alveolar nerve inside the mandible, supplying the lower jaw teeth and giving off its mental branch. (A) represents the upturned masseter muscle, and (C) the posterior belly of digastric.

Figure II has the mandible removed on the left side, presumably so as to show the hypoglossal and lingual nerves. The rest is confusing and not very helpful in enabling one to understand the anatomy of this area—presumably (E) is the anterior belly of digastric, (F) and (G) represent the two geniohyoid muscle bellies, and (A), (B), (and (C) the strap muscles.

Figures III to X are of little anatomical interest in the context of the eighteenth century, being taken from illustrations by Vesalius and Valverde.

In most of Berrettini's plates the nerves are emphasized, and stand out white from the dark shading of the other parts. For a date of 1618 the main figures are good; but the obvious Vesalian-type 'addenda' placed around them by Petrioli both detract from them and irritate the viewer.

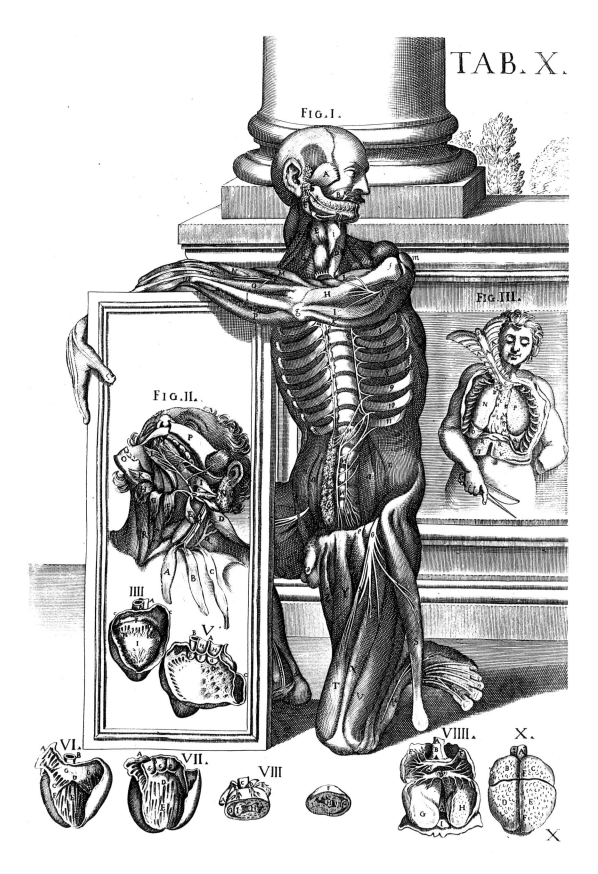

FIG. I.

TAB. X.

FIG. III.

FIG. II.

IIII

V.

VI.

VII.

VIII

VIIII.

X.

X

PLATE 66

Crisostomo Martinez, 1638–1694

In the years around 1490 Leonardo da Vinci included in his many interests a study of human proportions: 'When a man kneels down he will diminish by the fourth part of his height. When a man kneels with his hands to his breast, the umbilicus will be the middle of his height, and similarly the points of the elbows' and so on. Leonardo produced a drawing of a man with limbs extended, and enclosed within a circle and a square, his solution to the problem posed in a throw-away remark by Vitruvius in the first century BC that is recorded in his work on architecture. Leonardo was but one of a number of Florentine artists of the fifteenth century devoted to finding mathematical relations that would help them achieve a semblance of reality in their painting. It was but another facet of the study of perspective, a study which, initiated by Brunelleschi about 1425, had proved susceptible to geometric treatment in the hands of Masaccio, Uccello, Piero della Francesca, and others. L. B. Alberti provided the best theoretical basis for these attempts.

For many years Dürer also concentrated his attention on perspective and proportion, but gave up after many attempts to achieve perfection in representing bodily and facial forms by applying mathematical relationships between the parts. (A parallel, and more successful, endeavour had been to investigate the mathematical relationships between the notes of musical scales.)

The Fontainebleau school in France, as always influenced by things Italian, was also interested in the matter of perspective and in questions of human proportions. Jean Cousin wrote simple manuals on both subjects. His book *Livre de pourtraicture*, Paris, G. le Bé, issued first in 1560, was intended to be 'useful and necessary for painters, sculptors, architects, goldsmiths, embroiderers, joiners, and generally those who love the art of painting and sculpture'. This book contains woodcuts illustrating relatively simple rules. Our *Fig. 7.8*, from the 1671 edition, shows the proportions of the trunk. Some years later, in 1689, and from the same city, came a vastly more sophisticated engraving illustrating human proportions in an anatomical context (*Plate 67*). This very large copper engraving was in *Nouvelles figures de proportions et d'anatomie du corps humain*. The anatomist, the artist, and the engraver were one and the same person, a Spaniard, Crisostomo Martinez. The same print was reissued in Frankfurt and Leipzig three years later, re-engraved by Georg Bodenehr, one of a family of engravers and artists; and it is from this that our *Plate 67* is taken.

At the time when this print was published Martinez had been in Paris for about two years, and was in his early fifties. Previously he had lived his life in Valencia, where he had studied anatomy. About 1680 he had decided to produce a series of anatomical plates, and, to further the project, the Spanish Crown had funded his journey to Paris. His stay in France was however interrupted, for in 1690 he left under suspicion of spying. He died in Flanders shortly after.

About fifty years later, two more of the Martinez plates were printed, again in Paris, *Nouvelle esposition des deux grandes planches ... par Chrysostome Martinez, Espagnol, representant des figures ... de proportions et d'anatomie*, 1740. The editor was J. B. Winslow, whose book on anatomy,

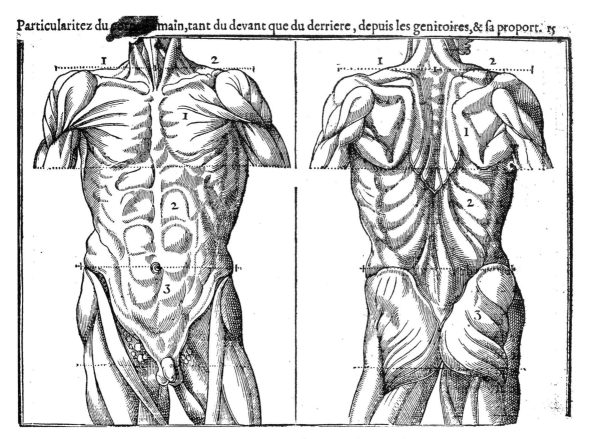

Particularitez du ███████ main, tant du devant que du derriere , depuis les genitoires, & fa proport. 15

7.8   J. Cousin's woodcut showing the proportions of the trunk from his *Livre de pourtraicture*, 1671.

1733, was illustrated only by a few engravings from Eustachio made two hundred years before.

Martinez had however progressed much farther than would be indicated from these three plates. Nineteen are extant, all of which were published in J. M. López Piñero's book on Martinez issued in Valencia in 1964 (second edition 1982). This work enables us to appreciate the remarkable achievements of this largely neglected anatomical scientist. Our plate of anatomical figures is extremely fine, but we may perhaps decide that the concentration on measurement and proportion is of doubtful utility—but how Leonardo would have appreciated the pictures! Martinez justifies his emphasis on measurement by a reference on a scroll above the architectural draughtsman's dividers shown at the bottom centre of the engraving to the Book of Ezekiel: Chapters 40 to 48 describe a complex vision in which a man 'with a line of flax in his hand and a measuring rod' shows the prophet the land of Israel, the temple, and the city, all of which are minutely described in terms of measurement. Whatever we might think about this, we surely should admire Martinez' ability to represent fine standing *écorchés*, showing the muscles, bones, and joints as if the body were transparent. We are reminded of Leonardo's term *corpo transparent*, which was however developed farther by Martinez, since his figures, unlike Leonardo's, did not rely on cross-sections.

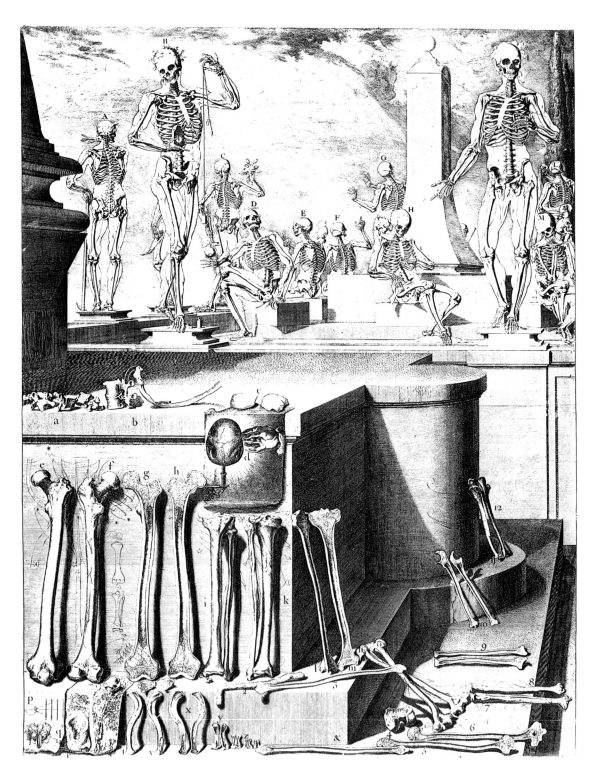

7.9   C. Martinez: skeletal groups c. 1685. Single-sheet engraving at Wellcome Institute Library.

In another Baroque engraving, Lamina XVII, Martinez shows groups of skeletons walking, sitting, and standing on masonry plinths and by monuments (*Fig. 7.9*). Each skeleton is seen as if viewed through a transparent body, so beautifully indicating the relationships of the bones to the surface markings. It may be noted that one of these skeleton figures holds a plumb-line, while another nearby is perhaps tossing an apple. Does this refer to the force of gravity, recently explained by Newton in his *Philosophiae naturalis principia mathematica*, London, 1687? Scattered below these standing and sitting skeletons are collections of bones placed in an orderly fashion on the stone steps of the monument. Some of these bones have been sectioned longitudinally to show the medulla and the cancellous bone. Martinez, as López Piñero shows, was an authority on the structure and function of bone, to investigate which he employed lenses. He must be regarded as a pioneer microscopist, for the first book on microscopy, Hooke's *Micrographia*, London, 1665, had only been issued some twenty years earlier.

Eustachio, Fabrici, Casserio, Berrettini, and now Martinez have this in common, that they set out to prepare copperplates for extensive treatises on anatomy, but died before the work was completed and published. To this number may be added Canano, who had, apparently, completed the engravings to show all the muscles of the body. While all issued a portion of their illustrations, the rest remained unpublished until long after the drawings or engravings had been completed. The gap for Eustachio was about 160 years, for Casserio, only 20 years or so, for Berrettini, 133 years, and for Martinez, 270 years. Fabrici's engraved plates of the paintings he commissioned are lost; only a few of the paintings have been reproduced. And Canano's prepared but unpublished plates will most likely never be printed, for they are lost.

The circumstances of a busy professional life, the complexity of anatomical structures to be illustrated, the difficulty of finding and the expense of employing patient and competent artists and engravers (how slowly the burin traces a line!), the demanding nature and costs of printing satisfactorily from plates as large as 70 × 50 cm, and the uncertainty of a sufficiently large market for the inevitably expensive product ... these are some of the shoals on which the enterprise may founder. It may legitimately be wondered what other plates of anatomical illustration may have been prepared in the years before 1700 that are now unknown, or are lost or unpublished. We must admire those anatomists, artists, engravers, printers, and publishers who successfully navigated these obviously troubled waters.

67 Skeletal and muscle figures to illustrate proportions by C. Martinez, Frankfurt and Leipzig, 1692. (Lamina XIX J. M. López Piñero, 1964.) Engraving (Wellcome Institute Library, from a single sheet bound with J. Remmelin, *Catoptrum . . .* , Ulm, 1619). 69.0 × 51.0 cm.

Like his rather crowded Lamina XVII—*Tabla grande de los esqueletos y huesos* (*see Fig. 7.9*), this plate emphasizes Martinez' interest in the relative proportions of the human body — as the scroll on the plinth shield states, after Ezekiel, 'mensura ista mensurabis'. At the same time, in the adult figures, he brings together bones and muscles in a most interesting manner.

In many cases the muscles are identified in the different views by very small numbers. Some of the muscle anatomy is not too accurate. For instance, in the posterior view of the thigh, gracilis and (presumably) sartorius just medial to it are curved too far posteriorly, and the hamstrings are not well drawn. The side-view of the calf and foot is an improvement, though it is a pity about the extensor retinaculum, which looks rather like a piece of felt laid over the tendons. However, the portrayal of pectoralis major and deltoid is good. In both the side and front views the rectus abdominis is over-conspicuous, and, in the latter, once again sartorius inclines posteriorly, above vastus medialis, at too high a level. In the posterior view, the position of the right scapula, with the arm raised from the side, is well captured; sad, though, are the single extensor tendons to each of the index and little fingers.

While a reasonable anatomical presentation for its date, the small child's skeleton—possessing rather too many teeth—presumably was included to point up the proportional differences between the child and adult—for example, the mid-point of the heel–vertex height is just below the iliac crest as opposed to the level of the pubic crest (or just below the femoral head) in the adult. Bearing in mind the great variations in anatomical build, and thus in the proportions of one part of the body to another in different individuals, too detailed mensuration might be thought counter-productive. In addition to Martinez, however, others have been interested in anatomical measurement, notably Leonardo and Dürer. Martinez was one of the first to examine and study the structure of bones, and illustrations of sectioned bones feature prominently in his work.

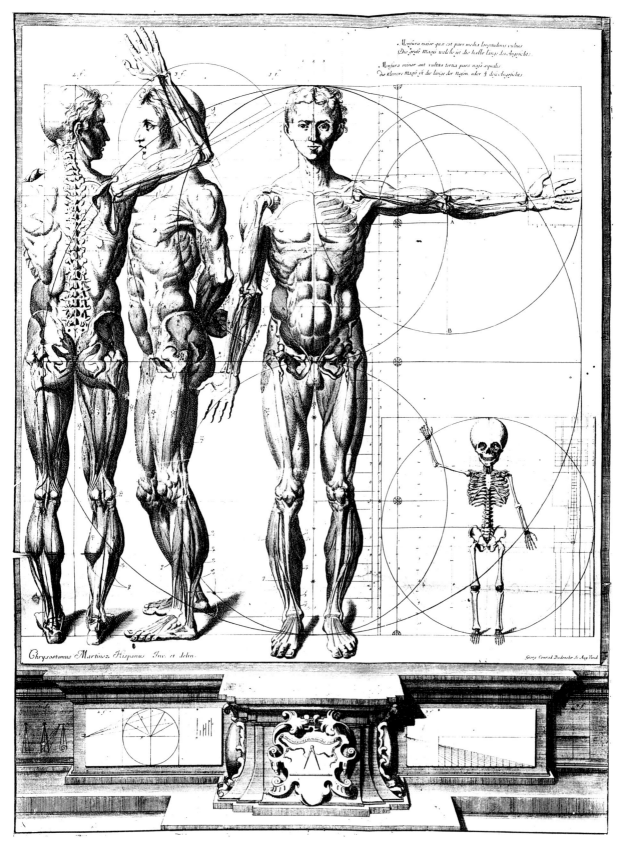

PLATE 67

Chapter 7: Selected reading

Briganti, G. (1962). *Pietro da Cortona o della pittura barocca*. Sansoni, Florence.

Cazort, M. (1987). On dissected putti and combustible chameleons. *Print Collector's Newsletter*, **17**, 197–201.

Cole, F. J. (1975). *A history of comparative anatomy*. Dover, New York (reprint of 1949 edition).

Duhme, L. (1980). *Die Tabulae anatomicae des Pietro Berrettini da Cortona*. Institut für Geschichte der Medizin, Cologne.

Dumaitre, P. (1964). Un anatomiste espagnol à Paris au XVIIe siècle: Chrysostome Martinez ... *Méd de France*, **154**, 10–15.

Glick, T. F. (1974). Crisóstome Martinéz. Dict. sci. Biog, **9**, 145–6.

Janson, H. W. (n.d.). Titian's Laocoön caricature and the Vesalian–Galenist controversy. In *16 studies*, Harry N. Abrams, New York.

Kemp, M. (1976). Dr William Hunter on the Windsor Leonardos and his volume of drawings attributed to Pietro da Cortona. *Burlington Mag.*, **118**, no. 876.

López, Piñero, J. M. (1982). *El atlas anatómico de Crisóstomo Martinéz grabador y microscopista de siglo XVII*. Archivo Municipal, Valencia.

Meyer, A. and Hierons, R. (1962). Observations on the history of the 'Circle of Willis'. *Med. Hist.*, **6**, 119–30.

Norman, J. M. (1986). *The anatomical plates of Pietro da Cortona* .... Dover, New York.

Premuda, L. (1971). Giulio Casseri. Dict. sci. Biog., **3**, 98–100.

Williams, E. (1968). *Gods and heroes: Baroque images of antiquity*.... Wildenstein, New York.

8

Anatomy in the Netherlands 1600–1800

The rise of medical science in the Low Countries

THE UNION OF UTRECHT in 1579 has been taken as the beginning of the effective independence of the United Provinces—the Dutch Netherlands—from the rule of Spain, the movement towards independence having been co-ordinated by the House of Orange, and in particular Stadtholder, Prince William the Silent. The population of the Netherlands trebled between 1550 and 1650. By 1700, Dutch companies, trading into the East and West Indies, had extended their empire to trading stations in South Africa, India, and Ceylon, as well as to many of the islands now united as Indonesia, to the Malayan coastline, to Nagasaki, and to parts of the east coast of South America; New Amsterdam had been transferred to the British in 1667, and renamed New York. At the beginning of the seventeenth century, the population density in the Netherlands (40 per square kilometre) was higher than that of other continental European countries with the exception of Italy (44 per sq. km). At the same time the homelands of the state were being increased by land claimed from the sea.

During the first hundred years of independence, years of almost constant political and military turmoil, there was a remarkable rise in Dutch commercial enterprise, from its beginnings as a Baltic trade in salted herrings, to a world-wide trade in every commodity. An archipelago of cities prospered, clustered on land that was either just above or just below sea-level, with Amsterdam emerging as the principal community. This city had a population of 30 000 in 1530, about 150 000 in 1650, and

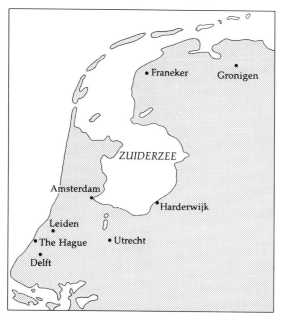

8.1 Map of the Netherlands.

200 000 by 1700. Most of the cities were predominantly Calvinist; but many of the villages remained Catholic, and there was considerable tolerance and co-operation, or at least a *modus vivendi*, between different religious sects, both during the period leading to independence and in the early years of the new trading nation. The universities were doctrinally Calvinist, but tolerated different opinions. Indeed questions of doctrine did not usually arise in the newer studies of the Universities: astronomy, physics, chemistry, botany, anatomy, and oriental studies were all subjects of importance to a state concerned with the welfare of its citizens, and particularly to a country which was both enlarging its land-mass and expanding overseas. Universities may have debated vigorously

Descartes' philosophical methods, and the orthodox curators of Leiden University might proscribe his teachings (as happened in 1647); but, for all this, the spirit of Leiden University and its medical school was Cartesian, and Descartes himself found an agreeable refuge for a time near Leiden, and a publisher there for his *Discours de la méthode ...*, 1637; his *De homine figuris ...*, published posthumously in 1662, applied his materialism to physiology. There was an 'extraordinary lack of religious prejudice or aggression in Holland ... compared to the rest of Europe. Issues of behaviour and belief that produced strife, accusations, even executions in England are notable by their rarity in Holland' (Alpers 1983).

The inhabitants of the new state did not turn in on themselves in narrow self-absorption; as citizens of a growing imperialist state, they welcomed foreigners. Half the Groningen professors in the seventeenth century were German in origin, and, while Leiden and other universities had a lower proportion, their professors were appointed from France, Scandinavia, the British Isles, Poland, and Hungary, as well as from Germany. The students, too, came from many countries. Since lectures were predominantly in Latin there were few language barriers in academic life. Foreigners, including religious refugees—Mennonites, Lutherans, Huguenots, and Jews— enriched the intellectual and commercial life of the Dutch cities. Scientific and technological studies were carried out in private houses as well as in the universities. In the sixteenth century individual traders in the Netherlands began to separate shop from private house. Antoni van Leeuwenhoek (1632–1723), prosperous draper and great microscopist, made his scientific observations in his house in Delft. Technology in the Netherlands emphasized instrumentation for surveying land and navigating ships. The construction of these instruments required accurate grinding of lenses and precise machining of the holders and stages required to position these lenses; such techniques could be applied to other uses, especially in biological and medical dissection and microscopy.

A flourishing book trade served to disseminate technical information in Latin, Dutch, French, and other languages. This had been consolidated by publishing handy reprints of classical, theological, or philosophical works that, for one reason or another, were banned in other countries. Dutch printing-houses also plagiarized books published elsewhere. A printing, publishing, and bookselling house that well exemplified the interdependence of commerce, science, and technology was the Bleau family, who specialized in maps, and whose multivolume *Atlas major ...*, 1650–62, became the standard by which others were judged. The founder of the house, who had worked with the astronomer Tycho Brahe, published his first map in 1604; by the time he opened his new shop in Amsterdam in 1637 he had become cartographer to the Dutch East India Company. The new printing-shop was visited in 1641 by John Evelyn, who reported, with exaggeration, that there was a room 'in which the copper plates are kept, from which the atlases ... and other choice books are printed and which must have cost a ton of gold'. There were nine presses for type and six for copperplate printing. It is not surprising that from such printing-houses there came, during the seventeenth and eighteenth centuries, a number of the finest technical books with copperplate engravings that have ever been produced. There were books of engineering, such as those on *wipmolen* (windmills) used for land drainage; and also large folio atlases of human and animal anatomy which have never been surpassed. An artist able to paint large canvases on classical themes might well be prepared to be engaged by other patrons as an illustrator of flowers and plants, or maps, or comparative and human anatomy. The orientation of Dutch cultural life was towards observation, representation, and description. There was a flowering of descriptive science, and a concomitant development of optical instruments. In this environment anatomical science, and anatomical illustration, prospered.

Some of the scientific activity in the Netherlands was informally organized outside the universities; groups of investigators met to report and discuss their findings. A 'Private College' in Amsterdam of Dutch, Danish, and German scientists flourished from 1664 to 1672, organized at the same time as on similar lines to the 'Invisible College', the precursor of the Royal Society of London. (There were other scientific societies developing, each with its own house style, in Italy, France, Germany, Denmark ...) Even earlier there were informal gatherings of experimenters—which in retrospect might be called research groups; in England the group around Thomas Willis in Oxford was one such. In the Netherlands there was a group of young men, originally pupils of Franciscus Sylvius (de le Boë), who experimented in the Harveian manner in the Botanic Gardens in Leiden, and later in the house of Johannes de Wale; included were the Dane, Thomas Bartholin, and Johannes van Horne, the son of one of the first directors of the Dutch East India Company. From these experiments, and those conducted later in Copenhagen, came Bartholin's discovery of the watery lymphatics, which resembled 'clear brooks winding over the plain'—a simile appropriate to the Low Countries. In his important publications, published in 1652–4, one may find an epitaph on the disenthronement of the liver as the central organ in cardiovascular and haematological physiology, the end of a 'sanguine empire'—a metaphor readily appreciated in the provinces that had successfully united against Spain.

Fredrik Ruysch (1638–1731)

Ruysch was born at The Hague, and, as a boy, was apprenticed to an apothecary. Even before he had passed the necessary examinations he opened a shop, for which he was reprimanded by the apothecaries' company. Soon after he had legitimized his position he travelled to Leiden and began a study of medicine at the university in 1661. He received his medical doctorate from Leiden in 1664. He was a student of Johannes van Horne, the Professor of Anatomy and Surgery. Others working under van Horne were Jan Swammerdam and Nicolaus Steno, a Danish student sent to the Netherlands by Thomas Bartholin. Later, in 1663, the researchers were joined by Regnier de Graaf. They conducted physiological investigations using live dogs, and, reporting on such experiments, Steno wrote: '. . . it is not without abhorrence that I torture them with such prolonged pain. The Cartesians take great pride in the truth of their philosophical system, but I wish they could convince me as thoroughly as they are themselves convinced of the fact that animals have no souls'. Ruysch preferred to work on human cadavers, at first studying the vascular distribution within the liver. Swammerdam had begun to perfect the then-current injection techniques. Injections were used for physiological purposes as well as for anatomical studies; Harvey himself (1651) had shown that one could demonstrate the pulmonary circulation by injecting fluids into the right side of the heart and finding that they passed through the lungs to the left side. The younger Dutch medical men were enthusiastic supporters of the Harveian doctrine. A number of variant injection methods were used: air was blown into vessels which were then dried in the sun and wind; fluids were injected, coloured appropriately—vermilion for arterial and various blue dyes for venous injections. Mercury, injected into the bronchi or into blood-vessels or lymphatic vessels, showed up the tubes as silvery trees. Warm fatty solutions were used which solidified when cool; these had the advantage that the fluid did not escape if the vessels were punctured during a subsequent dissection. At a later date, injections into the vessels were following by using corrosives which destroyed the tissue present, leaving casts of the vessels.

Following his studies on the liver, Ruysch was put to work by van Horne to study lymphatic vessels. He was asked to confirm the presence of valves in these vessels, in order to support van Horne's argument against the imaginative anatomy and physiology proposed by Louis de Bils, whose hypotheses required lymph to flow in both directions. Ruysch demonstrated the

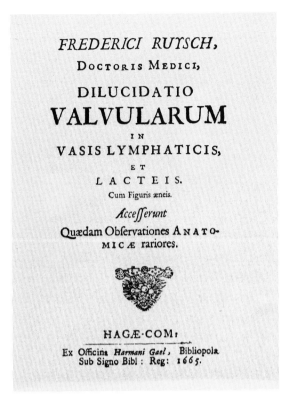

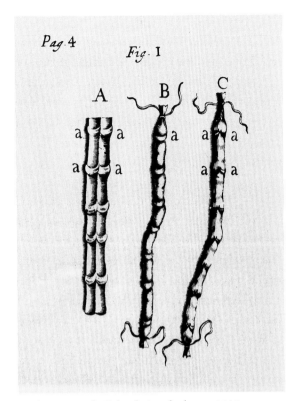

FREDERICI RUYSCH,

DOCTORIS MEDICI,

DILUCIDATIO

VALVULARUM

IN

VASIS LYMPHATICIS,

ET

L A C T E I S.

Cum Figuris æneis.

Accesserunt

Quædam Obfervationes ANATO-
MICÆ rariores.

HAGÆ-COM:

Ex Officina *Harmani Gael*, Bibliopola
Sub Signo Bibl : Reg: 1665.

Pag. 4   *Fig.* I

8.2a and b   Title page and figure of valves of the lymphatics, from Ruysch, *Dilucidatio valvularum*, 1665.

existence of the valves in front of de Bils, who retreated defeated from the encounter. This work was published in a small monograph *Dilucidatio valvularum in vasis lymphaticis ... 1665* (*Figs 8.2a and b*). Ruysch had already started medical work at The Hague, attending the sick during an epidemic of bubonic plague. In 1667, when he was twenty-nine years of age. Ruysch moved to the position of *Praelector* in Anatomy to the Surgeons' Guild in Amsterdam; he stayed there until he died at the age of ninety-two. In this post, and as city obstetrician, he lectured to surgeons and to midwives.[1] Ruysch also lectured on anatomy privately to foreign students— no visit to the Dutch anatomy schools was complete without a period with him. In addition, he later became forensic physician to the court of justice and Professor of Botany in the *Athenaeum Illustre*, which required him to give lectures on medical botany to apothecaries and others. Ruysch's son, Hendrik, and his daughter, Rachel—a professional painter of flower and fruit arrangements—both assisted in preparing some of his anatomical displays. Hendrik is shown, anachronistically as a young child, in the official painting by Jan van Neck (1682): 'Dr Ruysch's Anatomy Lesson' (*Fig. 8.3*). He is shown holding the skeleton of a baby—another

[1] The Dutch practice of taking seriously the education of midwives has continued. The Netherlands are fortunate, for midwives still maintain an exceptionally fine service, with maternal and infant mortality kept at the lowest levels.

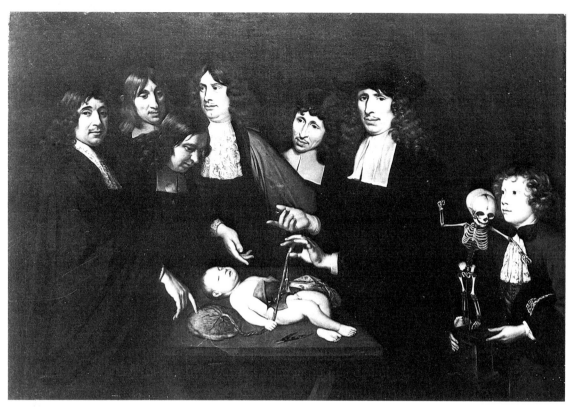

8.3 'Dr Ruysch's anatomy lesson.'

memento mori, so beloved in the Netherlands at that time. (An earlier portrait of Ruysch, again for the Surgeons' Guild of Amsterdam, was painted by Adriaan Backer in 1670. Rembrandt's 'Anatomy lesson of Dr Nicolaas Tulp' (1632) is an early painting in the same official series.)

During the sixty years and more that he worked in Amsterdam, Ruysch devoted most of his energies to the preparation of injected specimens, applying and developing the techniques that he had learnt as a student in van Horne's house. Using syringes of a type invented by de Graaf, he made injections of solidifying medium into the blood-vessels of human cadavers. His techniques and recipes he kept secret, but the injection fluids probably included talc, white wax (or suet), and cinnabar (that is, red mercuric sulphide). His clearing fluid was oil of lavender or turpentine, and his preserving fluid was possibly 67 per cent ethanol, to which black pepper had been added. The injections may have been made into bodies passively moved under warm water. Later workers condemned Ruysch's unethical secrecy: John Sheldon emphasized in 1784 that 'progress of the science has undoubtedly been much impeded by the mystery observed ... a mystery which deserves the severest censure ...'.

Injection methods were also exploited by other Dutch researchers. In 1671–2 Swammerdam sent to the Royal Society in London a preparation of the vessels of the uterus and its tubes injected with red wax. Later, combining microscopy and fine instrumentation, including microinjections, Swammerdam established the science of insect anatomy. During the period 1650–1800 injection was a principal tool for many anatomists and physiologists; as none was as well-known for this as Ruysch, injected preparations became known as examples of the 'Ruyschian art'.

What was the scientific return from Ruysch's years devoted to making injected preparations? Many anatomists had followed Galen in considering that there were many parts of the body devoid of a blood-supply. Ruysch was able to show that this view was largely mistaken, for in his preparations all could see minute blood-vessels in most of the organs of the body—even the periosteum of the tiny auditory ossicles and the walls of larger arteries had a blood-supply. So impressed was Ruysch with the profusion of blood-vessels shown by injections that he came to support the idea that many organs, including all the glands, were composed entirely of vessels, with no functional intervening parenchymatous tissue. The functions of an organ could be attributed to the particular pattern of arrangement of the blood-vessels, a pattern unique to that organ. This mechanistic, Descartian view was held to explain the different types of glandular secretions. Pores, beyond the limits of microscopical investigation, were shaped correspondingly to the shape of substances secreted. (Later Ruysch despaired of understanding secretion: 'only God knew how glands worked'.) Ruysch's views were widely adopted, for instance by Haller, and were still to be found in medical literature in the late eighteenth century. It is to be noted that van Leeuwenhoek came to quite different conclusions about capillary function as a result of microscopical observations, conclusions much more in accord with present-day understanding.

It is not so easy in our time to understand another aspect of Ruysch's professional life, namely his collection or 'cabinet' of anatomical preparations:

His museum, or repository of curiosities, contain'd such a rich and magnificent variety, that one would have rather taken it for the collection of a King than the property of a private man. But not satisfied with the store and variety it afforded, he would beautify the scene, and join an additional lustre to the curious prospect. He mingled groves of plants, and designs of shell-work with skeletons, and dismember'd limbs; and, that nothing might be wanting, he animated, if I may so speak, the whole with apposite inscriptions, taken from the best Latin poets. This museum was the admiration of foreigners: generals of armies, embassadors, electors, and even princes and kings, were fond to visit it.

This quotation is from Robert James, *Medicinal dictionary* ..., London, 1743. (The biography of Ruysch included in this encyclopaedic dictionary has been considered, on fragile stylistic grounds, to have been written by Dr Samuel Johnson. It is largely a translation of Bernard Fontenelle's *Éloge de Ruysch* ..., 1731.) In one such display (*Figure 8.4*) the construction starts from a wooden base on which are piled stones taken *post mortem* from the gall-bladder and the urinary tract. Actual and metaphorical vascular trees and branches sprout from the stony ground; a bird perches, and, high up, a four-month-old human fetal skeleton stands. 'Why should I long for the things of this world?' reads the text and 'Death spares no man, not even the defenceless infant'. On the either side, on separate plinths, are two other skeletons of a similar age, one holding a miniature sickle—ridiculously small for a symbol of death as a grim reaper; the other in a mourning stance, wiping a non-existent eye, an injected omentum serving as a handkerchief. 'Man that is born of woman is of few days, and full of trouble.' The engraving, by C. H. Huijberts, is said to be taken from 'life', that is, from an observed arrangement in Ruysch's cabinet, and not drawn from imagination. Ruysch's displays have been analysed in detail from both a scientific and a moral point of view by Luyendijk-Elshout (1970).

The engraving seems, in a post-surrealist, post-psychoanalytical era, to have the qualities of a dream, at the same time ridiculous and unpleasant. But to the burghers, to the nobility, and to the royal persons who visited Ruysch's cabinet, such assemblies were literally wonderful, serious and profound realities—at one and the same time scientific and moral. In another engraving the medical consequences of sin were similarly demonstrated: an infant's leg kicks the cranium of a prostitute, which shows syphilitic changes. This is a precursor of the nineteenth-century museums of syphilology open to the public, to promote both scientific curiosity and moral repugnance.

Preceding Ruysch's catalogue there had been a catalogue by Nehemiah Grew, 1681, of the Royal Society of London's collection of rarities. The seventeenth century's collections were the unfocused precursors of the great ones of William Hunter and John Hunter in the eighteenth century, collections donated to Glasgow University and the Royal College of Surgeons of England respectively.

There is little need to emphasize the persistence of the somewhat obvious theme of 'inevitable fate' in anatomical illustration, but seldom has it been expressed in such a whole-hearted, enthusiastic, and extravagant way. Swammerdam draws the same moral point in a treatise on the mayfly, whose imago lives only a few hours—this example of insecto-theology made a lasting contribution to entomology.

In 1715, Ruysch put his collection of approximately thirteen hundred specimens up for sale; and in 1717 Tsar Peter the Great purchased them for his *Kunstkammer* in St Petersburg. The price paid was 30 000 guilders, which in those days would have bought two houses in Amsterdam. Specimens from Ruysch's collection are still extant at Leningrad's Academy of Sciences. Although in his eightieth year, Ruysch immediately set to and gathered another collection, which at his death was sold to the King of Poland, John Sobieski. These royal attentions to anatomy were but marginally relevant to the progress of that science, and, not surprisingly, led to criticisms: 'A certain Professor of Physic very seriously advised him to renounce those novelties, and tread in the safe and beated paths of his predecessors ... [and] told him, that his conduct in that particular was inconsistent with the dignity of a professor; to all which Ruysch replied, in a noble and truly laconic strain, *come and see*' (James's *Medicinal dictionary*, 1743). This motto, not dissimilar to that of the Royal Society of London, was inscribed over the door to his cabinet. Peter founded his public museum on similar lines: 'I want people to look and learn'.

Govard Bidloo, with whom he argued in print, called Ruysch a 'subtile butcher'; Ruysch retorted that this was better than an infamous pimp—*Lánio subtilis, quam leno famosus*. Ruysch

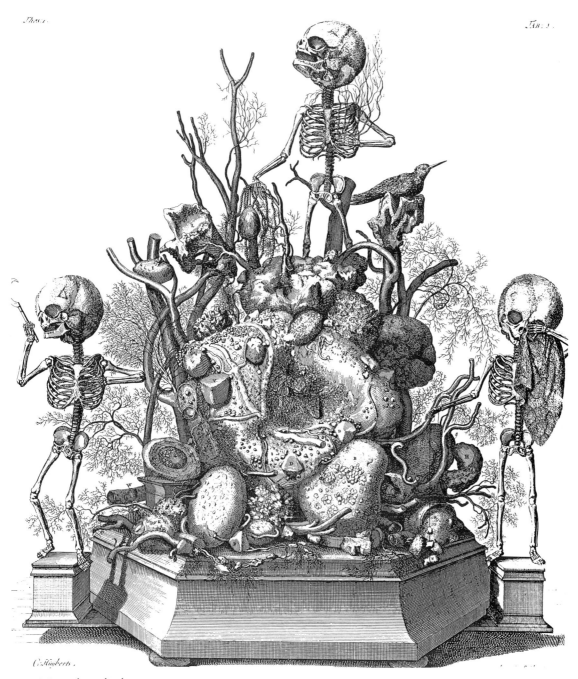

8.4 A Ruyschian display.

had equally vigorous arguments with others, but he could disagree politely: his younger friend Hermann Boerhaave and he published in the same volume a disputation, by an exchange of letters, as to whether or not the liver was made of vessels only. There is no doubt that Ruysch in many of his preparations produced artefacts by forcing fluids into his injected specimens at

ANATOMY IN THE NETHERLANDS: 1600–1800   295

pressures high enough to create false passages. His use of microscopes was perfunctory. Ruysch's attempts to answer physiological questions by purely anatomical means—the display of small vessels—may have contributed to the eighteenth-century failure to exploit Harveian methods. As our *Plate 68* shows, Ruysch was, however, a fine classical anatomist, and anyone who can demonstrate the vessels of the periosteum of the ear ossicles merits a certain amount of admiration. It was probably this side of Ruysch's work which was recognized by his election to the Royal Society of London and the Academy of Sciences in Paris.

The skill of Ruysch as an embalmer, who could prepare corpses in his house in Amsterdam so that 'they were so many prolongations of life ...' was attested to by the Tsar, who, it was said, was moved to embrace a displayed infant corpse—but this belongs to the history of undertaking, not anatomy.

Some books by F. Ruysch

1. After his dissertation, his first publication—and in the long run the most important scientifically— was his small book on the valves of the lymphatics: *Dilucidatio valvularum in vasis lymphaticis et lacteis*, The Hague, 1665. There was an edition in Dutch by Bidloo, Leiden, 1687.

2. Ruysch's arguments with Bidloo: *Responsio ad Godefridi Bidloi libellum ...*, Amsterdam, 1697.

3. There were published, from Amsterdam, separate volumes of Ruysch's letters on anatomical subjects: *Epistolae anatomicae problematicae ...*, 1696, etc. In 1722 there was a letter to Boerhaave discussing the nature of glands: *Opusculum anatomicum de fabrica glandularum ...*.

4. Beginning in 1691 with a preliminary account, a series of well-illustrated books was published based on Ruysch's collection, his 'cabinet' kept at his houses in Amsterdam: *Thesaurus anatomicus primus ...*, Amsterdam, Joannes Wolters, 1701 (in Dutch, *Het eerste anatomisch cabinet*). Ten volumes in this series were published, 1701–10, with two extra volumes as afterthoughts, 1724 and 1728; Ruysch was ninety years old when this last volume appeared. There were subsequent editions of the *Thesaurus* volumes. All these quarto books are well-illustrated by plates, some folding.

5. Ruysch's collected works, to date, were reissued with the accompanying plates as *Opera omnia anatomico-medico-chirurgica ...*, Amsterdam, 1721. This was updated in a new edition, again from Amsterdam, published posthumously in 1737, and, in the Dutch language, in 1744.

68   Two figures of the heart. Tabula IV from F. Ruysch, *Thesaurus anatomicus quartus*, 1704. The engraving occupies part of a folded sheet (Wellcome Institute Library). 21.5 × 16.0 cm.

The upper drawing is a human heart seen from the diaphragmatic surface, showing the coronary sinus (B) and the veins draining into it, together with its termination in the right atrium (D).

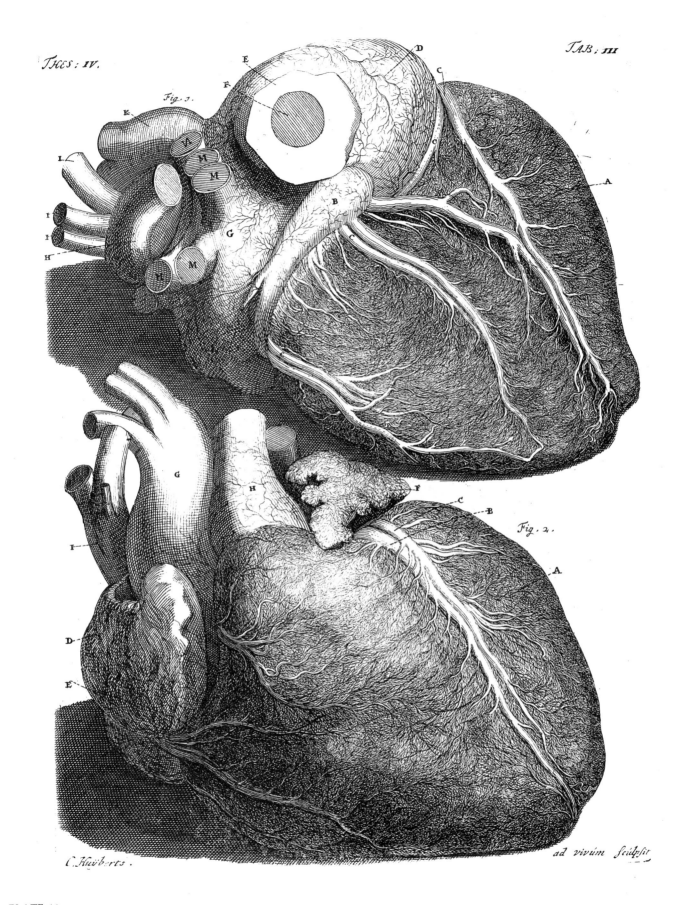

Fig. 1.

TAB: III

PLATE 68

C.Huÿberts.

ad vivúm Sculpsit

Fig. 2.

Also shown are the branches of the right and left coronary arteries, termed by Ruysch 'arteriae coronalis'.

The left atrium ('sacculus membranosus') is indicated by (G) and the pulmonary veins by (M), while (N) (reversed) is the right pulmonary artery. The somewhat displaced superior vena cava, (K),—'truncus ascendens venae cavae'—is shown entering the right atrium, while the aorta (H) and its three early branches are seen below and to the left. There is a curious portrayal of the inferior vena cava (F), cut as it passes through the diaphragm: it was termed by Ruysch 'truncus venae cavae descendens'.

In Figure 2, a sterno-costal view of the same heart, it would have been less confusing, where applicable, to have employed the same letters as were used in the upper figure. The left auricular appendage (F) is particularly well drawn, as are also the great cardiac vein (B) and the interventricular or descending branch of the left coronary artery (C). However, the pulmonary trunk (H) is placed to the left of the aorta (G), and not overlying it. It is passing strange that the position of the pulmonary trunk relative to the aorta should be thus drawn, when so much in both of the figures is excellent. One cannot conceive of any view of the normal heart that would produce such an appearance; yet a heart was surely in front of the artist (*ad vivum sculpsit*) whilst the figure was being drawn. It is also interesting that, while an anterior cardiac vein is featured, a much more sizeable vessel, the marginal branch of the right coronary artery, is not: the artery shown winding around the right border of the right ventricle is considered to be a diagonal branch of the right coronary artery.

69 Anatomical display. Tabula I from F. Ruysch, *Thesaurus anatomicus octavus*, 1709. Engraving on a folded sheet (Wellcome Institute Library). 38.2 × 40.0 cm.

This drawing, on a sheet which is folded a number of times, can best be described as a collection of pseudo-anatomical graffiti. In the background are arteries which closely resemble tree-stumps following a forest fire, together with fetal membranes, meninges, and scattered skeletal material, most of which offer a poor apology for actuality. There are fetal skulls of approximately six months (G and H), and another of four months (M): one fetal skull (E) has a crown of flowers arranged around it. The over-curvaceaous clavicles shown in the right-hand skeleton both appear to articulate with the humerus, and everywhere the carpal skeleton is shown solid. However, really it is pointless to comment on the anatomical content of this illustration. The whole production is an extravaganza, which has to be considered as the expression of a curious trait in the character of a most knowledgeable and experienced anatomist.

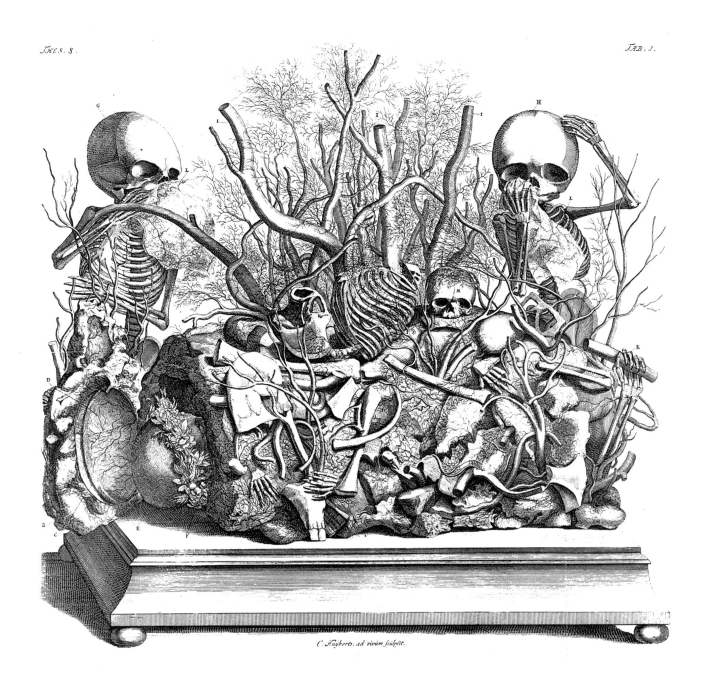

TAB. I.

C. Huyberts. ad vivim sculpsit.

PLATE 69

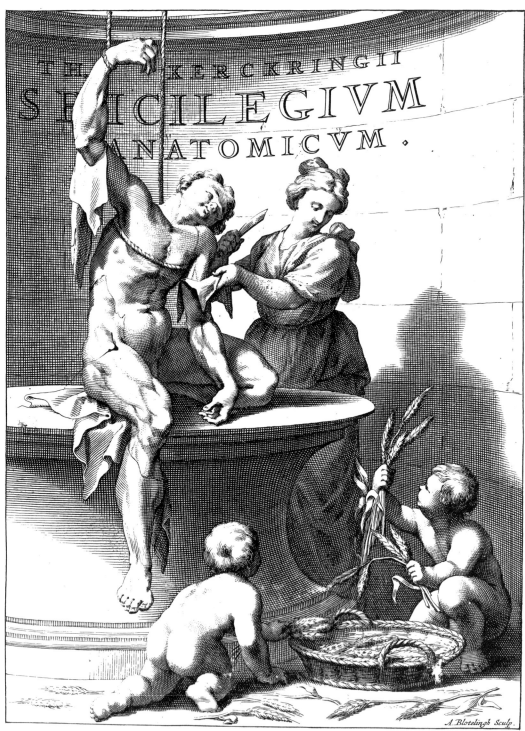

T[H]. KERCKRINGII

SPICILEGIVM

ANATOMICVM .

A. Blotelingh Sculp.

AMSTELODAMI, Sumptibus ANDREÆ FRISII, MDCLXX.

8.5 Title-page of Kerckring's *Spicilegium*, 1670.

Theodor Kerckring (1640–1693)

Embryology, including human embryology, and development, including insect metamorphosis, were both subjects of interest and study in the Netherlands during the later part of the seventeenth century. Swammerdam, van Horne, de Graaf, and Ruysch were among the investigators in these fields. Kerckring was yet another; his work on human development, and in particular that of the human skeleton, is illustrated here.

He was born to a German family living in Amsterdam. As a young man he studied Latin alongside Spinoza, and, later, medicine at Leiden under de le Boë (Sylvius). He was a friend of Ruysch. In 1678 he left Amsterdam and travelled to London; he had corresponded with Oldenburg, the Secretary of the Royal Society, and was made a Fellow early in that year. Further journeys took him to Paris and then Hamburg. His initial researches were published from Amsterdam: *Spicilegium anatomicum* ... [An anatomical gleaning], 1670. This title is represented symbolically on the engraved title-page (Fig. 8.5), which shows a male cadaver, suspended, being dissected by a classically-robed woman attended by two cherubs with stalks of corn. The engraver is given as A. Blotelingh. We know, from Cornelis Cort's engraving (1578) for instance (Fig. 8.6), that dissection was sometimes carried out on suspended corpses—a technique later used by Albinus to great effect. In the *Spicilegium* the anatomy of the fetal skeleton and its osteogenesis are among the subjects discussed and illustrated.

The following year (1671) another book by Kerckring, *Anthropogeniae ichnographia* ..., describes the early embryology of the human. This contains one plate showing development from one month of gestation onwards. The early figures are not convincing; the third-month embryo, shown inside a uterus opened like a flower, resembles a gingerbread man. But it is to be remembered that it was not until the twentieth century that the earliest stages of human embryological development were shown satisfactorily. Many Dutch scientists, including Kerckring, claimed to have discovered the human ovum—a 'discovery' described by William Cowper as one 'which the happy industry of the present age [had] made in the animal world'. In fact, it was the embryo within its decidua that they had seen, rather than the ovum. Kerckring, like his friend Ruysch, minimized the contribution that the microscope could make to medical science, so it is not surprising that his smallest embryos are pictured so sketchily. However his work on fetal osteogenesis was certainly more advanced than that of Coiter a hundred years earlier (see *Plate 52*, p. 227), and those of his contemporaries Ruysch and Bidloo (see *Plates 69 and 72*).

Like Ruysch, Bidloo, and others, Kerckring included in his publication vascular 'trees', but his figures have little symbolic content when compared with Ruysch. Later, when Kerckring had left the Netherlands to establish himself at Hamburg (1678), he collected together a 'cabinet' of anatomical preparations and other curiosities, as Ruysch, Albinus, and so many others were to do.

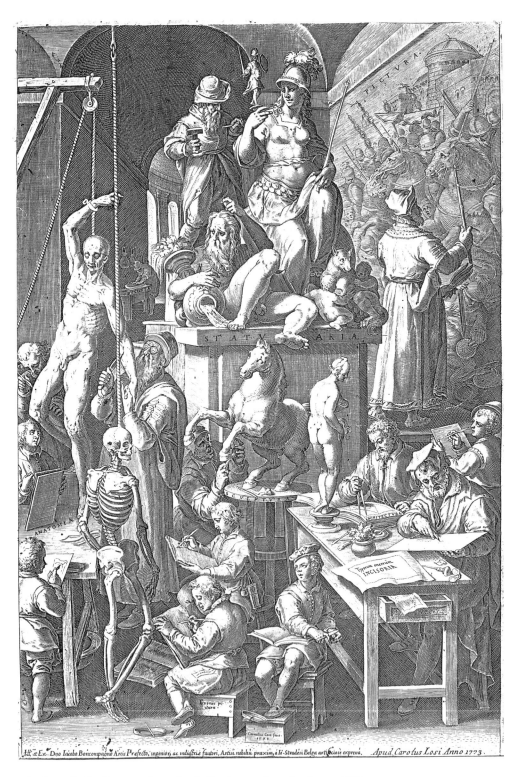

PICTVRA.

STATVARIA.

ANATOMIA.

ARCHITECTVRA.

INCISORIA.

Illmo et Exmo D^{no} Iacobo Boncompagno Arcis Præfecto, ingeniori, ac industriæ fautori, Artis nobilis praxim, à Io·Stradensi Belga artificiose expreßa.   Apud Carolus Losi Anno 1773.

8.6   Cornelis Cort's engraving, after J. Stradanus, of an Academy, 1578.

Some works by Kerckring

1. T. Kerckring, *Spicilegium anatomicum* ..., Amsterdam, A. Frisius, 1670. This work contained 100 observations on various anatomical and pathological subjects—polydactyly, the foramen ovale, the hepatic portal vein ... and, with a separate title-page, a section on the bones of the fetus.

2. T. Kerckring, *Anthropogeniae ichnographia, sive conformatio foetus ab ovo usque ad ossificationis principia* ..., A. Frisius, Amsterdam, 1671.

3. T. Kerckring, *Opera omnia anatomica* ..., C. Boutestyn, Leiden, 1717. The collected anatomical work of Kerckring.

70   The skeleton of a seven-month human fetus. Tab. XXXVII from T. Kerckring, *Spicilegium anatomicum...*, 1670. Engraving on a folded sheet between pages 272 and 273 (Cambridge University Library). 34.0 × 20.5 cm.

In this skeleton of a seven-month fetus, brandishing an admonitory finger, bone is clearly demarcated from cartilage by stipple, though the cartilaginous epiphyses appear rather crude. One notes that the carpus is shown simply as one solid piece of cartilage; that there are huge upper epiphyses of the ulna and/or lower epiphyses of the humerus; and that the tarsus, like the carpus, is solid cartilage (save for the calcaneus (P) and astragalus [talus] (O)). The explanation for this seeming crudity is that 'all major articulations are cartilaginous', and that this is what Kerckring intended to indicate by the stippled portions.

The skull correctly features an anterior fontanelle and also the frontal bone in two halves, but no lateral fontanelle is seen (neither does it appear in any of the other drawings in the book).

On the left lateral surface of the skull there is no indication of the greater wing of the sphenoid bone; this is, however, shown in a subsequent drawing of an eight-month fetus, though even then it is not labelled.

The vertebral column is a black mass in which it is impossible to make out any detail. The sternum is portrayed as being mainly cartilage, with four pieces of areas of ossification, which is correct for a seven-month fetus.

It is interesting that the ischium (L) is termed by Kerckring the 'os coxendicis'.

The use of stipple to indicate cartilage did not originate with Kerckring; as we have seen Coiter drew a skeleton of a six-month child showing stipple epiphyses, best seen in the lower limb and pelvis, nearly one hundred years earlier (see *Plate 52*, p. 227).

Kerckring was one of the earlier investigators of the development of ossification in the fetal skeleton, and writes about each bone individually. The smaller figures, II to VI, represent his views as to the appearance of the temporal bone, ear ossicles, atlas, axis, and scapula at a fetal age of seven months. In general these accord well with present-day views some three hundred years later. Indeed, an occasional centre of ossification that appears in the cartilage at the posterior margin of the foramen magnum, at about the sixteenth week of intrauterine life, and unites with the squamous part of the occipital bone before birth, is still known as 'Kerckring's centre'.

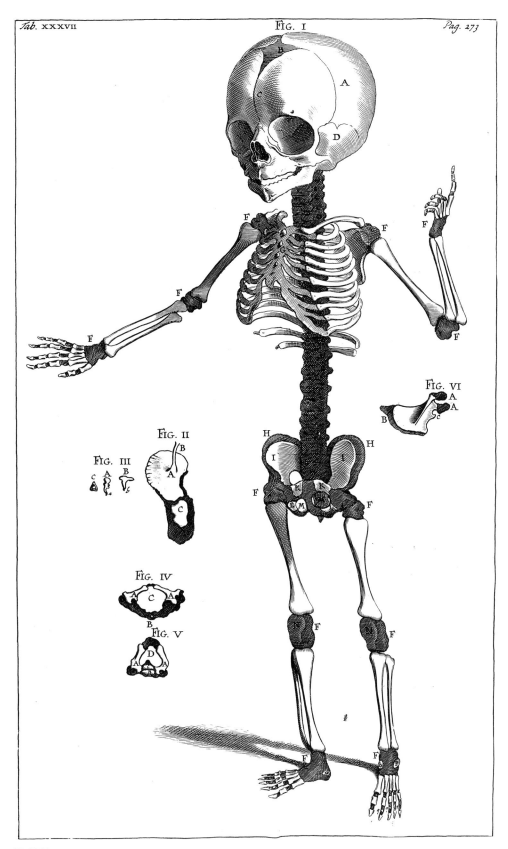

FIG. VI

FIG. II

FIG. III

FIG. IV

FIG. V

PLATE 70

The medical school at Leiden

The city of Leiden lies approximately twenty kilometres from The Hague and forty kilometres from Amsterdam. It has been a place of some importance since the thirteenth century, but it prospered during the first hundred years of the independent Netherlands for two reasons: it was a major centre for cloth weaving, and it was the site of one of the principal universities of Europe. The founding of the University was tied to the struggle for independence from Spain: the town was besieged from May to October in 1574 by the Spanish forces under the Duke of Alba, being only relieved when the dykes were opened and the countryside around was flooded, paralysing the enemy and allowing supplies and relief to come by boat to the city. Even the element of air collaborated: a storm dispersed the Spaniards, an event communicated as a national epic by historians, poets, and artists. Prince William of Orange, tradition has it, offered the valiant town the choice of relief from taxes for ten years or a university. (How many towns would today choose the second?)

The University opened its doors in 1575, William hoping that it would be a 'bastion and guardian of all the lands, and hence a lasting bridge not only between the lands themselves but also between them and the neighbouring provinces' and 'a sure and safe support of freedom and honest government not only in matters of religion but also in all things concerning the welfare of the common citizen'. From the first, Leiden University was European, and without effective religious restrictions. The second medical degree granted, in 1581, was to an Englishman, John James, later physician to Queen Elizabeth. Many of the early professors in the medical school were from Padua. Leiden at the height of its fame inspired the foundation of both the Edinburgh and Vienna schools of medicine, and these, in turn, many other medical schools of the world. In this way the spirit of Padua was dispersed widely. Among seventeenth-century professors were Pauw (whose work in anatomy we have already noted), Bidloo, Rau, de le Boë, Nuck, van Wale, and van Horne. In 1701 Hermann Boerhaave was appointed as a teacher, and the following year Bernard Albinus joined him as professor of theoretical and practical medicine. Under these two, the university became an incomparable centre of international medical education.

Boerhaave was born in a village near Leiden in 1668, and entered the University there when he was sixteen, receiving eventually a doctorate for studies in philosophy (1690), his thesis being on mind–body relationships. During this time he read extensively in the medical literature. After his degree he taught privately and continued his self-education in medicine, attending anatomical demonstrations but no lectures. He was given a medical degree in 1693 from Harderwijk, a small academy. In 1701, he was appointed Reader in medicine at Leiden; he also taught in the institutes of medicine (that is, physiology and other subjects basic to medicine). From that date onwards his fame began to spread across Europe both through students returning home and by a succession of texts such as the famous *Aphorisms* ... and a text on chemistry, first published by his pupils without his authority; he was forced to issue corrected versions.

From 1718 to 1729 Boerhaave held three of the five chairs in the medical school at Leiden—botany and medicine (to which he appointed in 1709), clinical medicine (1714), and chemistry (1718). His systematic approach to clinical teaching was developed in association with twelve beds; bedside teaching to complement lectures had already been in use in Leiden since 1636. In this also Leiden continued the Paduan tradition. Boerhaave established a pattern for 'ward-rounds' that was later copied in Edinburgh and elsewhere. In spite of his chemical interests—his text on chemistry was world-famous—he was not an adherent of the iatrochemical school. He was a widely read man, and fully conversant with contemporary scientific and philosophical ideas, Newton being particularly admired.

Since the search for first causes, for the essence of things (as Boerhaave stated in a lecture of 1715 at Leiden) had proved elusive and unprofitable, it seemed more reasonable to investigate those matters that we can experience directly. This approach limited the subject matter for enquiry, but its results might prove more valuable. Boerhaave was made a Fellow of the Royal Society of London and of the Parisian Academy of Science. His work was, however, that of a systematist rather than of a contributor of new knowledge. It has been unkindly said of him, by the Regius Professor of Physick at Cambridge, Clifford Allbutt, from the confidence of the year 1900, that he 'seems to have contented himself with hashing up the partial truths and entire errors of his time'.

Boerhaave died in 1738, his intellectual legacy being a medical school curriculum that gave equal weight to basic science and bedside teaching. His pupils included the Swedish systematist, Carl von Linné (Linnaeus), the polymath Albrecht von Haller (see later), Gerard van Swieten, one of the founders of the Vienna medical school, B.S. Albinus (also the subject of a later section), and a host of pupils from Europe and the New World, particularly from English-speaking countries, who represented a third of the total of about two thousand medical students registered at Leiden during Boerhaave's time.

Petrus Pauw's anatomy theatre at Leiden, built in 1597, was not only a place for didactic lectures and demonstrations of dissection, but was also in itself a 'cabinet', and hence a place for unspoken scientific and moral instruction. An engraving (Fig. 8.7) of 1610, for sale to visitors, shows elegant women and men inspecting the theatre and the curiosities it contained. With peculiar appropriateness it was housed, along with the University library, in a church. (The anatomy department continued to occupy it until 1822.) The architecture of the anatomy theatre was derived from Fabrici's anatomical theatre built three years earlier at Padua, except that it was lit by daylight streaming through the large windows rather than by candles, as was the one at Padua—so anticipating, one might think, the Enlightenment. Science is represented by articulated skeletons of birds, beasts, and human beings. A corpse is laid on the central table; a man pulls back the cover to show a visceral dissection. Impressive instruments are stored in an open cupboard. On the top of the cupboard reclines a *putto*, leaning on a skull and holding an hour-glass. The *memento mori* theme is also conveyed through human skeletons. Six of these hold staffs, each with a flagged motto telling of the impermanence of this life (for example,

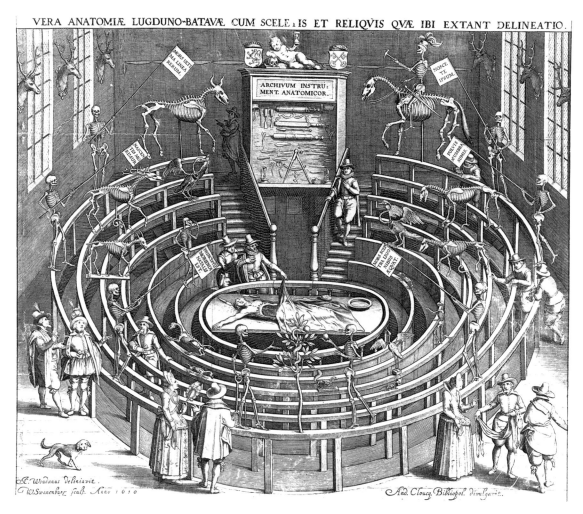

8.7   Anatomy theatre at Leiden, 1610.

Nascentes morimur—'to be born is to die'); another with a plumed helmet and sword by his side—Death himself—rides a skeletal horse triumphantly; and, centrally in the foreground, skeletal Eve passes the forbidden fruit across a snake-entwined tree to skeletal Adam, spade in hand. One of the two fashionable dressed women present is shown the flayed skin of a man, recalling to students of anatomy the illustration in Valverde and the title-page of Bauhin, and to classicists the unpleasant tale of pride shown towards Apollo by Marsyas, a pride punished by flaying. The other woman holds a fan with a central mirror—a traditional representation of vanity. The hundreds of students that came to Leiden to study returned to their native places with a knowledge of anatomy acquired in this theatre; it is probable that they also remembered the 'moral messages' so blatantly spelled out by the changing displays, though these were especially set up for visitors during the summer vacation. It has been said that dissections were accompanied by the playing of a flute to entertain anatomists, students, and visitors.

It may be helpful here to list Dutch universities that taught medicine and awarded doctorates in that subject, and to give the dates of their foundations: Leiden, 1575; Franeker, 1585; Groningen, 1614; Utrecht, 1636; Harderwijk, 1648. The *Athenaeum Illustre* in Amsterdam from 1641 also gave instruction in medicine.

Govard Bidloo (1649–1713)

Bidloo's grandfather was a leather merchant, his father a milliner in Amsterdam. Early medical experience was obtained during a surgical apprenticeship. He also studied in France and with Ruysch in Amsterdam; he translated Ruysch's book on the valves of lymphatics into Dutch. He obtained a doctorate from Franeker in 1682, having matriculated there only three days previously. During the period 1675–89, Bidloo was not only a medical man but also a man of the theatre, writing plays and the libretto of an opera for the New Amsterdam Theatre; some of these plays were still being performed half a century later. Bidloo, attached to the army, saw fighting in Flanders in 1685 with William of Orange against the French. His appointment as Professor of Anatomy at The Hague in 1688, in succession to Nuck, essentially put an end to his career in drama, but not to his connections with the army or with William, for in 1688–9 he travelled to England when that Prince became William III of England. Bidloo returned in 1690 to become supervisor of Dutch military hospitals; in 1692/3 he held a similar position in England. Bidloo cannot, obviously, have been able during this period to attend fully to his anatomical duties in The Hague. In 1694, presumably with the support of William, he became Professor at Leiden. There he had divided loyalties—to the House of Orange and to the medical school; in 1696 he was censured for absenteeism by the university authorities. In 1698, in a published letter to van Leeuwenhoek, he described for the first time animalcules (flukes) infecting the liver of sheep and other animals. He was in England again, and was appointed Royal Physician in 1701; and a year later attended William during his last illness, prescribing, for the infected dropsy that affected the King's feet and legs, a powder of crabs' eyes, flour, and cumin seed rubbed on with flannel, vapour baths, and a diet of strong beer—a regime which met with the disapproval of the doctors of the English court. Bidloo published an account of the last illness and death of King William. His association with rulers also included acquaintance with Tsar Peter the Great. That ruler had made a journey in 1697 to Western Europe to gain various technical experiences: gunnery at Königsberg; shipbuilding (at which he himself was highly experienced) at Deptford; and navigation at Venice. He saw the Ruysch anatomical cabinet in Amsterdam—a collection which, as we have seen, he subsequently purchased. Peter investigated anatomy with Bidloo in Leiden. Bidloo used his influence with the Tsar to obtain for his nephew, Dr Nicolaus Bidloo, a position as physician and director of Moscow's (which was also Russia's) first hospital.

From 1701 to his death in 1713, Bidloo was teaching—when he was actually in Leiden—at the same period that Boerhaave was attracting hundreds of students to the medical school;

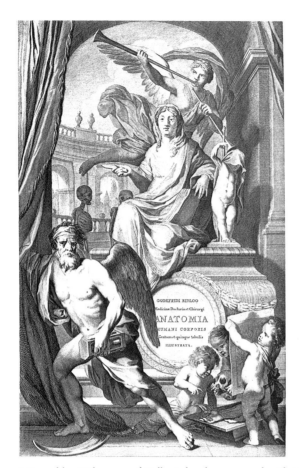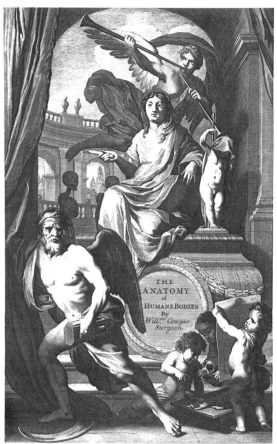

8.8a and b   Title-page of Bidloo's book, compared with title-page of Cowper's book.

there appears to have been little or no scientific association between them, or between Bidloo and Bernard Albinus, except that the latter's son, B. S. Albinus, was Bidloo's pupil. There is little doubt that Bidloo was an irascible man who argued with his medical colleagues both face to face and in print. No one seems to have been willing to give an oration at Bidloo's funeral.

In a work dedicated to the Royal Society of London and published in 1708, Bidloo argued correctly that the nerves were not tubes, as was generally thought. He was, for that period, advanced in his use of microscopes (he had correspondence with Leeuwenhoek), and he made anatomical preparations by injecting blood-vessels with an inert material, followed by maceration.

The work on which Bidloo's anatomical reputation stands is *Anatomia humani corporis* …, 1685 (*Fig. 8.8a*), It has been stated in print more than once that Bidloo's text to this work was not distinguished, and that the value of the book lay in the illustrations, a series of 105 folio copper engravings. Impressions of all the plates were incorporated into a book by William Cowper: *The anatomy of humane bodies* … 1698 (*Fig. 8.8b*). This matter is discussed later.

During the preparation of the drawings there must have been inadequate collaboration between anatomist and artist; it would appear that the former dissected the part and then left the artist to make the drawing without exercising sufficiently close supervision. Cowper, in his descriptive text to Bidloo's seventy-ninth plate, notes that 'the muscles adjacent to these parts … are here so confusedly exprest [that is, drawn], as no explanation of them can be asserted'. Quite different conditions of close collaboration between anatomist and artist had existed during the production of most of the Vesalian plates, and were later to exist when the plates of Albinus, Haller, and Soemmerring were prepared. Yet many of the Bidloo plates must take their place amongst the canon of great anatomical illustrations, and this is in no small measure due to the artist employed, Gerard de Lairesse. His name is fairly to be seen, along with that of the anatomist, on the letterpress title-page. (Vesalius alas, as we have noted, neglected a similar courtesy to his artistic collaborators in the *Fabrica*.) The drawings were well engraved in copper by persons unknown; the frontispiece portrait of Bidloo was done by Lairesse, and engraved by Abraham Bootteling, who may also have prepared some of the anatomy plates. Peter and Philip van Gunst have also been named as the engravers of some of the Bidloo–Lairesse plates.

Lairesse (1640–1711) was born at Liège, the son of a painter; three other brothers were also artists. He came under the influence of Bertholet Flameel (or Flémal), whose paintings show particular attention to architectural features, particularly porticoes and colonnades. Lairesse painted at Utrecht, where he was said to have been dissolute and poor. Fleeing justice after a duel, he went to Amsterdam, where, after a while, he was highly successful as a court and town painter, especially of historical and mythological subjects. Anecdotes of Lairesse abound: before beginning a painting he would, like Sherlock Holmes, play the violin to assist contemplation; for a wager, he painted a large canvas of Apollo and the Muses in less than one day … Lairesse is supposed to have completed 245 paintings. For the last twenty years of his life he was blind.

Lairesse's illustrations of Bidloo's anatomy are of two kinds: in one, the anatomical figures are given life—a skeleton, for example, emerges from a grave set in the midst of classical tomb architecture (*Plate 71*); in the other, the illustrations are of cadavers—dissected corpses recognizable as such, including the pins and blocks that prop up the dissected parts, sheets that wrap up surrounding areas, ropes that position the trunk, and, to emphasize an appearance of realism, a fly perched on the cadaver (*Fig. 8.9*). A large majority of the plates are of actual dissections, rather than anatomized figures in a landscape. Bernard Siegfried Albinus was later to use beautiful 'living' positions for his skeletons and muscle-men, poising them against classical backgrounds; while such anatomists as John and Charles Bell took the other route, and depicted the macabre realities of the dissecting room.

The one hundred and five plates took many years to produce, even for Lairesse. It seems the work started in 1676, and was not completed until about 1682. These were years in which Bidloo was producing plays in Amsterdam, obtaining his degree, and working as a surgeon. Lairesse and Bidloo were both members of the artistic movement in the Netherlands dedicated

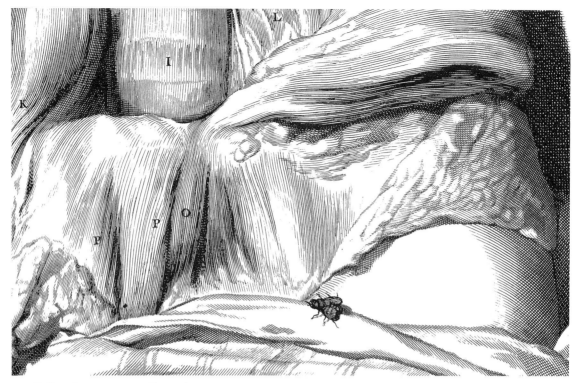

8.9 Bidloo–Lairesse, 1685: Fly on dissection.

to classicism in the theatre and in other arts. The cost of employing the engravers for such a large project must have been very high. It is perhaps not surprising that the Amsterdam publishers disposed of the plates, or impressions from them, to Cowper's publishers, when Bidloo's book was no longer selling well.

Most books of human anatomy published in the hundred and fifty years succeeding 1550 used modifications of the Vesalian figures. Until Bidloo's *Anatomia* was published in 1685 few books other than the Casserian-Spieghelian atlases contained illustrations that attempted to portray human anatomy in a quite different way. (We must remember, however, that the anatomical plates of Eustachio, *c*.1554, and Berrettini, *c*.1618, had been produced, but were not published until the eighteenth century.) Bidloo and Lairesse together should therefore take credit for their innovative approach, rethinking, from actual dissections, how to show the body not diagrammatically but naturalistically. In the plates of the skeletons, however, they used the traditional iconography of figures set in a landscape, adding, as Vesalius and others had done, tombs, fallen masonry, and plants symbolic of the inevitability of death. Remarkable as these Bidloo plates are, anatomists note their variable quality; some quite striking images are surprisingly inept scientifically, others are accurate representations of structure, but do not make a pleasing picture.

Some books by G. Bidloo

1. *Godefridi Bidloo Medicinae Doctoris et Chirurgi Anatomia humani corporis centum et quinque tabulis illustrata*, 1685. This is the title on the decorative engraved title-page; opposite is a portrait of Bidloo by G. Lairesse, taken from life—Bidloo was in his mid-thirties. It was published in 1685 at Leiden by J. à Someren, with J. à Dyk and the heirs to T. Boom. The page-size of the copy in the Cambridge University Library is 52 × 36 cm. On some of the finely printed plates, full-page, there are additional, innovative figures showing the microscopical appearance of some structures. The first three plates are of nudes: a man and woman from the front and from the back; these are pleasant enough drawings, but they in no way compare with those in Vesalius' *Epitome*. (An interesting copy of Bidloo's book was given by C. S. Sherington to F. S. Wesbrook, the first president of the University of British Columbia. It was signed by Gowland Hopkins and William Osler amongst others. It had originally been bought by the English architect Nicholas Hawksmoor in 1693.) Dutch-language editions were published from Amsterdam, 1690, and from Utrecht, 1728 and 1734.

   All the anatomical plates in the above book were incorporated, with a new and more extensive text, in *The Anatomy of humane bodies . . .*, Oxford, 1698 and Leiden, 1737. The English title was stuck over the Dutch one on the engraved title-page; the portrait of Bibloo was replaced by one of Cowper. Cowper added nine extra plates of his own devising in an appendix. He had had additional identification numbers and letters hand-drawn in ink on the plates, so that more structures could be pinpointed in his text than in Bidloo's original. (For further discussion on Cowper's book see Chapter 12.) Bidloo wrote an attack: *Gulielmus Cowper, criminis literarii citatus . . .*, Leiden, 1700. This was addressed to the Royal Society of London, of which both Bidloo and Cowper were Fellows. Cowper replied to this in a pamphlet published 1701. The Royal Society refused to arbitrate.

2. A work on anatomists in antiquity: *Dissertatio de antiquitate anatomes . . .*, Leiden, 1694.

3. Arguments against Ruysch's views are printed in: *Vindiciae . . . contra ineptas animadversiones Fred. Ruyschii*, Leiden, 1697.

4. Bidloo's work on the liver-fluke is: *Observatio . . . de animalculis in ovino aliorumque animantium hepate . . .*, Leiden, 1698 (also in Dutch same year).

5. In *Exercitationum anatomico-chirurgicarum, decades duae . . .*, Leiden, 1715 Bidloo includes his findings that nerve-fibres are solid, not tubular.

71 Skeleton emerges from the grave. Tabula 88 from G. Bidloo, *Anatomia humani corporis . . .*, 1685. Engraving (Cambridge University Library). 44.5 × 27.8 cm.

In this plate the inclination of the skull with regard to the cervical vertebral column would tax a contortionist. The vertebral column itself exhibits a slight uniform anterior concave configuration, and the sacrum is protrayed as being virtually vertical.

(M) is identified in the text as the clavicle, but it appears to articulate with the vertebral column. Even if it is meant as a rib, there are then only eleven on that side.

What certainly cannot be condoned is the skeleton of the right hand, which inexplicably is quite out of proportion to the rest. For example it is half the vertical height of the left femur, and in it the triquetral and pisiform bones are enormous.

The left femur appears very short and exhibits no anterior bowing: the trochanters are also poorly drawn.

A very incomplete dentition provides a touch of reality.

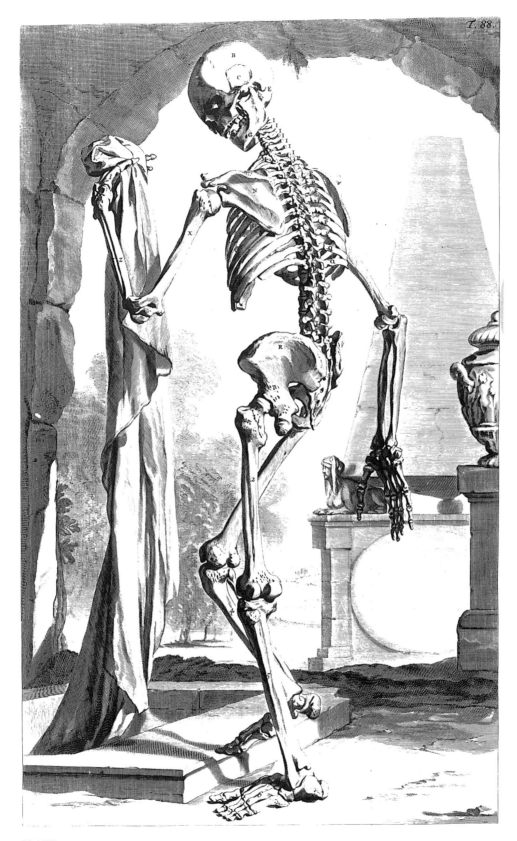

PLATE 71

72 Full-term fetal skeleton. Tabula 101 from G. Bidloo, *Anatomia humani corporis* ..., 1685. Engraving (Cambridge University Library). 44.3 × 27.5 cm.

This frontal view of the skeleton of a fetus of nine months is not anatomically impressive, the skull being far and away the best part of it. The scapulae are quite horrible.

The right clavicle, its medial extremity resembling a cobra's head, is shown as being continuous with an enormous cartilaginous acromion. The inclination of the ribs is all wrong for such a fetus, and it is instructive to examine the posterior parts of the ribs seen on the left side; for example, the rib visible just above the second costal cartilage. Traced downwards, the highest rib that this could represent would be the seventh; but the junction between the sixth and seventh cervical vertebrae (with which the head of the seventh rib articulates) does *not* lie above the manubrio-sternal angle, as it is shown here. The anterior parts of ribs four to six seem to arise posteriorly from a common stem.

The skeletal elements of the extremities and their epiphyses are very poorly portrayed, the latter a compound of ignorance and artistic 'fudging'; and the left ulna has a nasty twisted distal portion.

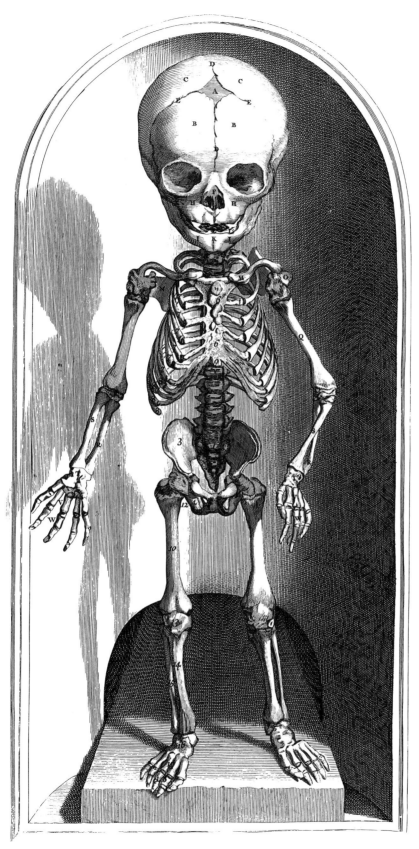

PLATE 72

73 Back of hand and forearm dissected. Table 70 from W. Cowper, *The Anatomy of human bodies ...*, 1698. This is impressed from the same copperplate as is to be found in Bidloo, 1685 (Tabula 70), but with the manuscript addition of eleven extra indicator letters. Engraving (Cambridge University Library). 47.4 × 33.0 cm.

This displays the muscles of the back or extensor aspect of the left forearm, together with the tendons on the dorsum of the hand.

The extensor retinaculum, whereby the tendons are 'held down' at the wrist, has been totally removed, and the tendons are held apart by divers odd small implements such as compasses.

While there are clearly two different muscle bellies and tendons (G, G)—that is, extensor carpi radialis longus and brevis—they were considered by Cowper to be a single muscle, 'radialis extensor'.

Other muscles include extensor digitorum (D), extensor carpi ulnaris (H), anconeus (I), flexor carpi ulnaris (L), extensor pollicis longus (C), extensor indicis (N), the extensor tendon to the little finger and extensor digiti minimi (K), and abductor digiti minimi (R).

The tendons labelled (O, O) are the present-day abductor pollicis longus and extensor pollicis brevis. With regard to these, in Cowper's day (and long after) the phalanges were termed 'internodes', and there were thought to be only four metacarpals, that of the thumb being considered to be its first internode. Hence the names for the two above muscles were 'extensores secundi et tertii internodii pollicis'. Later the long abductor became known as the 'extensor ossis metacarpi pollicis', before assuming its modern name: it is, in fact, both an extensor and an abductor of the thumb.

In this plate there is one definite error, namely the muscle labelled S, difficult to make out, but lying between C and the nearby E. This is referred to as the abductor pollicis. As (Q, Q) represent the interossei muscles, so (S) is the first dorsal interosseous; Cowper here is inconsistent, as he elsewhere terms this muscle the 'abductor indicis'—its function does, of course, include abducting the index finger.

The formation of the extensor expansion or 'hood' just distal to the metacarpophalangeal joints is not portrayed, although in an earlier part of the text the insertions of the lumbrical and interossei muscles are stated to be 'in conjunction with the tendons of extensor digitorum communis'.

This is a handsome, and, in the main, a carefully labelled drawing, which, for its period, was extremely accurate. The credit for the artistic anatomical accuracy, of course, belongs to Bidloo and Lairesse rather than to Cowper, who merely added additional alphabetical indicators to Bidloo's work.

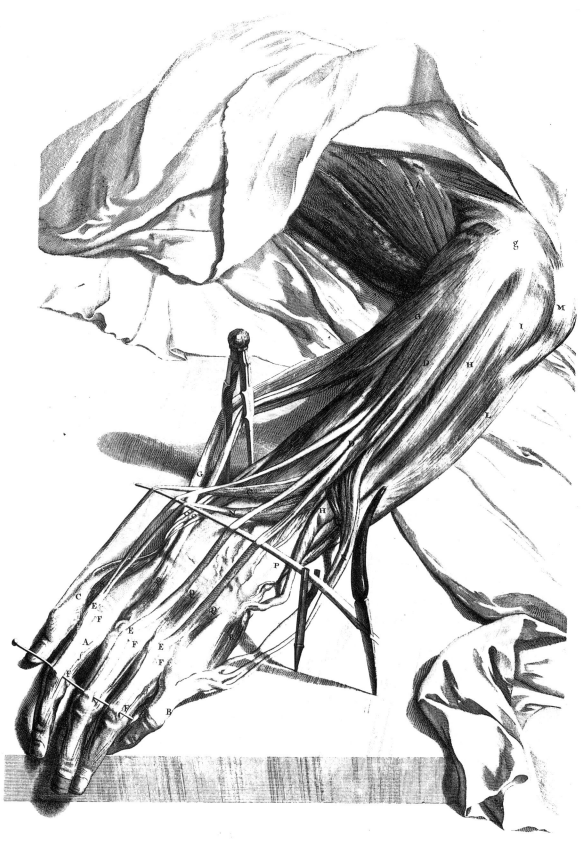

PLATE 73

Bernhard Siegfried Albinus (1697–1770)

Bernard Siegfried Albinus was the most prominent of an intellectual dynasty whose family name, Weiss, had been Latinized, according to humanistic ideas, in the sixteenth century. He was born in Frankfurt-on-Oder, now on the Polish–German border, where his father, Bernard Albinus (1653–1721), was Professor of Medicine. The father graduated in 1676 from Leiden, and the university persuaded him to return as a professor of theoretical and practical medicine in 1702, when his son was only five years old. The boy, a prodigy, entered the university of Leiden aged twelve, and spent the next nine years there studying under his father, his father's colleague, Boerhaave, and the anatomists Bidloo and J.J. Rau. Before taking his degree he left for Paris to work under Winslow and others, but was soon recalled in 1719 to substitute for Rau, who had fallen ill and subsequently died. Albinus received his medical degree in 1719 without sitting examinations, and, when his father died two years later, he was appointed to the chair of anatomy and surgery at the early age of twenty-four. One of his first publications was an inventory of Rau's collection of osteological and other specimens.

The remaining fifty years of his life were spent in Leiden. With Hermann Boerhaave as a colleague, friend, and collaborator for the first seventeen of these, he was responsible for maintaining the high standards and international reputation of the Leiden medical school. Albinus' personal life was quiet; until he was sixty-eight he lived with his two sisters. At that age he married a widow, and, surprisingly, the household apparently remained calm and amiable. His library of two thousand volumes included not only a thousand or more works on anatomy, medicine, and surgery, but also literary and philosophical works by Racine, Molière, Voltaire, Descartes, and Bacon. A work classified under anatomy was Venette's *Le tableau de l'amour conjugal*, 1740 edition. When Albinus died his widow married for a third time, and sold his house, which contained his library and museum arranged in fine free-standing bookcases; these may be seen as a frontispiece to the posthumous *Supellex anatomica ...*, 1774. His museum was catalogued by his brother Frederik Bernard Albinus. 'Cabinets of curiosities' were collected by most of the anatomists mentioned in this chapter, and by their contemporaries in Britain and on the Continent. Many scientific societies, including the Royal Society of London and the Royal Academy of Science in Paris, had their cabinets. A case of specimens is clearly illustrated in the engraved title-page of Ruysch's collected works issued in 1720 (*Fig. 8.10*). A history of such cabinets, the precursors of the later-eighteenth- and early-nineteenth-century museum, is given in a book edited by Impey and MacGregor (1985).

Albinus' scholarship was considerable: in 1734 he issued from Leiden an edition of James Douglas's bibliography of anatomy. This, the first modern bibliography of a medical subject, had been first published in 1715, and the Albinus edition was only supplanted by Haller's *Bibliotheca anatomica ...*, 1774–6. Albinus also edited a number of earlier medical writers, Vesalius in association with Boerhaave; Eustachio, Fabrici, and Harvey he edited himself. It was in 1744 that he published his fine edition of Eustachio's plates, with a new anatomical

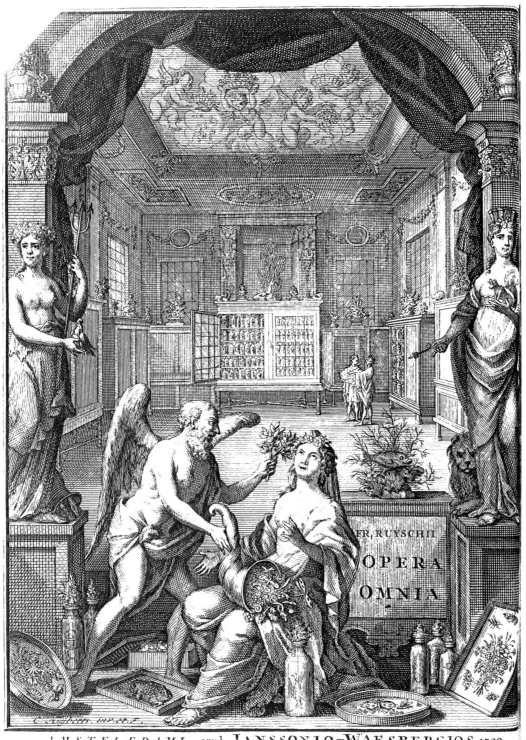

AMSTELÆDAMI apud JANSSONIO-WAESBERGIOS 1720.

8.10 Ruysch's museum, from *Opera omnia*, 1720.

commentary, copying carefully the illustrations prepared some two hundred years previously; this was not only of antiquarian interest, but also of practical use as a guide to anatomy. Each of these works had plates newly engraved on copper. The Vesalian woodcuts (from the *Epitome* and the *Fabrica*, not the *Tabulae anatomicae sex*) were beautifully translated to the softer medium; while they lost some of the dramatic vigour of the originals, they added a clarity and elegance appropriate to the eighteenth century. The Eustachian plates had a great influence on Albinus' own work. The master engraver for these illustrated books was Jan Wandelaar.

B. S. Albinus' work in anatomy was of a precision and care rarely matched in the history of anatomical illustration. Some time shortly before 1725, when in his late twenties, Albinus developed an ambitious plan to publish large-scale engraved plates of human anatomy that would surpass in excellence all previous anatomical illustrations. The work was not only to better the original illustrations of Vesalius and Eustachio, but also those in the perfected editions of these authors that Albinus himself edited. No major anatomist has applied himself so fully to anatomical illustration over so long a period as did Albinus. The first completed folio volume of his plan comprised 28 plates of the skeleton and muscles; it was not published until 1747: the engraving alone had occupied about eight years. Preliminary work had been published on the bones (1726), the muscles (1734), the vessels of the intestine (1736), and the fetal skeleton (1737). The only other parts produced were plates of the gravid uterus (1748–51), the bones (1753), and one plate to illustrate the thoracic duct, azygos vein, etc. (1757). The projected series on the viscera, blood-vessels, and so on did not materialize. As it developed the whole endeavour became so considerable that, in 1745, Albinus requested from the University administrators help in his teaching of medical students, so that he could concentrate on his anatomical researches. His youngest brother Frederik, who was a practising physician in Amsterdam, was appointed lecturer, then professor, in anatomy and surgery, so relieving Albinus of the heaviest burdens; Bernard Siegfried was appointed as a professor of medicine, and lectured mainly on physiology. Although pressed by the University to accept, he refused reappointment as Rector.

Albinus needed not only long hours free of teaching, but also subjects for dissection, and here he was less fortunate: he apparently had only one or two corpses each year, and sometimes these were only used for research with the permission of his students. Some of the early work was carried out in his house, but other dissections were performed in the old anatomy theatre built by Pauw.

Albinus had begun his attempt to produce the best anatomical illustrations with a confidence that stemmed from his upbringing by one of the world's finest anatomists (his father, Bernard Albinus), his training under Bidloo, Rau, and Winslow, his growing experience with the best available anatomy books during the preparation of his scholarly editions of their work, and years of teaching anatomy and publishing original work. The major publication that came from this bold plan was *Tabulae sceleti et musculorum corporis humani*, Leiden, 1747 (*Fig. 8.11*). In a preface to this book, Albinus gave an account of the work—*Historia huius operis*. Since his aims were so high, since to a large extent he achieved them, and since the resulting plates are among the very best in anatomical illustration, it is fortunate that we can follow in detail Albinus' own account of their genesis and execution. The following descriptions are given mostly in his own words, as translated into English in the excellent, but pirated, London edition, 1749.

Albinus explained how he was dissatisfied with the inaccuracies of the usual method of making, successively, drawings from skin to superficial muscles to deeper layers, and so down to the skeleton:

Which figures although they may be useful, nay extremely useful, yet they are deficient in many things ... I must pitch upon something that is common to [all human bodies] as the basis or foundation to build my figures upon. And this is the skeleton ... in most men at least, of whatever size or make, the muscles are connected and posited with the bones almost in the same manner; and in the same places.

He started with the skeleton, then added the muscles, so that '... the figures of the viscera might be referred to them; and to these ... the figures of the arteries, veins, nerves, etc. might likewise be referred'. He compared this method with architects laying foundations on which to build, and said that such a plan was used by Eustachio; and it is indeed the method recommended to artists by Leon Battista Alberti. But there was a paradox: in preparing the bones of the skeleton there is damage to cartilage and ligaments, and 'therefore when they are joined again, the articulations will not be so fit as they were before'. The skeletal inaccuracies of Vesalius, who also emphasized the bones as the basis of anatomical studies, were in part due to this problem. Albinus' solution was 'to prepare a fresh skeleton in such a manner, as to leave the ligaments of the joints entirely whole', but this would take time—three months' preparation and drawing for one specimen, during which the cartilages and ligaments would dry out or putrefy; so Albinus moistened them with water from time to time, pouring water into the joints through cuts in the capsule; and, to check putrefaction, he sprinkled the whole with vinegar. 'During the time that the first figure was a-taking off, a hard frost coming on, the whole skeleton was frozen, which was the best thing that could happen both for keeping it firm, and preventing

BERNARDI SIEGFRIED ALBINI

TABULAE

SCELETI

ET

MUSCULORUM

CORPORIS HUMANI.

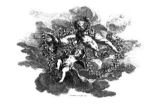

LUGDUNI BATAVORUM
Proſtant apud JOANNEM & HERMANNUM VERBEEK Bibliop.
CIƆIƆCCXLVII.

8.11 Title-page of Albinus, *Tabulae sceleti*, 1747.

the putrefaction.' When positioning the skeleton he used for reference 'a thin man, of the same size as my skeleton—and making him stand naked in the same position, I compared the skeleton with him, especially the hip-bone, spine, thorax, scapulae, and clavicles ...'. He came back to it repeatedly for some days, checking with the living subject. The frozen state of the skeleton was disturbed 'by the fire, which we were obliged to have always when the naked man stood; for he neither could nor would stand without it'.

The positioning of the skeleton—a standing one with most weight on the right foot, as can be seen in the plates—was achieved by a complex system of pulleys suspended from rings in the ceiling, a tripod placed on a table so the artist would not have to stoop, and a cord tied to the upper part of the spine, with another passed under the cheek-bones, and yet others to position the arms, legs, etc. By pulling on cords and using wedges the position of the naturally articulated skeleton could be adjusted to that of the naked man; naturally all of this took days.

... my next care was to have an exact figure [drawing] made of it. I foresaw that the figure would be very incorrect ... if it was taken off by merely viewing the original, as ingravers commonly do ... [to take measurements of every part] was an infinite task, nor could it possibly be done without some certain infallible rule to direct the ingraver.

Albinus solved the problem using two nets, or grids, of small cords. One grid was placed directly in front of the skeleton, and the other, with squares a tenth of those in the former, was positioned four 'Rhenish feet' away from the skeleton. The centre of both nets was opposite the middle of the left breast of the skeleton. '... the ingraver placing himself in the most proper situation near the skeleton ... endeavoured to make some point where the cords of the lesser [net] ... coincide to the eye with the corresponding decussating point in the cords of the greater one; and the part of the skeleton which was directly behind these points, he drew upon his plate ..., which was similarly marked out'. The engraver 'was to find out a proper place for viewing [the skeleton] through the [nets], by means of a fixed hole, and not very large; which by applying his eye to, he could see what parts of the skeleton answered to [the cords of the grid]'. 'According to this method then (which as it answered the intention, so it occasioned an incredible deal of trouble to the ingraver) a fore view of the skeleton was first drawn as it stood'; then back and side views were taken; after which the skeleton was disarticulated and the bones were cleaned completely, each one being then drawn to natural size, which served, he said, as practice for the artist.

Albinus deliberately chose a subject for the skeleton that met his ideals of proportion: '... elegant and at the same time not too delicate; so as neither to show a juvenile or feminine roundness and slenderness, nor on the contrary an unpolished roughness and clumsiness ... And I cannot help congratulating my good fortune' in getting such a good subject; yet even this had—so his aesthetics told him—imperfections. ... 'As therefore painters, when they draw a handsome face ... render the likeness the more beautiful [by removing blemishes]; so those things which were less perfect, [in the skeleton] were mended in the figures ... care being taken at the same time that they should be altogether just.' Albinus' illustrations do not therefore show warts and all, but are idealized representations of the skeleton of a man who embodied attributes appropriate to the ideal of a fine eighteenth-century gentleman—as may be seen, as he imperturbably stands in front of a massive rhinoceros.

Completing the skeletal figures, he passed on to the muscle-men: '... with the consent of my pupils, and whenever an opportunity offered besides, I traced [dissected] the muscles carefully, in order to observe their positions, connexion, figure, thickness, and substance.... In this manner I proceeded every year', preserving specimens in a 'proper liquor'. 'Thus prepared, and with firmer resolution, and more sanguine hope, I began to add the muscles to the figures of the skeleton in the year thirty-eight.' This was at least thirteen years after beginning the project. Albinus, and presumably his artist Wandelaar, were much influenced by the muscle-men plates of Eustachio, which they together produced so beautifully in a re-engraved form in 1744. Comparison of Eustachio plates (for example, Tab. XXXII) with Albinus' (for example, first muscle plate) shows similarity of general concept and detailed execution (*Figs 8.12a and b*).

Albinus describes how he made outline drawings of the skeleton, which were then impressed on a wax plate with a needle; subsequently correcting the reversal by taking an impression from this plate, he used it to engrave another waxed plate—the reversed image was itself reversed, and so corrected. This method, however, presented another obstacle:

In order that the figures may be well ingraved, it is necessary that the paper should be sufficiently macerated. But when the sheets thus wetted, *viz.* the original and the copy, are put into the press together, it happens that being squeezed between two cylinders (which kind of press the ingravers always make use of) they are not only pressed, but likewise extended; by which means the figures are rendered so much larger, that when the sheets are afterwards dried, they do not contract to their just dimensions.

The technology of printing from copper engravings in the Netherlands was, as we have seen, highly developed.

I took care too that the [plates] should be impressed as well as possible ... wherefore I both used the fittest paper, in which a great deal depends, and employed a very skilful and experienced workman.

At the end of it all, when the *Tabulae sceleti et musculorum* ... was completed, Albinus had some doubts: 'It is possible enough that I might have bestowed my labour, which in such a number of things was certainly very great, to a still better purpose'. The cost was not only in time and energy, but also in money. Albinus is said to have spent 24 000 florins on the production of the work, whereas he only paid 15 000 florins for his house in Leiden. However, he rallied, reassuring himself that accuracy and perfection were needed and necessary.

The memory of Albinus should be respected for the tenacity, taste, and scientific good sense with which he carried his part of his grand design to a successful, albeit incomplete, conclusion.

Albinus, in his account of the preparations of the illustrations, says:

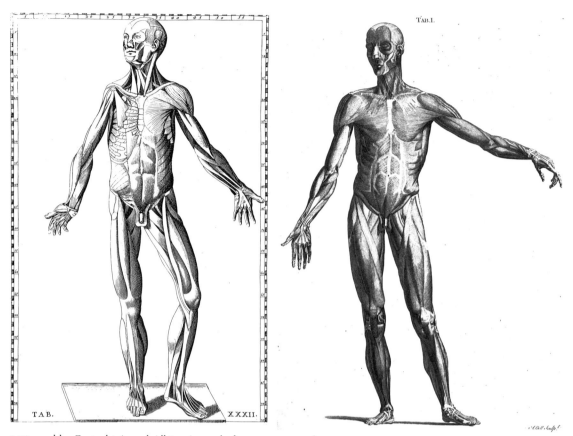

8.12a and b Eustachio's and Albinus' muscle figures compared.

I have not only studied the correctness of the figures, but likewise the neatness and elegancy of them. For this end I employed an artist very skilful, both in drawing and ingraving. And he happened to be one, which is very seldom the case, who was very fond of doing things in that way; which disposition I encouraged, by giving him whatever he demanded for his trouble.

Albinus goes on to describe how Wandelaar worked almost exclusively for him, mostly on the plates of this book, drawing and engraving everything. '... I was constantly with him, to direct him how every thing was to be done, assisting him in the drawing and correcting what was drawn. And thus he was instructed, directed, and as entirely ruled by me, as if he was a tool in my hands, and I made the figures myself.' Albinus compliments the skill and taste of the artist—using such words to describe his work as dignity, distinctness, force, grace, harmony, and perfection. The backgrounds to the figures—the wooded pools, the pastoral landscapes, the classical architecture—and the rhinoceros—are explained and justified; they serve to '... not only ... fill up the empty spaces of the tables and make them appear more agreeable; but likewise that ... the light and shades of the figures might be preserved, and heightened, and the figures themselves appear more raised or rounded ...'. It was suggested by Albinus that the plates be looked at through the cupped hand 'in the manner of a spy-glass'. Camper criticized the backgrounds that Wandelaar gave to the figures, but they do indeed confer a three-dimensional appearance. The English edition (1749) leaves them in; the plates were beautifully re-engraved by the famous Charles Grignion and others. The Edinburgh edition of Albinus (1777) left out the backgrounds, and the figures do indeed seem much flatter (*Fig. 8.13*).

Wandelaar and Albinus devised a method by which the beauty of the illustrations should not be impaired or bespotted with reference figures and numerals: same-sized, outline diagrams of each skeletal man and muscle-man were used for the key references: the text was merely an index to these references. This method, apparently invented by Albinus, was copied extensively by many authors of engraved anatomical plate-books during the following hundred years; it is still in use from time to time.

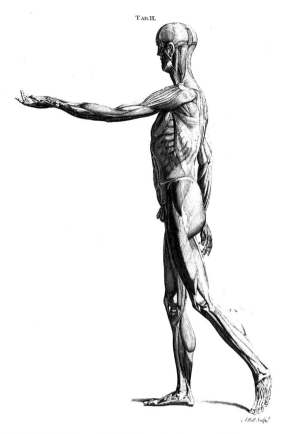

8.13 Tab. IX from the Edinburgh edition of Albinus, *Tables of the skeleton*, 1777.

The harmonious and close relationship between artist and anatomist lasted from 1721, when the two started to work together, until Wandelaar's death in 1754. Wandelaar lived in a part of Albinus' house for many years. It is said that when Wandelaar died, Albinus suffered a serious mental depression, from which he recovered but slowly. In justice, the life and background of Jan Wandelaar (1690–1759) should be allotted equal space to that of his friend and collaborator; but there is little that is known. He was a pupil of the artists Jacob Folkema and van der Gouwen, and of Gerard de Lairesse, who had worked for Bidloo. Wandelaar was employed on anatomical subjects not only in Leiden but also earlier in Amsterdam; he worked for Ruysch and for Arent Cant. He also engraved botanical illustrations which stood him in good stead when composing the foregrounds to the anatomical plates. His engraving techniques were learnt in Amsterdam from Folkema. Some wonderful chalk drawings by Wandelaar for Albinus' plates are in the University Library at Leiden.

The influence of the Albinus–Wandelaar plates on subsequent anatomical illustration has been profound, and continues to the present day. It extends not only to many anatomical texts, but also to three-dimensional representation—as in the wax models of anatomy at *La Specola* in Florence—and to anatomy for artists; a recent artistic anatomy has been based on Albinus' muscle-men. Stubbs, as we shall see, made use of the figures, as did Joseph Wright of Derby in one of his paintings. They were copied by Pierre Tarin (1753), by Andrew Bell (1798), by Loder (1803), and many other anatomists.

Some books by Bernard Siegfried Albinus

1. Albinus wrote no doctoral dissertation, but gave an inaugural lecture when he was twenty or twenty-one years old: *Oratio inauguralis de anatome comparata*, 1719.

2. We may group together Albinus' editions of the works of some of the most distinguished of his predecessors.

   a. *Andreas Vesali … Opera omnia anatomica et chirurgica*, 1725. This was with Herman Boerhaave.
   b. *Gul. Harvaeus. Exercitatio anatomica de motu cordis …*, 1736.
   c. *Fabricius ab Aquapendente. Opera omnia anatomica …*, 1737.
   d. *Explicatio tabularum anatomicarum Barth. Eustachii*, 1744.

3. There were a number of anatomical works published in quarto. These, illustrated principally by Wandelaar, included:

   a. *Index supellectilis anatomicae …*, 1725. The catalogue of Rau's museum.
   b. *Historia musculorum corporis hominis …*, 1734; a long work, with plates and outline diagrams, in the manner that Albinus had inaugurated, of the anatomy of the hand.
   c. *De arteriis et venis intestinorum hominis …*, 1736, with one fine plate of the vessels of the intestine.
   d. *Icones ossium foetum humani …*, 1737. In this work, more than 150 figures of separated fetal bones are shown on 16 plates, each with outlines.
   e. *Academicarum annotationum libri viii …*, 1754–68.

4. The four publications that were part of the grand scheme of anatomy—a complete survey of human anatomy—are given below. Each appeared in elephant folio—'forma atlant. maj.'. (Preparative manuscript work on other volumes is to be found at Leiden University and elsewhere.) They were printed by *Typographia Dammeana*, and published by Joannes & Hermannus Verbeek.

   a. *Tabulae sceleti et musculorum corporis humani*, 1747. This contains three skeletal plates, numbered 1 to 3 (front, side, and back), and nine plates of muscles, numbered 1 to 9 (seen from front, side, and back in various stages of dissection). All figures are set against elaborately-drawn landscape backgrounds. There are accompanying outline plates in the Albinian manner. There then follows sixteen plates, without outlines, illustrating the separated muscles, individually portrayed.
   b. *Tabulae VII uteri mulieris gravidae …*, 1748–51. Seven life-sized plates of the pregnant uterus and the contained fetus, and an eighth plate of the fetus alone.
   c. *Tabulae ossium humanorum*, 1753. Life-sized figures of all the bones of the body.
   d. *Tabula vasis chyliferi, cum vena azyga …*, 1757. A life-size figure of the thoracic duct, azygos vein, and intercostal arteries.

5. All the works listed above were originally published in Latin at Leiden, but some were reprinted in other places. Especially notable are the first London reprints, in 1749, of number 4a. above—in Latin; and (in a shorter version) in English, as *Tables of the skeleton and muscles of the human body*, H. Woodfall for John and Paul Knapton. The plates for these reprints were most carefully and elegantly re-engraved.

Plates 74 to 78 inclusive are from B. S. Albinus, *Tabulae sceleti et musculorum* ..., 1747 (private collection).

74 The skeleton seen from the side. Tabula III of the skeletal series. B. S. Albinus, 1747. Engraving. 54.8 × 38.6 cm.

The great care, already noted, that was taken in setting up the skeleton and also the muscle dissections is exemplified in this plate. Points of excellence include the appropriate curves of the vertebral column (all too rarely shown correctly); the transverse process of the atlas, and the strong bifid spine of the axis; the arrangement and configuration of the ribs; the tarsal skeleton; and the positioning of the patellae. Less good are the straightness of the femoral shafts; the 'separated' hip-joint; the size of the head of the left radius relative to the capitulum; and the backward tilt of the pelvic girdle with respect to the vertebral column. One might note that the greater sciatic notch is wide for a male skeleton.

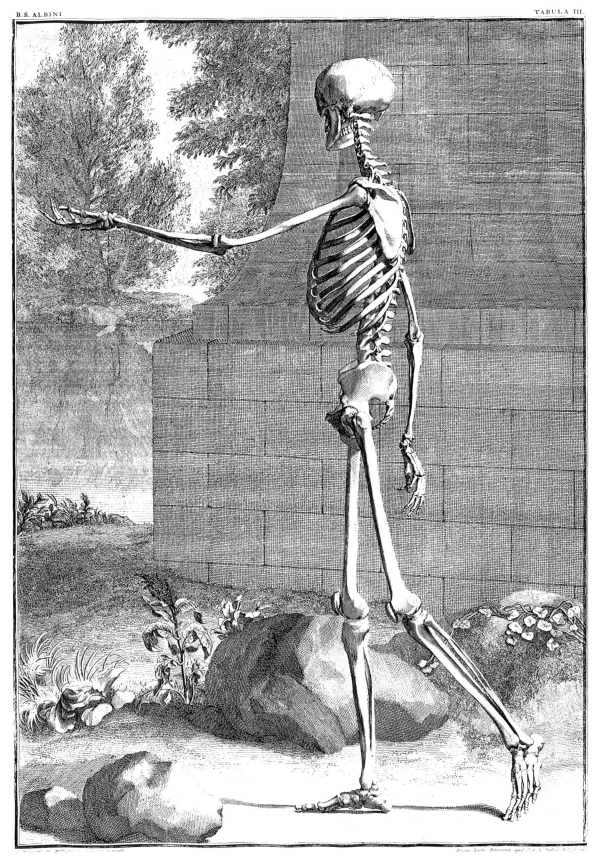

PLATE 74

75 Muscle-man seen from the front: Tabula II of the muscle series. B. S. Albinus, 1747. Engraving. 56.1 × 40.1 cm.

In this 'second stage' of the dissection certain of the more superficial muscles have been removed or cut short: for example, trapezius; platysma; pectoralis major and deltoid; brachio-radialis, pronator teres, palmaris longus, and extensor digitorum; the external oblique muscle of the abdomen (and its aponeurosis); sartorius and rectus femoris; and tibialis anterior. Excellently portrayed are the linea alba (it is not just a white line); the arch at the origin of the right flexor digitorum superficialis, the thenar, hypothenar, and lumbrical muscles; and pectoralis minor.

Less good are the abnormal medial rotation of the left thumb; the broad insertion of extensor hallucis (and the supplementary insertion shown is rare); the tibialis posterior tendon, which hardly inserts at all into the navicular bone; and the arrangement of the lower fibres of the internal oblique passing over the spermatic cord.

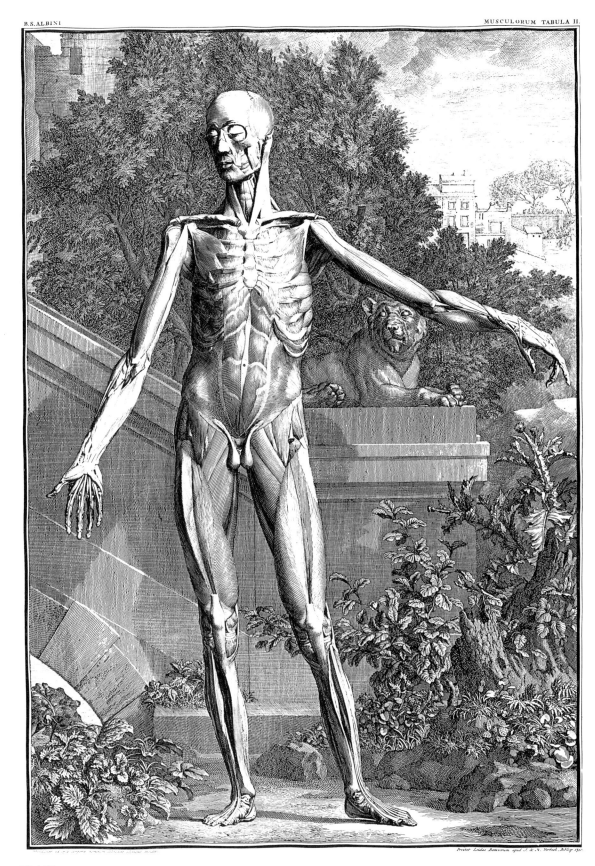

PLATE 75

76 Muscle-man seen from the front: Tabula IV of the muscle series. B. S. Albinus, 1747. Engraving. 56 × 40 cm

In this 'fourth stage', the human figure stands out remarkably well from the ornate background.

Revealed are the deep muscles in the palm, adductor pollicis, and the interossei. The supinator muscle is best seen in the left forearm; subscapularis, longus cervicis, and scalenus medius are also featured.

The origin of the adductor magnus appears to extend too high on the pubic bone, the strong tendon of psoas major is poorly depicted, and the bulging peroneus brevis is displeasing. The diaphragm is notoriously difficult to draw well; however, it is excellently shown in Albinus' separate muscle drawings later in his book.

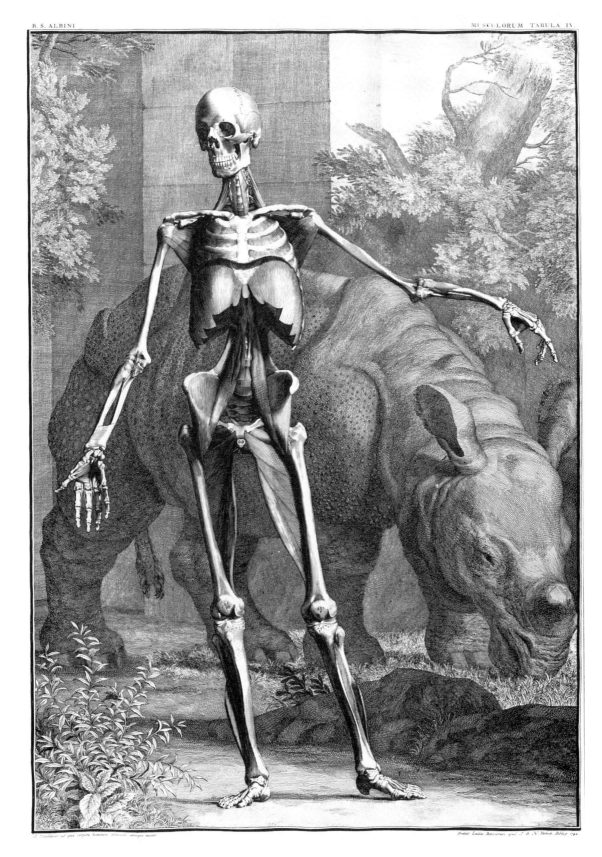

PLATE 76

77 Muscle-man seen from the back: first stage, an *écorché*. Tabula V of the muscle series. B. S. Albinus, 1747. Engraving. 56.0 × 39.7 cm.

The posterior 'first stage' shows the superficial muscles. So much is good (for example, gluteus maximus inserting into the ilio-tibial tract; the triangle of auscultation in the angle between latissimus dorsi and trapezius; the extensor tendon 'hoods' of the right hand) that one can forgive the two bellies of gastrocnemius extending to the same level, the too-short tendon of semi-tendinosus, the inclination of the postero-medial fibres of gluteus medius, and the too distal extent of the extensor carpi radialis brevis tendon in the right hand.

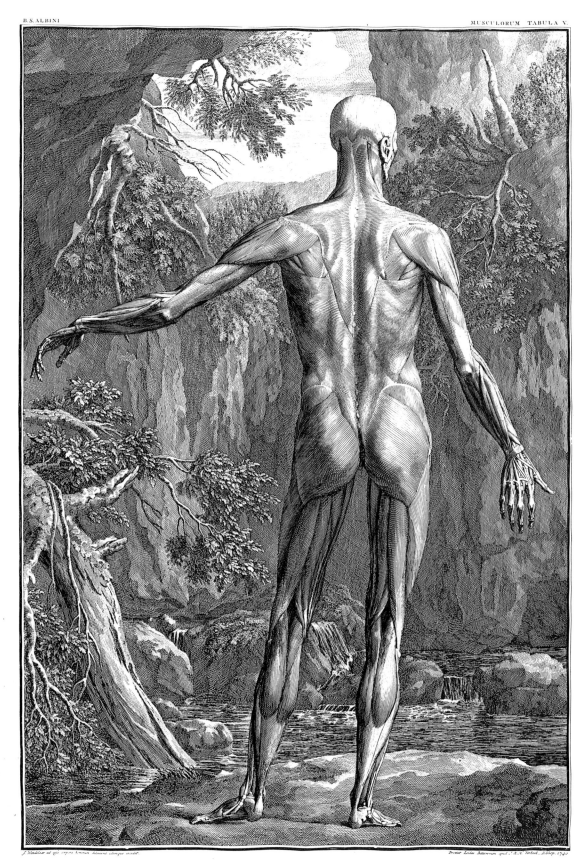

J. Wandelaar ad ipsi corporis humani lineavit elimque incidit.

Prostat Lugduni Batavorum apud .' S. & J. Verbeek, Bibliop. 1749.

PLATE 77

78 Muscle-man seen from the back: Tabula VII of the muscle series. B. S. Albinus, 1747. Engraving. 56.4 × 40.1 cm.

The last error referred to above has been rectified in this drawing, which represents the 'third stage' of dissection from the back. Once again, there is much to admire: the right popliteus muscle; the 'curvaceousness' of semimembranosus; longissimus capitis in the neck, and the 'beef-to-the-heel' portrayal of flexor hallucis longus. Weak are the obturator internus muscle, and the impression given that part of semispinalis capitis is taking origin from a cervical spine.

As mentioned earlier, Albinus included in this book excellent drawings, over three hundred in total, both of separate muscles (not excepting stapedius and tensor tympani!) and also of muscle groups. They remind one strongly of Canano's approach of more than two hundred years before (see (*Plate 21*, p. 95), though understandably the illustrations of Albinus are more accurate and more clearly drawn.

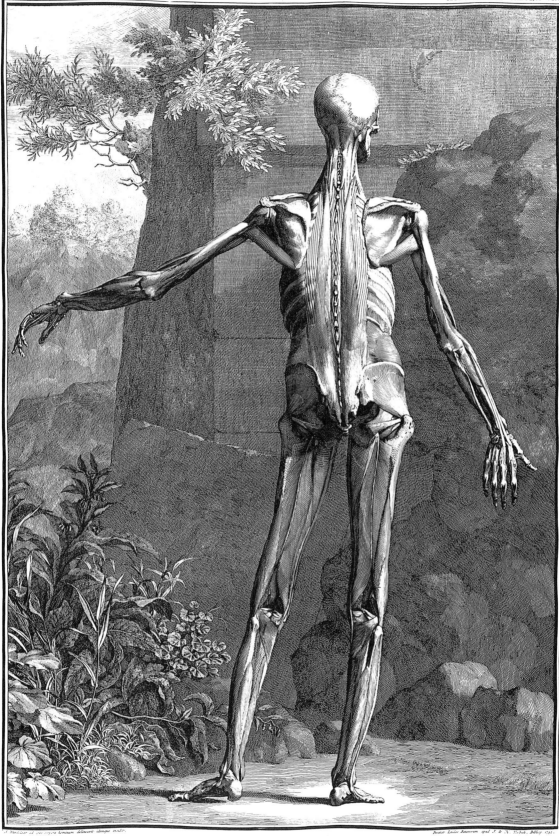

PLATE 78

Petrus (Pieter) Camper (1722–1789)

Camper was a native of Leiden, his father being a minister of religion who had worked in the Dutch East Indies. He entered the University when he was twelve years old, eventually taking his medical degree in 1746. He had studied with B. S. Albinus. Shortly after graduation he journeyed to London and enrolled in William Smellie's midwifery class. On this occasion, he remained in England for more than a year. Camper's first academic appointment was in 1750 at the University at Franeker, in Friesland, which had only four medical students when Camper arrived. The institution was more popular by the time he left to take up a chair at the *Athenaeum* in Amsterdam in 1755. As had obtained with his predecessors in this post, Tulp and Ruysch, there was an official 'Anatomy of Prof. Petrus Camper' painted, in this case by Tibout Regters. Camper's final appointment was as Professor at Groningen, 1763–73.

For periods from 1761 to 1763 and from 1773 onwards he lived at his country house near Franeker, but involvement in political affairs became more pressing, and he finally had to move to The Hague when he was made a State Councillor; he died in that city.

Camper had acquired a taste for foreign travel as a postgraduate, and continued to make journeys to medical and scientific centres. He revisited Smellie in London in 1752, contributing drawings for Smellie's *A sett of anatomical tables ...*, 1754 (*Fig. 8.14*). Other visits were made, particularly during the 1770s and 1780s, to France, Germany, and England. The journals of his travels in England 1748–85 were published, and much later translated into English in 1939. A portrait medallion of Camper was included in Josiah Wedgwood's series of 'Illustrious Moderns' made at Etruria towards the end of the eighteenth century.

Camper's name appears in the histories of a number of subjects: surgery, obstetrics, forensic medicine, comparative anatomy, public health, veterinary medicine, hygiene, and physical anthropology, as well as human anatomy. A few examples of his contributions to some of these may be listed:

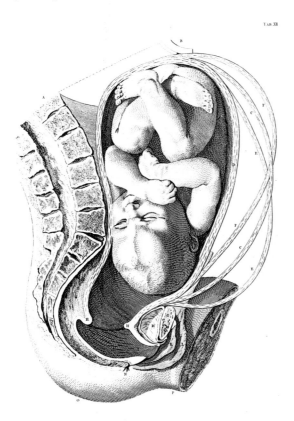

8.14 Camper's drawing of Tab. XII in Smellie's *A Sett*, 1754.

studies on hernia, including those published posthumously by his pupil Soemmerring.

post mortem recognition of stillborn babies.

the anatomy of the orang-utan, with particular attention to vocalization and the adoption of the upright posture; the anatomy of bone air-sacs in birds; studies on hearing in whales. The Dutch maritime empire enabled Camper to have access to live and dead specimens of apes, elephant, rhinoceros, and other exotic animals.

studies on cattle plague and on inoculation against small pox.

investigations on the deformities of the foot produced by ill-designed shoes. (Soemmerring was to extend this type of investigation to the baleful effects of tight corseting.)

work on physiognomy that led to a publication in which he showed, *inter alia*, that drawing faces to a geometric formula produced proportions that were at variance with reality; Camper included, in a lecture to the Art Academy of Amsterdam, a geometric measurement of a facial angle—one of the first measurements to be made in physical anthropology.

Camper had maintained and developed his natural ability as an artist from boyhood, when his talents were encouraged by study under Karl (Carel) de Moor, father and son; he illustrated his own works.

Albinus and many of his predecessors—Vesalius, for instance—had had the artist represent a perspective view taken from one observation point; the Dutch master, it will be remembered, had Wandelaar view the skeleton, etc. through a spyhole. Camper wished to have the part drawn from multiple equidistant viewpoints, as in an architectural drawing. Soemmerring, an admirer of Albinus but an ardent pupil of Camper, was perhaps the most famous of subsequent anatomists to sympathize with Camper's methods.

Some books by Petrus Camper

1. Camper published, as was then required, his theses for doctoral degrees at Leiden in science and medicine in 1746. They were on aspects of vision.

2. There were inaugural lectures for his chairs at Franeker (1751), Amsterdam (1755, and again in 1758, when he achieved a new professorship) and Groningen (1763). These were of a general, philosophical nature.

3. His most considerable scientific work in anatomy is *Demonstrationum anatomico-pathologicarum. Liber primus continens brachii humani fabricam et morbos*, Amsterdam, J. Schreuder and P. Mortier Jr., 1760. These very large plates on the upper limb were followed by a second volume, on the pelvis, published in 1762. The plates, some of which had accompanying outline diagrams, were engraved by J. v. d. Schley from Camper's own drawings. There were no more in this projected series, but Camper's pupil, S. T. Soemmerring, after Camper's death, published *Icones herniarum*. Camper's plates for these anatomical and pathological books take their place alongside the illustrations prepared by the artists Lairesse and Wanderlaar for the anatomists Bidloo and Albinus. Together the achievements of these atlases represent, both scientifically and aesthetically, a high point of Dutch civilization in the eighteenth century.

4. There were publications in the broad field of art, anatomy, and medicine:
   a. *Epistola ad anatomicorum principem magnum Albinum*, Groningen, 1767. Albinus and Camper disputed as to the best means of reproducing three-dimensional anatomy on the plane of a paper sheet.
   b. Two works in Dutch, Utrecht 1791 and 1792, edited by Camper's son, A. G. Camper. The second was translated into English by T. Cogan, MD as *The connexion between the science of anatomy and the arts of painting, drawing, statuary, etc . . .*, London, 1794. The chapters of this book were taken from lectures given by Camper before the Academy of Graphic and Plastic Arts in Amsterdam, for which he received a gold medal: it contained 17 plates.

79 Dissections of the upper limb, Book I, Tabula I of P. Camper, *Demonstrationum . . .*, 1760. Engraving (Cambridge University Library). 56.4 × 37.9 cm.

In Figure I a small inferior cervical sympathetic ganglion can be seen, with connections to an elongated first thoracic ganglion which is positioned between scalenus anterior and longus cervicis.

The cut phrenic nerve has, curiously, been swung out laterally from its correct position on scalenus anterior. The axillary nerve is rather unimpressive, and seems to give rise to the lower subscapular. Only one medial cutaneous branch (cut short) arising from the medial cord is shown.

It is unfortunate, in Figure II, that the stipple technique employed makes the nerves appear more like arteries than the arteries themselves. The mode of origin of the lateral thoracic artery, an upward loop, is certainly erroneous, and the whole axillary area is confusing; it might have been better to have eliminated the veins from this crowded area.

The palmaris longus is shown inserting entirely into the flexor retinaculum at the wrist, and the thin nerve seen crossing the hypothenar muscles is unusual, to say the least. It is identified in the accompanying line diagram of the drawing as 'rami ulnaris externi conjunctio cum interno'. It is clear (from Figure III) that it is a branch of the dorsal branch of the ulnar nerve. The general anatomy of the palmar structures is accurate.

In Figure III, the nerves are now white and look like nerves—for example, the dorsal branch of the ulnar and the superficial radial. One would prefer, however, to have the tendons of abductor pollicis longus and extensor pollicis brevis restrained by a continuation of the extensor retinaculum. The tendon of extensor indicis is not in evidence, but the fibrous bands between the extensor tendons are well portrayed, as is the insertion of the extensor digitorum on to the index finger and also the first palmar interosseous joining the extensor expansion.

The drawings stand out pleasingly from the plain background; they are easily comprehended, and are in the forefront of mid-eighteenth-century anatomical illustrations.

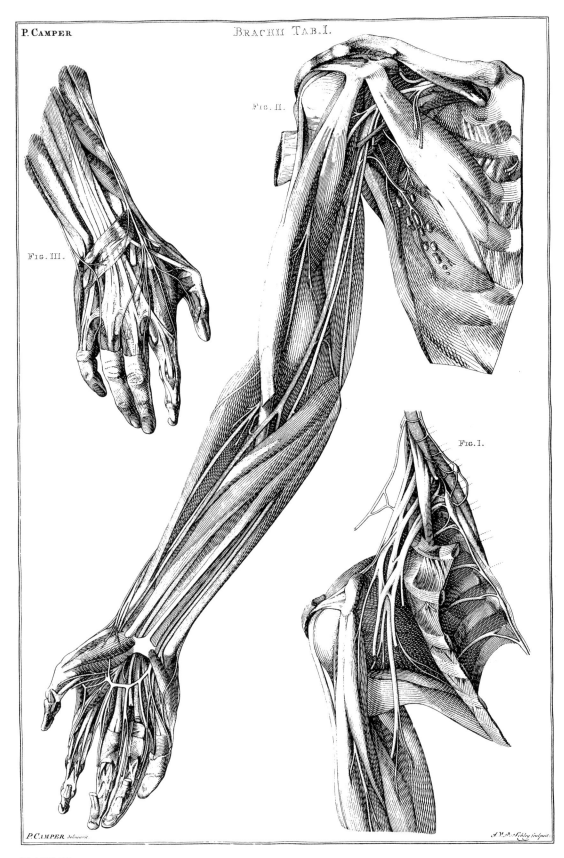

Fig. II.

Fig. III.

Fig. I.

P. CAMPER *delineavit*

J. V. D. Schley sculpsit

PLATE 79

Chapter 8: Selected readings

The rise of medical science in the Low Countries

Alpers, S. (1983). *The art of describing: Dutch art in the seventeenth century.* ... University of Chicago Press.

Braudel, F. (1981–4). *Civilization and capitalism in the fifteen and sixteenth centuries* (trans. S. Reynolds). Harper and Row, New York.

Clair, C.. (1976). *A history of European printing.* Academic Press, London.

Huizinga, J.H. (1968). *Dutch civilization in the seventeenth century.* ... Collins, London.

Impey, O. and MacGregor, A. (ed.) (1985). *The origin of museums: the cabinet of curiosities in sixteenth- and seventeenth-century Europe.* Clarendon Press, Oxford.

Lindeboom, G. A. (1984). *Dutch medical biography, a biographical dictionary of Dutch physicians & surgeons, 1475–1972.* Rodopi, Amsterdam.

Parker, G. (1979). *The Dutch revolt.* Penguin, Harmondsworth.

Schama, S. (1987). *The embarrassment of riches: An interpretation of Dutch culture in the golden age.* Collins, London.

Schupbach, W. (1982). *The paradox of Rembrandt's 'Anatomy of Dr. Tulp'.* Wellcome Institute for the History of Medicine, London.

Frederick Ruysch

Ackerknecht, E. H. (1971). Mannerist anatomy: Frederik Ruysch and his collection. *Image (Med. Illust. Roche),* **43,** 27–32.

Cole, F. J. (1921). The history of anatomical injections. In *Studies in the history and method of science,* (ed. C. Singer), **2,** pp. 286–343. Oxford University Press.

Cole, F. J. (1975). *A history of comparative anatomy* ... [Chapter XXV on Ruysch]. Reprint of 1949 edition. Dover, New York.

Hazen, A. T. (1939). Johnson's life of Frederic Ruysch. *Bull. Hist. Med.,* **7,** 324–34.

Houtzager, H. L. (1982). Frederik Ruysch. *Europ. J. Ob. reprod. Biol.,* **13,** 199–201.

Lindeboom, G.A. (1975). Frederik Ruysch. *Dict. sci. Biog.,* **12,** 39–42.

Luyendijk-Elshout, A. M. (1964). *Frederik Ruysch: Dilucidatio valvularum in vasis lymphaticis ...,* with an introduction. B. de Graaf, Nieuwkoop.

Luyendijk-Elshout, A. M. (1970). Death enlightened: A study of Frederik Ruysch. *JAMA,* **212,** 121–6.

Mann, G. (1964). Museums: the anatomical collection of Frederik Ruysch at Leningrad. *Bull. Cleveland Med. Lib.,* **11,** 10–13.

Ruestow, E. G. (1980). The rise of the doctrine of vascular secretion in the Netherlands. *J. Hist. Med.,* **35,** 265–87.

Theodor Kerckring

Bayle, A. L. J. and Thillaye, A. J. (1855). Théodore Kerckring. *Biog. méd;.* **2.** 137–8.

Parker, R. G. (1983). Academy of fine arts ... by Cornelis Cort. ... *J. Hist. Med.,* **38,** 76–7.

The medical school at Leiden

Brockbank, W. (1968). Old anatomical theatres and what took place therein. *Med. Hist.*, **12**, 371–84.

Doolin, W. (1941). *Wayfarers in medicine* [Chapter VII: *The anatomists in art*, includes material on group portraits of Amsterdam surgeons]. William Heinemann, London.

Lindeboom, G. A. (1959). *Bibliographia Boerhaaviana.* ... E. J. Brill, Leiden.

Lindeboom, G. A. (1970). Hermann Boerhaave. *Dict. sci. Biog.*, **2**, 224–8.

Lindeboom, G. A. (1970). Medical education in the Netherlands 1575–1750. In *History of medical education*, (ed. C. D. O'Malley). University of California Press, Berkeley.

Mulder, W. J. (ed.) (1984). *Guide to the Museum of Anatomy and Embryology.* ... Leiden: University Hospital.

Smith, R. W. I. (1932). *English-speaking students of medicine at the University of Leyden.* Oliver and Boyd, Edinburgh.

Underwood, E. A. (1977). *Boerhaave's men at Leyden and after.* Edinburgh University Press.

Witkam, H. J. (1980). *Catalogues of all the chiefest rarities in the publick anatomie hall of the University of Leiden.* H. J. Witkam, Leiden.

Govard Bidloo

Beekman, F. (1935). Bidloo and Cowper, anatomists. *Ann. med. Hist.*, NS **7**, 113–29.

Dumaître, P. (1982). *La curieuse destinée des planches anatomiques de Gérard de Lairesse.* Rodopi, Amsterdam.

Gysel, C. (1986). Aspects odonto-stomatologiques de L'Anatomia de Bidloo (1685). ... *Méd. et Hyg.*, **44**, 2212–3.

Herrlinger, R. (1966). Bidloos Anatomia: Prototyp barocker Illustration? *Gesnerus*, **23**, 40–7.

van der Pas, P. W. (1978). Govard Bidloo. *Dict. sci. Biog.*, **15**, 28–30.

Rosenberg, J., Slive, S., and ter Kuile, E. H. (1966). *Dutch art and architecture: 1600 to 1800.* Penguin, Harmondsworth.

Russell, K. F. (1959). The anatomical plagiarist. *Med. J. Australia*, **1**, 249–52.

Willemse, D. (1975). *The unknown drawings of Nicolaus Bidloo, director of the first hospital in Russia.* D. Willemse, Voorburg, Netherlands.

B. S. Albinus

Elkins, J. (1986). Two conceptions of the human form: Bernard Siegfried Albinus and Andreas Vesalius. *Artibus et historae*, **14 (VII)**, 91–106.

Gysel, C. (1977). B. S. Albinus (1697–1770). La croissance et les dents. *Rev. Belge Méd. Dent.*, **32**, 163–94.

Hale, R. B. and Coyle, T. (1979). *Albinus on anatomy.* Watson-Guptill, New York.

Hilloowala, R. (1986). Bartolomeo Eustachio: his influence on Albinus and the anatomical models at La Specola, Florence. *J. Hist. Med.*, **41**, 442–62.

van der Pas, P. W. (1978). Bernard, Bernard Siegfried, Christiaan Bernard, and Frederick Bernard Albinus. *Dict. sci. Biog.*, **15.** 3–6.

Punt, H. (1980). An historical evaluation of perspective aids particularly in the anatomical illustrations of B. S. Albinus (1697–1770). *Hist. Ophthal. intern.*, **1**, 217–26.

Punt, H. (1983). Bernard Siegfried Albinus (1697–1770). 'On human nature': anatomical and physiological ideas in eighteenth-century Leiden. B. M. Israel, Amsterdam.

Petrus Camper

Lindeboom, G. A. (1971). Peter (Petrus) Camper. *Dict. sci. Biog.*, **3**, 37–8.

Nuyens, B. W. T. (1939). *Petri Camperi itinera in Angliam 1748–1785*. No. 15 of *Opuscula selecta Neerlandicorum de arte medica*. Amsterdam.

Rooseboom, M. (1954). Wedgwood medallion of Petrus Camper. *Bull. Hist. Med.*, **28**, 553.

9

The classical tradition develops in Germany

Albrecht von Haller (1708–1777)

ANYONE attempting to place von Haller and his anatomical work in perspective is inevitably overwhelmed by the extraordinary diversity of this man's scientific and literary energy and productivity.

He was born in Berne, Switzerland, his family belonging to the Reformed Church of the Protestant humanist, Huldreich Zwingli. A prodigy, especially in languages, Haller entered the University of Leiden, where he was deeply influenced by Boerhaave's ideas. He learned his anatomy under the young B. S. Albinus. When he was only eighteen years of age he received his doctorate, with an anatomical dissertation relating to the salivary glands, based on work he had started earlier in Tübingen University.

Haller then began his *Wanderjahre*, the customary European journey. He travelled to London, 1727, where he met Fellows of the Royal Society, including anatomists William Cheselden and James Douglas, and Sir Hans Sloane, who had succeeded Isaac Newton as President that same year. Sloane was President also of the College of Physicians, and physician to George II. Haller then journeyed to Paris, studying with the Danish anatomist Winslow. Later, in 1728, he began a course of lectures on anatomy in Basle, as Vesalius had done two hundred

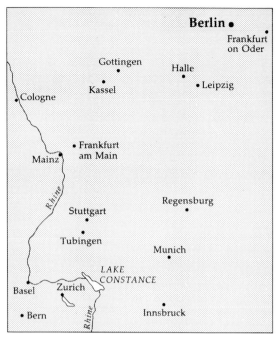

9.1 Map of Germany

years previously. At Basle he studied mathematics, and also botany in the field, or rather on the mountains. From 1729 he remained in Berne for eight years, attempting to establish himself as a physician, without great success. But he continued his scientific studies, with publications on the diaphragm, on Siamese twins, and on botany.

Haller also wrote poetry: his poem *Die Alpen*, 1732, is an early Romantic work describing the simple life of mountain-dwellers amongst the grand picturesque scenery of the Alps; before Haller the mountains had been noted principally as impediments to trade, and frightening. From 1734 Haller gave demonstrations in an anatomy theatre that had been constructed in the city at his urging; but there was no salary for this.

In 1736, he was appointed Professor of Anatomy, Surgery, and Medicine at the University of Göttingen in Hanover. He had applied for this post, but was appointed only when the chosen man died. Göttingen was a new university, which finally opened in December 1737. It had been founded by the Elector of Hanover—George II of England—to rival the prestigious University of Halle nearby, established in 1694. The appointments of Göttingen were under the control of a Baron Münchausen (no less!), who wanted as professors men whose teaching would 'lead neither to atheism nor naturalism, neither assail the fundamental articles of evangelical religion, nor introduce enthusiasm, nor any evangelical Papacy ... but sober diligent scholars'. Haller's attitude and talents certainly agreed with this job description. Münchausen encouraged and protected Haller as he carried out his various projects.

The move to Göttingen at the age of twenty-eight started tragically with the death of his wife, leaving him with three children. He remarried in 1739, but his second wife died in childbirth. He married a third time. One might have imagined that in these circumstances there would have been more than enough work for Haller in the foundation of a new medical school intended to rival Halle, if not Leiden itself. But in these years, Haller not only established the curriculum, in which he taught anatomy, physiology, and bedside clinical medicine, but also set up the library, established a botanical and medicinal garden, and helped to start the Royal Society of Sciences of Göttingen, of which he became President. He was President of the College of Surgeons, and physician to George II while the latter was in Hanover. He started and edited the journal *Göttingische gelehrte Anzeigen*. For his work he was elevated to the nobility as a Baron, and was elected as one of the great council of Berne. But what must amaze the lesser breed of medical academics and administrators that exist nowadays is his ability to carry out, at the same time, important scientific work, and to publish his investigations in literally hundreds of papers. This was the principal creative period of Haller's scientific life.

In 1753 Haller travelled with his family on a visit to Berne, his native city, where he applied for and was awarded a minor government post. He stayed in Berne, resigning unexpectedly his chair at Göttingen, not even returning there to remove his library or household belongings. (His wife went later, without him, to arrange this.) His motivation for this abrupt move is uncertain. Haller could be an irascible, opinionated man; and his life in the university community was probably not smooth.

He remained in Berne or nearby for the rest of his life, achieving a more important position as manager of a salt-works. He was an exceptionally good administrator, controlling this municipal enterprise—a small world—benignly, efficiently, and profitably. He continued to write voluminously, and to observe and experiment on a very wide range of subjects. His studies on normal human anatomy did not continue for lack of subjects for dissection. Leaving aside his work on a fine herbal of Switzerland, his writing on economic and philosophical matters, and his literary output (three novels were written in this last period at Berne), his publications in medically-related subjects may be grouped under the headings of physiology and anatomy; embryology and teratology; and bibliography. The last group included an exposition and discussion, in more than a thousand pages, of Boerhaave's *Methodus studii medici* ..., Amsterdam, 1751, and an attempt to create an annotated listing of all the important work of medical interest, a vast compendium, a *Bibliotheca medica*. The botanical (1771–2), surgical (1774–5), and anatomical (1774–6) parts of this latter were completed, and published along with one on practical medicine 1776–88. They contain a description of over 50 000 volumes. A *Bibliotheca physica* is in manuscript in the State Library in Berne. Haller was a confident systematizer and assiduous compiler, at a time when many other scholars were beginning to turn to classification, systematics, and the construction of encyclopaedias.

In his studies on embryological development Haller was a preformationist, or, as it was also called, an 'evolutionist': structures were already present in the egg before it was stimulated by the spermatozoon; from these the embryo evolved as development preceded.

Haller wished to have his work in anatomy and physiology considered as complementary—structure and function going hand-in-hand. The structure of the diaphragm and the anatomy of the intercostal muscles must be investigated if the mechanisms of respiration were to be understood, and it was also necessary to know whether air was present in the pleural cavity or not. Haller made discoveries in each of these areas, exemplifying his ideal of a living anatomy, *anatomia animata*. His work, still unrecognized, on lymphatics was in the same mode. William Harvey's anatomical exercises or experiments and Haller's living anatomy have this much in common. But one looks in vain in amongst the thicket of Haller's verbosity for what one finds in Harvey's *De motu cordis* ..., succinct and clear arguments, based on precise, thought-through, crucial experiments and observations.

Studies on the heart and its circulation, the irritability of muscles and the sensibility of nerves, the fine anatomy of connective tissues—these studies and many more were summarized in what has been regarded as the first modern physiological textbook, an eight-volume work: *Elementa physiologiae corporis humani* ..., 1757–66. Haller's development of Glisson's ideas on irritability and his own ideas on sensibility were based on simple experiments that, in retrospect, can be faulted fundamentally. These concepts of the properties of muscles and of nerves, respectively, were subjected to argument, but also to unjustified theoretical elaboration, as in the medical system constructed by John Brown of Edinburgh. (Brunonian theories seemed to fill a contemporary need, particularly in the academic climate of German medicine in the latter part of the eighteenth century.)

Haller's correspondence was voluminous: there are 67 bound volumes of letters addressed to him. Probably no scientist, before or since, has published so many papers—some thousands. Haller suffered throughout his life from migraine headaches and insomnia, the latter exacerbated by the quantities of strong tea he consumed. He took opium to relieve these distressing ailments, and became addicted. Dispassionate scientist that he was, he published a paper on his experiences as an addict.

No attempt will be made to list Haller's chief publications, for reasons which must be now obvious. His individual studies were published over the years in many journals and books; where appropriate, they were illustrated by plates. In classical gross anatomy the main work was *Icones anatomicae ... 1743–56*. What is illustrated in this work is intended to represent normal anatomy, and to Haller normal was defined mathematically rather than aesthetically or idealistically: it was defined as the most common, not as the most beautiful. Since anatomical arrangements—the branches of specific arteries, for instance—are subject to a certain variability, a single illustration must choose which variant to show. Haller chose to depict the commonest variant, and in order to be able to do so, he had to dissect and take careful note of many cadavers. This approach is usually the one taken by present-day anatomists; but the idealistic view was adopted, as we shall see, by Soemmerring.

The engravings of the *Icones anatomicae* ... were based on dissections carried out at Göttingen. The subjects chosen did not follow a logical plan; however there was no overlap with the illustrations in Albinus' work. (One thinks what a wonderful grand anatomical atlas could be made by combining Albinus', Haller's, and other eighteenth-century plates.) In Haller's work there are no backgrounds—the tradition of placing anatomized persons against a landscape background, seen early in Berengario, Vesalius, and Casserio, had been continued through to Albinus. In a more restrained age of 'solid, diligent scholars', not subject to wild 'enthusiasms', a straightforward presentation seemed more proper. Albinus justified his elaborate settings on grounds of usefulness—they projected the figure into prominence. Even though his work was carried through with elegance and (in spite of rhinos and so on!) with visual restraint, Albinus was severely criticized. Since Albinus few anatomists have placed their figures in landscapes. Some continued to draw realistically the context and surroundings of a dissecting room; most abstracted their figures, showing the parts against an unencumbered plain page. This meant, of course, that the *memento mori* theme was no longer in evidence. For most of his work, as we have seen, Bidloo adopted these views; for the skeletons he returned to an earlier tradition, by showing them emerging with winding-sheets from the tomb (see *Plate 71*, p. 315).

There were, of course, reasons of economical practicality involved too: if the background to the anatomy was to be as complex as that drawn by Wandelaar for Albinus then an exceptionally skilled artist would need to be employed for long and costly months of work. The figures themselves were becoming more complex, as more detail was shown and identified—to engrave intricate detail against an intricate background would have proved not only confusing, but also extremely expensive. Indeed anatomical details in the Albinus–Wandelaar plates are only identifiable because of the accompanying outline plate. Many of the plates in Haller's *Icones* are similarly uninterpretable save for the outline plate; and this itself may be so complex that on it literally hundreds of parts may be shown identified by numbers, often not too clearly. This

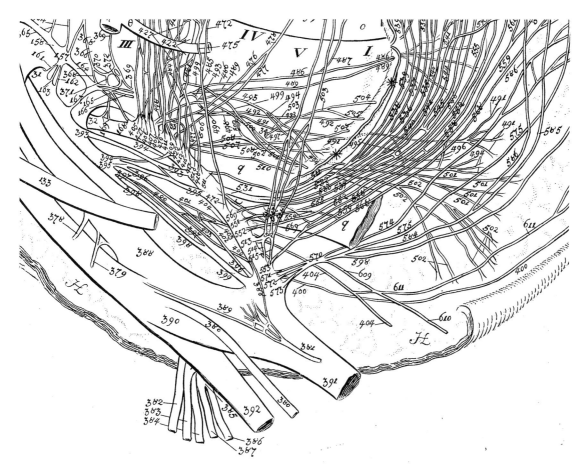

9.2   Detail from Walter's outline drawing accompanying our *Plate 83*.

technique was continued by many later anatomists. The outline drawing to one of Walter's plates of the nerves, our *Plate 83*, illustrates this point (see *Fig. 9.2*).

When the finest branches of veins, arteries, and nerves are shown in an anatomical illustration, the detail can only be relevant to the actual specimen in front of the anatomist and his artist, for one is often (but not always) at a level of considerable variability: at this detail, the pattern of small veins, within a more-or-less regular pattern of larger vessels, is not constant, but peculiar to each individual. It is not then possible to choose between variants on a numerical basis, and what is shown can have little didactic value. We shall have cause to return to these considerations later.

The work from which our *Plates 80 and 81* are taken is *Icones anatomicae.* . . . It was issued 1743–56 from Göttingen in a series of large folio plates collected into fascicles, or small 'bundles'. The whole work, issued by van den Hoeck and dated 1756, was dedicated to George II. The work was reissued 1781–82.

The first plate chosen (*Plate 80*), the arteries of the whole body, is from a drawing made in Göttingen in the years 1750–1 by J. P. Kaltenhofer; it was engraved by J. van der Spyk in Leiden in November, 1754. Accompanying this plate is an outline figure, and this was engraved by Carl Sepp in Amsterdam in 1756. One can appreciate the patience needed to produce this, or any other anatomical atlas, containing copper engravings. The dissections were made six years before the final engraving was completed. Printing and publication, by the firm of Abram van den Hoeck, followed the same year, 1756.

The second illustration chosen (*Plate 81*) was also drawn by Kaltenhofer, but was engraved by I. C. Schrader, of Göttingen. Kaltenhofer was the artist for most of the plates, the other artist was a medical doctor, G. J. Robin, who also drew for Haller's botanical works.

The influence of Dutch anatomists, illustrators, engravers, and publishers is evident in this work by Haller: the subjects chosen may be seen to complement those of Albinus, Haller's anatomy teacher; the drawing and engraving, as in Wandelaar's work, were quite precise and unambiguous; many of the engravers were from the Netherlands, and the publisher was of Dutch origin.

80 The arteries of the body. Fasciculus VIII, Tabula I of A. Haller, *Icones anatomicae* . . . . Engraving (Wellcome Institute Library). 56.5 × 44.4 cm. This plate is from the last *fasciculus*, published in 1756.

In this frontal full-figure of a male baby at term, the large head with adult features and virtually no neck gives the impression of a 'manikin'.

In the book from which this illustration was taken there is, opposite to the drawing, a line-diagram which is lettered and numbered for structure identification. This contains some 65–70 indicators for the left wrist and hand alone, which is surely ludicrous!

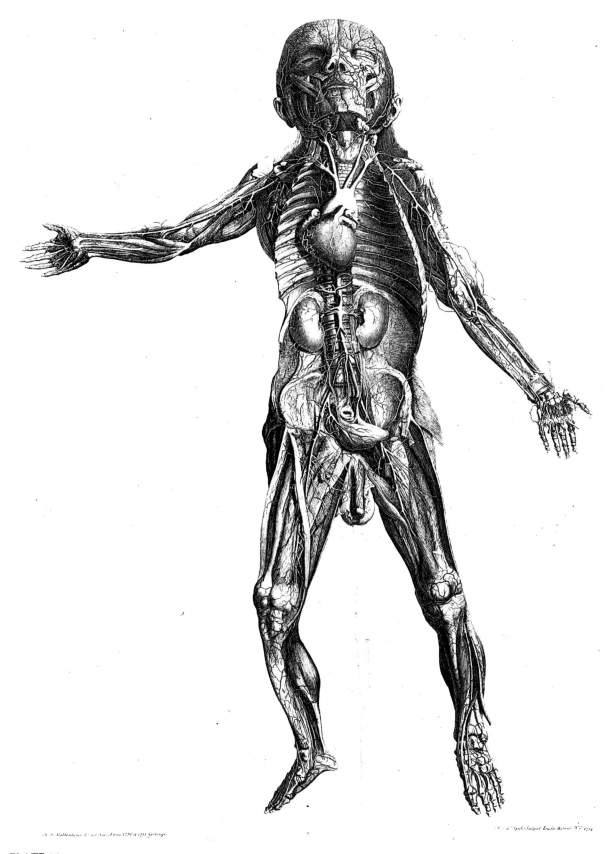

PLATE 80

The figure, designed to show the arterial system of the whole body, features a number of peculiarities.

The heart is situated too far to the right side, and the right and left auricular appendages closely resemble well-fed worms—or leeches.

There is no proper pulmonary trunk—indeed, at first sight, it seems as though the right ventricle is directly connected to the under-side of the aortic arch. The left pulmonary vessels appear just superior to the left auricular appendage, and close examination shows that the artery *could*, perhaps, be traced to the right ventricle, which would leave the interconnecting vessel as representing a patent ductus arteriosus, but of inaccurate origin. It passes understanding why the correct relationship of the pulmonary trunk to the aorta was not made crystal-clear.

The external carotid artery passes anterior to the digastric muscle on the right side but posteriorly (correctly) on the left. In the abdomen the testicular arteries are clearly portrayed, but the coeliac axis and the superior mesenteric artery seem to have been 'stuck on' to the aorta as an afterthought, and the common iliac arteries are very long and thin. The distribution of the internal iliac artery seems to be mainly to the urinary bladder.

If the course of the femoral artery was not known to the viewer it would be difficult to determine it from this plate. With regard to the right femoral artery, one could be excused for believing it to peter out on the medial side of the knee-joint.

The arteries best portrayed are the left profunda femoris, testicular, superficial temporal, and facial, and also the arteries of the upper limb, though in the latter case the scale renders these difficult to make out.

81 The arteries of the upper limb. Fasciculus VI, Tabula III, Fig. IV of A. Haller, *Icones anatomicae.*... Engraving (Wellcome Institute Library). 42.0 × 24.8 cm. In this *fasciculus*, published 1753, there are four other plates, the arteries of the arm, hand and pectoral region, and the muscles of the arm.

This figure, of the anterior aspect of the right arm, is mainly concerned with muscles and blood-vessels, much less so with nerves.

The cephalic and basilic veins are well drawn, though the latter shows very exaggerated valve swellings. In general the structures are drawn accurately, although the proximal portion of the limb is somewhat confusing because of the perspective. Interestingly, the omo-hyoid (A) is referred to as the 'coraco-hyoideus', even though it is not attached to the coracoid process. The dotted indicator lines are, in most cases, very difficult to follow to their destination even in the original plate, and the whole plate suffers from being over-detailed and over-labelled. The combination of Roman capital letters, italic capitals, small letters, and Greek letters may perhaps have been less confusing to anatomists of the eighteenth century than to those of the

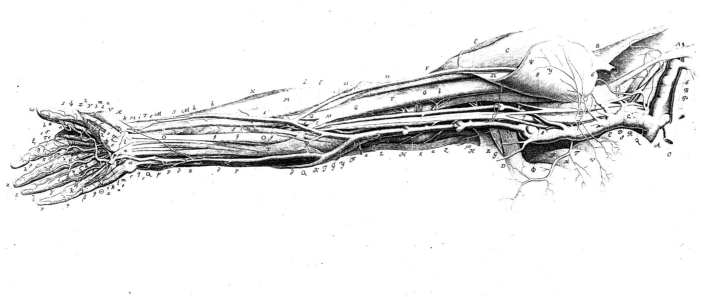

Fasciculus VI.   Tab. III.
Fig. IV. Brachium dextrum, anterius visum.

Kaltenhofer del.   Schrader sc.

PLATE 81

present day. Identification is rendered more difficult because the key, covering four pages, is placed elsewhere in the book.

Although the median and musculo-cutaneous nerves are readily identifiable, the ulnar nerve is nowhere to be seen—at the very least it could surely have been shown accompanying the ulnar artery in the forearm. Haller, however, was remarkably coy about nerves in general; very few are portrayed in his *Icones*.

The main strengths of this illustration are its accuracy, clarity (*pace* the lettering), and the realism of the blood-vessels; the superficial palmar arch and its distribution are especially good.

Johann Gottlieb Walter (1734–1818)

In the second half of the eighteenth century the most remarkable anatomical illustrations were copper engravings showing in great detail the anatomy of a particular body system: the arteries, the nerves, the lymphatics, and so on. Most often only one region was shown. The publications typically contained one or more anatomical plates, each with its lettered and numbered outline or index diagram of the same size. The text could be restricted just to the naming of the indexed parts. The lifetime research of many anatomists was to display the precise details of structures already known in general.

Analysis always underlies anatomical investigation; no anatomist looks at the parts he dissects in a naïve manner. He has preconceptions as to their structure and function based on his own experience and his understanding of the sciences of morphology and physiology currently available. Looking at the structures of the neck he thinks in terms also of the function of arteries, veins, nerves, muscles, and so on. From the time that Harvey's ideas on the circulation gained general acceptance, anatomists have always considered the branches of the external carotid arteries, for instance, as conveying blood at high pressure from the left ventricle of the heart to the structures they supply—to the thyroid gland, the neck muscles, and so on. The muscles are not considered merely as of such a shape and position, but in terms of their ability to contract, and so bring insertion and origin closer together, contributing to a movement around one or more joints. In a similar way there was no significant detailed anatomy of the lymphatics until investigators understood, in at least an elementary way, how this system was organized functionally. When the role of the lymphatics as absorbent vessels was expounded in the mid-eighteenth century a series of well-illustrated anatomical monographs appeared. Again, following Haller's discussions on the irritability of muscles and the sensitivity of structures, there were detailed investigations into innervation. Contraction of the gut or the heart-muscle in response to both direct and indirect stimulation had to be understood in relation to their nerve-supply. Questions about what structures were innervated could be answered by patient dissection, and were relevant to important physiological, and even, in eighteenth-century terms, philosophical problems. Indeed much about the relationship of autonomic nerve-supply and visceral activity still remains perplexing; but, as now, so earlier, it is well understood that the relevant structures must be defined as completely as possible. In the eighteenth century the definition had to be mainly morphological, and at the level observable with the unaided eye. The nerves that went to the heart and the viscera must be described, not in general, but in every particular. And what better way of describing them than to picture them? So anatomists such as Haas, 1781, or Walter, 1783, or Charles Bell, 1803, or Swan, 1830, or Lee, 1849 and 1851, throughout patient long-drawn-out hours dissected the branches of the vagal and sacral parasympathetic and the sympathetic nerves, and their intricate plexuses as they ramified to the heart, stomach, and so on.

The dissections then had to be drawn, without error and without distortion. It was fortunate that the technology of intaglio printing from engraved copperplates had been so perfected. Precise drawings could by these means be reproduced in a manner more perfect than in the sixteenth-century woodcut or the nineteenth-century lithograph. One prerequisite for such monographic illustrations was an anatomist with young eyes (lenses or microscopes were not usually employed; illumination by lamps was less than satisfactory); with patience and persistence; and with the experience and ability to distinguish the finest nerves from fibrous connective tissue—the Royal Society of London was thrown into turmoil early in the 1800s when an investigating committee accused, unjustly it seems, Robert Lee of falsifying nerve branches in the abdomen. Also required was an accurate draughtsman who could, with instruction, see as if through the eyes of the anatomist. We have described how Wandelaar and Kaltenhofer came to be in this position with Albinus and Haller respectively. Theoretically the ideal situation was when anatomist and illustrator were one and the same person: Scarpa (see Chapter 10) was one such. Next, there was needed an engraver, who might have to work for weeks, if not months, on a single plate. At the end of the eighteenth century there was an army of engravers stationed throughout Europe, each man or woman capable of superb work. In addition, there were printers able to take perfect impressions from the very large copperplates. Finally there had to be sufficient money to pay artists and engravers and the costs of printing, including the expensive sheets of heavyweight paper. Publishing these monographs was sometimes not a viable venture; they had to be subsidized out of the anatomist's own pocket, as in the case of William Hunter's atlas of the gravid uterus, or by what amounted to research grants from funds made available by learned societies in the form of prizes (as in Mascagni's plates of the lymphatics), or, as we shall see, by direct publication grants.

The work of J. G. Walter is here taken to exemplify this classical, elegant period of precise anatomy, which reached a high level in the German states in the period from 1770 to 1800; in particular note will be taken of his *Tabulae nervorum thoracis et abdominis*, 1783, published with the support of the Royal Academy of Sciences in Berlin.

Walter was born at Königsberg, now Kaliningrad, studied in the University there, and completed his medical training at Frankfurt-on-Oder (MD, 1757). He went to Berlin to work under the elder J. F. Meckel at the Medical–Surgical College. He learned injection techniques from N. Lieberkühn. Appointed second professor of anatomy in 1762, he took the senior chair

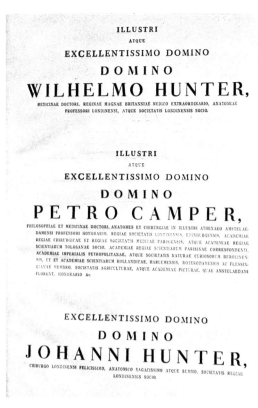

ILLUSTRI
ATQUE
EXCELLENTISSIMO DOMINO
DOMINO
WILHELMO HUNTER,
MEDICINAE DOCTORI, REGINAE MAGNAE BRITANNIAE MEDICO EXTRAORDINARIO, ANATOMIAE
PROFESSORI LONDINENSI, ATQUE SOCIETATIS LONDINENSIS SOCIO.

ILLUSTRI
ATQUE
EXCELLENTISSIMO DOMINO
DOMINO
PETRO CAMPER,
PHILOSOPHIAE ET MEDICINAE DOCTORI, ANATOMES ET CHIRURGIAE IN ILLUSTRI ATHENAEO AMSTELAE-
DAMENSI PROFESSORI HONORARIO, REGIAE SOCIETATIS LONDINENSIS, EDINBURGENSIS, ACADEMIAE
REGIAE CHIRURGICAE ET REGIAE SOCIETATIS MEDICAE PARISIENSIS, ATQUE ACADEMIAE REGIAE
SCIENTIARUM TOLOSANAE SOCIO, ACADEMIAE REGIAE SCIENTIARUM PARISINAE CORRESPONDENTI,
ACADEMIAE IMPERIALIS PETROPOLITANAE, ATQUE SOCIETATIS NATURAE CURIOSORUM BEROLINEN-
SIS, UT ET ACADEMIAE SCIENTIARUM HOLLANDICAE, HARLEMENSIS, ROTERODAMENSIS AC FLESSIN-
GIANAE MEMBRO, SOCIETATIS AGRICULTURAE, ATQUE ACADEMIAE PICTURAE, QUAE AMSTELAEDAMI
FLORENT, HONORARIO &c.

EXCELLENTISSIMO DOMINO
DOMINO
JOHANNI HUNTER,
CHIRURGO LONDINENSI FELICISSIMO, ANATOMICO SAGACISSIMO ATQUE SUMMO, SOCIETATIS REGIAE
LONDINENSIS SOCIO.

9.3 Dedication page from Walter's *Tabulae nervorum*, 1783.

in 1774, aged forty years, when Meckel died. He was also interested in obstetrics, devising an operation for symphysectomy in cases of difficult labour due to disproportion. His clinical obstetrical work was carried out at the Berlin Charité Hospital.

During his career, Walter worked also towards creating a museum of anatomical and other preparations, collected from a total of 8000 dissections he is said to have made. This museum was catalogued by his son F. A. Walter in 1796. J. G. Walter's papers on various anatomical subjects—normal anatomy, 'monsters', the lactiferous tubules, the veins of the head—were collected in *Observationes anatomicae*, 1775 (*Plate 82*)—a German translation, 1782. The work was dedicated to Frederick II of Prussia—Frederick the Great. In 1803 his successor purchased Walter's museum for a very large sum of money, so acquiring for that state one of the finest collections in the world. (The son, F. A. Walter, became the royal physician.)

Another work by Walter was published in 1778. Written in the form of a letter to William Hunter, it described in Latin and in German the vessels of the eyes.

The *Tabulae nervorum thoracis et abdominis*, 1783 was a masterful production: a very large folio of four plates on heavy paper. The first two plates were dated 1771, the other two, 1778. The short scholarly introductory text was followed by seventeen pages naming the parts shown on each plate and indexed on an accompanying same-sized outline diagram. The plates, plus the diagram plates, show the distribution of the autonomic and other nerves of the thorax, abdomen, and pelvis. In a copy at the Wellcome Institute Library the pages of text are followed by blank leaves. To each of these has been attached the outline plate, and then, in turn, the actual anatomical plate. When folded out these pairs of illustrations can be seen as the book is opened to the relevant pages of text. It must be noted, however, that this arrangement, convenient in one sense, is cumbersome in another: the page size is so large that a clear table of nearly six feet is required to examine the book in this way. Anatomy plates in elephant folio were evolving into such mammoth sizes that the genus was liable to extinction.

The book was dedicated to William Hunter, Petrus Camper, and John Hunter (in that order) (*Fig. 9.3*). Anatomical science was not confined within nationalistic or linguistic borders. In 1791 the Royal College of Physicians of Edinburgh made Walter a Fellow. Linné (Linnaeus) and Haller had also received this honour in 1771 (Jenner in 1806); but there were few other non-Scots. In 1804 Walter's plates were published in London, re-engraved from the originals. The preface stated:

Among the numerous cultivators of human anatomy in the present day, is to be reckoned the justly celebrated John Gottlieb Walter, whose indefatigable zeal, industry and application, enabled him to unravel the intricate distribution of the thoracic and abdominal nerves; to expose their ganglia, and to trace their ramifications and junctions, with unprecedented exactness.

The original production was described in glowing terms, 'but the expense attending the purchase, and the difficulty of obtaining a copy, have operated greatly to the detriment of this division of anatomy'. The hope was that the re-engraved plates in smaller versions would 'not be found inferior to the original'. To an extent these hopes were fulfilled; but naturally enough, when comparison is made, the superior qualities of the Berlin originals may be seen.

Walter's artist for this, and many other of his published plates, was J. B. G. Hopffer, and his engraver was J. H. Meil; they were able to show all the smallest branches of the nerves in near-life-sized illustrations. On the outline index diagram hundreds of structures, including all these twigs, were identified by number or letter, and these, in turn, were all named in the text. For the first plate there are more than six hundred and fifty references (*Fig. 9.2*). The problem associated with representation of such fine detail, a problem we have noted before, is that it shows a pattern of distribution in one individual only; at this level of detail, in these autonomic nerves, the pattern of branching will not be exactly similar in other individuals.

Books by J. G. Walter noted above:

1. *Observationes anatomicae*, Berlin, 1775.
2. *Epistola anatomica ad ... Wilhelmum Hunterum ... de venis oculi ... de arteria centrali retinae*, Berlin, 1778.
3. *Tabulae nervorum thoracis et abdominis*, Berlin, 1783.
4. *John Gottlieb Walter's Plates of the thoracic and abdominal nerves, reduced from the original ...*, London, John Murray 1804.

Note also:

5. F. A. Walter, *Anatomisches Museum, gesammelt von Johann Gottlieb Walter*, Berlin, 1796; and *Walters ... Leben und Werke*, Berlin, 1821.

82 The veins of the head and neck from Caput 4, Tabula 1 of J. G. Walter, *Observationes Anatomicae*, 1775. Engraving (Wellcome Institute Library). 36.5 × 25.0 cm.

This plate shows a head and neck viewed from the right side, and on the following page in the book is a line drawing with some 30 letters and 216 numbers as an aid to identify the structures illustrated.

The anatomical arrangement of the veins of the head and neck varies greatly from individual to individual, so that it might be considered that to illustrate the superficial veins of the region in such detail as in this plate serves no very good purpose.

The majority of the known veins are certainly present, yet the clinically important anastomosis between the facial veins and the veins of the orbit is nowhere suggested. However, this is a beautifully produced plate, and much can be learned from it, although the basic pattern of the venous drainage of this area is difficult to determine from a study of it.

Tab. I.

Venarum Capitis et Colli.

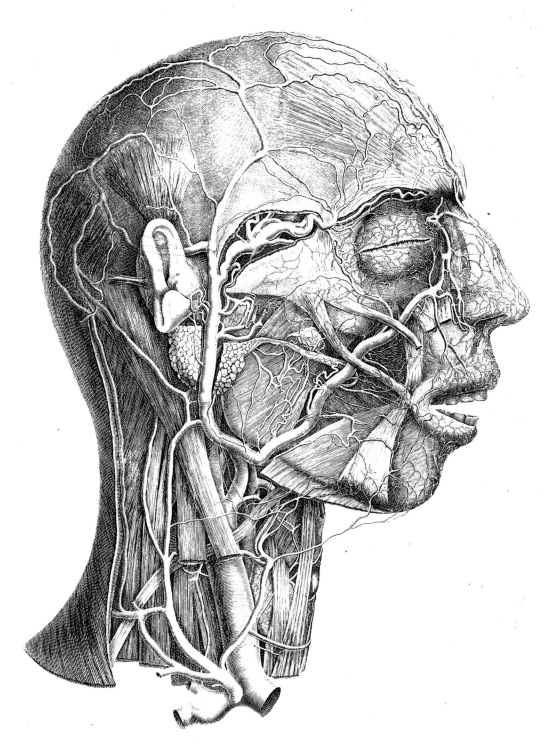

J. B. G. Hopffer ad nat. delin.

C. C. Glaßbach Filius sculps. Berolini

PLATE 82

83 The thoracic and abdominal nerves. Tabula 1 of J. G. Walter *Tabulae nervorum ...*, 1783. Engraving (Cambridge University Library). 56.0 × 41.5 cm.

Preceding this Tabula there are two line-diagrams of the illustrations, with letters and numbers again indicating various structures, together with an explanatory text identifying the same. For Figura I, the lettering comprises both capital and lower case, together with 8 letters from the Greek alphabet and numerals extending from 1 to 614. The smaller Tabula II fortunately only employs A to D, I to V and a mere hundred and fifty or so numbers!

In the larger figure, the displacement anteriorly of the right kidney, together with the ureter and renal vessels, has resulted in the inferior vena cava being displaced forwards and to the left (no doubt the lumbar veins were considered expendable), so that the aorta, the nerve plexus upon it, and the lumbar arteries can be visualized. The drawings of the bladder, the vagina, the uterus with its too-substantial round ligament, and the ovary are rather poor.

It is interesting that the right kidney is shown with two renal veins, the inferior one receiving a large right ovarian vein. The thoracic duct, alongside the thoracic part of the aorta, is large, and the arrangement of the right crus of the diaphragm, with a large elongated aperture for the greater splanchnic nerve, is unusual.

The *raison d'être* of this plate is, of course, its portrayal of the nerves. The tenuous nature of the sympathetic chain is excellent; the splanchnic nerves also. It does appear, however, that the phrenic nerve largely supplies the superior surface of the diaphragm.

The lumbar nerves are shown forming the (cut) femoral and obturator nerves, with the latter receiving a *very* small contribution from the fourth lumbar nerve. Arising from the first lumbar nerve, and passing downwards and forwards to the round ligament of the uterus and the pubic symphysis, is a slender nerve that is termed 'external spermatic'. This would appear from the text to represent the genito-femoral nerve (which actually arises from the first and second lumbar nerves); if so, its distribution is somewhat inaccurate.

A rather large nervus furcalis of the fourth lumbar nerve is shown joining the fifth to form the lumbo-sacral trunk, though this is not identified as such. This latter is then shown combining with the sacral nerves to form the sciatic nerve and the latter's two components, the tibial and common peroneal (referred to as the major and minor sciatic).

The profuse nervous elements illustrated in the adipose tissue of the buttock are largely imaginary. To produce this plate (and the diagrams!) must have required hours of very pernickety prior dissection and skilled draughtsmanship, and so much in it is good that it is a pity that such devotion to detail has nevertheless let the imagination run amok at times. It is admirable more for its clear presentation, than for its overall anatomical accuracy.

Figure II is perhaps somewhat unnecessary, purporting in the main to show the inter-connections of the two sympathetic trunks, their conjunction and termination.

I.G.WALTER

NERVORUM THORACIS ET ABDOMINIS TAB. I

FIGURA I

FIGURA II

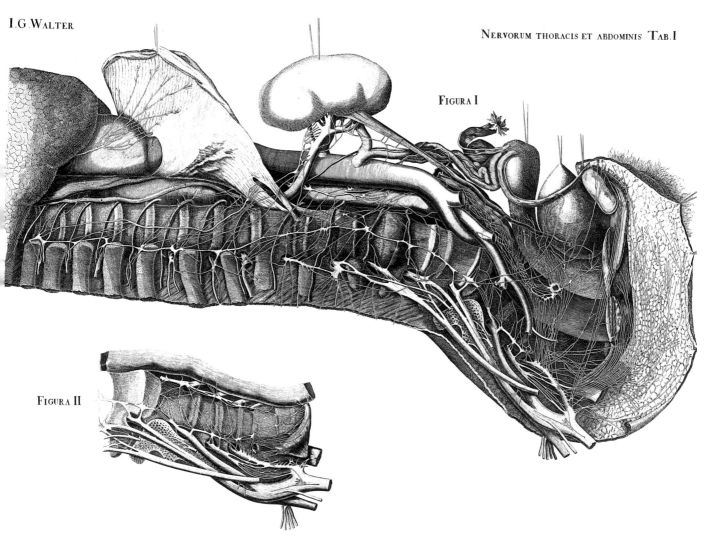

I.B.G Hopffer ad nat ddin 1777. I.H Mal Sen fculp

PLATE 83

Samuel Thomas von Soemmerring (1755–1830)

Soemmerring was born in Torun (Thorn), an old Hanseatic town in Poland; his father, a German-speaking Lutheran who had studied at Leiden, was the town physician. Samuel Thomas received his medical doctorate in 1778 from the University of Göttingen, where his mentor in anatomy was H. A. Wrisberg. In spite of discouragement from his father, he had already decided to become an anatomist, and in pursuit of further education travelled to the Netherlands to visit Petrus Camper, where he was impressed by the complete skeleton of an elephant. He then went to London, where he met the Hunters, Cruikshank, and Sheldon, and to Edinburgh to see Alexander Monro *secundus*. From his formal medical education and through his travels, Soemmerring came under the influence of Albinus: at Göttingen, through study in a school where anatomy had been established by Albinus' pupil, Haller; and more directly through Camper and Monro, who had themselves studied under that great anatomist. Soemmerring was able to repay some of his indebtedness to one of his teachers by publishing in 1801 the Camper illustrations of the anatomy of hernias, *Icones herniarum . . .*, Frankfurt, drawn by Camper himself in 1779, at about the time the two men met. He also paid homage to William Hunter by publishing, as an addendum to the illustrations of Hunter's late-gestation fetuses, a series showing the external form of embryos and fetuses at earlier stages.

In 1779 Soemmerring was appointed anatomist at the Caroline College at Kassel, a town about forty kilometres from Göttingen. In 1784 he moved to Mainz, where he remained as Professor of Anatomy until his resignation in 1797; he then sold his anatomical collection to pay his debts, and practised for a while as a physician in nearby Frankfurt-on-Main. In 1805 he was persuaded to continue his southward migration to join the Bavarian Academy of Science at Munich, where he received the civil distinction of knighthood. For the last ten years of his life, von Soemmerring returned to medical practice in Frankfurt. During these changes Soemmerring remained a correspondent to the *Göttingische gelehrte Anzeigen*, writing reviews and articles on anatomy and related subjects. He took over this responsibility from Haller himself. He also, with Wrisberg and Meckel, produced a new edition of Haller's text on physiology.

From the beginning Soemmerring had a particular interest in the anatomy of the brain and in graphic representation of nervous structures. His graduation dissertation, dedicated to his father, concerned the base of the brain: *De basi encephali . . .*, Göttingen, 1778. This was issued by Haller's publishers, Abram van den Hoeck. The illustrations were drawn by Soemmerring himself. In this work, he explained a method of describing the cranial nerves in twelve (rather than ten) pairs, a method that is still used today. He was largely responsible for this system's replacing Thomas Willis's, introduced originally in 1664.

The most unusual of Soemmering's works on neuroanatomy was *Ueber das Organ der Seele* [Concerning the organ of the soul], Königsberg, 1796. In this, with other strictly anatomical matters, he gives a good description of the sympathetic nervous system; but he included also metaphysical speculations, in accord with current *Naturphilosophie*, making the suggestion that

the cranial nerves end in relation to the ventricular system of the brain, and convey in this
way sense-impressions to the cerebro-spinal
fluid, which can thus co-ordinate them. This
book of romantic physiology was dedicated
to Immanuel Kant; but this metaphysician
rebuked the author for unjustified theorizing.
Goethe, a correspondent, thought he should
have published the work under a different
title. Soemmerring had indeed revived a most
ancient idea, that one of the ventricles constituted an organ of *sensorium commune*. This
concept, already formulated in the fifth
century BC, persisted well into Renaissance
times. Descartes located the soul in the pineal
gland on equally hypothetical grounds.

Soemmerring was interested in other old
scientific ideas, or at least in what were
regarded as such in eighteenth-century European thought. At Kassel, Soemmerring had
been a Freemason and a Rosicrucian, and had
involved himself in alchemy and spiritualism.
He had an intense emotional involvement
with Georgius Forster, and they, with
Johannes von Müller, founded a secret society
to make gold (they lost money), to commune
(probably without success) with the dead, and
to reach states of religious ecstasy, which they
may have achieved.

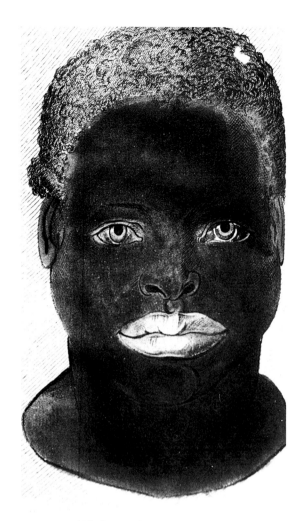

9.4 Face of black man, from Soemmerring's paper
comparing the anatomy of black and white people,
1785.

His books following the work on the soul are much more restrained in speculation. Soemmerring's interests spanned the centuries, for he made contributions to the development of the
electric telegraph. Towards the end of his life he spent much time studying sunspots.

A further interest of Soemmerring while at Kassel was that of comparative physical anthropology. In a nearby village there was a community of negroes, and he had the opportunity of
carrying out autopsies on some of them. He pointed out certain structural differences, but wrote
that black and white people were of the same species. His paper was illustrated by two rather
fine hand-coloured plates of a handsome black man, full-face and side-face (*Fig. 9.4*). He was
one of the first in a very long line of nineteenth- and twentieth-century white anatomists and
anthropologists to provide observations and measurements that purported to identify human

races, theoretical concepts which some developed into elaborate systems justifying philosophical and political racism.

Other anatomical work included an essay in what might be called social anatomy: *Ueber die Schädlichkeit der Schnürbrüste*, 1788. This described how fashionable corsets, tight lacings, and so on caused anatomical deformities of the thorax and abdomen and their contents. Fashions that deliberately deform structures and impair function have been, in most civilizations—and still are—imposed on women by society. Since Soemmerring was becoming a well-known anatomist in the German-speaking world, his documented studies had an effect in mitigating the wilder extremes of fashion.

In contrast to these studies on anatomical deformation, Soemmerring attempted in his illustrations of normal anatomy to show every structure in its most perfect form. This approach developed that of Albinus, and inevitably led to a dilemma: there should be painstaking care to ensure veracity, yet the illustration should show the structure in its Platonically ideal form, which, Soemmerring added, must needs be correspondingly beautiful. About truthfulness, he wrote: '... even the best representation never attains to nature's perfection in respect of minuteness and variation ... it seems only fair to demand that every possible effort should be made to approach nature as nearly as possible ...' The hard work that he and his artist, Koeck, put in was obviously productive of accurate anatomical illustrations. But the anatomists 'should always select the most perfect and therefore most beautiful specimen for the model of their descriptions'. Anything that the dissector described anatomically as a normal structure must be beautiful. John Keats, a medical man, in his 'Ode on a Grecian Urn', 1815, expressed that same fallacy: Beauty is truth, truth beauty—that is all / Ye know on earth, and all ye need to know'. Soemmerring recognized some difficulties in reconciling these two aims—truthfulness to nature, and representation of the ideal form. 'With this in mind' he wrote 'One is all the more bound to recommend the imitation of the masterpieces of the great Albinus, works of Attic perfection.' This was only one of many acknowledgements that Soemmerring gave to the Dutch master. A very practical homage was made when Soemmerring deliberately set out to complement Albinus' elegant skeletal men with companion illustrations of the skeleton of a woman (*Plate 84*). Albinus had specifically deplored the lack of a female skeleton. The subject that Soemmerring chose was that of a young and handsome woman who had died aged twenty years. In preparing the final drawings the artist, Christian Koeck, was directed to compare other specimens of skulls, etc., that were judged to represent ideal form, and to make comparisions both with ancient sculpture and with living models.

Above all I was anxious to provide for myself the body of a woman that was suitable not only because of her youth and aptitude for procreation, but also because of the harmony of her limbs, beauty, and elegance, of the kind that the ancients used to ascribe to Venus.

Soemmerring prepared the skeleton from the cadaver of a twenty-year-old woman from Mayence; she had had one child.

Soemmerring, while acknowledging the importance of scientific accuracy, justified to himself an illustration of a female skeleton whose perfection would never actually be encountered. The result is indeed beautiful, but inevitably insipid, just as it would be if the illustration represented an 'ideal' shape of legs, hips, breasts, neck ... As we have noted previously, there is always, in anatomical illustration, a tug of war between the desire to represent the actual dissected part of one individual cadaver and representation of the *normal*; it was Soemmerring's view, or fallacy, that the anatomist could arrive at normality by knowing the beautiful. It is the view, or fallacy, of many present-day anatomists that the normal has a meaning which may be defined statistically.

Perhaps the peak of Soemmerring's work as an anatomist was a series of well-illustrated monographs on the organs of the senses: eyes, ears, tongue, and nose (*Plate 85*). Just as Albinus worked closely with Jan Wandelaar, so Soemmerring's anatomical illustrations were the product of a collaboration between anatomist and artist. Christian Koeck, a Mainz craftsman and artist, developed his talents to a very high level during this collaboration, probably because Soemmerring himself was sufficiently skilled as a draughtsman to understand the problems of anatomical drawing. Koeck's early work was done during Soemmerring's Mainz period, and the anatomist provided room in his house for the artist to live; save for an unsuccessful period in Moscow, Koeck stayed with Soemmerring until he died, in 1808.

It may be of interest to list alphabetically some of the anatomists whose plates Soemmerring recommended in his multivolume, but unillustrated, *De corporis humani fabrica* ..., 1794–1801; this list indicates the view of a professional well able to judge the best available anatomical illustrations in the years around 1800. Amongst those mentioned were Albinus, Bidloo, Camper, Cruikshank, Haller, William Hunter, Meckel, Monro, Scarpa, Vicq d'Azyr, and Walter.

84 Female skeleton—the only plate—in S. T. Soemmerring, *Tabula sceleti feminini juncta descriptione*, Frankfurt, Varrentrapp and Wenner, 1797. Engraving (Wellcome Institute Library). 48.0 × 30.5 cm.

This large engraving, which has been folded in half, was the outcome of Soemmerring's desire to illustrate the 'perfect woman' through the medium of her skeleton. From it one may deduce that his perfect woman was tall, long-legged, most likely slim of build, and with a full dentition.

From a strictly anatomical viewpoint, however, some imperfections may be noted. Amongst these are the scoliotic vertebral column, the poor congruity between the head of the femur and acetabulum, the infero-lateral inclination of the coracoid processes, the odd configuration of the junction of the first costal cartilage and the manubrium, and the peculiar transverse processes of the seventh cervical vertebra. Three 'floating' ribs on each side are featured instead of the more usual two.

The limb bones are well portrayed, and the correct positioning, in an erect skeleton, of the patellae, the majority of the ribs and cartilages, and the arches of the foot, and the placing of the tip of the coccyx, the upper surface of the pubic symphysis, and the tip of the greater trochanter on the same horizontal plane, are all commendable.

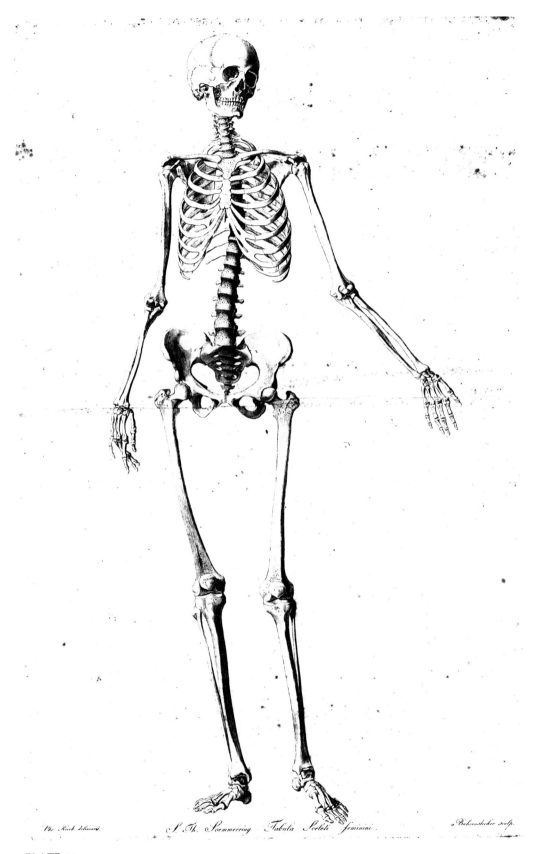

S.Th. Soemmerring Tabula Sceleti feminini.

PLATE 84

85 Sagittal section through the skull showing the organs of smell. *Tabula prima* from S. T. von Soemmerring, *Abbildungen der menschlichen Organe des Geruches*, Frankfurt, Varrentrapp and Wenner, 1809. Engraving (Wellcome Institute Library). 32.0 × 23.0 cm.

In this sagittal section, just left of the mid-line, the nasal septal cartilage, the vomer, and the ethmoid (with a somewhat club-like crista galli) are seen above the mouth cavity. The frontal sinus is prominent, but the sphenoidal sinus is rather small.

The specimen employed for this drawing was an immature one, as the basi-occiput is not yet synostosed with the basi-sphenoid.

The falx cerebri is nicely presented, with the opened superior sagittal sinus. The rendering of the tentorium cerebelli makes it difficult properly to visualize its form: however, it is never easy to draw this in an illustration with this particular perspective.

Visible through the opening bounded by the free edge of the falx cerebri are faint middle meningeal vessels, or their grooves, superimposed on a rather fanciful interpretation of the appearance of the skull bones in this region.

The pituitary gland can be seen in its fossa, and just above this are the optic chiasm, the olfactory tract, and the cut-off stub of the internal carotid artery.

The stumps of all the cranial nerves are shown, though the trigeminal is too small when compared with the oculomotor nerve above and the stato-acoustic below. The varied inclinations of the nerves make it difficult to comprehend just where the brain stem would actually lie. The spinal accessory nerve is seen ascending posterior to the hypoglossal rootlets, though it is drawn so that it appears to peter out before it reaches the jugular foramen. The rather worm-like structure postero-inferior to it is a poor representation of the vertebral artery, and the cut spinal cord is rather stylized when compared with the drawing as a whole.

In the tongue genio-glossus and genio-hyoid are well displayed, above the thin horizontal mylohyoid muscle. With regard to the larynx it must be said that the sectioned anterior plate of the cricoid cartilage is tiny, though the true and false vocal folds and laryngeal sinus are nicely portrayed.

Posterior to the soft palate can be seen the opening of the Eustachian tube and the salpingo-pharyngeal fold.

Overall this is a commendably clear drawing of an area of anatomy that is difficult to portray in but two dimensions.

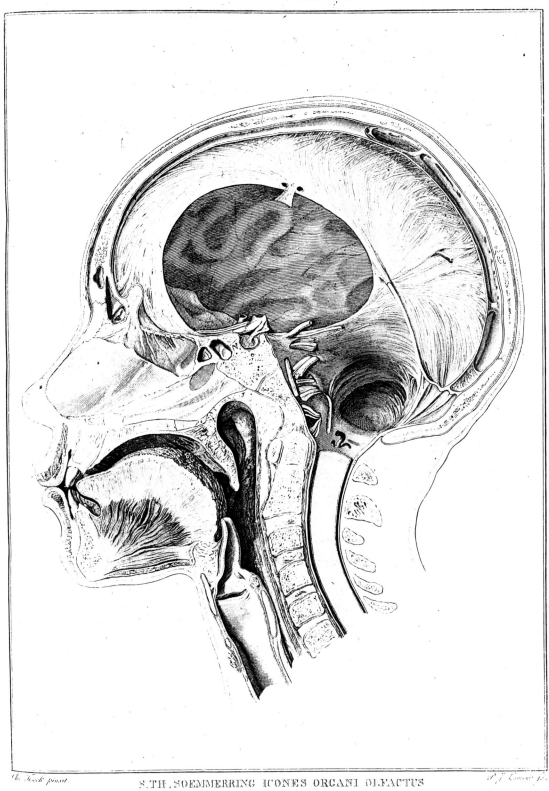

S.TH.SOEMMERRING ICONES ORGANI OLFACTUS

PLATE 85

Chapter 9: Selected reading

Geyer-Kordesch, J. (1985). German medical education in the eighteenth century.... In *William Hunter and the eighteenth-century medical world*, (ed. W. F. Bynum and R. Porter). Cambridge University Press.

Mann, G., (1964). Medizinische-naturwissenschaftliche Buchillustration in 18. Jahrhundert in Deutschland. *Marburger Sitzungsberichte*, **86**, 3–48.

Albrecht von Haller

Bayle, A. L. J. and Thillaye, A. J. (1855). Albert de Haller. *Biog. méd.*, **2**, 361–6.

Gloor, B., (1958). *Die künstlerischen Mitarbeiter an den naturwissenschaftlichen und medizinischen Werken Albrecht von Hallers*. Paul Haupt, Berne.

Hintzsche, E. (1972). (Victor) Albrecht von Haller. *Dict. sci. Biog.*, **6**, 61–7.

King, L. S. (1966). *First lines of physiology by the celebrated Baron Albertus Haller, M. D...* [Reprinted from the 1786 Edinburgh edition] with new introduction. Johnson Reprint Corporation, New York.

Temkin, O. (1936). *A dissertation on the sensible and irritable parts of animals by Albrecht von Haller*. (London, J. Nousse, 1755). The Johns Hopkins Press, Baltimore.

Temkin, O. (1964). *The classical roots of Glisson's doctrine of irritation. Bull. Hist. Med.*, **38**, 297–328.

Johann Gottlieb Walter

Dezeimeris, J. E. (1839). Jean-Théophile & Frédéric-Auguste Walter. *Dict. hist. méd. ancienne moderne*, **4**, 360–2.

Gurlt, E., Wernich, A., and Hirsch, A. (1934). Johann Gottlieb Walter. *Biog. Lex. der hervorragenden Ärzte ...* **5**, 835.

Samuel Thomas Soemmerring

Bast, T. H. (1924) The life and work of Samuel Thomas von Sömmerring. *Ann. med. Hist.*, **6**, 369–86.

Bayle, A. L. J. and Thillaye, A. J. (1855). Samuel-Thomas Soemmerring. *Biog. méd.*, **2**, 774–6.

Hintzsche, E. (1975). S. T. Soemmerring. *Dict. sci. Biog.*, **12**, 509–11.

Schiebinger, L. (1987). Skeletons in the closet: The first illustrations of the female skeleton in eighteenth-century anatomy. In *The making of the modern body: sexuality and society in the nineteenth century* (ed. C. Gallagher and T. Laqueur) University of California Press, Berkeley.

10

Italian anatomical engravings circa 1800

F OR TWO hundred years from 1521 to 1713, much of Italy was under Spanish domination—the Venetian Republic being a notable exception. The influence of the Holy Inquisition on cultural life was widespread, the most notorious example of intellectual repression being the examination of Galileo Galilei, a process now—more than three hundred years later—publicly recanted by the church authorities. The repressive influence was least evident in Venice, where the Inquisition was under the supervision of state authorities.

Marcello Malpighi (1628–94), at Bologna, was the most prominent of the Italian biological scientists cast in the mould of William Harvey. Scientific societies— the earliest being the short-lived *Accademia di Cimento* (that is, 'Academy of Experiments') at Florence (1657–67)—perpetuated an experimental and observational approach to natural phenomena, always with a certain amount of apprehension. The *Accademia degli Inquieti* at Bologna, 1690, continued until it was eventually merged with the *Istituto delle Scienze*, 1714, and the combined Institute with the University in 1803. Its attitude was summarized in the statutes: 'It should be considered as a fault to support those things which cannot be derived by direct observation or verified by experiments or demonstrated by positive ratiocination'.

The domination of Spain was removed at the Peace of Utrecht (1713), when

Archduke Charles of Austria became Emperor, and large areas of Italy came under his influence. Most of the period between the Peace of Aix-la-Chapelle, 1748, and the invasion by French forces, 1796, was a time of peace in Italy. In Lombardy, centred on Milan (which was under the control of the Emperor), and in Tuscany, centred on Florence, which was under the Habsburg Duke of Tuscany, this was also a period of reform, initiated and carried through by the rulers with little active encouragement from the inhabitants. The reforms included more equitable taxation; the concomitant prosperity of the country benefited the universities and medical institutions. For instance, the dissolution of more than a third of the 290 monasteries for men in Lombardy in 1768 profited hospitals, orphanages, and the University of Pavia (Milan did not have a university of its own until the twentieth century). In Tuscany, Duke Leopold I spent a great deal of money on biological and medical research at the Royal Imperial Museum of Physics and Natural History that he established in Florence.

The names of distinguished researchers in north Italy whose academic appointments coincide with this period of growth include:

G. B. Morgagni, student Bologna; professor Padua, 1715
L. Galvani, student and professor, Bologna, 1762
F. Fontana, student Padua and Bologna; professor Pisa and Florence, 1765/6
A. Scarpa, student Padua; professor Modena, 1772, and Pavia, 1783
A. Volta, student and professor Pavia, 1778
P. Mascagni, student Siena; professor Siena, 1779, Pisa, 1801, and Florence, 1803

The flowering of Italian medical science in the second half of the eighteenth century stems from interrelated political, social, and economic causes, but was rooted in pre-existing attitudes: the Vesalian tradition was still alive at Padua, and the Malpighian attitude to experimental sciences persisted at Bologna. The pathologist G. B. Morgagni, who spent more than fifty years as professor at Padua, was custodian of both inheritances, having been a pupil of Valsalva at Bologna. Valsalva was himself taught by Malpighi.

In the medical schools, reform of the curriculum was common during this period. The students were brought into close relationship with the patient, and encouraged in careful bedside observation; when patients died, post-mortem examinations had to be made to show the seats and causes of disease; in anatomy, the following attitude was expressed in a 1773 curriculum for the University of Pavia:

Lectures must not be pompous, academic speeches; they should, on the contrary, be a description and a simultaneous inspection of the parts of the human body, carried out on cadavers. Students must be led to the habit of dissection, and they must practise the fine cutting or injection methods. These operations must be done by the teacher and repeated, under his control, by the most promising students, so that they will learn to operate.

In these curricula may be seen influences originating from the Leiden school as it developed under Boerhaave and Albinus, and the Viennese school, founded by Boerhaave's pupil, van Swieten.

Illustrations from the works of two internationally known anatomists, Scarpa and Mascagni, appear in our book, along with a plate from a little-known man, the Bolognese Antonio Cattani. The anatomical studies of Valsalva, Morgagni, Galvani, and Volta were overshadowed by their work in other fields.

Antonio Scarpa (1752–1832)

The scientific work of Scarpa was carried out in three medical schools: at Padua, where he was a student (MD 1770, aged eighteen years) and an amanuensis to his teacher Morgagni; at Modena, where he was appointed Professor of Anatomy (1772, aged twenty-one years); and at Pavia, where he was Professor of Anatomy (1783) and later of other subjects. The medical school at Pavia, like that at Padua, was of ancient foundation (1361); but that at Modena was founded 1678–83 by Duke Francis II of the Este family, which ruled the city under the protection of various external powers from the thirteenth to the nineteenth centuries.

As a young man at Modena Scarpa published *De structura fenestrae rotundae auris* ..., 1772. The membranous labyrinth, including the utricle and saccule, was first described in this work, and the endolymph named. During the eleven years Scarpa was working at Modena the city was in a relatively quiet period; the Duke, who had sided with the Spaniards, and the Empress Maria Theresa were reconciled by the Peace of Aix-la-Chapelle, 1748.

In 1781, Scarpa was granted study leave, and went to Paris and London, meeting among others the anatomists Vicq d'Azyr and William and John Hunter. He worked with John Sheldon, drawing for him two of the illustrations for *The history of the absorbent system, part the first* ..., London, 1784; the other parts were not published. Scarpa, Joseph Banks, William Blizard, James Douglas, William Heberden, and John Hunter are included in the subscription list of this book by Sheldon, who was at various times in his life teacher of anatomy, surgeon, balloonist, innovative Greenland whaler, and editor of Lieberkuhn. (When visiting London Petrus Camper also drew for Sheldon.) After his sabbatical leave, Scarpa was invited to the medical school at Pavia, an appointment made in 1783 by Emperor Joseph II. Among likely reasons for the move were: prestigious colleagues, among whom were Spallanzani, Professor of Natural History, and Volta, Professor of Physics; greater opportunities—a new anatomy theatre designed by Giuseppe Piermarini; and a new curriculum that encouraged, as Spallanzani wrote, 'a spirit of observation' in the young student.

Shortly after his appointment, Scarpa travelled with Volta to Vienna, where he visited the army medical school, and also to Prague and other Central European cities. He stayed at Pavia for the remainder of his life, practising surgery especially in the fields of ophthalmology and orthopaedics, teaching both anatomy and surgery, dominating the medical school, living in grand style, collecting old masters, and cultivating his own gardens. He was a formidable, domineering director of the medical school 1815–18. In the 1803 curriculum, human anatomy was taught in each of the last four years of both the medical and surgical streams.

Political instabilities came to Pavia, and other Italian cities, with the advance of the republican French forces in 1797, which made the Po valley an area for the clash of French, Russian, and Austrian armies on and off until after the Congress of Vienna, 1815. There were also uprisings in support of or against the French. The formation of the Transpadane Republic, centred on Milan, and the Cispadane Republic, including Bologna (united later to form the Cisalpine Republic), put the cities of Pavia and Bologna and their universities under new rulers. It is said that Scarpa in Pavia and Galvani in Bologna refused the oath of allegiance and were dismissed. Scarpa was reinstated in 1805 by Napoleon himself when he visited Pavia.

All Scarpa's publications were finely produced, often at considerable expense to himself, and each was scientifically innovative. The list of subject areas shows Scarpa's concern for practical medicine and surgery: orthopaedics (shoes for club-feet); ophthalmology (operations for cataract, acknowledging previous work by Cheselden); the anatomy and therapy of hernias and of aneurysms; the anatomy of auditory and olfactory organs; and hermaphroditism.

The illustrations to Scarpa's works were prepared with the greatest care; they were boldly drawn and clearly engraved. Two works especially may be taken to show the excellence of Scarpa's anatomical plates: *Tabulae neurologicae ad illustrandam historiam anatomicam cardiacorum nervorum ...*, Pavia, 1794; and *Sull' aneurisma riflessioni ed osservazioni anatomico-chirurgiche*, Pavia, 1804. The former work (dedicated to the Royal Society of London) included seven large plates, and the latter (a prize essay of 1798 dedicated to the Vice-President of the Italian Republic) ten plates, many with key outline diagrams. These illustrations were often drawn by Scarpa himself, and show his mastery of both anatomy and draughtsmanship. Technical drawing in architecture, engineering, and anatomy sometimes not only achieves its primary purpose, but, passing beyond the transmission of information, reaches an excellence akin to that of commissioned fine art. Scarpa's work is of this quality. Until 1794 various engravers from Milan, London, Vienna, and Florence were employed to put Scarpa's ink drawing on the copperplates; in that year, Scarpa employed and trained Faustino Anderloni, one of a family of engravers, whose work comes to match the achievement of the anatomist-illustrator. In later publications Anderloni, presumably closely watched by Scarpa, made both the drawing and the engraving from Scarpa's preparations. The paper used for the impressions, the inks, and the presswork were of a quality appropriate to contemporary fine printing in Italy, headed by the Bodoni presses in Parma. The plates of Scarpa and Anderloni must stand among the finest anatomical illustrations ever produced.

Some of Scarpa's works, orginally in Latin, were published also in other languages; those in Italian were also translated. A work on the structure of bone, 1799, appears in English as *A treatise on the minute anatomy of the human bones.* English libraries received Scarpa's work in other languages, including Latin, French, and Italian. Scarpa's collected works were issued in Italian: *Opere del Cav. Antonio Scarpa . . .* , Florence, V. Batelli 1836–9.

86 The nerves of the heart. Tab. 3 from A. Scarpa, *Tabulae neurologicae* ..., 1794. Engraving (Wellcome Institute Library). 47.8 × 41.9 cm.

This view of the right neck and thorax, drawn by Scarpa himself, includes certain arteries as well as nerves. The well-marked swelling at the origin of the internal and external carotid arteries, the carotid sinus, is probably the earliest illustration of this structure: it is, however, neither labelled nor commented on. Note that the superior thyroid artery is shown very large—larger than the inferior.

This beautiful plate must have resulted from many very painstaking dissections. Opposite it, in the book, is an outline drawing with letters, Greek letters, and numbers; there is, earlier in the book, an explanatory text for this plate, comprising some nine pages.

The numbering of the cranial nerves differs from later usage; the vagus is referred to as the eighth, and the hypoglossal as the ninth. The latter has been cut shortly after it has been crossed [*sic*] by the occipital artery; the spinal accessory nerve likewise, just lateral to levator scapulae.

The facial nerve and its initial distribution are well illustrated. Oddly, the upper cervical nerves are cut off at the border of levator scapulae, giving the impression they wind around it.

The nerve descending from the upper trunk of the brachial plexus (the suprascapular) was termed 'nervus supraspinatus' by Scarpa. The artery just below it must surely represent the suprascapular artery, but it pursues a strange course, inferior to the coracoid process!

The 'ganglion cervicale superioris nervi intercostalis' [superior cervical ganglion] is rather small, while a structure, lying midway between scalenus anterior and the common carotid artery, and just medial to the vagus, is identified as the 'ganglion cervicale medium nervi intercostalis'. This, though drawn too large, is shown giving off its thick cardiac branch, as well as a branch that hooks around the subclavian artery to join with branches arising from the 'ganglion cervicale imum' and from the 'thoracicum primum ganglion': these latter branches represent the present-day ansa subclavia.

The rami communicantes to the cervical spinal nerves can be clearly seen, as also the phrenic nerve, though this is artificially separated from the 'pulled away' heart.

The cardiac ganglion and plexus, called by Haller the 'plexum cardiacorum nervorum', are shown just to the right of the ascending aorta, lying on the right pulmonary artery. The anterior pulmonary plexus is portrayed lying on the left main bronchus. Both are seen to receive branches from both the vagus and the sympathetic system. The nerve plexuses on the right and left coronary arteries are impressive.

This illustration may be compared with the similar one by Swan, reproduced later in this book as *Plate 108*, p. 511.

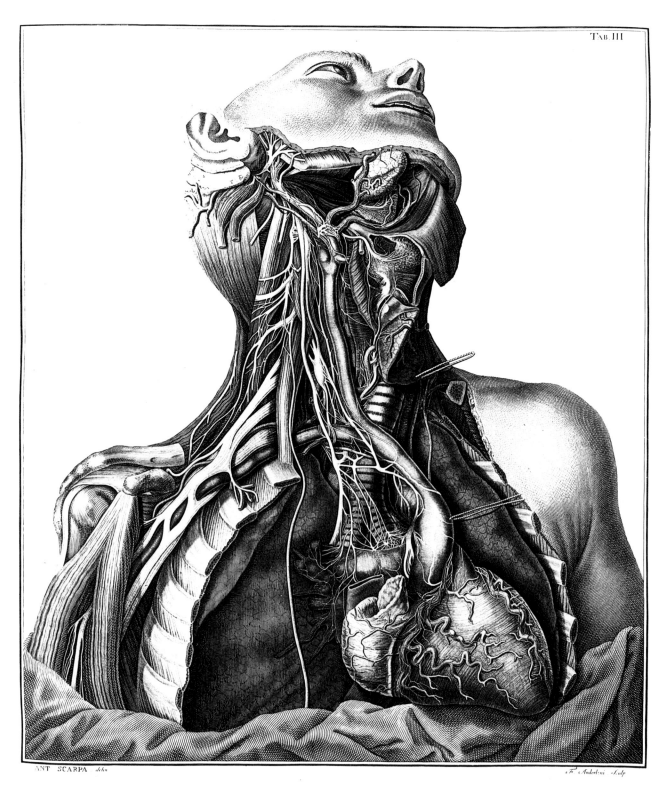

Tab III

ANT SCARPA delin   F. Anderloni Sculp

PLATE 86

87 The arteries of the face, neck, and upper arm. Tav. V in A. Scarpa, *Sull'
aneurisma riflessioni ed osservazioni anatomico-chirurgiche*, Pavia, Bolzani, 1804.
Engraving (Wellcome Institute Library). 59.0 × 44.5 cm.

As might be expected from the book's title this illustration portrays the pectoral region, axilla
and upper arm, neck and lower face, dissected primarily to show the arteries, not the veins or
nerves. In the book a key line-diagram faces it, employing 112 numbers as well as capital and
lower-case letters.

The carotid sinus swelling, at the bifurcation of the common carotid artery, is again well
drawn, although, as in *Plate 86*, the superior thyoid artery is rather too large. The inferior
thyroid artery, together with the superficial transverse cervical and suprascapular arteries, is
seen arising from the thyrocervical trunk; the ascending cervical branch of the inferior thyroid
artery is larger than usual.

In the neck, the facial and lingual arteries (and a submandibular artery) are shown arising
from a common trunk, which, although not usual, is not too uncommon. There is also an artery
arising from the external carotid which seemingly passes direct to the sterno-mastoid muscle,
in addition to the usual sterno-mastoid branch of the occipital artery. The deep cervical artery
is well defined, but not the superior intercostal artery; these may well have had separate origins
in this specimen, as indeed they often do.

The arteries in the axilla are pleasing, particularly the subscapular artery with its circumflex
scapular branch and its continuation to latissimus dorsi as the thoraco-dorsal artery. The anterior
circumflex humeral artery is somewhat large; but the rendition of the profunda brachii, ulnar
collateral, and ulnar and radial recurrent arteries is very good.

Although in black-and-white, this figure gives a much better impression of the arteries than
many that employ colour.

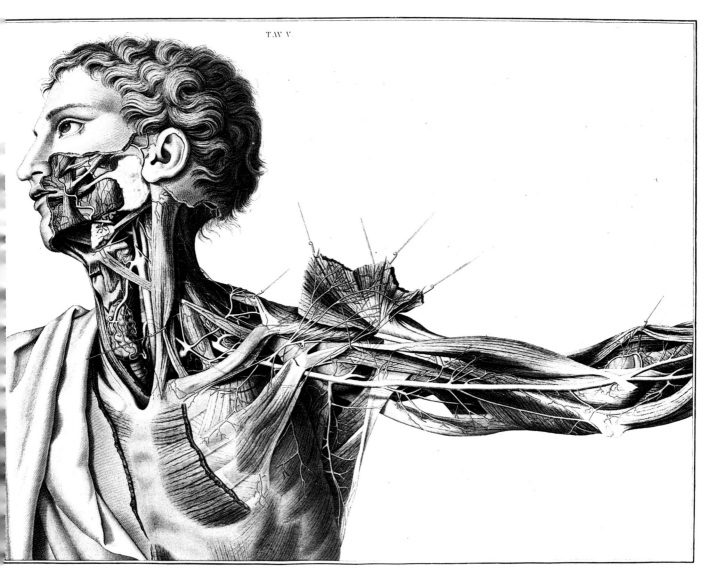

TAV V.

Antonio Cattani

In 1780, from the Bologna press of Antonio Cattani and Antonio Nerozzi, *presso Volpe*, there was published, in large folio, a work on the anatomy of the bones and muscles of the human head, hand, and foot: *Osteografia e miografia della teste, manie piedi*. The twenty plates had been issued previously one by one, at intervals of forty days, and were obtainable by subscription. This information is conveyed on plate 13, an illustration of a skull resting on a book (as in the Lairesse–Bidloo plate), which was issued 16 November 1778. The illustrations were apparently drawn by Cattani, and at least some of them were engraved by him. The explanatory text to the figures was placed at the lower part of each engraving, and was in fine engraved calligraphy.

88 Muscles and tendons of the dorsum of the foot. Tav. XVIII from A. Cattani, *Osteografia e miografia ...*, 1780. Engraving, with etching (Wellcome Institute Library). 33.0 × 22.2 cm.

Underneath this illustration can be found a key to the structures indicated in it. The lower (lateral) number 18 lies on the tendon of peroneus tertius: as this tendon does not extend to a digit, it cannot logically be considered a part of 'extensor grande delle Dita'.

The positioning of the peroneus brevis tendon (21) is rather awkward; if the ankle were to be dorsiflexed from the position shown the tendon would seem to pass through the talo-fibular joint! There is nothing to indicate the peroneal retinaculum, and the tibialis anterior tendon (16) is placed too far medial; it looks as though it is going to an insertion on the *plantar* aspect of the foot! The muscle bellies of extensor digitorum brevis and extensor hallucis brevis (19 and 20) are rather too strap-like and separated.

For the last quarter of the eighteenth century the portrayal of anatomy in this drawing leaves much to be desired, no matter how visually attractive it is.

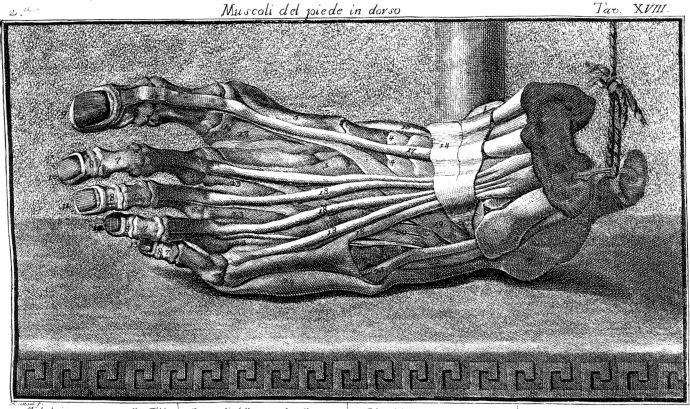

PLATE 88

1. Malcolo interno spettante alla Tibia
2. Malcolo esterno spettante alla Fibola
3. Osso del Calcagno
4. Osa del Tarso
5. Le 5. osia del Mettatarso
6. Internodj della p.ª fila o sia fallange
7. Internodj della seconda fila
8. Inter.ᵐᵒᵈⁱ della 3.ᵃ fila coper.ᵗⁱ in par.ᵗᵉ dall' unghie
9. Dito Pollice
10. Dito vicino al pollice
11. Dito Medio
12. Dito vicino al minino
13. Dito Minino
14. Ligamento Anulare
15. Tendine d' Achille o corda magna
16. Tendine del Muscolo Tibiale antico
17. Tendine dell' Estensor lungo del Pollice
18. Estensor grande delle Dita
19. Estensor breue del Pollice
20. Estensor breue delle Dita
21. Tendine del Peroneo 2.ᵈᵒ
22. Tendine del Peroneo i.ᵒ o sia lungo
23. Muscoli interossei
24. Muscolo Abduttore

in Bologna presso la C.

Paolo Mascagni (1755–1815)

Mascagni was a Tuscan by birth and education, and in Tuscany he remained. He attended the University of Siena, a school of ancient foundation (1203) that trained doctors and lawyers. Having obtained his medical degree, Mascagni became assistant to Pietro Tabarrini, the Professor of Anatomy. Mascagni was appointed to the vacant chair at the death of Tabarrini in 1779, and devoted the remainder of his life to anatomical studies, renouncing the practice of clinical medicine. He was at Siena from 1779 to 1801, went then to Pisa, and finally to Florence in 1803.

While he was still an assistant to Tabarrini, Mascagni's research was on lymphatics, preparing specimens like so many others by injecting mercury, wax, or glue into the peripheral lymph vessels to outline them as they passed centrally. The ten years either side of 1780 were periods of active research on the anatomy of human lymphatics. Three major illustrated works appeared in London: J. Sheldon's *The history of the absorbent system* ..., 1784; W. Hewson's volume, in which the human lymphatics were described: *Experimental inquiries. Part II* ..., 1774; and W. C. Cruickshank's *The anatomy of the absorbing vessels* ..., 1786. In Germany, Walter (1775) and Soemmerring (1779); in France, Sabatier (1780); and in Italy, Scarpa (1783) were others writing on this subject, while the controversy between the two Scots, William Hunter and Alexander Monro, had been at its height a few years earlier.

The injection technique which Mascagni used most extensively depended on cannulating a number of lymph vessels successively, filling each by the weight of mercury in an upright wide-base glass tube which acted as a reservoir, and which was drawn out to a fine pipette bent at a right angle, the point of which was inserted into the small, fragile lymph vessels. As many as twenty or more separate cannulations were made in the hand in order to fill the lymphatics of the upper limb. Mercury-injected specimens prepared by Mascagni may be seen, to this day, in a dried state, at the Physiocritical Institute of Siena.[1] Radiographs of these preparations are closely similar to lymphangiograms made today by injecting non-toxic radio-opaque fluids into peripheral lymphatics of healthy living subjects. Mascagni patiently traced lymphatics in the limbs and in other parts; of particular note was his description of the superficial and deep lymphatics of the lungs and their drainage pathways to the hilar lymph nodes. Mascagni used bodies of patients who had died of dropsy (or, for the lungs, of consumption) in whom the lymphatics would be dilated. He showed that peripheral lymphatics did not originate in blood-vessels, and that lymph always passed through at least one lymph node on its way centrally.

The French Academy of Sciences was in the habit of offering prizes for research on subjects specified by them. For the year 1784 the subject was lymphatic vessels. Mascagni, then aged twenty-nine, decided to compete, and submitted an entry, printed both in French and Italian:

---

[1] The *Accademia dei Fisiocritici* in Siena, founded by P. M. Gabrielli in 1691, built a natural history museum in 1816. This building contains many of Mascagni's preparations and his library.

Prodome d'un ouvrage sur la système des vaisseaux lymphatiques, Siena, 1784. It arrived late in Paris, and could not be considered for the regular prize; but the examiners thought so highly of it that an additional prize was awarded. The *Prodrome* was itself an ambitious undertaking, and was followed by the substantive work *Vasorum lymphaticorum corporis humani historia et ichnographia*, Siena: P. Carli 1787 (*Fig. 10.1*). Its dedication was to Leopold, Grand Duke of Tuscany; the artist was Ciro Sancti.

All subsequent work on the naked-eye anatomical distribution of the lymphatics was a refinement on that done during 1770–90— discoveries that could only be transmitted to others through illustration. Mascagni's contributions to these advances were as great as any. The publication *Vasorum lymphaticorum corporis humani* ... made Mascagni internationally renowned, for the book was both the best available and widely distributed (see *Fig. 10.2*).

Mascagni's last years at Siena were troubled, for, as one of Siena's prominent citizens, he was swept up into the political turmoil of the French-inspired Tuscan republican government in 1797; he was made Super-

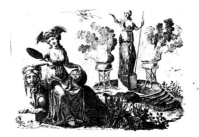

VASORUM LYMPHATICORUM
CORPORIS HUMANI
HISTORIA
ET
ICHNOGRAPHIA
AUCTORE
PAULO MASCAGNI
IN REGIO SENARUM LYCEO
PUBLICO ANATOMES PROFESSORE.

SENIS
Ex Typographia PAZZINI CARLI
MDCCLXXXVII.
SUPERIORUM PERMISSU.

10.1 Title-page of Mascagni's *Vasorum lymphaticorum*, 1787.

intendent of Arts, Sciences, and Charitable Institutions at Siena. This post was forced on him, according to his autobiography written some years later. On the return of the Grand Duke following the invasion by Austrian and Russian troops, Mascagni was arrested and imprisoned for some months. Following political change, he was released and appointed to Pisa, and a year later Florence, where he held, at a high salary, a number of chairs concurrently. He was also responsible for teaching art anatomy. A volume of plates of anatomy for art was prepared, and, as we shall see, published shortly after his death.

At Florence, Mascagni collaborated in the project to produce anatomical wax models of all the systems of the body. Life-sized models were made under the scientific direction of Felice Fontana, and, until 1805, under the technical direction of Clemente Susini. The young Grand Duke Leopold, it is said, had an antipathy to the use of cadavers in anatomical teaching, and

TAB. XVIII.

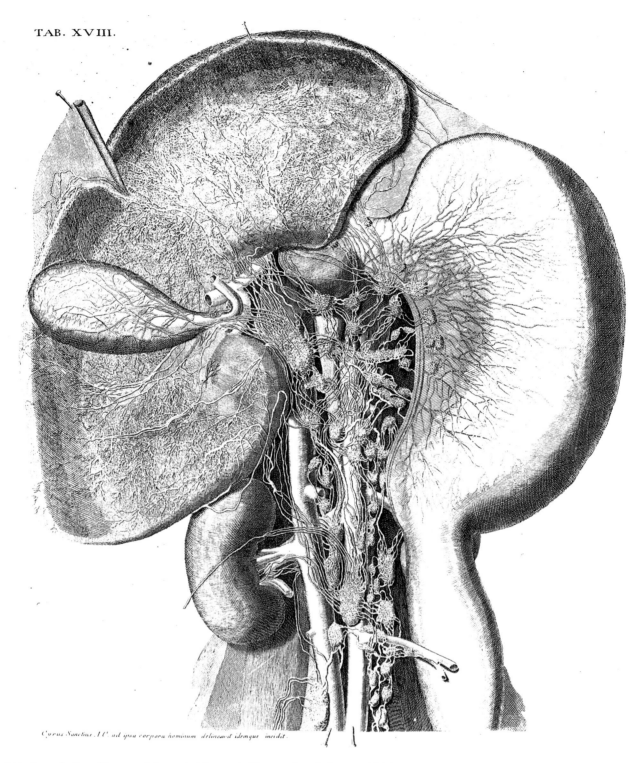

Carus Sanctus A C ad ipsa corpora hominum delineavit idemque incidit.

10.2 Lymphatics of liver and stomach. Mascagni, *Vasorum lymphaticorum*, 1787.

hoped to obviate this necessity by providing detailed, true-to-life, models. The work began in 1770. Precise water-coloured drawings of these models were also prepared, showing in detail each model from a number of viewpoints.

But the project to which Mascagni devoted much of his time, his effort, and in the long run his money, was a *Universal anatomy* based on life-sized illustrations of the entire human body. To aid him he had the help of Sienese and Florentine artists, particularly Antonio Serantoni, whom Mascagni employed for many years. Very large copperplates were engraved, two or three for each representation; the impressions could be put together to create life-sized portraits.[2]

The technology of engraving was sufficiently developed and elaborated by the end of the eighteenth century to be able to cope with the demands of anatomists for accurate, precise representation. Engravers could imitate chalk or crayon drawing, and could use stipple methods to shade broad areas. Multiple plates used successively with different inks could produce a range of colouring in the final print. These techniques were all time-consuming.

Mascagni, like others, underestimated the time and labour required to finish such a task. He died in 1815 aged sixty years.

His family inherited many plates, drawings, and notes relative to this endeavour, an endeavour that had proved so costly that he had had to mortgage his estate. Choulant explained the complex situation that resulted.

Mascagni apparently had three main projects in hand: an illustrated anatomy for sculptors and painters; a prodromal work to the large anatomy on the structure of living organisms, what we would now call an introduction to the tissues of animals and plants; and the great *Universal anatomy* itself.

The first work was quite rapidly prepared for publication, and issued as *Anatomia per uso degli studiosi di scultura et pittura, opera postuma di Paolo Mascagni*, Florence, G. Marenigh, 1816 (*Figs. 10.3 and 10.4*). The plates were drawn and some were engraved by Antonio Serantoni. Barnardino and Aurelio Mascagni, relatives of the anatomist, had supervised its production, and Francesco Antommarchi (sometimes Antonmarchi), a pupil and an anatomical colleague of Mascagni, had edited it.

The second work—the *Prodromo*—came out three years later: *Prodomo della grande anatomia; seconda opera postuma di P. Mascagni* ..., Florence, G. Marenigh, 1819. Antommarchi, described here as anatomical dissector at the Hospital of Santa Maria Nuova, was again the editor, working for the trustees of the Mascagni legacy—Barnardino and Aurelio had died in the interim. There was a second edition, published 1831 from Milan, revised, re-edited, and re-engraved.

The publication of the third work presented formidable difficulties. First, the undertaking

---

[2] J. L. Borges tells the apocryphal story of an Emperor of China who, dissatisfied with the small scale of the maps his geographers produced for him (even though they were large), insisted that they 'map', in the western desert, his realms at the scale of 1:1!

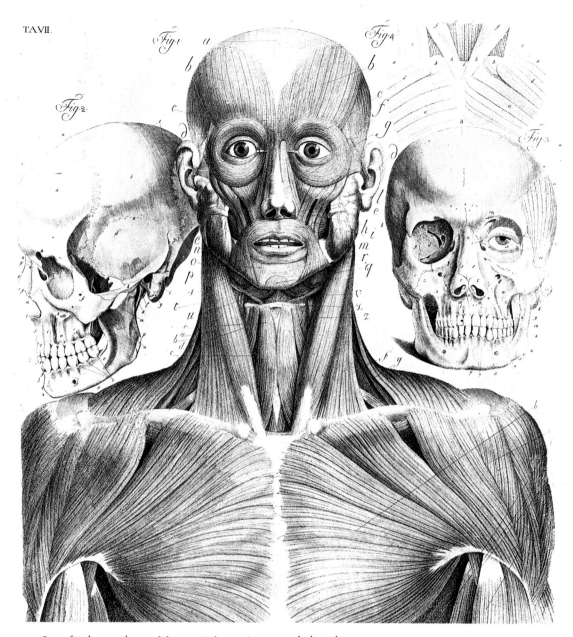

10.3 Superficial musculature. Mascagni, *Anatomia per uso degli studiosi*, 1816.

required a substantial capital outlay. Secondly, the editor entrusted with the first two works, Antommarchi, a Corsican, had been appointed Napoleon Bonaparte's physician, and had left for St Helena early in 1819. Thirdly, the trustees of Mascagni's anatomical legacy had argued with Antommarchi—the publication of the first two posthumous works had not provided money, as was the intention. And lastly, by the 1820s a new printing technique, lithography, had arrived, which was possibly more suitable for the realization of Mascagni's plans.

Such considerations go some way to explain the subsequent issuing of the *Universal anatomy* in two separate, competing publications: an official one, published in Pisa, 1823–32, in nine parts; and a pirated one, published by Lasteyrie and his successor in Paris, 1823–6. These two will be considered separately.

The official publication consists of a volume of text: *Anatomia universa, XLIV tabulis aeneis juxta archetypum hominis adulti, accuratissime repraesentata ...*, Pisa, N. Capurro, 1823, *typis Firmini Didot*. Alongside this text are the plates, in a separate volume *Anatomiae universae P. Mascagni icones*, same place and publisher. The editors for this work were three professors from the University of Pisa; they had purchased the plates from the owners. Firmin Didot, printer, was a master type-designer of this period, a member of a family who over a hundred and twenty-five years had helped to purify the 'language' of typography.

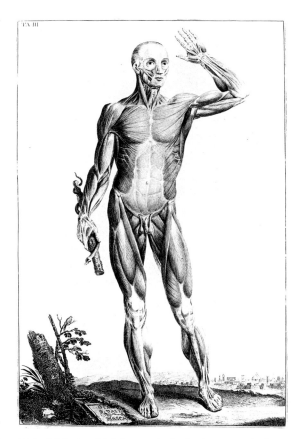

10.4 Male *écorché*. Mascagni, *Anatomia per uso degli studiosi*, 1816.

In most copies, the figures of the impressions of Mascagni's plates are highly coloured. Each has been printed in black ink in the usual way; but it appears that they have also been separately impressed by at least one other plate prepared in the 'crayon' manner with a reddish-brown ink to depict the muscles (a similar technique had been used in the volume on art anatomy). The printed sheet has then been coloured by hand in red, blue, and so on, the conventional colours for arteries, veins, and other structures. The pigments are exceptionally bright and laid on thickly, an incredibly laborious procedure. Some of the colouring follows the engraved outlines and cross-hatching of vessels and so on, but in other places the colours must have been put on free-hand from a master copy, since there are no printed guidelines. Antonio Serantoni is listed on some plates as having been responsible for the drawing, engraving, *and colouring*. (Elsewhere Serantoni is described also as a modeller in wax.)

The anatomy is shown life-size; a full-length dissected figure, seen from the front for instance, is accommodated in three plates. To each coloured figure there is an accompanying outline plate, with references to identify the structures. The total collection therefore was 88 plates,

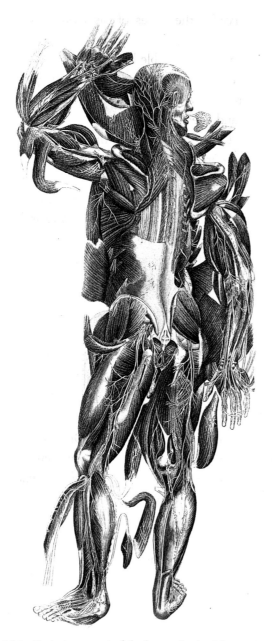

wonderfully printed on heavy paper, each page measuring approximately 95 × 68 cm (3 feet 3 inches by 2 feet 3 inches). The vast book cannot be safely lifted by one normal person, and can only be opened on a table at least a yard wide and two long. A *Universal anatomy* has been produced, but in book form is unusable. The pages may, alternatively, be separated and pinned to a wall to form standing figures, in which case the viewer should be provided with steps to inspect closely the anatomy of the head, and be prepared to kneel in order to inspect the structure of the feet. But who would dare to use such a fine work in this way.

Antonio Serantoni, realizing that the cumbersome Pisa edition of the Universal anatomy was practically useless, prepared an edition in smaller format—in folio!—that was published from Florence, 1833 (*Fig. 10.5*). This incorporated many changes.

There can be few examples of copperplate printing more magnificent in scope or scale; but, as we have stated, the work is almost unusable. Moreover, an unaffected, restrained style of anatomical illustration such as is found in Scarpa's drawing is here ignored, and we have such a mannered treatment that the extravagance distracts the eye from the purpose of conveying information; this is seen especially in the fantastical treatment of muscles, whereby they have been detached from their insertions and brought out beyond the bodily contours—a convention also adopted in some of Vesalius' muscle-men, 1543. This creates an unreal or surreal effect. Although the anatomy is by an acknowledged master, and most carefully thought out, nothing could be less true to nature than these figures. One wonders whether the decision to demonstrate human anatomy in this way was taken primarily by the artists concerned, or by Mascagni himself; and, if the latter, whether it was taken at a time when he was taking too much opium.

10.5 Posterior aspect of the human body. Mascagni, *Anatomia universale*, Florence, 1833.

Certainly a quite different attitude to anatomy pervades the plates of his work on lymph vessels.

Mascagni's *Universal anatomy* remains one of the most remarkable books (if it can be called a book) of scientific illustration ever produced, and even if it was a failure from the point of view of anatomy, as we have argued, it was a failure on the grandest scale, one that enriches us by the extravagant imagination of its conception and execution.

We now return to the other printing of Mascagni's *Universal anatomy*, to the 'pirated' edition.

During his life, Mascagni delayed issuing the work in the hope that printing technology would so far develop that entirely satisfactory coloured prints could be produced. In the first twenty-five years of the nineteenth century such a technique was being developed. Invented in the 1790s, lithography was in frequent commercial use in the 1820s, particularly in Paris. The entrepreneurs there were Lasteyrie and Engelmann. It was the former who issued the 'pirate' edition of the *Universal anatomy*. The editor was Dr Antommarchi, the editor of the other two posthumous works by Mascagni, the man who had had a falling-out with Mascagni's heirs, the physician who was Napoleon's last doctor at St Helena.

Antommarchi obtained his medical degree at Pisa in 1808, and his doctorate in surgery in 1812. He was appointed Mascagni's prosector in anatomy in 1813. When Mascagni died in 1815, Antommarchi was charged with arranging and editing the unfinished anatomical material, which included the plates for the *Universal anatomy*, already engraved by Serantoni. Before he was able to publish this work, he was designated successor at St Helena to Dr O'Meara, who had got into conflict with the Governor there, Hudson Lowe. Cardinal Fesch, Napoleon's uncle, and therefore a fellow Corsican of Antommarchi's, had recommended him. On his journey through Europe to embark from Gravesend to St Helena, Antommarchi carried with him copies of the *Prodromo* and impressions of thirty or so of the plates for the *Universal anatomy*. He showed them to royalty and to fellow scientists, who were suitably impressed; the newspapers carried reports.

Napoleon knew that his new physician had edited Mascagni's *Prodromo*, and he had heard tell of the new, remarkable illustrations. So, shortly after his arrival, Antommarchi was asked to show them to the former Emperor. According to the account that Antommarchi wrote later, Napoleon spent hours inspecting the engravings: 'Deux heures d'anatomie pour un homme qui n'a jamais pu supporter la vue d'un cadavre!' Antommarchi claimed that Napoleon told him to go to Europe and publish the plates—funds would be provided, science would be advanced.

After the death of Napoleon in May 1821, Antommarchi assisted at the autopsy, where he interpreted the Emperor's 'bumps' along phrenological lines. He then left for Rome; and then the following year went to Paris, probably with the idea of publishing the Mascagni figures. His contract with the owners of the Mascagni property had been annulled. He met with the Comte de Lasteyrie, and together they decided to reproduce the *Universal anatomy* in lithography, copying the figures from the impressions Antommarchi had taken when he left for St Helena. The work proceeded quickly, for they knew from a prospectus that the official *Universal anatomy* was to start publication, as it did, the next year, 1823. The lithographic artist employed was Pedretti. Remarkably the first of a total of fifteen parts was ready in Paris also in 1823, demonstrating the clear advantage of lithography in terms of speed—an engraver making new plates would have completed the task in years, not months. The first part of the Parisian edition was for sale actually earlier than that of the Pisan edition, and the former completed publication by 1826, while the latter was not complete until 1832. The plates in the two editions are not exactly the same, since in both changes had been made to the original designs; Antommarchi had prepared a few entirely new plates. The size of the pages and images in the two editions was similar.

The 'pirated' Parisian edition was entitled, in full, *Planches anatomiques du corps humain exécutées d'après les dimensions naturelles, accompagnées d'un texte explicatif par F. Antommarchi, publiées par le Comte de Lasteyrie, éditeur*, Paris, 1823–6. Antommarchi's and Lasteyrie's names are prominent, but nowhere is the name of Mascagni to be seen on this title-page—a grave injustice and error. Neither does the name of the original artist, Serantoni, appear.

The Pisan and the Parisian editions of what are essentially the same anatomical illustrations differ in so many respects, and the differences anticipate and demonstrate the remarkable changes that anatomical illustration was to undergo with the advent of lithography. The 'official' engraved plates were of the older order, produced slowly and expensively over years, putting the family of the anatomist into debt. The Parisian lithographic plates were of the newer age, produced from start to finish in a matter of months, and costing much less, perhaps even turning a profit for Antommarchi, if not for Lasteyrie. The title-pages show the differences: the title-page to the Pisan edition is relatively formal, restrained, elegant, and orderly; the Parisian one employs many different and exaggerated letter-forms, being flowery, extravagant, and romantic. The one, an élitist work; the other, the result of entrepreneurship, an industrial enterprise, undercutting the competitor and ruthlessly exploitative.

89 The lymphatics of the lower trunk. Tab. XIII in P. Mascagni, *Vasorum lymphaticorum corporis humani ...*, 1787. Engraving (Wellcome Institute Library). 42.3 × 28.5 cm.

This illustration shows the lymphatics of the dorsum of the penis, testes, front of thigh, iliac crest, and kidneys, together with iliac and aortic lymph glands, the cisterna chyli, and the formation of the thoracic duct. On the facing page of the book is a lettered and numbered outline drawing; there is also a Latin explanatory text earlier in the book.

The superficial and deep inguinal glands and their intercommunications are shown: perhaps the lymph gland lying medial to the femoral vessel in the femoral canal is that later known as Cloquet's gland, though the larger and more lateral glands seem to send most vessels into the abdomen.

TAB. XIII.

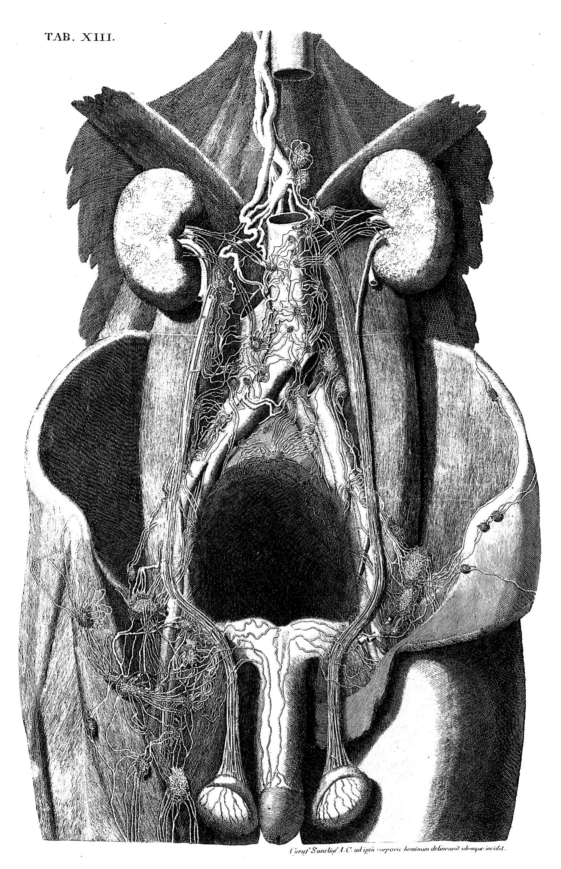

Cyrus Sanctus A.C. ad ipsa corpora hominum delineavit idemque incidit.

PLATE 89

Clearly shown, particularly on the left side, is the drainage of the testes to the lateral and pre-aortic lymph nodes at the level of the lower pole of the kidney.

The formation of the cisterna chyli from abdominal lymphatics is very variable; even so the latter here seem too high when the positioning of the diaphragm is considered.

The representation of the kidney lymphatic plexus is presumably the capsular plexus, with the peritubular drainage vessels seen emerging at the hilum *en route* to aortic lymph glands. The common iliac lymph nodes, in particular, are nicely portrayed.

90 Viscera of abdomen and thorax. Viscera Tabula III in P. Mascagni, *Anatomiae universae ... icones*, 1823. Engraving (Wellcome Institute Library). 76.8 × 56.3 cm.

The Royal Society of Medicine, London, possesses a book containing forty-four grandiose and very colourful Mascagni plates. The pages of this book measure 97 × 68 cm, and, in a heavy binding, it requires two people to move it. Each of the plates has a facing outline diagram with numbers and letters as identifiers of the various structures. No explanation of these appears in the book itself, but one can be found in a (thankfully) smaller volume, *Anatomia universa, XLIV tabulis aeneis ...*, 1823.

Collections of these Mascagni plates, each sheet separate and unbound, exist in a number of places—for example, the Countway library in Boston and the library of the Wellcome Institute for the History of Medicine in London. While we would dearly have liked to present a composite photograph of one of the 'exploded' muscle sets (on three separate sheets the combined height of these figures is 190 cm, or 6 feet 3 inches!) we have settled on another of Mascagni's flamboyant plates, one featured on but a single page, which belongs to the Wellcome Institute Library.

The drawings of the hearts and also those of the larynx and trachea are of no great moment, but the main figure presents some interesting features, quite apart from its colourful presentation. As might be expected of Mascagni, the lymphatic system is given considerable prominence— thoracic duct, tracheal and hilar lymph nodes, axillary nodes, and those alongside the internal jugular vein are all well featured.

Below the diaphragm the antero-lateral abdominal wall has been peeled back and the viscera viewed through the peritoneum. The liver, part of the stomach, the spleen, and coils of intestine can be seen, though there is no evidence of a greater omentum. The (cut) left ribs extend too caudally—the spleen here would lie on ribs 8, 9, and 10. On the left side (anatomical right) is seen the rectus abdominis muscle, together with the right inferior epigastric vessels. The rectus sheath is nowhere featured, although its posterior portion would lie deep to the left inferior epigastric vessels. To remove it (and the transversalis fascia) and yet leave the peritoneum intact

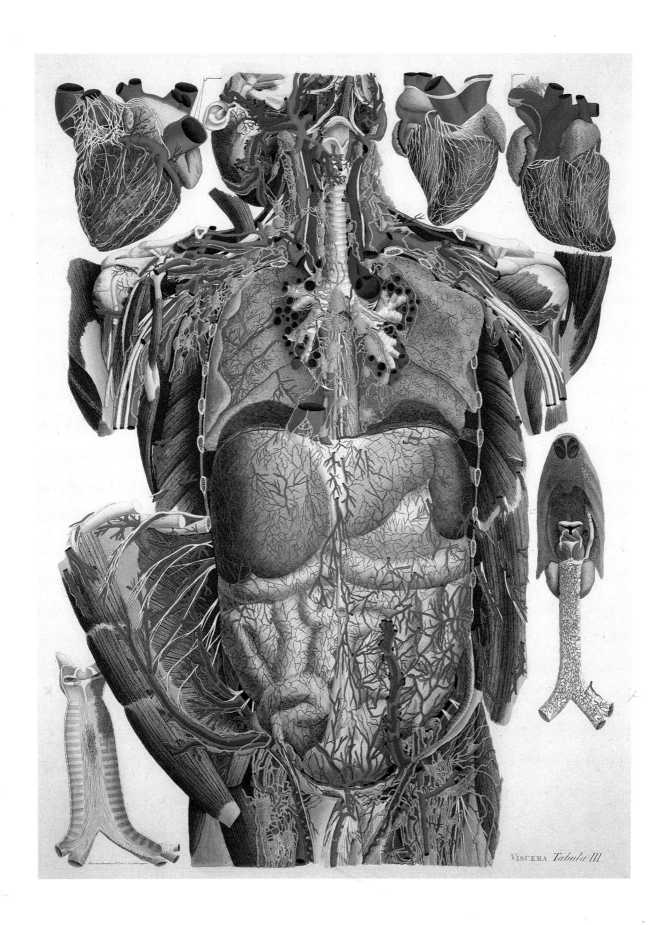

VISCERA *Tabula III.*

indicates a high degree of dissecting determination and skill! The right spermatic cord appears to pierce the peritoneum, carrying a sleeve of the latter for some distance.

In the axillary region the anatomy of the brachial plexus and its nerves is obscured by the more colourful blood-vessels. A number of the veins, both here and elsewhere, have little white lines in them to indicate valves.

The structures in the hilum of the lung seem to have been extended into the lung tissue for some distance (ten branches of the left pulmonary artery, thirteen of the right); yet the drawing gives little inkling of this. The bifurcating or trifurcating branches from the common carotid branches are extravagant in size—for example, the superficial temporal artery.

The attraction of these large anatomical plates is visual, because of their size and riot of colour. The anatomy shown is frequently undistinguished—certainly it hardly merits the chore of moving such a large book and then finding a table big enough to enable it to be opened. Uncharitable though it may seem, it is likely that the enormously lengthy and tedious task of producing such plates was in reality an essay in futility in the anatomical sense. But what wonderful wallpapers they would make!

Chapter 10: Selected reading

Allodi, F. (1955). *La storia . . . dei linfatici del cuore nelle opere di Paolo Mascagni*. L. S. Olschki, Florence.

Azzaroli, M. L. (1975). *'La Specola': the zoological museum of Florence University*. L. S. Olschki, Florence.

Bertelli, R. (1961). Paolo Mascagni (1755–1815). *J. cardiovasc. Surg.*, **2**, 414–21.

Belloni, L. (1970). Italian medical education after 1600. In *The history of medical education*, (ed. C. D. O'Malley) University of Californa Press, Berkeley.

Cazort, M. (1982). Wax anatomical models as teaching devices in eighteenth century Bologna and Florence. *Drawing*, **4**, 5–8.

Choulant, L. (1962). *History and bibliography of anatomic illustration*. Ed. M. Frank. Hafner, New York. (Reprint of 1945 edition.)

Dumaître, P. (1981). *Les planches anatomiques d'Antommarchi*. *Clio Med.*, **16**, 13–23.

Franceschini, P. (1975). Antonio Scarpa. *Dict. sci. Biog.*, 136–9.

Hearder, M. and Waley, D. P. (ed.) (1966). *A short history of Italy*. Cambridge University Press.

Kortan, H., Lesky E., and Wächter, O. (1968). *Anatomiae Universae Pauli Mascagnii Icones: Dokumentation*. Academy of Fine Arts, Vienna.

Ricci, C. (1972). *L'Accademia dei Fisiocritici in Siena*. L'Accademia dei Fisiocritici, Siena.

Zimmerman, L. M. and Veith, I. (1967) *Great ideas in the history of surgery* [pages 386–93 on Scarpa]. Dover, New York.

11

Early British anatomical illustration to 1750

Thomas Willis (1621–1675)

IN 1669 the Danish neuroscientist Nicolaus Steno (Niels Stensen) wrote: '... in anatomy, no diagrams [that is, anatomical illustrations] are more imperfect than those of the brain'. They are nevertheless useful to aid the memory, or for those whose 'aversion to blood prevents them from satisfying their curiosity by inspecting natural specimens ...'. But 'it would be better to have no diagrams than false or imperfect ones'. For exact illustrations 'a good draughtsman is as necessary as a good anatomist'. Steno goes on to describe a particular difficulty of brain research: '[with] other parts of the body, to obtain a diagram, it is sufficient to make one preparation; the brain on the contrary, subsides, after preparation before the diagram is drawn, so that it is necessary to draw plans of several brain preparations to obtain a single diagram ...'. Steno's book *Discours ... sur l'anatomie du cerveau* Paris, 1669, was published during his stay in that city; it contains four plates with drawings showing sagittal and transverse sections of the brain, the first three of which have parallel accompanying outlines, anticipating the Albinian manner; but these are unlabelled (*Fig. 11.1*). The brain stem is well shown, and the cerebral convolutions, drawn characteristically as coils of intestines, are, even so, more realistic than those of previous authors.

A few years earlier Thomas Willis in Oxford had faced up to the same need for anatomical illustration of the brain during preparative work for his *Cerebri anatome ...,* London, 1664 (Fig. 11.2). An English translation was made by a minor poet, Samuel Pordage, and published with *The remaining medical works [of Willis] ...,* London, 1681. Willis also realized the need of competent draughtsmen, and he found them in his scientific colleagues, Christopher Wren and Richard Lower. In some preparations it seems that he may have been able to overcome the problem that Steno noted by a form of partial fixation produced by perfusing the cerebral circulation with spirits of wine; certainly the resulting plates of the brain resemble in many respects modern formalin-fixed preparations.

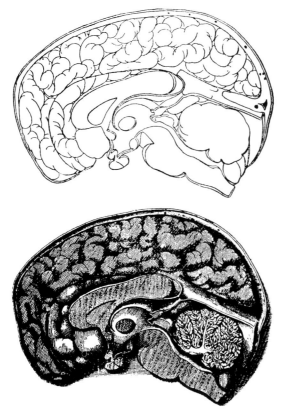

11.1 Hemisected brain from Steno's *Discours*, 1669.

The son of a royalist farmer, Willis received his bachelor's degree in 1639 from the University of Oxford, and his medical qualification at the age of twenty-five years in 1646—that was the year when royalist Oxford was surrendered to the parliamentary forces, so effectively ending the Civil War. He began the practice of medicine in Oxford and in the surrounding towns and villages. He visited Abingdon, for instance, once a week, where he was prepared to prescribe for unseen patients on the basis of a recounted medical history and by 'casting waters'—diagnosis from the appearance of a specimen of urine. Later in the course of twenty years' medical work in Oxford he became well-known, much consulted, and consequently prosperous; with other physicians he established consulting rooms, and what amounted to a small hospital, at 'The Angel' on the south side of the High Street, not far from Magdalen Bridge. In 1667, at the time of his move to London, Willis was among the wealthiest men in Oxford.

Willis's name, and that of Dr William Petty, teacher and later Reader in anatomy at the University, became widely known in 1650 owing to a bizarre event: a young woman, Ann Green, had been hanged in Oxford for killing her illegitimate new-born child (the child had probably been stillborn). Her body was brought to the rented rooms of Petty for dissection. Although she had been suspended for half an hour, and although her friends had pulled on her feet to hasten the end of her sufferings, it was realized that she was breathing. Someone stamped on her chest a number of times, possibly a sort of external cardiac massage. Petty, with Willis, used contemporary but probably irrelevant procedures—bleeding, enemas, sensory stimulation … they then put her in bed with another woman to warm her. She recovered fully in the succeeding days, and successfully petitioned for a pardon. A broadside wryly commented: 'Thus 'tis more easy to recall the dead / than to restore a once-lost maidenhead'. Naturally enough in popular esteem Petty and Willis were thought to be fine practical doctors. Less sensationally, but probably in the long run more effectively, Willis's practice prospered because of the sober and painstaking care he gave his patients.

In learned circles, Willis became known as a medical writer after the publication of a book *Diatribae duae medico-philosophicae* … 1659, which contained discussions on fevers, especially epidemic fevers—these he regarded as derangements of a process analogous to fermentation. Rather than this and other speculative and pedestrian work, we now remember Willis's observational and experimental studies as a member of the various groups of Oxford *virtuosi* during and after the Cromwellian period. These experimentalists often followed the Harveian anatomico-physiological approach to the investigation of biomedical phenomena. It may be remembered that Harvey was Charles I's physician, and resided in Oxford with the royalists, becoming head of Merton College for a brief period, 1648–9. The Oxford natural philosophers often investigated mathematics,

CEREBRI ANATOME:

CUI ACCESSIT

NERVORUM DESCRIPTIO

ET USUS.

STUDIO

THOMÆ WILLIS, ex *Æde Christi* *Oxon.* M. D. & in ista Celeberrima Academia Naturalis Philosophiæ Professoris *Sidleiani.*

LONDINI,

Typis *Ja. Flesher,* Impensis *Jo. Martyn* & *Ja. Allestry* apud insigne Campanæ in Cœmeterio *D. Pauli.* MDCLXIV.

11.2 Title-page of Willis, *Cerebri anatome,* 1664.

physics and chemistry, and questions of astronomy in rooms—proto-laboratories—at Wadham College. Biological and medical questions were also at the centre of discussions and experiments in private rooms of physicians and others in Oxford. With Willis were William Petty—that is until his appointment in Ireland, 1652, Thomas Millington, Christopher Wren, and, in particular, the physician Richard Lower. From 1654 Robert Boyle was also one of the company of natural philosophers, having taken rooms in the High Street.

The *virtuoso* might find himself engaged both in physical and in biological experiments, working at times individually, at times in a group. Thus Wren was involved in individual work in mathematics and the recording of meteorological information, and in collective work on blood-vessel perfusion and blood-transfusion. Willis spent much time with chemical experiments and the preparation of chemical remedies; but his work in these fields seems to a present-day reader late medieval rather than early modern; he recognized five rather than four elements—earth and water, but also sulphur, salt, and spirits. Some of his chemical remedies Willis kept secret, and their sale proved profitable, both in Oxford and later in London.

Following the restoration of the monarchy in 1660 Willis was appointed Sedleian Professor of Natural Philosophy. This was an appropriate appointment for the times, since Willis was known as a faithful royalist (his father had died in the cause, and he himself had been in the militia in Oxford). Moreover he had faithfully adhered to the Church of England; Anglican religious services had been conducted, secretly but regularly, at the Willis household throughout the period of the Commonwealth. The Sedley Chair had been established earlier in the century to emphasize Aristotelian philosophy, but Willis's twice-weekly lectures were in the realm of Baconian new philosophy, particularly as exemplified by studies on the structure and function of the nervous system. A careful record of his lectures was made by John Locke on the basis of earlier notes by Richard Lower—a remarkable conjunction of anatomy and physiology, psychology and philosophy. Dewhurst recently transcribed and edited these notes: *Thomas Willis's Oxford Lectures*, Oxford, 1980; much of the above account is from Dewhurst's book. Willis's own description of his work on brain anatomy may be used to amplify this account.

In the preface of *Cerebri anatome ...*, addressed to the reader, Willis described how, as Sedleian Professor, he was charged to 'comment on the offices of the senses, both external and also internal, and of the faculties and affections of the soul, as also of the organs and various provisions of all these ...'. He therefore produced 'some not unlikely hypotheses', which developed into a systematic argument, a doctrine. But these pleasant constructs were, after more serious consideration, seen to be a 'poetical philosophy and physick neatly wrought ...', but lacking in reality. So he resolved on a new course, relying only on 'nature and ocular demonstrations'. In this spirit, then, Willis 'betook [himself] wholly to the study of anatomy: and as I did chiefly inquire into the offices and uses of the brain ... I addicted my self to the opening of heads especially ...'. He acknowledged the colleagues who collaborated with him: the 'most learned physician and highly skilful anatomist, Doctor Richard Lower'; 'no day almost past over without some anatomical administration [dissection]; so that in a short space there was nothing of the brain ... that seemed not plainly detected, and intimately beheld by us.' Willis notes that Lower drew some of the figures; among these may be the remarkable diagram showing the autonomic nervous system in the neck and thorax (*Fig. 11.3*). He also acknowledges Dr Thomas Millington and Christopher Wren, doctor of laws and (by then) Savilian Professor of Astronomy. The latter was thanked for delineating 'with his own most skilful hands many figures of the brain and skull ...'.

In the book Willis described first his methods for dissecting the brain. In Chapter VII, the functional anatomy of the arterial circle at the base of the brain—the circle of Willis—is discussed (our *Plate 91*): 'if by chance one or two [of its constituent arteries] should be stopt, there might easily be found another passage instead of them ...'

This he confirmed by ocular demonstrations:

… I have squirted oftentimes into either artery of the carotides, a liquor dyed with ink, and presently the branches on either side, yea and the chief shoots of the vertebrals, have been dyed with the same tincture: yea, if such an injection be sometimes iterated by one only passage, the vessels creeping into every corner and secret place of the brain and cerebel, will be imbued with the same colour.

To exploit Harvey's concepts of the circulation in such ways was one of the innovative achievements of the Oxford school. It seems that to Christopher Wren must go much credit for this particular experimental approach. It was a pity that this technique of vascular injection should have been the only one exploited later in this century by investigators such as Ruysch.

Willis's *Cerebri anatome* is dedicated to the Archbishop of Canterbury. Even a devout and orthodox Anglican, whose faith had been tried and not found wanting in the difficult days of the Civil War and in the Commonwealth, felt it necessary to defend himself against possible accusations of errors. The first accusation, but not perhaps of prime importance, was that he had slain so many animals of all kinds; the

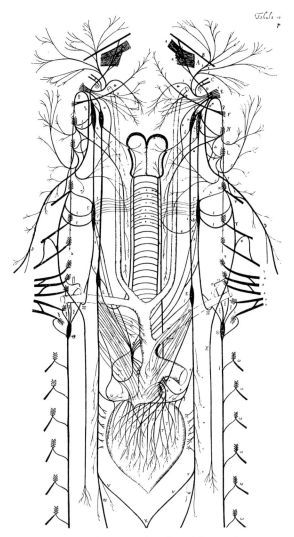

11.3 Diagram of nerves of neck and thorax from Willis' *Cerebri anatome*, 1664.

second, and certainly significant, was that he might be charged with atheism—'it hath been a long while accounted as a certain mystery and school-house of atheism to search into nature, as if whatever reasons we grant to philosophy, should derogate from religion …'. He defended himself in terms similar to those that anatomists had used in the previous century, and were to use for the next two hundred years and more: he was of the opinion of those who looked into nature 'as into another table of the divine word, and the greater Bible: For indeed, in either volume [of nature or of the Bible] there is no high point, which requires not the care, or refutes the industry of an interpreter; there is no page certainly which shows not the Author, and his power, goodness, trust, and wisdom'. Willis thus argued that he had as much right to study carefully the book of nature as had divines to study the scriptures. It was in this same spirit Willis went on to write two other parts to his study on brain structure and function: one on pathology, *Pathologiae cerebri ...*, 1667; and the other on psychology and neuropsychiatric subjects, *De anima brutorum* 1672.

91 The base of the brain. Figura prima from T. Willis, *Cerebri Anatome ...*, 1664. Engraving (Wellcome Institute Library). 17.0 × 15.3 cm.

Thomas Willis will always be associated with the arterial anastomosis at the base of the human brain which bears his name—the Circle of Willis, parts of which had been described earlier by Falloppio, Casserio, and Wepfer. It was therefore thought fitting that the figure illustrating this should be chosen as representative of his many anatomical illustrations. It is of interest that the drawing was made by Christopher Wren, designer of many famous architectural gems, not least St Paul's Cathedral in London. Wren was often present at Willis's dissections of the brain, and used 'to confer and reason about the uses of the parts' (Samuel Pordage's English translation, 1681).

In this plate the white (or unhatched) parts include the olfactory bulbs (D), the optic nerves (E) together with the optic chiasm and tracts, the mammillary bodies (Y), and, more caudally, the pons, the medulla, and the origins of the cranial nerves. With regard to the cerebral hemispheres (A) one might comment that the portrayals of the gyri and sulci are reasonably accurate; but the main interest in the plate is the configuration of the arteries.

The two vertebral arteries (TT) are rather small, and, although the anterior spinal artery (also T) is shown between them, from the text it is clear that Willis considered this latter as part of the ascending vertebral arterial system. It is strange that, although the basilar artery is shown dividing into the right and left posterior cerebral arteries, the superior cerebellar artery, which should be seen just behind the oculomotor nerve (F), is absent. He makes it clear in the text that he considered the internal carotid arteries to divide into anterior [anterior cerebral] and posterior [posterior communicating] branches—'the anterior branches of the carotides go away united, [here referring to (R) the anterior communicating artery] moving forward into the fissure

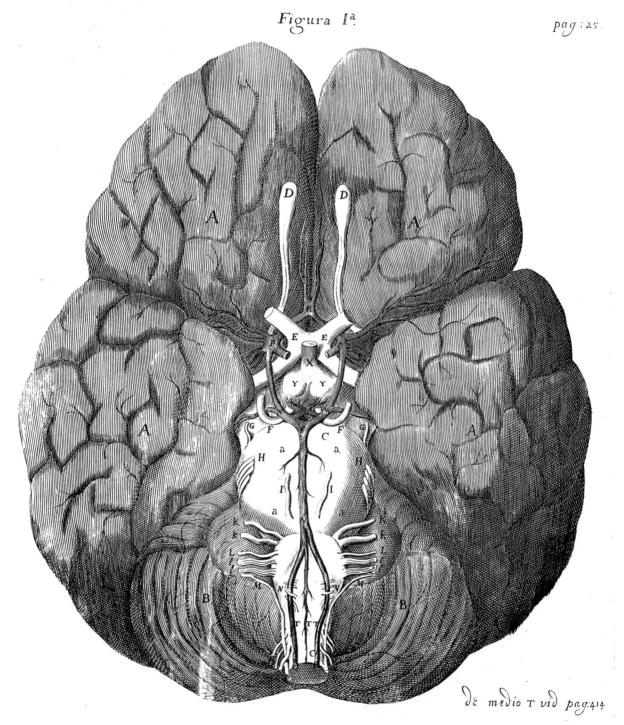

PLATE 91

or cleft of the brain' and 'the posterior branches of the carotides united, [at S] and meeting with the vertebral trunk [basilar artery]'. The usually large middle cerebral artery (here represented by an unusual leash of vessels) is referred to as 'a branch of it [internal carotid] going in between two lobes of the brain'.

With regard to the more caudal cranial nerves, Kk are termed 'the auditory or hearing nerves and their two processes on either side of them the seventh pair', and Ll 'the wandring pair, or the eighth pair consisting of many fibres'—the facial, vagus, glossopharyngeal, and cranial accessory were not recognized as separate nerves. The spinal accessory nerves (M) are referred to as 'the spinal nerves coming from afar to the origine of the wandring pair', while (N), the hypoglossal nerves, are 'the ninth pair consisting also of many fibres ...'.

Contemplating the figure one can understand why the word 'circle' originated as a descriptive term for the carotid–vertebral anastomosis. The first to attach Willis's name to the 'circle' (more accurately polygon) was Haller, in the eighteenth century. However, with the exception of the anterior communicating artery, the circle had been previously illustrated, seventeen years before Willis, by Vesling in his *Syntagma*, 1647.

The figure itself is beautifully drawn, not surprisingly considering who was the artist, and the cranial nerve roots are accurately shown (except for the abducent, (I), here rather sketchy), even if Willis was partially deceived as to their numbering and functional significance.

As to what Willis considered the function of the 'circle' to be, in the text he states that, while in part it serves thoroughly to mingle the blood, more importantly it enables the blood-flow to overcome a stoppage in one part, for example: '... if the carotides of one side should be obstructed, then the vessels of the other side might provide for either province. Also as to the vertebral arteries, there is the same manner of provision made. Further, if both the carotides should be stopped, the offices of each might be supplied through the vertebrals, and so on the other side the carotides may supply the defects of the shut up vertebrals.'

John Browne (1642–1702)

After service in the Navy, Browne established himself as a surgeon in Norwich. In the mid-1670s he moved to London, and become 'sworn chirurgeon to the King', that is surgeon in ordinary to Charles II. (Later he held this far from prestigious position to other monarchs.) In 1678 he published a book on cancers, *A compleat treatise on preternatural tumours* ... and another entitled *A compleat discourse of wounds* ... By that time he had also produced a manuscript of an illustrated monograph on the muscles of the human body (MS129.b.22, Royal College of Surgeons of England). The work however was not printed and published until 1681: *A compleat treatise of the muscles....* This book contained thirty-seven full-page copper engravings, many of which were drawn by unknown artists in a strangely effete baroque style, but well engraved by Nicholas Yeates. The book was reissued in 1683, in which year Browne was, on the

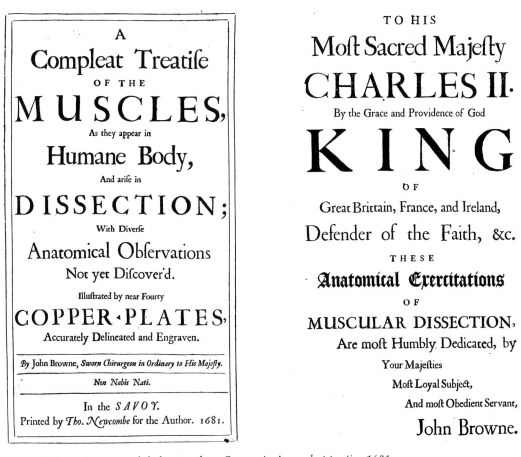

A
Compleat Treatife
OF THE
MUSCLES,
As they appear in
Humane Body,
And arife in
DISSECTION;
With Diverfe
Anatomical Obfervations
Not yet Difcover'd.
Illuftrated by near Fourty
COPPER·PLATES,
Accurately Delineated and Engraven.

By John Browne, Sworn Chirurgeon in Ordinary to His Majefty.

Non Nobis Nati.

In the *SAVOY.*
Printed by *Tho. Newcombe* for the Author. 1681.

TO HIS
Moft Sacred Majefty
CHARLES II·
By the Grace and Providence of God
KING
OF
Great Brittain, France, and Ireland,
Defender of the Faith, &c.
THESE
𝕬𝖓𝖆𝖙𝖔𝖒𝖎𝖈𝖆𝖑 𝕰𝖝𝖊𝖗𝖈𝖎𝖙𝖆𝖙𝖎𝖔𝖓𝖘
OF
MUSCULAR DISSECTION,
Are moft Humbly Dedicated, by
Your Majefties
Moft Loyal Subject,
And moft Obedient Servant,
John Browne.

11.4a and b   Title-page and dedication from Browne's *A compleat treatise,* 1681.

recommendation of the King, and, it seems, against the wishes of the Governors, appointed surgeon to St Thomas's Hospital.

In 1684 Browne continued his career as a medical writer by issuing *Adenochoiradelogia: or an anatomick–chirurgical treatise of glandules and strumaes, or King's-Evil-swellings* ... Browne had assisted in the ceremony of touching for the King's Evil, or scrofula—names then given to diseases of lymph nodes, often tubercular in origin. As Browne described, more than 4000 persons a year were on average touched by the King in the period from 1660 to 1682. Samuel Johnson was touched by Queen Anne in 1712, when he was an infant.

In 1685 Browne published, in the Royal Society's *Philosophical Transactions,* a letter describing the clinical history and post-mortem appearances of a young soldier with liver cirrhosis and ascites. This was an early description of the pathology of this condition. In the last year of his life came Browne's book *Somatopolita ...,* London, 1702, reissued as *The surgeons assistant,* 1703.

Browne's most successful work was his treatise on the muscles, already mentioned; our *Plate*

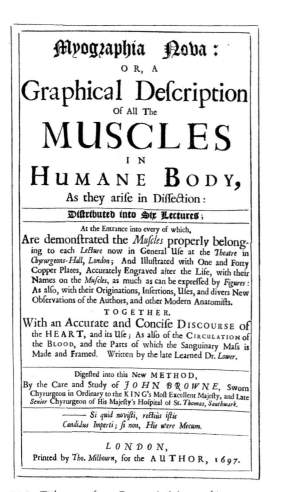

11.5 Title-page from Browne's *Myographia nova*, 1697.

92 is from this book. It appeared in a total of five editions in the English language (1681, 1683, 1697, 1698, and 1705, all from London), four in Latin (1684, London, 1687 and 1690, Leiden, and 1694 Amsterdam), and one in German (1704, Berlin). The form of the first edition is as follows:

a fine portrait of Browne, aged thirty-nine;

the title-page and a dedication to the King (*Fig. 11.4 a and b*);

A copyright, or royal warrant 'granting unto the said John Browne the sole privilege of printing the aforesaid treatise with its copper figures; and strictly charging, prohibiting and forbidding all our subjects to copy or counterfeit any the sculptures or description aforesaid ... or to import ... any copies or exemplars of the same reprinted beyond the seas within the term of fifteen years ...';

a second dedication to the Duke of Albemarle;

an imprimatur from two royal physicians, including Charles Scarburgh, and five officers of the College of Physicians;

a Latin address to that Royal College;

five letters of recommendation from prominent physicians;

an address 'To the ingenuous and studious reader';

a list of 247 subscribers, including the name of Sir Thomas Browne, the noted Norwich physician, antiquary, 'metaphysical' essayist, and person of equable temperament—an acquaintance of our Browne, but not apparently a relative;

a list of all the muscles described in the book, in the order in which they arise in dissection;

a list of the names 'of the authors concerned in this muscular discourse'; this includes many that we have dealt with;

the text in 205 pages, with each muscle being given a separate page, and 37 full-page copper engravings;

and finally, before the Index, a Table showing which muscles are involved in particular movements—for example, 'The leg is contracted by sartorius, gracillis, seminervosus, semimembranosus, biceps'. This Table is from Scarburgh.

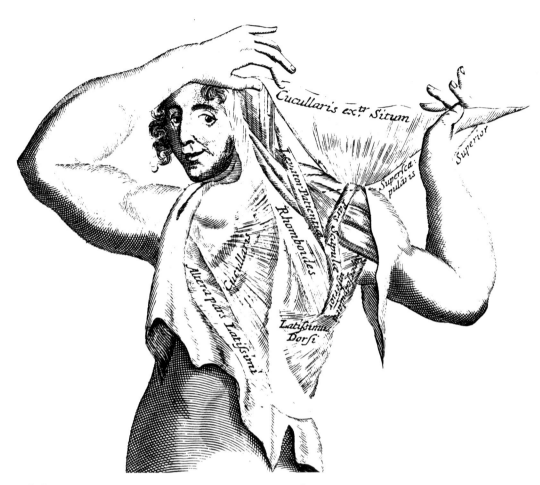

11.6 Labelled superficial back muscles from Browne's *Myographia nova*, 1697.

One can see that such a manageable, even if rather confusingly organized, book of somewhat more than two hundred pages could have been of assistance to students and practitioners of anatomy, surgery, or medicine, and might have well served painters and sculptors. The work was popular in England and north Europe.

We must now indicate briefly the sources and the qualities of this text and its illustrations.

The text of the manuscript of 1675, corrected by Browne, was directly derived from William Molins, *ΜΥΣΚΟΤΟΜΙΑ: or, the anatomical administration of all the muscles of an humane body* ..., London, 1648, reissued 1676 and 1680. The text in Browne's published book is but slightly modified from Molins. The text in later editions, including those published under a new title *Myographia nova* ..., 1697 (Fig. 11.5), was further modified—not, however, for the better.

The illustrations were taken more or less directly from other sources, principally from the plates of Casserio, the edition used being that published in Frankfurt, 1632. For example, the

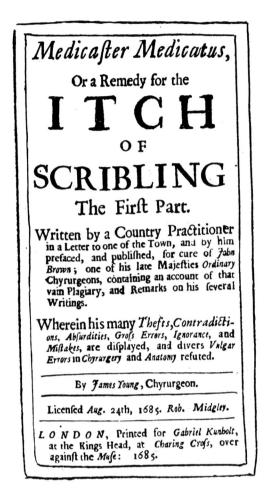

11.7 Title-page from Younge's *Medicaster medicatus*,
1685.

Casserian figure showing the muscles of the lower limb in a drawing of ambling legs (see our *Plate 62*, p. 267) is directly and clearly copied in this book, but with a simplified landscape; the figure from Casserio that exhibits the anatomy of the penis (see our *Fig. 7.3*, p. 261) is transferred, in Browne's engraving, from a treed landscape to a luxurious bed, the positions of the arms altered, the legs drawn very poorly, and the male member enlarged extraordinarily. The copyist has some flair for the extravagant, but his capabilities were of a much lower order than those of Casserio's artists. In these, and in some other plates, the same lettering in the same places was used as that found in Casserio. In editions of Browne's book from 1697 on, the full name of each muscle is engraved on the muscles shown—an original idea, apparently by Molins, taken up by Browne (*Fig. 11.6*). These editions also contain an acknowledged, posthumous work by Richard Lower.

Nowhere in his book does Browne acknowledge his indebtedness to Molins or to Scarburgh.[1] Nowhere is it stated that the majority of the plates are re-drawn and re-engraved after Casserio. Browne implicitly claims the credit, and, as we have seen, the copyright, for text and illustrations, which rightly belong to Molins, to Scarburgh, and to Casserio and his artists.

Of course, Browne's plagiarisms were uncovered, notably by James Yonge (1646–1721). He, like Browne, established himself after service in the Navy as a provincial practitioner. He rose to be Mayor of Plymouth, and was well known also in London—as a medical writer (on amputation, wounds to the head, and so on), as an authority on trade with Newfoundland, and as a contributor to the *Philosophical Transactions*. He corresponded with Hans Sloane, and Millington, and was made F R S and a licentiate of the Royal College of Physicians. His exposé of Browne was published as *Medicaster medicatus, or a remedy for the itch of scribling . . .*, London, 1685 (*Fig. 11.7*).

[1] Scarburgh is acknowledged in the 1697 edition, but only in a general way.

Struggling unsuccessfully to understand the meaning of some of Browne's introductory pages, one is grateful to read Yonge's trenchant remarks: 'in a barbarous and confused manner, [Browne] attempts to give us an account of Steno's mathematical hypothesis of muscles and musculary motion ...'. Yonge continues:

The Table which he saith do give the names of the muscles as they arise in dissection, is verbatim from Mr. W. Moline's Myotomia, as are all his descriptions throughout the book word for word. His cutts are taken from Casserius Placentius, and Spigellius ... His Table shewing the [muscles involved in various movements] is a verbatim transcript from Dr. Scarboroughs, and yet such is the ingratitude and dishonesty of this thief, that he no where owns it ...

There is no need for us here to detail Browne's plagiarisms. Nor will we go through the long-drawn history of Browne's dismissal from his position of senior surgeon at St Thomas's Hospital. The interested reader may read a fine account of these matters in K. F. Russell (1959; 1962).

The influence of Casserio's illustrations of muscles as reproduced by Browne—sometimes well, more often ill—continued into the eighteenth century; Browne's figures were again reprinted, re-engraved, in J. J. Manget, *Theatrum anatomicum*, Geneva, 1716 and 1717.

92 Superficial muscles of the back. Tab. XIIII from John Browne, *A compleat treatise ...*, 1681. Engraving (private collection). 25.3 × 16.7 cm.

This figure, despite the rural background being more in keeping with the English origin of the book than those of the others it contains, gives a rather 'kitschy' impression. This Browne plate has been chosen because, though derived from a Casserian figure, it is not a straight copy from Casserio, as many of Browne's other plates are. Additional dissection has been done, for example trapezius has been reflected, and the identifying letters are Browne's own. It portrays a bucolic male with protuberant abdomen, prominent buttocks, over-developed calves, and grinning face, holding the right trapezius ('cucullaris') rather coyly aloft. The left trapezius and right latissimus dorsi are accurately drawn, but the two rhomboids (DD) are not good (they are *much* better depicted in the next figure in the book), and it is obvious that the upper part of the right trapezius (BB, c, d, e) lies between rhomboid minor and levator scapulae (C), an anatomical absurdity. The scapular muscles are difficult to understand; and this is the more surprising because the accompanying text is remarkably accurate—the credit for this, however, belongs to Molins, not Browne.

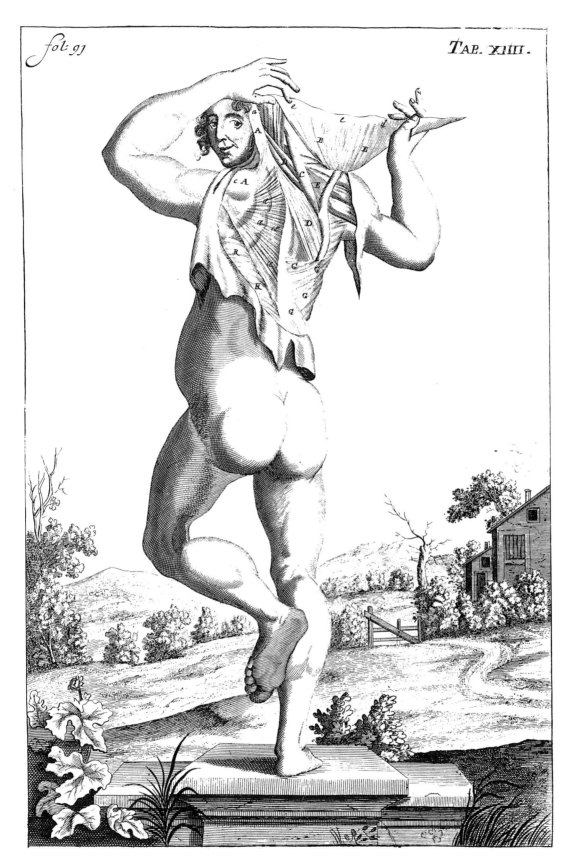

TAB. XIIII.

PLATE 92

William Cowper (1666–1709)

It has been the fate of Cowper, surgeon, to be best remembered as a plagiarist, and as the anatomist whose name has been applied to the male urethral glands, redescribed by him in 1697. His own writings, however, show Cowper to have been intelligent, reliably informed, and, on many occasions, original.

A brief biography would state that he was born in the small country town of Petersfield in Hampshire, England; apprenticed to a London surgeon at the age of sixteen years; admitted as a Barber-Surgeon in 1691; elected a Fellow of the Royal Society (to whose *Philosophical Transactions* he contributed). He then continued in surgical practice, scientific writing, and teaching until his early forties, when congestive cardiac failure necessitated an early retirement to the vicinity of his birthplace, where, shortly afterwards, he died.

The main facts relating to his plagiarism are these: he wrote a new text to illustrations that had previously appeared, as we have seen, in a book by the Dutch anatomist, Govard Bidloo, of which a Latin edition had been issued in 1685, a Dutch one in 1690 (see Chapter 8, p. 313). Cowper's publication, *The anatomy of humane bodies* ..., Oxford and London in 1698, gave no prominent acknowledgement either to Bidloo or to his artist, Lairesse. The most foolish aspect of this borrowing without permission or proper acknowledgement may be seen by comparing the nearly identical engraved title-pages of the two works. The English publishers had simply covered Bidloo's name with a pasted cut-out on which Cowper's had been printed. It is not certain how the blame should be apportioned—to Cowper, to his Oxford printers, to his London publishers, or to Bidloo's Amsterdam printers and publishers, who handed over impressions of the plates or the plates themselves. It was, however, inevitable that the deception would be discovered, and that Bidloo would be enraged. His attack on Cowper, directed to the Royal Society, was published in Leiden in 1700: *Gulielmus Cowper, criminis literarii citatus. . . .* This occasioned a milder rejoinder from Cowper two years later. The Royal Society refused to be drawn into the argument. It may be noted here that Bidloo had met Cowper in London, possibly in 1692, and was shown anatomical preparations.

F. J. Cole (1949) has pointed out that plagiarism was roundly condemned by many authors of the time (not excluding Cowper), but that nevertheless it was widely practised.[2] Publishers retained the right to sell the printed sheets of a work to any who applied, and the purchaser was permitted to publish under quite a different imprint. This was the case with the Cowper plagiarism, though here, at least, the text was original, and longer, than Bidloo's. Cowper added an appendix of nine plates, two of them drawn by Henry Cook; the other seven were probably by Cowper himself. All nine were engraved by an immigrant artist from Antwerp, Michael van der Gucht (1660–1725).

---

[2] Cowper, in *Myotomia reformata*, 1724, condemned Browne for his plagiarisms and then continued: 'Originals are few and rare; mankind finding it much easier to transcribe and steal, than to invent and improve . . .'.

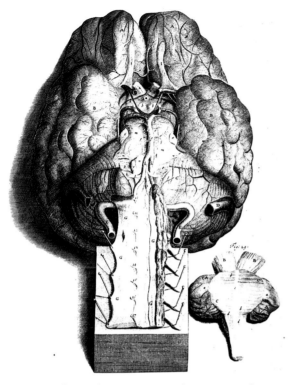

THE
ANATOMY
OF
HUMANE BODIES,
WITH FIGURES
DRAWN AFTER THE LIFE
BY SOME OF THE BEST MASTERS IN EUROPE,
AND CURIOUSLY ENGRAVEN IN ONE HUNDRED AND FORTEEN COPPER PLATES,
ILLUSTRATED WITH
LARGE EXPLICATIONS,
CONTAINING MANY NEW
ANATOMICAL DISCOVERIES,
AND
CHIRURGICAL OBSERVATIONS:
To which is Added an Introduction Explaining the
ANIMAL OECONOMY,
WITH A COPIOUS INDEX.
By WILLIAM COWPER.
REVISED AND PUBLISH'D
By C. B. ALBINUS.
PROFESSOR OF MEDICINE, ANATOMY, SURGERY AND PRACTICE,
In the UNIVERSITY OF UTRECHT.
The Second Edition.

LEYDEN,
Printed for JOH. ARN. LANGERAK,
And to be had in LONDON from Meſſ'ʳ INNYS and MANBY at the Weſt End of St. Paul's.

11.8   Base of brain from Cowper's *The anatomy of humane bodies*, 1698.

11.9   Title-page from Cowper's *The anatomy of humane bodies*, 1737.

These additional plates have been called perfunctory; but we differ from this opinion. The plate showing the base of the brain (*Fig. 11.8*) and that of the fetal arteries (*Plate 93*) are unusual and interesting. The two *écorché* plates are carefully and elegantly carried out. They were drawn from casts, of 'plaister of Paris', made from prepared cadavers; they would have made the work as a whole more useful for artists, and, perhaps, anatomists.

In the second edition of *The anatomy . . .*, 1737 Cowper's address to the reader acknowledges that:

These figures were drawn after the life, by the masterly painter G. de Lairess, and engravd by no less a hand, and represent the parts of the humane bodies far beyond any extant; and were some time since publish'd by Dr. Bidloo, now Professor of Anatomy in the University of Leyden. I have added above seven-hundred references, all of which are letter'd with a pen in the several figures . . .

Cowper in this edition reviews current anatomical and experimental findings related to human and, occasionally, animal structure and function, with some original contributions. The second, Leiden, edition (*Fig. 11.9*) was prepared by Cowper, but was edited by C. B. Albinus and published posthumously by J. A. Langerak, publisher also of some of B. S. Albinus' anatomical atlases and such influential works as A. C. Thebesius' *De circulo sanguinis in corde . . .*, 1716. The title-page of Cowper's book indicates that it was also available in London from Messrs Innys and Manby; they were printers and publishers for the Royal Society.

The dedication of the book is 'To the Right Honourable Charles Mountague' (1661–1715), a public man, supporter of William of Orange, President of the Royal Society, and an associate of John Locke and Isaac Newton.

Each of the two introductory sections of Cowper's *The anatomy of humane bodies . . .*: (*To the reader* and *The introduction explaining the animal oeconomy*) gives a list of significant discoveries in anatomy and physiology:

The present and last age, have been industrious in making discoveries in the animal machine, by detecting the structure of the heart, and artifice of the circulation, the origin and course of the lymphe-ducts, the several salival glands and their channels, the texture of bones, and medullary cells, the mucilaginous glands of the joints, the organs and process of generation, the organs of the external senses, in reforming the myology . . .

It can be seen that, after referring to the animal machine, Cowper selects the findings of Lower, Harvey, Aselli, Nuck, Wharton, de Graaf, Malpighi, Leeuwenhoek . . . as of major significance.

In *The introduction . . .*, Cowper lists 'the discoveries which the happy industry of the present age had made in the animal world . . .'. They are:

'the doctrine of the circulation of the blood' (1628: Harvey)

'the unity of the veins and arteries' (1661: Malpighi)

'the origin and distribution of the chyle and lympha' (various authors, beginning 1627: Aselli)

'the ovaria in females' (1672: de Graaf)

'the embriunculi [spermatozoa] in the masculine seed' (1667: van Leeuwenhoek)

A list prepared today of the contributions to basic medical science in the seventy years from 1628 might not be too different. The excitement of that period is well expressed by Cowper when he adds to this list the 'multitude of other curious observations we daily make by the help of microscopes, mercurial injections, and such like methods'. Microscopes and injections of one kind or another were major experimental tools of anatomists and physiologists for much of the eighteenth century.

Other anatomical and physiological matters were discussed by Cowper; but the above five subjects were selected by him as illustrating major scientific advances of his time. In each subject he has reviewed the literature well; he has moreover taken pains to give full acknowledgement to his predecessors and contemporaries, usually choosing authorities that we, even with the different perspective of hindsight, would also choose. Cowper attempts some independent observations and experiments. He recognizes when he is speculating; and he conjectures reasonably from the information available. His attitude to science is well expressed in a sentence from his other major book, *Myotomia reformata* ... (1724 edition):

One great mistake has obstructed the advancement of true knowledge, and that is a general opinion, that the senses are gross and ignoble, and that abstracted contemplations are the perfection of human nature, and so it comes to pass that man's mind is fed and pleased with chimaera's and shadows, instead of true substantial knowledge, which is only to be learnt from the true physical examination of things by sense and experiment.

This Baconian approach to medical sciences, shown in both his anatomy and his muscle book, was entirely appropriate for a surgeon and a Fellow of the Royal Society. It was the view of Hooke, and presages that of another scientific surgeon, John Hunter (1728–93).

The texts of both Cowper's *Anatomy* and his *Myotomia* were firmly within the new experimental science propagated by the Royal Society, which encouraged and appreciated Cowper. His work may be contrasted with that of another popular anatomy of about the same date—Thomas Gibson's *The anatomy of humane bodies epitomized* ..., London, 1682. Gibson (1647–1722) was a Fellow of the 'King's College of Physicians, London' but *not* of the Royal Society. He studied at and received his M D from the University of Leiden, unlike Cowper and other Barber-Surgeons, who had been trained by apprenticeship. The fourth edition of Gibson's *Anatomy*, 1694, almost contemporary with Cowper's, contains illustrations that truly are perfunctory. While his anatomical descriptions are well written—they are said to have been derived largely from Read's manual of anatomy, 1634—the physiological comments are scholarly and frequently speculative, but rely on cited authority, not on experiment.

After examining the informed text of Cowper's book, of which most of the plates were originally reproduced without permission or acknowledgement, one can more readily understand why its author was nevertheless well regarded in medical and scientific circles both in London and in Leiden. The Secretary of the Royal Society, Dr James Jurin, and the great Dr Richard Mead produced the second edition of Cowper's excellent book on muscles. An English-language edition of his book on anatomy was issued from Leiden, edited by C. B. Albinus and spoken for by Boerhaave and Haller, two dominant figures of European medicine. Written in the vernacular, but also translated into Latin (and published by the same firm) for those who did not speak English, the work was widely distributed, and served well at least two generations of medical men, introducing them to the findings of gross and microscopic anatomy, while at the same time propagating the attitudes of experimental enquiry.

Cowper's major wholly original publication was *Myotomia reformata: or, a new administration of all the muscles of humane bodies* ..., London, 1694. This was dedicated to, among others, Edward Tyson, physician and admirable comparative anatomist, who in 1698 dissected a young chimpanzee during his demonstrations in anatomy before the Barber-Surgeons. Cowper was to assist him in illustrating the publication on the anatomy of these apes, *Orang-outang* [sic], *sive Homo sylvestris, or the anatomy of a pygmie* [sic], London, 1699.

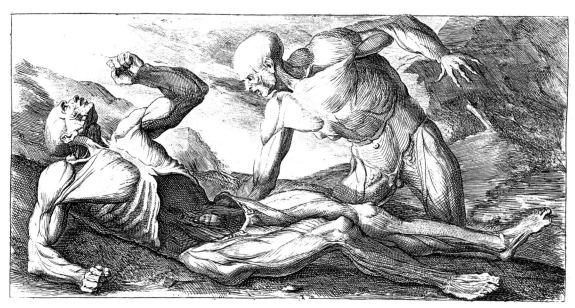

11.10 Two muscle-men from Cowper's *Myotomia reformata*, 1724.

The first edition of *Myotomia* was a modest octavo volume. It begins with a history of myology which even now would be worth reprinting. Cowper writes systematically of the muscles of the body, from Chapter 1: *Of the muscles of the abdomen*, to Chapter 36: *Of the muscles of the four lesser toes*. An appendix discusses the penis, and the manner of its erection. In this edition there are ten plates containing eighteen figures. The second edition, published thirteen years after Cowper's death, is a much grander volume, a beautifully produced folio, with more than sixty plates: our *Plate 94* is taken from this 1724 edition. Richard Mead's 'advertisement' describes how the

author had finished the plates of this book a little before his death, and was preparing to put in order the text, when he found his weakness, occasioned by frequent fits of an asthma, which had brought him into a dropsy, to grow upon him so fast, that he should not be able to complete his design ... [Cowper] delivered his papers into my hands, and desired me ... to take care of the publication of the book.

Mead persuaded Dr James Jurin to sort out Cowper's text, and had Dr Henry Pemberton, editor of Newton's *Principia*, 1726, write an essay on the physics of 'muscular motion'. In spite of these delays, the book as published in 1724 was, Mead stated, more complete than any other produced in English or in any other language up to that time.

As Cowper explains:

The outlines of some of these figures are drawn after Rafael, Sir Peter Paul Rubens, Guido Reni, Mons. Le Fage; but the muscling is done after several human subjects, and not copied from any anatomical book whatever.

Cowper thought the figures of the more superficial muscles would be of use not only to surgeons but also to 'those who bend their studies to the admirable arts of sculpture and painting ...'—arts which Cowper had studied, and in which he was proficient.

There are many conceits in the production of this remarkable book(*Fig. 11.10*). Not the least interesting are the decorative initial letters; for example, a letter G in Chapter VIII: *Of the muscles of the eye-lids*, is decorated with a drawing of these muscles (*Fig. 11.11*).

Cowper's name has long been associated with the epithet *plagiarist*; it is time we also noted his contributions to didactic, investigative, comparative, and surgical anatomy.

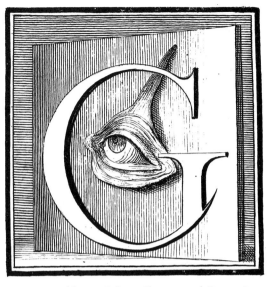

11.11 Initial letter G from Chapter 8 of Cowper's *Myotomia reformata*, 1723.

93 Fetal arterial system. Third table of Appendix to W. Cowper, *Anatomy of humane bodies . . .*, 1698. Engraving (Cambridge University Library). 54.2 × 31.3 cm.

The Appendix consists of 'muscle-men' and 'divers parts of the humane bodies which are either omitted or not well exprest' in the main portion of the book. This large folded diagram is of the arterial system of the fetus injected with wax and then dissected.

One fears that considerable artistic licence was involved in producing such a diagram from a cast; it is reminiscent of similar portrayals of the arterial system that had appeared some two hundred years earlier.

Errors and misinterpretations abound. Thomas Willis would surely have gnashed his teeth to see 'his' circle so abused; the right brachial artery is clearly shown trifurcating (only the radial branch receives a symbol, perhaps because it 'makes the pulse'), and no palmar arches are depicted; the aorta and ductus arteriosus appear as twin vessels, and the origin of the coronary arteries is bizarre. The internal pudendal arteries (60) receive short shrift—they might as well be called the penile arteries; the common carotid arteries do not divide into internal and external branches (how could this be not noticed?), but instead sprout wild arteries from a common trunk.

However, enough is enough; one has to be satisfied with the correct portrayal of the (large) umbilical arteries (56), even if the urinary bladder receives a poor blood-supply.

Figures 4 and 5 are microscopial renderings of the veins and arteries in the fin of a fish. Figure 6 purports to show the origin of a lymphatic vessel (c), while Figure 7 (perhaps best ignored) is said to depict 'the manner of the origin of the excretory ducts'.

It can truthfully be stated that Cowper, bereft here of Bidloo, did little to immortalize himself with these illustrations: to this end his eponymous glands must suffice.

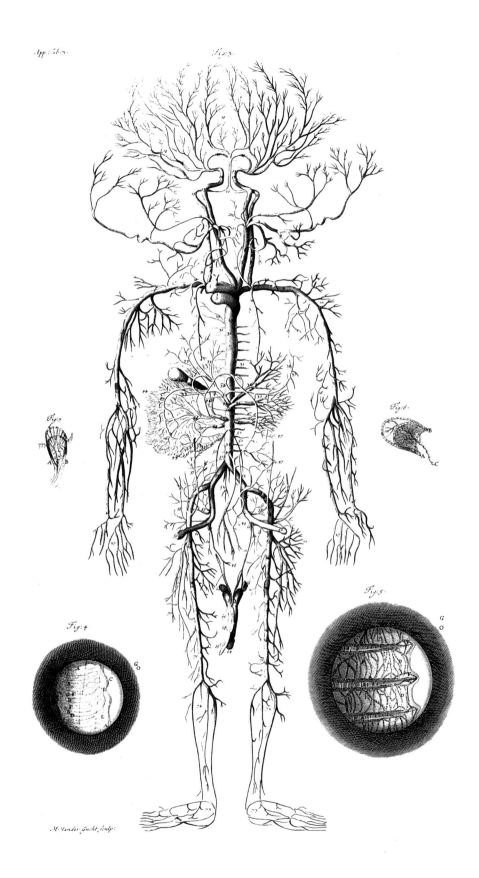

PLATE 93

94 Superficial musculature. Table XXI from W. Cowper, *Myotomia reformata . . .,* 1724. Engraving (Cambridge University Library). 26.5 × 19.7 cm.

This is the first of two drawings designed to show the facial musculature, the dissection shown here being more superficial than the one following it.

The thin sheet of muscle fibres (18), termed 'quadratus genae' (although the name 'platysma' was used by Galen) is shown covering most of the neck, spreading down over pectoralis major; this latter muscle is not labelled, and its relation to the platysma is not made very clear. One might consider that *all* was the platysma; for example, in the text, (19) is listed as platysma 'over the buccinator', but one would not look for it to do this, nor for it seemingly to cover the masseter, shown between the parotid gland (H) and (19). Evidently Cowper considered the platysma to be more extensive than in fact it is now considered to be.

The appearance of the various facial muscles is very much as they would be seen at a dissection—more true to life than many of the more modern renderings. However, the occipitalis appears to be continuous with the sternomastoid, and is rather too prominent, as is also (D), termed 'elevator auriculae'.

Apart from the over-emphasis of the platysma this is a most strikingly honest and accurate drawing; it is of interest to compare it with a similar drawing by Charles Bell (see *Plate 105* p. 497) some seventy-five years later. One particularly admires the rendering of the deltoid (L), the slips of serratus anterior (P), and biceps brachii (O).

TAB.XXI.

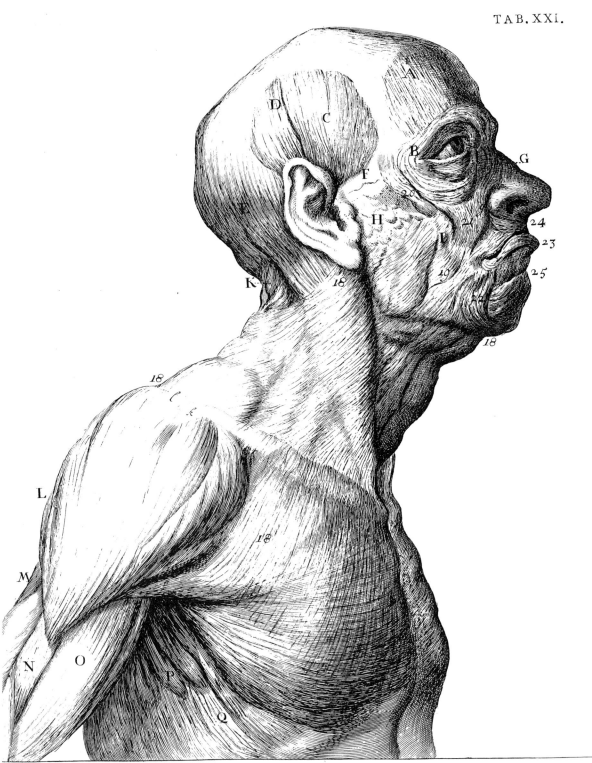

18. *Quadratus Genæ, seu Quad.Colli*.
19. *Buccinator Quadrato Genæ tectus*.
20. *Zygomaticus*.
21. *Elevator Labiorum*.

22. *Depressor Labiorum*.
23. *Orbicularis Labiorum*.
24. *Elevator labii superioris proprius*.
25. *Depressor labii inferioris proprius*.

PLATE 94

William Cheselden (1688–1752)

During the first years of the eighteenth century, there were in London at least three centres of anatomical investigation and training: classes were given by George Rolfe in his house; James Douglas was active; and Cowper was at work until he retired in 1709. However, from 1711 and for the next twenty-five years, another surgeon, William Cheselden, became the foremost teacher of anatomy in the metropolis.

Cheselden was born to a farming family, owners of a small estate in Burrough on the Hill near Leicester, in the midlands of England. At the age of fifteen he was apprenticed to James Ferne, a surgeon at St Thomas's Hospital. (Payments of from £150 to £400 were made to such a master surgeon when a young man was indentured.) He is said to have learned his anatomy from William Cowper, 'with whom he resided'.

In 1711 Cheselden, only a few months after he had taken his examinations and had been admitted to the Barber-Surgeons' company, advertised a course of instruction in anatomy consisting of 35 lectures, five a week for seven weeks. The course was to be given four times a year, with no work being done during the hot summer months of June to August, when prolonged dissections were not possible. 'First we teach the osteology; after that the enterology in brutes, then in humane bodies together with the muscles as they arise in dissection and in both comparative and

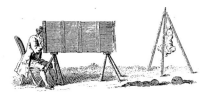

THE

ANATOMY

OF THE

HUMAN BODY.

BY

W. CHESELDEN,

Surgeon to his Majesty's *Royal Hospital* at CHELSEA
Fellow of the ROYAL SOCIETY.
And Member of
The *Royal Academy of Surgeons* at PARIS

THE Xᵀᴴ EDITION

with FORTY COPPER PLATES
Engrav'd by *Ger: Vandergucht*.

LONDON.

Printed for W. Johnston, Hawes, Clarke, Collins,
J. Dodsley, R. Baldwin, W. Nicoll and T. Cadell.

——— 1773. ———

11.12 Title-page from Cheselden's *The anatomy of the human body*, 1773.

humane anatomy.' The prospectus for the course was published: *Syllabus sive index humani corporis* ..., London, 1711.

When Cheselden was twenty-five, he published the first edition of a book for his classes, one that was to stay in print in Britain until 1792; this was *The anatomy of the humane body*, 1713. The format was a modest and handy octavo, illustrated at first with 23 plates; in the 1740 edition there were 40 plates. The originals had been engraved by various artists, but the 1740 plates were all re-engraved by Gerard van der Gucht. Some of the figures were taken from James Douglas's projected osteology, and the debt to Douglas is acknowledged in the book. *The anatomy of the humane body*, which until 1750 also contained the syllabus of Cheselden's lecture course, was not too expensive—five shillings a copy for two of the early editions, later nine shillings on small paper, fifteen shillings on large. There were arrangements whereby earlier editions could be returned by students with credit towards the later issues. Many thousands of copies were probably printed before 1749, when Cheselden sold the copyright to two London bookseller-publishers. This property was still sufficiently valuable for shares to have been sold in 1771 and again in 1778. *Figure 11.12* shows the title-page of the tenth edition, 1773.

However, Cheselden's career was not restricted to the teaching of anatomy: in 1718 he was appointed a surgeon to St Thomas's Hospital. His work there included amputations, operations for cataract, and, after a probationary period of two years, removal of bladder-stones. It was in these last two fields that Cheselden achieved pre-eminence as a surgeon. His ophthalmology patients included Alexander Pope, who appreciated his advice. Pope, recognizing his own physical disabilities, wrote:

Weak tho' I am of limb and short of sight,
Far from a lynx, and not a giant quite,
I'll do what Mead & Cheselden advise,
To keep these limbs, and to preserve these eyes.

OSTEOGRAPHIA,

OR THE

ANATOMY

OF THE

BONES.

BY WILLIAM CHESELDEN

SURGEON TO HER MAJESTY;

F. R. S.

SURGEON TO ST THOMAS'S HOSPITAL,

AND MEMBER OF THE ROYAL ACADEMY OF SURGERY AT PARIS.

LONDON MDCCXXXIII.

11.13 Title-page from Cheselden's *Osteographia*, 1733.

Cheselden's anatomical and surgical proficiency in devising and carrying out novel ways of cutting for bladder-stone was outstanding. He took, it was said, from thirty seconds to three minutes to complete the removal of a stone, with an overall death-toll in 213 operations of 30, that is, a rate of less than 15 per cent. The record of this enumeration of the results of surgical intervention was an early example of quantitation in clinical medicine; Cheselden was elected a Fellow of the Royal Society in 1721, and may well have been influenced by the statistical work of the Society under the Presidency of Isaac Newton. (James Jurin, secretary of the Royal Society in the early 1720s, was demonstrating statistically the effectiveness of smallpox inoculation.)

Cheselden in nineteen years at St Thomas's took sixty-four pupils, charging twenty-four guineas a time. He also had at least six apprentices, who paid increasingly large amounts for this privilege. New hospitals were being established, and Cheselden became associated with some of these; about 1724, he joined the Westminster Infirmary; in 1733 he was a lithotomist, and later a governor, of St George's. In 1737 or 1738, Cheselden left these positions to reside at The Royal Hospital, Chelsea, a home for the custodial, and incidentally medical, care of old soldiers. While in semi-retirement as the surgeon to this hospital, he continued in private practice, but operated less frequently.

Cheselden was a prime mover and perhaps the chief orchestrator in the separation of the Surgeons from the Barber-Surgeons in 1745, a separation that appears to have been accomplished with less rancour than one might have expected. It is possible that Cheselden had determined to effect this since his earliest years as an anatomist, when the Barber-Surgeons censored him for conducting private dissections in competition with the official anatomies at their Hall.

From his professional work, Cheselden became wealthy, charging rich patients as much as £500 for an operation. He used his excess income in interesting ways. Even as early as 1714, he had sufficient funds to invest £1000 in South Seas Stock; in 1728 he put up a similar amount to form a company that built a wooden bridge at Fulham, up-river from Lambeth and Chelsea. He also used his money for charity. He was a contributor to the Foundling Hospital, and gave sums towards the building of a hall for the new Surgeons' Company. In 1733, Cheselden published an anatomical book that, unlike his earlier, popular volume was not intended to have a wide sale or to make a substantial profit; in the event the book is said to have incurred an expenditure of more than £1500. The work was *Osteographia, or the anatomy of the bones*, published in 1733 in London with no printer, publisher, or bookseller named; the work was to be obtained from Cheselden directly (*Fig. 11.13*). This book, reviewed as 'the most magnificent work of its kind now extant', may be described in Cheselden's own words. In the remarks *To the reader* he wrote:

Every bone in the human body being here delineated as large as the life ... I thought it useless to make long descriptions, one view of such prints shewing more than the fullest and best description can possibly do; and for this reason ... the mechanical contrivancies of the bones are rather treated of than their shapes.

He tried out various methods for reproducing the configuration of the bones in a two-dimensional format, eventually deciding to make use of the camera obscura, as illustrated on the title-page:

I contrived (what I had long before meditated) a convenient camera obscura to draw in, with which we corrected some of the few designs already made, and finished the rest with more accuracy and less labour, doing in this way in a few minutes more than could be done without in many hours, I might say in many days ... my engravers, Mr. Vandergucht and Mr. Shinevoet ... knew too well the difficulties of representing irregular lines, perspect-ive, and proportion, to despise such assistance, always declaring that it was impossible to do these things so well without.

Concerning the camera obscura, Cheselden writes in chapter eight:

About six inches within that end where the drafts-man sits, is fixed the table glass, upon the rough side of which he draws with a black-lead pencil, which he afterwards traces off upon paper; towards the other end, in a sliding frame, is put the [convex] object-glass, which being moved backwards or forward, makes the picture bigger or less, and the inside of the case is made black to prevent reflections of light.

John Belchier, surgeon and pupil of Cheselden, reviewed the book in the *Philo-sophical Transactions*, November, 1733. He is the man arranging the skeleton on the tripod in the illustration on the title-page to the *Osteographia*.

The book was issued with two sets of plates, each set consisting of 56 folio plates, 'one set unlettered to shew them in their full beauty, and one set lettered for explanations' (see *Figs. 11.14a and b*). The original sketches for the plates are owned by the Royal Academy, and are on loan to the Royal College of Surgeons of London.

The finished drawings and the engraving and etching of 53 of the 56 large plates of human osteology:

were done by Mr. Gerard Vandergucht, and how great an artist he is, the open free stile in which these plates are etched and engraved, and the inimitable manner of expressing the different tex-tures of the parts sufficiently show.

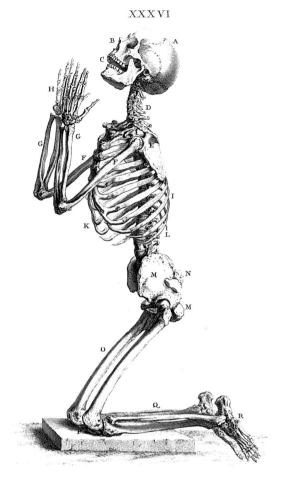

TABLE XXXVI.

THE fide view of the fceleton of a very robuft man, put into this attitude to reprefent the figure in a larger fcale.

A *The bones of the cranium.*
B *The bones of the face.*
C *The jaws.*
D *The fpinal proceffes of the vertebræ of the neck.*
E *Scapula.*
F F *Os humeri.*
G G *Radius & ulna.*
H *The bones of the hand.*
I *The ribs.*
K *The cartilages of the fternum.*
L *The fpinal proceffes of the vertebræ of the loins.*
M M *Os innominatum.*
N *Os facrum.*
O *Os femoris.*
P *Patella.*
Q *Tibia and fibula.*
R *The bones of the feet.*

11.14 a & b Lettered plate of praying skeleton (above) with explanatory key (below) from Cheselden's *Osteographia . . ., 1733.*

The small plates, except two, and three of the larger plates were engraved by:

Shinevoet who left Holland, his native country, on account of misfortunes ... his manner of etching, though wonderfully neat and expressive, and well suited to such things as he was mostly employed in, is nevertheless much inferior in stile to that of Mr. Vandergucht.

Cheselden described his role in the preparation of the plates:

The actions of all the sceletons ... were my own choice: and where particular parts needed to be more distinctly expressed on account of the anatomy, there I always directed; sometimes in the drawings with the pencil, and often with the needle upon the copper plate.... The expressing the smoothness of the ends of the bones by engraving only with single lines, while the other parts were all etched, was also my contriving ...

Cheselden had made an effort to train himself as a draughtsman, but it is not certain how much he contributed to the actual drawings. Cheselden's original intentions were to prepare a complete work on human and comparative anatomy:

when I begin this work I intended a whole system of anatomy adorned with the comparative, in three volumes in this manner, provided I found any encouragement.

It is to be regretted that Cheselden was unable to complete his plans.

In 1735, John Douglas published an attack on Cheselden entitled, *Animadversions on a late pompous book, intituled, Osteographia....* Included in this pamphlet are criticisms of the pretensions of Cheselden as an artist, who, Douglas said, could not be compared with William Cowper in this respect.

John Douglas had been Cheselden's predecessor as lithotomist at the Westminster Infirmary, and probably felt he had been unjustly supplanted. Douglas was himself preparing an *Osteographia anatomico-practica*, which was advertised in 1735, but never saw the light of day. Cheselden seems, however, to have remained on friendly terms with James Douglas, the brother of John, and the subject of the next section.

95 Child's skeleton. Table 33 from W. Cheselden, *Osteographia ...,* 1733. Engraving (private collection). 37.8 × 22.9 cm.

This portrays the skeleton of a nine-year-old boy, with his left arm resting negligently on a horse's skull, the latter being included so as to indicate scale, or show the size of the boy.

The lower remnant of the frontal or metopic suture is present. The angulation of the ramus of the mandible is correct; but the arrangement of the 'teeth' is obscure. The caption states: 'C, the jaws in which the teeth are newly changed'; as the bone of the anterior portions of both mandible and maxilla seem to extend to the margins, one gets the impression of sockets rather

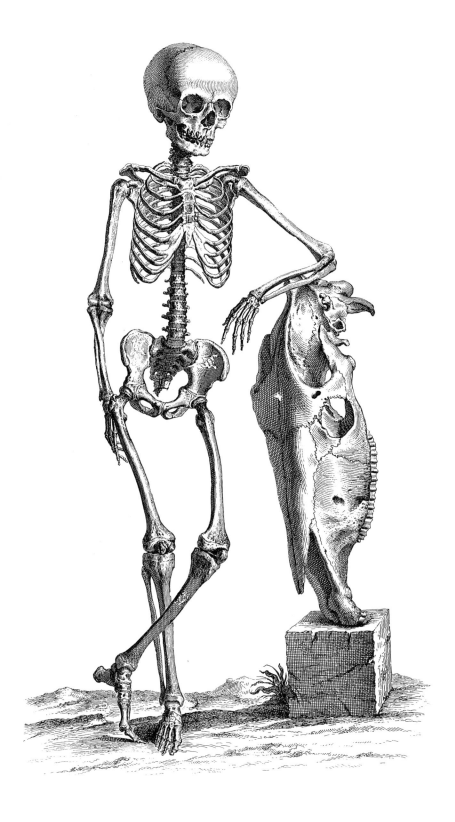

PLATE 95

than teeth. Both incisors, first premolar, and first molar of the permanent dentition would be expected to have erupted by this age.

There is a suspicion of a bicipital groove on the right humerus, but no real greater tuberosity is shown. The coracoid processes point too laterally, no doubt owing to the scapula's being positioned too far dorsal on the chest wall. The anterior aspect of the proximal part of the right ulna is rather too massive.

The clavicles articulate inaccurately too low on the manubrium; and, probably as a result of this, the first and second ribs (particularly on the left side) both appear erroneously to articulate with the manubrio-sternal joint cartilage. The rib interspaces, particularly the upper ones, are too wide, and the ribs themselves are too thin; the tenth rib is 'floating'.

The vertebral column has an unpleasing 'straight' look about it, and the gap between the iliac crest and rib border is ludicrously large. The drawing of the sacrum is not felicitous, and one receives little impression either of the concavity of the false pelvis, or that the true pelvis is basin-shaped.

The right tibial medial malleolus is inaccurately shown extending more distally than the lateral; and the tarsal skeleton in both feet is crudely drawn. The articulation between the femoral head and the socket formed by the triradiate cartilage is very awkwardly portrayed.

96 'Praying' male skeleton. Table 36 from W. Cheselden, *Osteographia . . .*, 1733. Engraving (private collection). 40.2 × 25.5 cm.

This is the skeleton of 'a very robust man', posed so that the drawing could be on a larger scale than would be possible if the skeleton were shown in the erect posture. The pose also affords an opportunity to illustrate the cervical, dorsal, and lumbar curves of the vertebral column.

No suture is seen in the zygomatic arch, and, as in *Plate 95*, not a great deal of care has been taken in portraying the teeth—they all look much the same. The inferior ramus of the mandible now possesses a mental foramen, which was not shown in the boy's skeleton.

The medial ends of the clavicle are now placed in their correct, seemingly unstable, position with regard to the manubrium; and, again accurately, only the second rib articulates at the well-defined manubrio-sternal angle.

The left humerus displays both greater (not very distinct) and lesser tuberosities, with a well-marked groove between them for the tendon of the long head of biceps. The forearm bones are, however, too 'wavy', as also are the ribs. Once again the tenth rib is floating (this seems an *ideé fixe* of Cheselden's; all his skeletons, both young and old, feature this); and the eleventh rib is surely a great deal too long.

Something, alas, appears very wrong in the area of the pelvic girdle. The lower lumbar part of the vertebral column is placed far too anteriorly with regard to the ilium, and what one can see of the sacrum suggests it to be inclined almost horizontally backwards. The upper part of

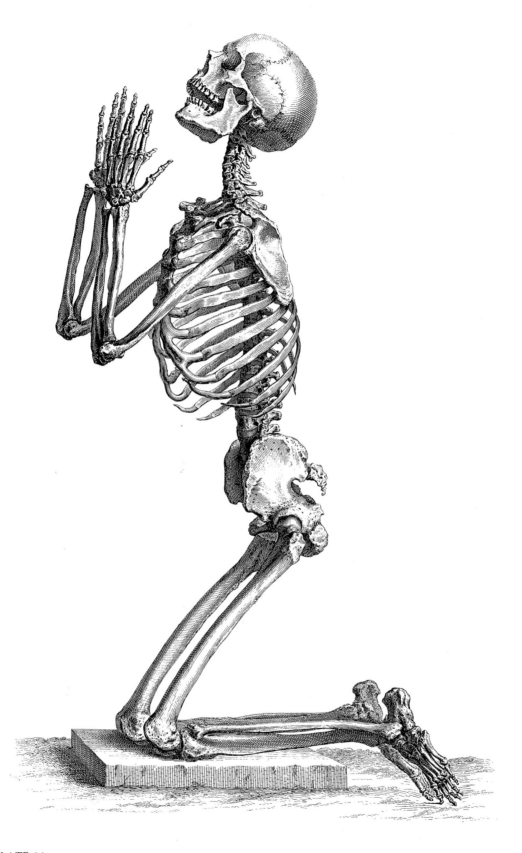

PLATE 96

the pubic symphysis, the ischial spine (shown with the end chipped off), and the tip of the coccyx certainly do not lie on the same horizontal plane, as they should do.

The anterior bowing of the femur is well illustrated, and the large and small radii of the femoral condyles (particularly the left) are well suggested. The depiction of the carpal and tarsal bones is better than before, although the talo-navicular articulation is inaccurate (it looks like a wavy plane joint); and the fifth metatarsal is over-curved.

It should be stated that in others of Cheselden's illustrations there are good and accurate portrayals of the carpal and tarsal bones. Indeed, in several drawings, the articulations between the clavicle and ribs and the manubrium and sternum are correctly shown. It may be that, for some reason, he was not too concerned with the true appearance of the bones in his whole-skeleton plates. For example, the sacrum is very poor indeed in all of them. Nowhere is there to be found a really decent drawing of this bone; where it is best depicted (in his Plate 12) it is composed of six segments, instead of the much more usual five.

To many, perhaps the most fascinating section of the *Osteographia* is that devoted to remarkable drawings of numerous diseased bones and joints.

James Douglas (1675–1745)

James Douglas was born at Baads, near Edinburgh. His medical education was on the continent of Europe, partly at Utrecht. He graduated MD in 1699 from Rheims, and returned to practise in London, becoming first a licenciate and then, in 1721 an honorary Fellow of the (London) College of Physicians. He was a notable obstetrician—Alexander Pope wrote of his 'soft obstetric hand'; and he eventually became a Physician Extraordinary to Queen Caroline, wife of George II. He had probably been associated with Paul Chamberlen in his obstetrical practice during the period 1700–12. He was elected FRS in 1706.

Douglas was a physician in the humanist tradition, with extraordinarily wide and scholarly interests: he contributed to botanical science and to etymology and linguistics, and formed a notable collection of editions of Horace; above all he was an assiduous and careful anatomist. His most popular anatomy book concerned muscles: *Myographiae . . . a comparative description of all the muscles in a man and in a quadruped . . .*, London, 1707. Eight editions in English were published, from London, Edinburgh, and Dublin. The *Myographiae* was to be the first of a six-part work to complete the anatomy of the whole person; but only the first volume was issued. Douglas's bibliography of anatomy, in Latin, was published from London: *Bibliographiae anatomicae . . .*, 1715; it was also issued in Leiden in 1734, an edition prepared by B. S. Albinus.

The anatomically accurate work *A description of the peritonaeum . . .* by Douglas was published in London by J. Roberts in 1730, with other editions: Helmstad, 1733 and Leiden, 1737. The author was considered by John Freind, in *The history of physick . . .*, 1725–6, to have been the first to give us any true idea of the peritoneum. The work was the result of painstaking dissections done to aid his brother, the surgeon John Douglas, in developing a high operation for the removal of bladder-stones.

Douglas was one of the first to set up private classes in anatomy in London. He took these classes in his own house, first near Fleet Street, then in Bow Lane, Cheapside, then in Covent Garden, and, finally, further west in Red Lion Square. An advertisement issued before 1707 described the syllabus—or objectives—of the course: *An account of what Dr. Douglas obliges himself to perform in a course of human and comparative anatomy.* The syllabus was also included as an appendix to Douglas's *Myographiae.* Not only were dissections performed during the course and dried preparations shown, but injections were also made with wax and mercury into the excretory ducts of glands.

The results of Douglas's researches were included in eleven books and in a number of papers in the Royal Society's *Philosophical Transactions,* but these published works represent merely the visible part of his literary activity. A number of other works were prepared, but never published, even though manuscripts often reached an advanced stage of completion, with illustrations drawn, and engraved at great expense, and proof-prints taken.

One of Douglas's projected, but unpublished, works was an *osteographia,* which had reached a preliminary stage as early as 1713, and a secondary stage in 1717, with revisions made over the rest of his life. Douglas was early interested in the skeleton, and was Gale lecturer for the Barber-Surgeons on this subject in 1712. The work was advertised at the back of his botanical book, *Lilium sarniense ...,* 1725; it was to contain 'all the bones in an adult human body, drawn and engraved by the best masters in a great variety of instructive views, and all as large as life ... this great work will follow as speedily as the business of his profession can permit'. Prints of sixty engravings for this *osteographia* exist in the (William) Hunterian Collection in Glasgow University; some of the accompanying text is also preserved, including a fine history of osteology, listing all previous osteological illustrations known to Douglas. In 1727 he prepared an account of the book for the Royal Society; Douglas promised to give the 'weights and dimensions of every bone in one sceleton with the chemical analysis of the whole ...'—quite proper investigations in the context of the Royal Society's interest in quantitation and medical chemistry. Douglas's proposed introduction, in the Hunterian papers, states that he will include:

1. Each single bone of the entire body, and one of such as are double, separated from all the rest, as large as the life, and in all different views ...

2. All the articulations of bone designed for manifest motion ... [see *Fig. 11.15*]

3. The natural situations of all the other bones with respect to one another whose motion is more obscure ...

4. The compages or system of all the bones in different views of the sceleton.

He also proposed to show the structure of the interior of bones (see *Plate 97*).

William Hunter, in his *Two introductory lectures,* 1784, seventy years after Douglas had completed half the book, described the anatomical plate-books of the bones: 'We have had four

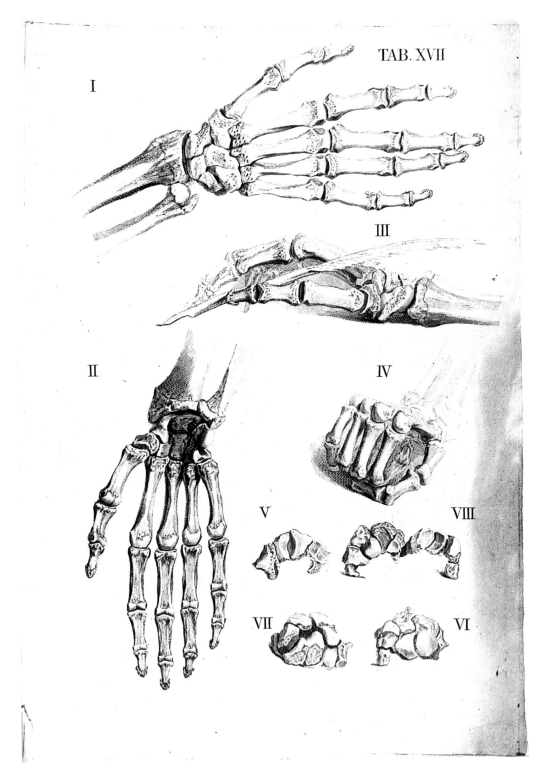

11.15 Bones of the hand from James Douglas's MS drawings *c.* 1715.

large folio books of figures of bones, viz Cheselden's, Albinus's, Sue's and Trew's, besides one which was long expected from my old master and friend, Dr James Douglas, and, which I wish to have time to publish, as the plates are all in my possession'. Hunter had made corrections to the proofs pulled from Douglas's plates. Hunter did not complete this project, but one set of plates was sent to B. S. Albinus—both Douglas and Hunter knew the Dutch anatomist.

Another work that Douglas prepared, but did not publish, was 'Gyneciorum prodromus or an introduction to the knowledge and cure of the diseases incident to women and the improvement of the practice of midwifery'. To accompany this work, Douglas had drawn many anatomical illustrations, similar to those in the atlases of Smellie and of Hunter; one, for instance, of the external female genitalia is very similar to Smellie's figure. Others are of babies *in utero*—six months to full term; there is a careful drawing of the relaxed pubic symphysis during parturition, showing the fetal head dilating the cervix; and there are drawings of dissections of the muscular (*Plate 98*) and vascular systems of the fetus.

James Douglas received a grant to pursue these studies on the bones and the reproductive system: 'his Majesty has been graciously pleased by a gratuity of five hundred pounds, to encourage and enable Dr. James Douglas ... to communicate the observations and discoveries he has made in anatomy, both human and comparative ...'. It was not the only time that a grant has been well used by medical scientists, who have then failed to communicate their results.

Undoubtedly Douglas's books on the bones and on the gravid uterus would have stood comparison with the plate-books of Cheselden and Hunter respectively. It is indeed probable that these latter were, in some important respects, derived from Douglas's work.

Some early drawings for Douglas of the anatomy of bones were by François Boitard (1670–1715), who had also worked in France and Holland. His son, Louis Pierre Boitard, contributed very clear drawings. Others were also French—Claude Dubusc, Charles Dupuis, and Bernard Baron. The first two had been brought over to England to engrave the Raphael cartoons, and the last named was employed by Dr Richard Mead to engrave the *Story of Ulysses* from designs by Rubens.

Both Michael van der Gucht (1660–1725) and his son, Gerard (born 1697) engraved for Douglas as well as for William Cowper and for Cheselden. A medical man, James Parson (1705–70), worked for Douglas as his assistant and artist from 1736. He was a careful and accurate artist, employing—like most others working for anatomists in the eighteenth century—coloured crayons (sometimes black or red, and white crayon on grey paper) for the drawings from which the engraver worked.

97 The mandible. *Tabula octava de osse maxillae inferioris.* James Douglas, MS figures, *c.*1715 (DF7(49) Hunterian collection, Glasgow University Library). 33.4 × 27.7 cm.

The mandible featured on the left is most likely to be from a young person, as there is no indication of either of the third molar teeth; the letter (F) embraces both premolars and molars. The angle of the mandible is somewhat everted, suggesting a male bone.

In the upper drawing the mental foramen is correctly positioned midway between the premolar teeth; but it is placed rather too posteriorly in Figure III.

In the right (IV) the mandibular foramen, lingula, and mylohyoid groove and line are excellent. The mandibular canal and root-sockets of a full dentition are shown in V; compact and cancellous bone-structure is well demonstrated in the lower two drawings.

Nowadays James Douglas is best remembered by the eponymous 'pouch of Douglas' (recto-uterine pouch) and the 'semilunar fold of Douglas', where the posterior rectus sheath becomes formed only by transversalis fascia and peritoneum. However, the latter was never described by Douglas; and, as to the former, in his *Description of the Peritonaeum*, he writes:

where the peritonaeum leaves the foreside of the rectum, it makes an angle, and changes its course upwards and forwards over the bladder; and a little above this angle there is a remarkable transverse stricture or semioval fold of the peritonaeum, which I have constantly observed for many years past, especially in women.

This description is as close as Douglas comes to a description of 'his' pouch (the 'angle'). It is odd that the first use of the term 'pouch of Douglas' was seemingly late in the nineteenth century.

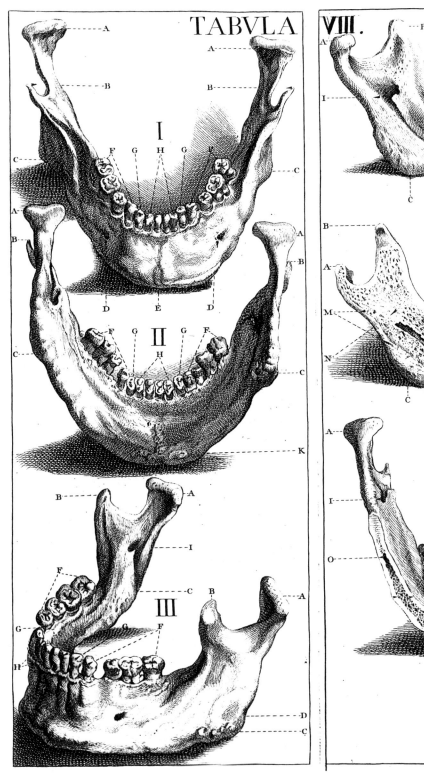
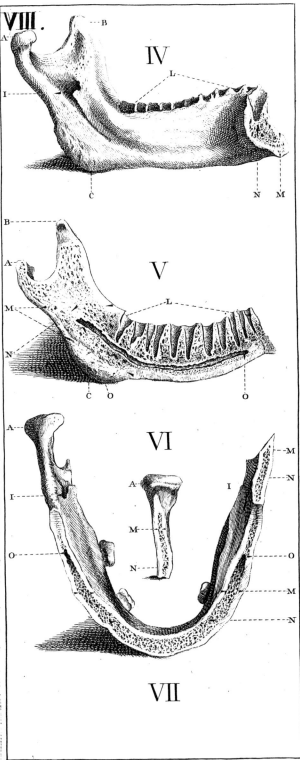

TABVLA VIII.

I

II

III

IV

V

VI

VII

PLATE 97

98 Fetal *écorché*. Tab. 13. James Douglas, ᴍs figure, *c*.1715 (DF86 (12) Hunterian collection, Glasgow University Library). 26.5 × 21.7 cm.

This is a most unusual drawing of a skinned fetus—'In this I have showed the muscles that lye next to the outer integuments . . .'.

Impressions of blood-vessels (not very accurate) can be made out on the skull, together with a very faint frontalis muscle. The orbicularis oculi, temporalis, and masseter muscles, together with a small stylized parotid gland, can clearly be seen. However, the ear is peculiarly positioned, as is the uppermost part of sterno-mastoid. The deltoid, infraspinatus, and teres muscles are shown lying between trapezius and latissimus dorsi. The shoulder, drawn forwards and medially, enables a part of the rhomboid major muscle to be viewed. On the lateral side of the abdomen lies the external oblique, with some of its serrated origin.

The tendons of the extensor muscles of the forearm are well portrayed, including the twin tendons to the little and index fingers, and also the tendon of abductor pollicis longus crossing those of the radial wrist extensors.

In the buttock region gluteus maximus and medius are featured, together with tensor fasciae latae inserting into a (displaced) ilio-tibial tract; in the thigh are the vasti and hamstrings, with the biceps femoris tendon (rather thin) inserting into the head of the fibula. The muscles of the anterior compartment of the leg, together with the peronei and superficial muscles of the calf, can also be seen. One notices that the little toe is longer than the fourth.

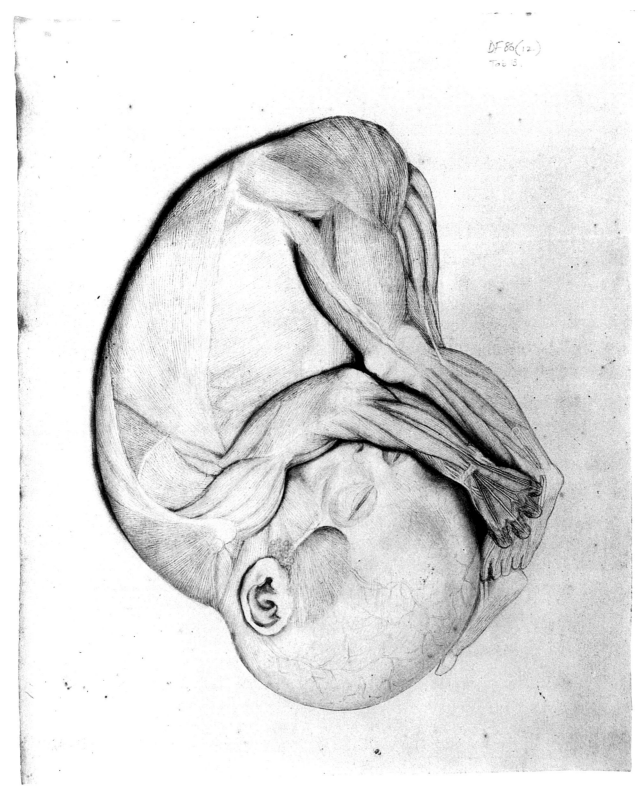

PLATE 98

Alexander Monro primus, *1697–1767*

The University of Edinburgh was given its first charter as the town college in 1583; but its school of medicine was not finally established until 1726. Edinburgh surgeons had supported the practical study of anatomy much earlier; a surgeons' hall and anatomy theatre had been built at the end of the seventeenth century. A public dissection was made in 1703 on the corpse of David Mylles, hanged for incest with his sister. In 1705, a teacher of anatomy was appointed by the town—Robert Eliot; he dissected a human subject once every two or three years. The person who was to dominate Edinburgh anatomy for the first forty years of the medical school was, however, the first Alexander Monro.

Monro's father, John Monro (1670–1740) was born in Edinburgh, where he was apprenticed to surgeons. He completed his medical education at Leiden, staying there two years. He was a British army surgeon for some while, and then returned early in the new century to Edinburgh, where he set up as a surgeon-apothecary, later becoming Deacon (or President) of the Surgeons. (Many Edinburgh surgeons practised also as apothecaries.) From this and other important civic responsibilities he was instrumental in creating the circumstances in which the Edinburgh medical school was established. John's son, Alexander, had been born during the time the family was residing in London. He was apprenticed as a young man to his father, and attended courses in anatomy given by Eliot and his successors. He completed his education in London, where he attended various courses, notably those given by Cheselden. Using Vesalius as a guide, he dissected on his own account. While in London, he was part of the Scottish medical fraternity there: when he acquired a severe suppurative infection from a dissection wound he consulted James Douglas. During this period, he sent to Edinburgh several anatomical preparations, which John Monro, always assiduous in promoting his son's welfare, divided between the College of Physicians there and the Edinburgh Barber-Surgeons. (The barbers and surgeons separated in 1722.) The Museum of the Royal College of Surgeons of Edinburgh has to this day a mahogany case containing a skeleton inscribed 'These anatomical preparations were gifted to the Incorporation of Chirurgian Apothecaries of Ed. by Alexr. Monro 1718'.

Alexander Monro then spent time on the continent of Europe; in 1718 in Paris, attending courses in botany and chemistry at the *Jardin du Roi*, and in medicine, surgery, and 'accouchemens' at the Charité and the Hôtel-Dieu; and in Leiden, where he was under Boerhaave for instruction in chemistry and clinical medicine. While in the Netherlands, he visited Ruysch, who as usual demonstrated his baroque anatomical preparations.

Alexander Monro returned home to Edinburgh in the autumn in 1719, and, after examination, was admitted as a surgeon. His father insisted that he gave public lectures immediately, and brought along the President and Fellows of the College of Physicians and the Deacons and Brethren of the Surgeons to hear the first lecture. The groundwork having been so well prepared, the Town Council appointed Alexander as the Professor of Anatomy at the University early in 1721. Monro, however, continued to teach at Surgeons' Hall until 1725, when he transferred to the University buildings, ostensibly to guard his anatomical preparations from Edinburgh inhabitants—mobs had gathered from time to time, incensed at grave-robbing and the unfounded suspicion that live persons were being dissected. In 1726, four other professors in medical disciplines were appointed to the University—and the medical school was under way.

Alexander Monro's course was given annually between October and April for the next forty years. According to Monro's manuscript (auto)biography, the first course was organized as follows:

1. Preliminary discourses, among which was comprehended the history of anatomy from its rise to the then present time.
2. The demonstration of the human bones according to the account of them afterwards printed.
3. The muscles and bowels of a human subject.
4. The blood-vessels and nerves of another subject—after each demonstration he endeavoured to explain the uses and functions of the organs, so far as coud be deduced from the fabrick immediately befor exhibited, and remarked what diseases they were subject to, with some account of their symptoms and the method of cure in each.
5. A sketch of comparative anatomy ... This part was greatly subservient to the following one.
6. Physiological discourses on the more abstruse parts of the animal oeconomy, these were accompanyed with the demonstration of the more subtile structure of the organs then talked of.
7. All the chirurgical operations performed on a human body, with an account of the diseases which made these operations necessary.
8. The application of Laques bandages and other chirurgical dressings.

Monro kept a list of students who attended the courses, and towards the end of his life 4464 names were on the list. He received fees from each student, in addition to £15 per annum stipend from the university. His private practice as a surgeon-apothecary was also profitable. Early in his career, Monro considered becoming a physician, but had decided that he would make more money if he were to remain in the surgeons' camp. In 1756, when Alexander Monro had been Professor of Anatomy for more than thirty years, and had taken his son into anatomy and so secured the succession, he accepted an honorary MD degree from the University, becoming a Fellow of the College of Physicians of Edinburgh. Soon after, he relinquished the practice of pharmacy and surgery.

With Cheselden's support, he became a Fellow of the Royal Society of London when he was twenty-six years old. His fame in France was such that in 1742 he was appointed a foreign member of the Royal Academy of Surgeons of Paris, founded in 1731. His most popular book was on osteology. His fame rested on some fifty papers, on his classes in anatomy, and on his many books.

There is an extant copy of a contemporary biography of Alexander Monro; the manuscript was written in the third person, but the text, which presents the professor in an adulatory light, is probably by Monro himself (Erlam 1953–5):

Soon after beginning to teach Mr. Monro observed how much his students for want of an accurate enough osteological treatise were at a loss to follow him rightly in the demonstrations of the bones; without an exact knowledge of which the other parts of anatomy can not be understood, he therefore compiled his Anatomy of the bones ...

The book *The anatomy of the humane bones*, 1726, was issued in Edinburgh, the publisher being his friend and a scientific colleague, William Monro; the London agent was T. Longman, booksellers 'at the Ship in Pater-noster-Row'. To the second and subsequent editions were added an account of the nerves, a commentary on Boerhaave's views on the motions of the heart, and a description of the human *receptaculum chyli* and thoracic duct. Twenty editions were published, the last in 1828. Monro did not include illustrations in his book, relying on the reader to have access to those in Eustachio's anatomy, illustrations prepared two hundred years previously, or, later, those in Cheselden's *Osteographia ...*, 1733.

In 1759, in Paris, a magnificently illustrated edition of Monro's osteology was published, translated and edited by J. J. Sue, père, (1710–92), a distinguished anatomist and professor of that subject at the Royal Academy of Painting and Sculpture and the Royal Schools of Surgery in Paris, Fellow of the Royal Society of London, and author of a number of anatomy texts. (One of Sue's descendants was Eugene Sue (1804–57), author of *Les Mystères de Paris* and *Le Juif errant*.) The 1732 Edinburgh edition was used for Sue's volume, and lead to Monro's comment "Tis pity Mr. Sue had not the latest edition of the English copy that all justice might have been done to his original author'—a mild enough comment of Monro's, considering the whole enterprise was apparently unauthorized by him. A contemporary French critic writes 'Cet ouvrage est un chef-d'œuvre tout concourt: papier, caractères, burin, frontispices, vignettes, cul de lampe [tail-piece], etc.'. And Monro himself said that the plates are '... very elegant figures of the bones with their explications' and called the work 'most sumptuous'. This work was issued some twenty-six years after Cheselden's *Osteographia* and twelve years after Albinus' *Tabulae sceleti et musculorum*.... As may be seen in the second plate of the *Traité d'ostéologie ...* (our *Plate 99*), the old tradition of posing standing figures against an elaborate background was continued. The thirty-one figures were reproduced twice, in a manner somewhat similar to that used by Albinus in his edition of Eustachio, 1744. Below some of the plates the names of engravers are indicated—Gobin, Aubert, and others. Our *Plate 99* was engraved by Jardinier, and the drawing is by Tarsis (Tharsis in other plates).

Plate number four of Monro–Sue's osteology is a front view of a standing female skeleton (*Fig. 11.16*). This, as Schievinger (1987) explains, is an early depiction of a woman's skeleton in an anatomical work, the first probably being the highly unsatisfactory one in Bauhin's *Theatrum anatomicum*, 1605. It should be noted that this latter is, in fact, a reversed and slightly altered copy of the skeleton in Platter's *De corporis humani ...*, 1583, (see our *Plate 54*, p. 231).

The Monro–Sue skeleton plate was published a quarter of a century before the fine idealized one by Soemmerring (see *Plate 84*, p. 369). Schiebinger in her stimulating paper (1987) argues that it was only in the eighteenth century that scientists and others began to be interested in skeletal female–male differences, and to pay particular attention to the smaller skull and more commodious pelvis said to be characteristic of women, a view used to assign to women a primary destiny as bearers of children. Schiebinger also raises the question of the role of a remarkable French woman anatomist in editing the *Traité*. She argues that it was Marie-Geneviève-Charlotte Thiroux d'Arconville who not only translated Monro's text, but also supervised the making of the anatomical illustrations, having them 'redone many times in order to correct the slightest fault'. This is explained in the introduction to the *Traité*, an introduction that is reprinted in a collection of d'Arconville's works. She, apparently, wished to remain anonymous, and was content to have attributions in the book ascribed to her colleague J. J. Sue. D'Arconville had studied anatomy at the *Jardin du Roi*. It is ironical that if this illustration was supervised by d'Arconville, the plate showed a skull disproportionately small and a rib-cage that Soemmerring might have considered as distorted by tight-lacing! Barclay, as late as 1829 in *The anatomy of the bones of the human body*, Edinburgh, reproduced this female skeleton rather than that of Soemmerring.

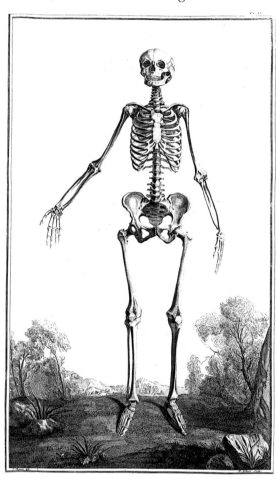

11.16   Female skeleton from Monro-Sue, *Traité d'ostéologie*, 1759.

In Edinburgh there was a project to produce an illustrated anatomy under Monro's direction:

The anatomical figures in the common systems of that science being generally very indifferent, P.[rofessor] M.[onro] recommended Eustachius's Tables to his students, but as these were not so elegant as what were in some modern books, and many parts discovered in the two preceding centuries were not there represented; while the well executed modern figures such as these of Cheselden, Albinus etc. were sold at too high a price for the greater number of students to purchase and at no rate such a collection cou'd be had as wou'd comprehend a compleat system of anatomy, the students at Edinburgh prevaild on a number of physicians and others to join with them in solliciting their Professor to direct such a system of figures with their explications as wou'd be most assistant to their studies and cou'd be sold at a moderate price.

Monro then writes how the work was begun and the plates issued as they were produced; but the publisher, being apprehensive that the work would be plagiarized,

woud publish no more till all that were intended were finished. The figures of all the remaining muscles and of the bowels were engraved in the order directed by P.M. [Professor Monro], but so inaccurately that he woud not add the letters nor give any explication 'till they were corrected, befor this was executed the bookseller became bankrupt, and further progress was not made in the work tho' advertised in the medical Essays.

It is a great pity that Munro had not the pertinacity to carry out this project on his own.

99 Oblique view of standing skeleton. Volume II, Pl. II in A. Monro [*primus*], *Traité d'osteologie* ... J. J. Sue's edition, 1759. Engraving (Wellcome Institute Library). 44.2 × 26.3 cm.

This adult skeleton is stated to be that of a man five feet six inches in height, reduced to some fourteen and a half inches in the drawing. (Actually the drawing of the skeleton is $16\frac{1}{2}$ inches in height.) There is also a line-diagram (recto, previous folio) of the illustration, which is labelled with letters and explanatory numbers. Unfortunately, the key to the forty-two numbers on the diagram refers to only seven of them.

It is not really an illustration for appreciation of skeletal details. For instance the cervical vertebrae are 'fudged', as are the phalanges of the toes, and, to a lesser extent, the carpal bones. One gets the impression that this plate was meant more for display, setting the scene so to speak, rather than for real skeletal accuracy. This latter is attempted, mainly very successfully, in drawings, later in the book, of separate bones and portions of the skeleton. Indeed, the mode of treatment of the subject matter is very similar to that of Cheselden.

The three-quarter side-view pose enables the skull-bones of the right side to be visualized; also both the front and back of the hands, although this has little point to it.

The styloid process of the radius is underemphasized, while the anterior bowing of the right femur is exaggerated; the clavicle gives little impression of its essential curvaceousness. In addition, the head and neck of the mandible are curved more posteriorly than they should be,

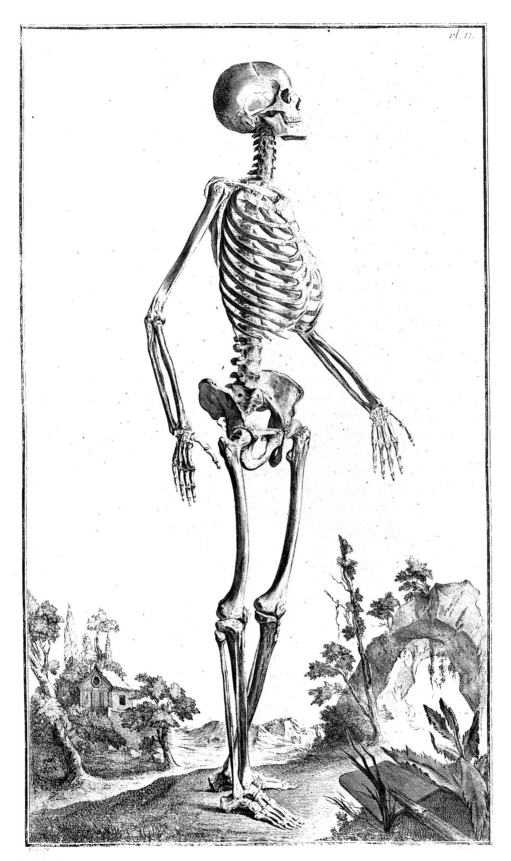

PLATE 99

and the pubic bones seem to join rather like a V —there is no curving of their superior rami. For its date this is not a very impressive skeletal drawing.

Chapter 11: Selected reading

Thomas Willis

Dewhurst, K. (1980). *Thomas Willis's Oxford Lectures*. Sandford Publications, Oxford.

Feindel, W. (1965). *Thomas Willis. The anatomy of the brain and nerves*. McGill University Press, Montreal.

Gibson, W. C. (1969). The medical interests of Christopher Wren In *Some aspects of seventeenth-century medicine and surgery*. University of California Press, Los Angeles.

Gunther, R. T. (1925). *Early science in Oxford*, Vol III, for the Subscribers, Oxford.

Meyer, A. and Hierons, R. (1965). On Thomas Willis's concept of neurophysiology. *Med. Hist.*, **9**, 1–15.

Scherz, G. (1965). *Nicolaus Steno's Lecture on the anatomy of the brain*. Arnold Busck, Copenhagen.

John Browne

Russell, K. F. (1959). John Browne, 1642–1702 ... *Bull. Hist. Med.*, **33**, 393–414 *and* 503–25.

Russell, K. F. (1962). A list of the works of John Browne (1642–1702). *Bull. med. Libr. Assoc.*, **50**, 675–83.

William Cowper

Beekman, F. (1935). Bidloo and Cowper, anatomists. *Ann. med. Hist.*, N S **7**, 113–29.

James Douglas

Brock, C. H. (1974). James Douglas of the pouch. *Med. Hist.*, **18**, 162–172.

Brock, C. H. (1977) The rediscovery of James Douglas. *The Bibliotheck*, **8**, 168–76.

Brock, C. H. (1979). James Douglas (1652–1742), botanist. *J. Soc. Bibliography nat. Hist.*, **9**, 137–45.

Thomas, K. B. (1964). *James Douglas of the pouch and his pupil William Hunter*. Pitman, London.

William Cheselden

Cope, Z. (1953). *William Cheselden 1688–1752*. E. and S. Livingstone, Edinburgh.

Nicolson, M. and Rousseau, G. S. (1968). *'This long disease, my life': Alexander Pope and the sciences* [sections on Cheselden]. Princeton University Press.

Russell, K. F. (1954). The Osteographia of William Cheselden. *Bull. Hist. Med.*, **28**, 32–49.

Alexander Monro primus

Anderson, R. G. W. and Simpson, A. D. C. (ed.) (1976). *The early years of the Edinburgh Medical School*. Royal Scottish Museum, Edinburgh.

Erlam, H. D. (1953–5). Alexander Monro, *primus* [The MS 'Life of Dr. A[r.] Monro Sr.']. *Univ. Edinburgh J.*, **17,** 77–105.

Finlayson, C. P. (1971). Alexander Monro (*Primus*). *Dict. sci. Biog.*, **9,** 479–84.

Schiebinger, L. (1987). Skeletons in the closet: The first illustrations of the female skeleton in eighteenth-century anatomy. In *The making of the modern body: sexuality and society in the nineteenth century.* University of California Press, Berkeley.

Wright-St Clair, R. E. (1964). *Doctors Monro: a medical saga.* The Wellcome Historical Medical Library, London.

12

British obstetrical atlases of the eighteenth century

IN THE third quarter of the eighteenth century, three major obstetrical atlases were issued in England. The authors—Smellie, 1754; Jenty, 1757; and William Hunter, 1774—employed for the majority of their illustrations the same artist, Jan van Riemsdyk. Van Riemsdyk also drew illustrations for Thomas Denman *A Collection of engravings* ... [on obstetrical subjects], 1787. These books indicate the rise of the profession of man-midwife, which, by the end of that century, had captured much of the lucrative practice of obstetrics in England.

The rise of the man-midwife

For centuries women in childbirth had been assisted by those neighbours, friends, and relatives who had themselves borne children. Women widowed and with children to support could turn to few remunerative jobs; but midwifery many could do well. There was little competition from medical men, who were for the most part excluded from the room when delivery was in progress. Many midwives were resourceful not only in normal labour but also in difficult cases. Practice among ordinary families brought in only modest sums, but midwifery for the well-to-do could be quite remunerative: Mrs Hester Shaw in the middle years of the seventeenth century acquired an estate worth more than £3000 by her work as a midwife.

From as early as the 1500s the midwives of London were required to be licensed by the ecclesiastical authorities, and those who met this requirement—it certainly was not all—used the licence to inspire confidence. But there were few opportunities in Britain for a formal education in midwifery; generally, women would train themselves by associating with a more experienced midwife. In Paris, where obstetrics had been developed more fully, there were, at least by the beginning of the eighteenth century, opportunities for women to be educated formally in the subject.

Traditionally, midwives did not use instruments in case of difficult birth. However, when the mother died, they were under some obligation to extract the child by Caesarean section in order to baptize it. In difficult cases of prolonged labour, and when the family could afford it, the midwife would call in a surgeon—who often could do little but destroy the child and extract its body piece by piece.

A new attitude to the male practitioner of obstetrics was seen in the seventeenth century, and the change was accelerated in the next. Medical men were called in to the birth rooms, not only as a last resort, but also during normal labour. This practice, regarded as fashionably French, was adopted by the 'quality', and spread to the middle class and eventually to artisans and tradespeople. Such male practitioners were called men-midwives (a word noted as early as 1625) or, more pretentiously, 'accoucheurs'. Men-midwives, when they had been well trained, could occasionally save mother and child when the average midwife could not, for medical men had the use of a new instrument—the obstetrical forceps; moreover, they had available new knowledge of obstetrical anatomy, unavailable to most midwives.

The invention of the obstetrical forceps has a somewhat obscure history. In seventeenth-century England, forceps were employed by one family, Huguenot in origin, Chamberlen by name, who kept to themselves the secret, to their financial advantage. The first of the family to use the forceps was Peter Chamberlen, who died in 1631. When labour was protracted, and one of the Chamberlens was called in, he would produce the forceps, and, under a sheet, would put them in place around the presenting part of the baby and effect accelerated delivery. The family secret was kept more or less intact for some hundred years, but by the early years of the eighteenth century forceps were being more widely used. But not without criticism from laymen, other physicians, and, more particularly, female practitioners of midwifery. The complaints have a familiar sound: that the procedures adopted by the obstetrician were determined more for his own convenience and remuneration than for the obstetrical needs of his patient.

Probably more important for the general improvement of obstetrical practice was the new knowledge of the anatomy of the birth canal and the mechanics of parturition; it was here that the medical profession made its greatest contribution. William Hunter, in the dedication of a book to King George III, described his subject as illustrating 'one part of science [obstetrical anatomy] hitherto imperfectly understood, and ... the foundation of another part of science [midwifery], on which the lives and happiness of millions must depend': obstetrical anatomy is the foundation for midwifery.

Some physicians and surgeons well-trained in anatomy investigated, in labour rooms and by dissections, the way in which the baby's head was engaged in the pelvis; how the uterine contractions on the baby assisted it to pass down the birth canal; how the child rotated; and how presentations other than occipito-posterior could be managed. Although the training of medical men in this respect was often grossly deficient, it was possible to obtain instruction in these basic aspects of the birth process. Smellie, Hunter, and, probably, Jenty trained hundreds of men; and there were others in London teaching obstetrics in the middle years of the eighteenth century. English midwives, however, had to make what arrangements they could to familiarize themselves with the anatomy and physiology of parturition.

It is difficult to determine whether the newer knowledge of the birth process, and of obstetrical forceps and the indications for their use, and a growing understanding of many obstetrical problems, made any impact demographically as this knowledge spread through the publication of books for midwives and for medical men. Certainly those practitioners and teachers of obstetrics that were able to refer to Smellie's atlas would have a sounder understanding of their subject. Smellie's books would reach only a few of the male and, very rarely, female practitioners. That of Jenty, and especially the expensive volume by William Hunter, would have an even more restricted distribution. Nevertheless, these books would be seen by some of the most influential persons concerned with obstetrics, and they in turn would reflect the newer knowledge in their teachings, writings, and practice. At the end of the century Margaret Stephens was, in her book *Domestic Midwife...*, 1795, teaching obstetrical anatomy and requiring her midwife pupils to read Smellie.

At the splitting of the Barber-Surgeons Company in 1745 the Surgeons excluded men-midwives from holding high office; and so it came about that a number of practitioners were working in obstetrics, but holding a licence from the College of Physicians. When William Hunter received his doctorate in medicine from Glasgow, he gave up his membership in the Company of Surgeons, applied successfully for a licence from the College of Physicians, and practised as a prescribing physician and as an obstetrician. This anomalous position did not please the College of Physicians, for they voted to exclude him from a Fellowship, in spite of his Royal appointment and aristocratic connections. He could not claim Fellowship as a virtual right, as he would have been able to do had his degree been from Oxford or Cambridge.

Some of the men-midwives had their training as apothecaries. A hundred years before the time of Smellie and Hunter, Willughby complained of apothecaries who, 'leaving the beating of their mortars, turn doctors, as also taking it upon them to be men-midwives'.

Against this turbulent background of medical and obstetrical life in mid-eighteenth-century London, Smellie, Jenty, and Hunter practised and prepared their books for publication.

William Smellie (1697–1763)

William Smellie was born at Lesmahagow, a few kilometres south-west of Lanark, an ancient Lowlands town in Scotland, about forty kilometres from Glasgow. He was apprenticed to an apothecary in Lanark. After appropriate examinations by the Company of Barber-Surgeons in London in 1720, Smellie then joined the Royal Navy as a surgeon's mate, a not-uncommon route for further education taken by apprentices to surgeon-apothecaries. His subsequent professional life of nearly forty years was spent half in Lanark (1722–39) and half in London (1739–59), where he established a wide reputation as a man-midwife, a teacher of obstetrics, and a anatomist of parturition.

Smellie's mid-life education in 1739 included study of obstetrics in Paris and a period with Frank Nicholls, physician at St George's Hospital. He was assisted by a Scottish obstetrician, Alexander Stuart, FRS, also of St George's, to establish a practice, and, in 1741, to set up a private school in this subject. For his course of lectures given from his own home Smellie charged three guineas. He used obstetrical 'dolls'—leather-covered skeletons—and the bones of the female pelvis to demonstrate the rotations of the child in the birth canal. In a printed description of his *Course of lectures upon midwifery...*, 1742, he states that he explains in the clearest manner how to deliver women 'in all the variety of natural, difficult, and preternatural labours, perform'd on different machines made in imitation of real women and children'. Itemized at the auction of Smellie's effects after his death were 'a variety of anatomical preparations, illustrating the theory of mid-wifery ... [and] exquisite artificial machines, in imitation of the living subjects...'. Smellie's clinical methods and his teaching were attacked by the Bostonian physician, William Douglass, in two pamphlets published in London in 1748, the first entitled, *A letter to Dr. Smellie, shewing the impropriety of his new invented wooden forceps; and also the absurdity of his method of teaching and practising midwifery*. Smellie's popularity as a teacher was not apparently disturbed by this attack, for medical men from Britain and the Continent came in large numbers to study with him; he trained nine hundred pupils between 1741 and 1751. For example, David Schultz, sent to London by the Swedish government to learn about inoculation, took the opportunity to study under Smellie, and, on his return, became the first professor of midwifery in Sweden. Another person who worked with Smellie was, as we have seen, the Dutch anatomist Petrus Camper.

Smellie summarized his experience of obstetrics in *A treatise on the theory and practice of midwifery*, London, 1752. In this he described, perhaps for the first time accurately, the mechanical-anatomical aspects of the birth process in each of the common, and some of the rarer, presentations of the child. He described improvements he had made in the obstetrical forceps, and, perhaps more important, clinical indications for their use. (Smellie had an 'original portrait in oil of the late celebrated Dr. Chamberlaine'.)

As a supplement to *A treatise on the theory and practice of midwifery*, Smellie published two volumes of case histories—the first in 1754 and the second in 1764, five years after he had returned to Lanark into retirement at the age of sixty-two. In preparing the text of his work, Smellie had the assistance of a fellow Scot, his friend the novelist Tobias Smollett, who had himself started on a medical career only to abandon it for literature. The obstetrical writings of Smellie had a wide distribution, being, for example, advertised in newspapers in Boston, New York, and Philadelphia.

Smellie's obstetrical atlas was:

A sett of anatomical tables, with explanations, and an abridgment, of the practice of midwifery, with a view to illustrate a treatise on that subject, and collection of cases. London, 1754.

This book was printed for the author and published by him in an edition said to be of only 100 copies. A second edition, where *Sett* had been respelled *Set*, was issued in 1761 (the spelling error was noted in the Errata in the first edition). By 1800 the work had appeared in all formats from folio to duodecimo, the plates usually re-engraved from the original illustrations; it had been published in London, Edinburgh, Paris, Nuremberg, Amsterdam, Boston, and Worcester, Mass. The plates were also included in some editions of Smellie's *A treatise on ... midwifery*. The publications of these obstetrical plates had been announced three years previously in the *Treatise*. In a review of this work van Riemsdyk was referred to as 'a very able artist ... In point of design and anatomical exactness, we may venture to pronounce them to be superior to any figures of the kind hitherto made public'. In a second edition, Smellie writes of the 'great care and expense' of producing these large figures; certainly the engraving of this number of plates must have taken a considerable amount of time and cost much money.

Smellie's personal copy of the first edition of *A sett...*, with emendations in his own handwriting, may be seen in Lanark at the Lindsay Institute: Smellie had bequeathed his books to the Grammar School there, which he had attended.

Although not published until 1754, twenty-two of the plates for *A Sett...* were ready by 1752, but, as Smellie says, 'I soon saw that a further illustration and consequently an addition to that number was necessary'. Seventeen additional plates were engraved.

William Hunter lodged with Smellie when he came to London. Some time before 1752, both Smellie and Hunter were employing the same artist, van Riemsdyk. In Smellie's ninth plate, the reader is instructed to 'Consult Mr. Hunter's elegant plates of the gravid uterus'—a specimen plate could be seen at Hunter's house; this, however, was not published in book form for another twenty years, when it appeared with others in William Hunter's *The anatomy of the human gravid uterus exhibited in figures*, 1774. By the time Smellie retired to Lanark in 1759, Hunter, with his fine bedside manners and circle of aristocratic friends, had taken a large share of the wealthy practice of obstetrics in London. Smellie, who was usually called to care for working class women during difficult labour, had a much rougher presence; Elizabeth Nihell referred to Smellie and his 'delicate fist of a great horse-godmother of a he-wife'. But probably Smellie had the greater and more lasting impact on the science of midwifery. The two differed not only in style, but in obstetrical practice and experience; Hunter, who attended many aristocratic, normal deliveries, very rarely used forceps, and was all for masterly inactivity. 'There are two times at the time of labour which I am frightened at (all the other I don't care a sixpence for); one is a flooding and the other, convulsions', that is, partum haemorrhage and eclampsia. The association of Hunter with Smellie's work continued after the latter's death; Hunter bought Lot 39 at the 1770 Soho sale of Smellie's effects; 'twenty-five original drawings, fram'd and glaz'd'; these were the van Riemsdyk originals. They are now in the Hunterian Collection at Glasgow University.

Eleven of the thirty-nine illustrations in *A sett* ... were from originals by Smellie's former pupil Petrus Camper, and these are now in the Royal College of Physicians of Edinburgh; and two by 'another hand', probably Smellie himself. All the others were by van Riemsdyk. Our *Fig. 12.1* shows 'in what manner the head of the foetus is helped along with the forceps as artificial hands, when it is necessary to assist with the same for the safety of either mother or child'; it was by 'Dr. Camper Professor of Medicine at Franequer in Friesland'.

The reason for publishing the plates was to produce a graphical epitome of obstetrical anatomy, '... to shew every thing that might conduce to the improvement of the young

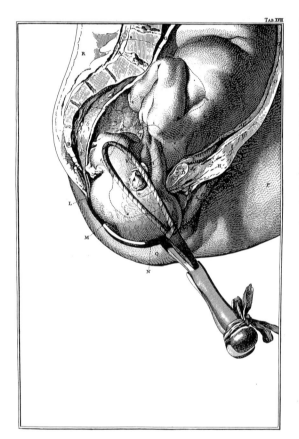

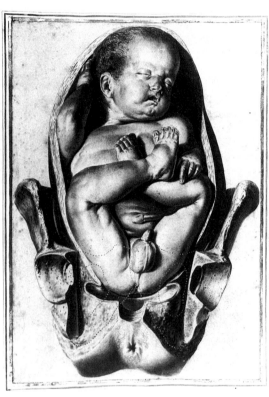

12.1 Application of obstetrical forceps, Smellie, *A sett*, 1754.

12.2 Breech presentation. J. van Riemsdyk's original drawing for Smellie's *A sett*, 1754.

TAB X

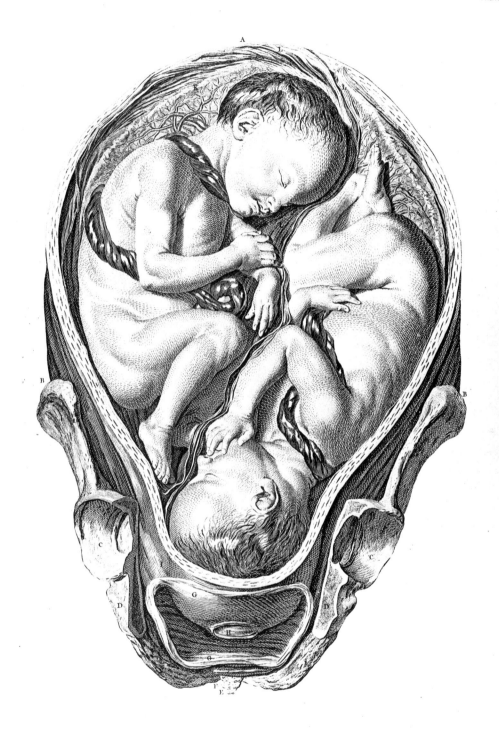

12.3   Twins *in utero*, Smellie, *A sett*, 1754.

practitioner ...'. He was minded to publish this work of anatomy and applied anatomy

finding that most of the representations hitherto given of the parts inservient to uterine gestation and parturition were in many respects deficient, I have been induced to undertake the following tables, with a view to supply in some measure the defects of others, and at the same time to illustrate what I have taught and written on the subject.

The anatomy was to be drawn in a 'strong and distinct manner'.

We have chosen to illustrate plate thirty, drawn by van Riemsdyk and engraved by Charles Grignion (our *Plate 100*). This picture of one type of breech presentation shows very well the abilities of van Riemsdyk and his engraver to give a rounded, spatial appearance to the figure. The original drawing is in the Hunterian Collection (D1.1.27, no. 21) (our *Fig. 12.2*), and may be compared with Grignion's engraving (our *Plate 100*). On the facing page of this engraving in the book is a résumé of methods of managing such presentations. Smellie's *Tenth Table* shows a front view of twins *in utero*, in the beginning of labour (*Fig. 12.3*).

100 Breech presentation. Tab XXX in W. Smellie, *A sett of anatomical tables with explanations...*, 1754. Engraving (Cambridge University Library). 48.5 × 33.5 cm.

In this forward-facing breech presentation, the anterior part of the uterus has been removed to show the fetus. Of all the drawings in Smellie's book, it best exemplifies the ability of the artist to convey a vivid three-dimensional impression. Interestingly, out of a total of thirty-nine, it is the only plate depicting fetal external genital organs.

To an extent the anatomical shortcomings of this drawing may be explained by reference to the preface, where Smellie writes 'the situation of parts, and their respective dimensions being more particularly attended to, than a minute anotomical investigation of their structure', ('anotomical' is a typographical error, and is corrected in the Errata section at the end of the book).

The stylized depiction of the vaginal orifice and the appearance of the maternal pelvic bones are almost identical with those appearing in several of his other plates, and were therefore presumably employed rather as a common template. Even so, it is curious that they are not more anatomically accurate, particularly in view of his obvious knowledge in this respect, as shown both by earlier illustrations in the book and in his text.

Anatomical purists may grumble about the crudely-drawn infant scrotum and penis, the 'tubular' umbilical cord, and the awkward appearance of the big toes (also, what happened to the amnion?); but such criticisms pale on overall consideration of this early drawing, a remarkably lifelike impression of a fetus *in utero*.

TAB.XXX

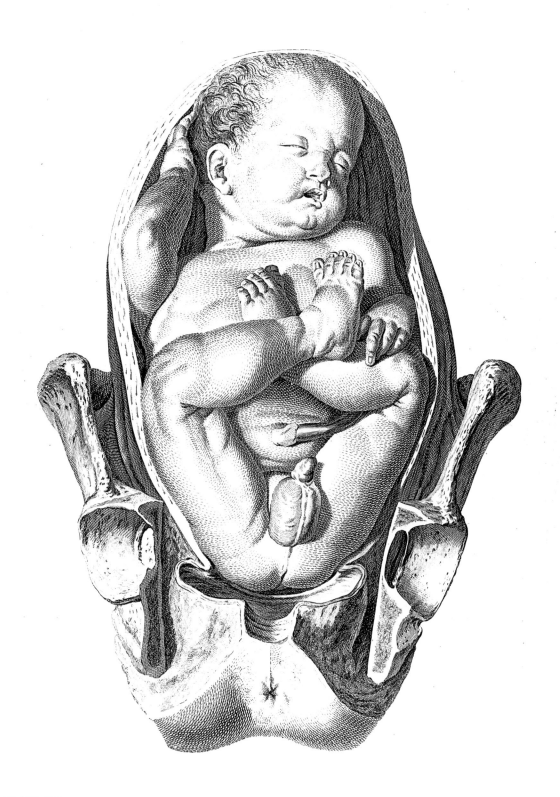

PLATE 100

Charles Nicholas Jenty

In 1757, three years after Smellie's obstetrical plates, Charles Nicholas Jenty published in London his volume of the anatomy of pregnancy:

The demonstrations of a pregnant uterus of a woman at her full term. In six tables, as large as nature. Done from the pictures painted after dissections by Mr. Van Riemsdyk. London: Printed for, and sold by, the author, at his house in Fetter-Lane, and all the eminent booksellers in Europe. 1757.

The six plates are life-size; the sixteen pages of text are octavo. The title is ambiguous; the pictures, not the dissections, were by van Riemsdyk.

Almost all that is known of Jenty comes from his published work. He was born, date unknown, in France, and educated in Paris as a surgeon; the dedication of the above text is to the members of the Royal Academy of Surgery at Paris and reads:

Gentlemen ... I would not have you imagine, that because I am, at present, settled in a foreign country, I have so far forgot myself, as not to remember my native place, where I received the first elements of my profession from some of your most learned members ...

The same year in which he published his obstetrical plates he issued: *A course of anatomico-physiological lectures on the human structure...,* in which he excuses his text, saying that his writings 'are not so well penned, as if they came from an English hand...'. The probability is that by 1757 he had been in England some years, and had been teaching anatomy from his house in Fetter Lane. On 4 August 1757, Jenty presented to the Company of Surgeons of London four large anatomical prints, coloured, glazed, and framed, which they accepted with gratitude, inviting Jenty to dinner five days later. These prints were probably from another Jenty publication in that same busy year of 1757:

An essay on the demonstration of the human structure, half as large as nature, in four tables, from the pictures painted after dissections, for that purpose. London: Printed for, and sold by, the author, at his house in Fetter-Lane, and all the eminent booksellers in Europe. 1757.

A Latin edition, *Testamen de demonstranda structura humana...,* was issued at the same date and place. The four plates in this book are even larger than the obstetrical ones.

About this time Jenty gave a paper to the Royal Society, published in the *Philosophical Transactions,* 1758: *A remarkable case of cohesions of all the intestines....* He may have been engaged in surgical as well as anatomical practice. By April, 1762, Jenty was a surgeon's mate with Lord Loudoun's expeditionary force to Portugal in the Seven Years War. He received five shillings a day. (John Hunter was a full surgeon to this force, and received ten shillings.) On discharge, he stayed in Portugal for a while, but then moved to Madrid, possibly lecturing on anatomy and surgery. A surgical work in Spanish appeared under Jenty's name in 1766. No more is known of him after this date.

The large plates in Jenty's two volumes were printed in 'mezzotinto', a technique invented in the seventeenth century, but most unusual in anatomical illustration. It had been employed, as we shall see (Chapter 14) by Ladmiral and the Gautier family: they used the mezzotint process to produce colour prints. Jenty himself considered, but rejected, using coloured prints, as he writes in his preface to *An essay*. . . . Instead he suggested that his prints should be coloured afterwards by hand: 'Gentlemen may have these mezzotinto prints, coloured after the original pictures, of different degrees of perfection, according to the price allowed to the colourer'. Jenty argued that mezzotints were well-suited for colouring:

as this method is softer, and capable of exhibiting a nearer imitation of nature than engraving, as artists themselves acknowledge that nature may admit of light and shades, well blended and softened, but never did of a harsh outline: So it must be confessed, that these prints may want the smartness which engraving might have contributed; but the softness which they possess, may approach nearer to the imitation of nature, when coloured, than any engraving possibly could, merely thro' the unavoidable delineation of the outline.

In the mezzotint process used in Jenty's work, the whole of a copperplate is roughened by a toothed rocker to produce a fine velvety covering of minute depressed stipples and raised burrs. If the plate were now inked and wiped, as in any intaglio process, it would print an all-over black. White highlights, shadings, and lines are obtained by removing the burr and smoothing the plate appropriately. This method has been termed the 'black art',

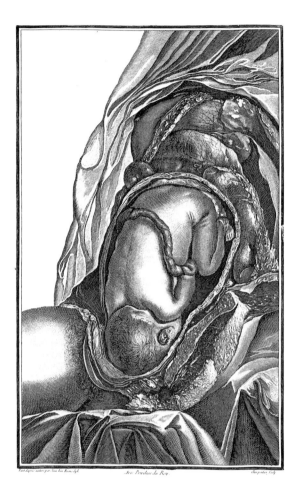

12.4 Fetus *in utero*, Jenty, *Demonstration de la matrice*, 1759.

and was used in Britain to reproduce the work of such artists as Morland. The three-dimensional appearance of these mezzotints is quite unlike that of an engraving, as may be seen when the original Jenty plates are compared with the re-engravings for the Paris edition, 1759 (compare *Plate 101* and *Fig. 12.4*). Similar immediacy of appearance did not appear in anatomical illustration until the development of lithography in the 1820s. It was fortunate that Jenty chose to use this method when it was reaching its highest technical competence in Britain, and that he used some of the finest artists for his plates—Edward Fisher and Richard Purcell of the McArdell school, working in Dublin and London.

As in the obstetrical atlas of Smellie, all but one of the illustrations from which these mezzotinters worked were made by Jan van Riemsdyk. The original drawings were in coloured crayon.

In the early 1760s original anatomical drawings prepared by van Riemsdyk for Jenty were sent to the Pennsylvania Hospital in Philadelphia by the Quaker physician, John Fothergill, whose contact there was William Shippen, jun., a pupil of the Hunters who was shortly to become Professor of Anatomy and Surgery in Philadelphia. A total of eighteen coloured drawings, framed and glazed, were sent, and with them cases of anatomical casts and a skeleton.

The influence of Jenty's obstetrical plates was not insignificant, for they were republished in London by the author, 1758, and issued also in a Latin–German edition in Nuremberg, dated 1761. Parisian editions, with plates conventionally engraved, were issued in 1759 and 1763–4. There was also a Dutch edition, Amsterdam, 1793.

101 Uterus opened to show fetus. Tabula IV in C.N. Jenty, *Demonstratio uteri praegnantis mulieris cum foetu . . .*, 1761. Engraving (Wellcome Institute Library). 59.0 × 42.6 cm.

Mention has been made earlier of the quality of Jenty's illustrations. Dramatic, certainly, is the impact of this one, showing the opened uterus, the stretched cervix (R) with the fetal head partially in the vagina (U), the pubic symphysis (Z) cut through, the right part of the pelvic girdle removed, and portions of the maternal small and large intestines shown surrounding the uterus. The folds of a sheet touchingly frame the whole.

The convoluted nature of the umbilical cord, shown crossing the back, is particularly well portrayed, and the typically 'hunched up' appearance of the fetus is excellently conveyed. The placenta, shown within the upper part of the uterus, is rather a caricature of the real thing.

Neither maternal pubic nor fetal hair are very lifelike in their appearance, and, anatomically, the drawing of the infant's ear is regrettably little short of disastrous. It must be said that this drawing, dated 1757, from London, is not one of van Riemsdyk's best.

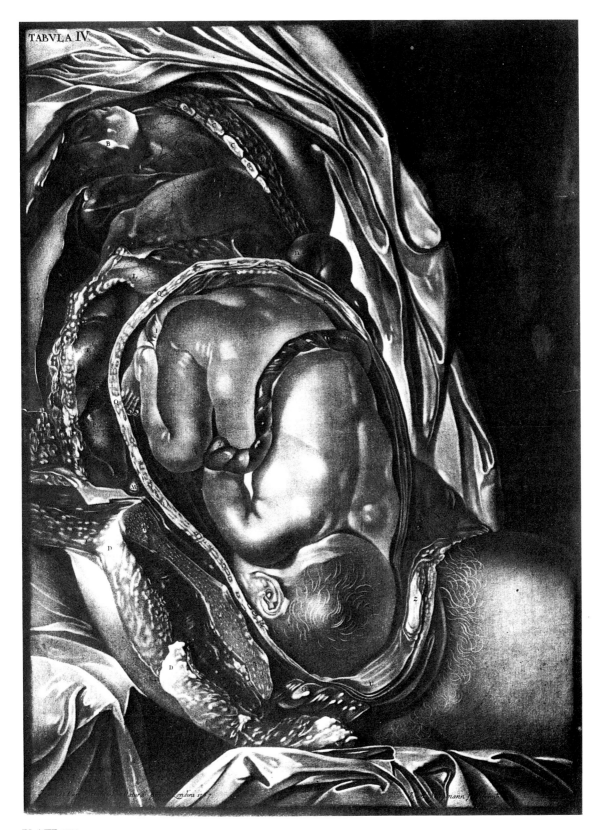

PLATE 101

William Hunter, 1718–1783

To the medical profession, William Hunter has been overshadowed by the towering reputation of his younger brother John, the comparative anatomist and surgeon.

William was the seventh child of the owner of a small estate in the countryside near East Kilbride, south of Glasgow and some thirty-five kilometres from Lanark, the home town of Smellie. He attended Glasgow College (or University) for five years; his intention was to study for the Church, but he could not bring himself to subscribe to certain tenets. Instead in 1737 he joined William Cullen (1710–90), a practitioner in nearby Hamilton, as an assistant and pupil; Hunter spent his next three years with Cullen—the most happy years of his life, he later said. (Cullen was later Professor of Chemistry, then of Medicine, first at Glasgow, then Edinburgh.) Hunter attended the lectures of Alexander Monro *primus* in Edinburgh, and then travelled in 1740 to London to lodge with Smellie, at that time practising from his house in Pall Mall. There was a prominent Scottish medical fraternity in London: the Union of the Kingdoms had been in 1707, but the rebellion, or unsuccessful independence movement, of 1715 was soon to be followed by that of 1745. Hunter once gave a toast at a club which met at the British Coffee House—a meeting-place of Scots: 'May no English nobleman venture out of the world without a Scottish physician, as I am sure there be none who venture in.'

Hunter had brought an introduction from the Glasgow printer, Robert Foulis, to another Scot, James Douglas, who was well established (see Chapter 11, p. 431). Douglas offered him the posts of tutor to his son and assistant in his dissecting rooms, which Hunter was delighted to accept. Hunter also attended Frank Nicholls's classes in anatomy at St George's Hospital, founded ten years previously. (Hunter later credits Nicholls with major advances in techniques for preparing injected specimens.) Hunter continued to lodge with the household after the death of James Douglas the next year. He is said to have become engaged to Douglas's daughter, who, however, died in 1744 of consumption.

William Hunter developed a practice as a surgeon and man-midwife, disliking the former work, but being most successful as an obstetrician. In 1746, when he was twenty-eight, he advertised to the general public:

On Monday, the 13th of October, at 5 in the evening will begin a course of anatomical lectures to which will be added the operations of surgery with the application of bandages, by William Hunter, surgeon. Gentlemen may have the opportunity of learning the art of dissection during the whole winter season in the same manner as at Paris. Proposals to be seen at Mr. Millar's bookseller opposite to the end of Katharine Street in the Strand.

Hunter's school in the disreputable environs of Covent Garden and Drury Lane became famous, for his capabilities as a lecturer were attested to by all who heard him. Later, many eminent persons, including Adam Smith, Edmund Burke, and Edward Gibbon, went out of their way to attend his lectures. He prepared his lectures so skilfully that he could convey detailed, accurate information over the space of two hours without tedium. His lectures were accompanied by demonstrations of injected and preserved specimens.

Hunter in 1763–4 proposed to the government of the day that a national school of anatomy and medicine should be started in London; a letter shows that Hunter looked forward to having Cullen and Joseph Black from Edinburgh join in this venture, which he would have endowed with a large sum.

[Hunter asks] to be allowed a proper piece of ground, that he may forthwith lay out six, or even seven thousand pounds, in erecting a building fit for the purpose under any condition that may be agreeable to the King.

The proposal was not adopted.

In 1747 William Hunter was made a member of the Corporation of Surgeons, founded two years earlier at the break-up of the Barber-Surgeons. From 1748 he was for a year or so surgeon–accoucheur to the Middlesex Hospital, and then, for ten years, to the British Lying-In Hospital. Accompanying Douglas's son, he visited anatomical centres in Paris and in Holland, where he met both B. S. Albinus and Haller. Hunter received the doctor of medicine degree from Glasgow when he was briefly in Scotland in 1750, and somewhat later discontinued his work as a surgeon, attending only medical and obstetrical cases. (After 1750, 'Dr. Hunter' usually refers to William, and 'Mr. Hunter' to John.) When he returned to London, William Hunter left Mrs Douglas's household, and set up his consulting rooms and anatomy school in Jermyn Street. From then on, he established himself as the fashionable accoucheur of London. He became a friend of many of the chief figures in mid-Georgian London, William Pitt the elder, Horace Walpole, numerous members of the aristocracy, and eventually Queen Charlotte, the young wife of George III. Hunter became physician-extraordinary to the Queen in 1762. For her first delivery, he waited in an ante-room while the baby was delivered by a woman midwife. After the birth, he was called in to inspect the baby and the placenta. The *Annual Register* for 1762 records 'August 12—The Queen was delivered of a prince [later George IV] by Mrs. Draper; Dr. Hunter was in waiting in case of his help being wanted'. The Queen had fifteen children, and Hunter probably attended later deliveries, an indication of the growing propriety and acceptance of men-midwives. His rise to such a dominant position was not without criticism, both from the midwives themselves and from others in the medical profession. His former teacher at St George's, Frank Nicholls, was much against the new fashion of employing men-midwives. Although he was granted a licence by the College of Physicians on the strength of his Glasgow degree, Hunter was, as we have seen, rejected when proposed for a Fellowship in 1771; the work of an accoucheur was too manual and too reminiscent of surgeons to be acceptable to physicians. He was, however, elected a Fellow of the Royal Society in 1767.

His practice brought him a large income, and he was able in 1767 to give his introductory lecture in a new anatomy school built to his designs in Great Windmill Street, with magnificent rooms for dissection, teaching, and the preparation of specimens, and a fine museum, as well as lodgings for himself. There exist a number of manuscript notes of Hunter's lectures written by students at the Windmill Street School. The course in 1775 consisted of the following lectures: 80 on anatomy, 3 on anatomical techniques, 15 on operative surgery, 12 on midwifery. A number of bodies were dissected during the course.

Hunter died in 1783, a few days after he had, despite the urging of friends, given an introductory lecture to a course in anatomy—'If I had strength enough to hold a pen,' he said, 'I would write how easy and pleasant a thing it is to die.'

William Hunter disputed with some contemporaries concerning priorities in anatomical discoveries: with Monro *secundus*, about who first described the absorbent functions of the peripheral lymphatics (Hunter must be given priority); with Percival Pott concerning the anatomy of congenital hernia; and most sadly, with his brother. Ten years younger than William, John had arrived in London in 1748, a craftsman woodworker, without any useful academic or professional education. William appointed him an assistant; his abilities as a dissector and anatomist were apparent from the very first. In 1761, for reasons of health, John sailed with an expeditionary force to France and Portugal. On his return, he set up a school on his own, and came to dominate surgery and comparative anatomy in London. William's arguments with John had to do with the contributions each had made to unravelling the placental circulation. The two brothers had contrasting styles—William, a persuasive, smooth talker with impeccable manners towards his aristocratic clientele; John, abrupt, outspoken, and uncompromising to the generality of Londoners. John assisted in many of the dissections for his brother's book on the gravid uterus, and his help is gracefully acknowledged.

William Hunter was not a prolific writer. The only substantial text he published was titled '*Medical Commentaries Part I*. Containing a plain and direct answer to Professor Monro Jun, interspersed with remarks on the structure, function, and diseases of several parts of the human body. London, 1762.' A supplement was published two years later, with arguments against Percival Pott.

The book for which William Hunter is chiefly remembered is:

The anatomy of the human gravid uterus exhibited in figures. Printed at Birmingham by John Baskerville, 1774. Sold in London by S. Baker and G. Leigh, in York-Street; T. Cadell in the Strand; D. Wilson and G. Nicol, opposite York-Buildings; and J. Murray, in Fleet-Street.

This title was preceded, on the same page, by the title in Latin: *Anatomia uteri humani gravidi tabulis illustrata*.... Each illustration is faced by a description, in Latin and in English, of that illustration. The work is dedicated to the King.

The life-history of this publication is known, which—because of the book's inherent interest and its superb quality, and because it serves as an example of the co-operation required to produce an anatomical plate-book—deserves consideration here at some length.

In the course of Hunter's obstetrical practice and his work in his private anatomy school he would rarely have had the opportunity to dissect the body of a pregnant woman. The first such opportunity was in 1750; as Hunter describes in his preface:

A woman died suddenly, when very near the end of her pregnancy; the body was procured before any sensible putrefaction had begun; the season of the year was favourable to dissection; the injection of the blood-vessels proved successful; a very able painter, in this way, was found; every part was examined in the most public manner, and the truth was thereby well authenticated.

The 'very able painter' was van Riemsdyk. Over the next few months, van Riemsdyk completed ten life-size drawings, in red crayon (chalk) which were 'publicly exhibited'; Hunter used them in his lectures. Very great care was taken to represent every part just as it was found. Hunter stated that not so much as one joint of a finger had been moved to show any part more distinctly, or to give a more picturesque effect. The drawings were made by van Riemsdyk as soon as the dissections were completed, for Hunter demanded work done from immediate observation, not from recollection. From the sketches, finished drawings were completed; and from these the engravings were made. Each stage of many of the illustrations may still be seen in the Hunterian Collection at Glasgow University.

Because of a favourable reaction to the superb illustrations, Hunter decided to publish an illustrated anatomy of the gravid uterus, and 'the work was immediately put into the hands of our best artists; and subscriptions were received'. The best artists here referred to are engravers, 'ingenius artists'; Hunter thanks particularly Mr Strange, 'not only for having by his hand secured a sort of immortality to two of the plates, but for having given his advice and assistance in every part with a steady and disinterested friendship'. This may be interpreted to mean that Robert Strange supervised the work of what eventually was a team of eighteen engravers, many of them Frenchmen, or British with French training. The labour in making precise copper engravings of detailed work may extend over several months. Strange is said to have spent six months engraving one of the plates. The cost of such work was obviously considerable; Strange was paid 100 guineas for one plate. In 1752 Hunter advertised that a plate could be inspected at his house in Little Piazza, Covent Garden, and that names could be put on a subscription list there or at a bookshop in the Strand. Hunter goes on to describe progress:

In the mean time a second subject was procured; which, though the weather happened to very unfavourable, afforded a few supplemental figures, of importance enough to be taken into the work. And before the engravings were finished, a third subject occurred very opportunely, which cleared up some difficulties, and furnished some useful additional figures.

The original plan having been only to publish the first ten plates ... in this branch of anatomy, to be added whenever good opportunities should be offered, the author now began to entertain hopes of being able to give a much more compleat work. He foresaw that, in the course of some years, by diligence he might procure in this great city, so many opportunities of studying the gravid uterus, as to be enabled to make up a tolerable system; and to exhibit, by figures, all the principal changes that happen in the nine months of utero-gestation.

As it turned out, however, progress was quite slow, with Hunter doing little or nothing towards completing the book in the next ten years, a busy period when he was becoming the fashionable accoucheur of the Town. Sixteen plates were probably completed before 1754, the remaining fifteen produced between 1764 and 1772 (two plates were not by van Riemsdyk). A total of thirteen subjects were illustrated, five full-term. By 1772, the book had been twenty-two years in production; but a plan to have the book printed from a press located in Hunter's new establishment in Great Windmill Street was not realized. At that period in England, a few wealthy gentlemen were privately printing works for limited distribution—Horace Walpole's press at Strawberry Hill is the most important example, and Hunter and Walpole were well acquainted. Hunter's brother, John, also had a press in his establishment.

A printer was finally engaged, John Baskerville at Birmingham. And the choice was fortunate, for Baskerville would combine, in this book as in others, the conoisseurship of a private passion for fine book-production with a professional and commercial experience of printing acquired through three decades. How were Hunter, the client, and the printer, Baskerville, brought together? One man who was a correspondent and an adviser to both was Benjamin Franklin. Franklin, a hard-working printer in Philadelphia before becoming a statesman, was in England from 1757 to 1762 and from 1764 to 1775. He had been consulted by Baskerville, who in 1768 wished to dispose—lock, stock, and barrel—of his printing business. Franklin was also, in 1771, a mutually-agreed arbitrator between Hunter and his former assistant and partner, William Hewson, when the two fell out, ostensibly over the ownership of anatomical preparations.

Hunter recognized that Baskerville did elegant work; but he was particularly pleased with his attention to details of ink, and of the paper, 'a leaf of his press-work [being] an excellent preservative of the plates between which it is placed'. Few other printers have had such complete control over their work as Baskerville, for he designed and produced the type, was responsible for the paper, formulated the ink, and supervised every aspect of the presswork.

The resulting book, so long in gestation and so expensive, was finally ready in 1774; it was an élitist book, attention having been given, without regard to cost, to the accuracy of the anatomy and the quality of illustration, engraving, and printing.

Hunter was now faced with the problem of selling the book. The list of persons holding the work for sale included the influential names of some of the chief booksellers of London. A subscription list had been opened twenty years before, and money had been handed over; but many subscribers must have given up hope (or the ghost) in the interim. New advertisements for the book appeared just prior to the publication date, November 1774; the cost was six guineas. It was re-advertised, misleadingly, in 1777: 'This day is published, in one large volume folio, price six guineas in boards. The Anatomy of the Human Gravid Uterus...'. By 1784, after Hunter's death, it was sold at a remaindered rate of three and a half guineas. The work was, however, subsequently reprinted from the original plates and reissued three times. It was reproduced in facsimile by the Sydenham Society in 1851.

William Hunter had written but not published a number of other texts, including a history of printing; among these manuscripts was one designed to accompany the gravid uterus plates. This was published a decade after his death, edited by his nephew, Matthew Baillie: *An anatomical description of the human gravid uterus, and its contents*, London, 1794.

In his atlas of obstetrical anatomy, Smellie had intended to provide a guide to the young practitioner; Hunter's objective and accomplishment was, though of the highest precision and integrity, less practical: it was a book of *anatomy*. Baskerville's typography had the effect of imposing a restrained elegance, entirely suitable to William Hunter's style, upon the shocking images of dissected corpses of pregnant women.

Hunter had the opportunity to observe, in the house of his wealthy clients and friends, fashions in fine art. Robert Strange helped develop his tastes as a collector of paintings, drawings, prints, and ancient coins. It was not surprising, then, that the first professor of anatomy at the Royal Academy, 1768, should be William Hunter, a connoisseur, and, by all testimony, the finest anatomy teacher in London. Zoffany pictured Hunter lecturing to the Academy and its President, Sir Joshua Reynolds. William Hogarth visited Hunter's dissecting rooms and drew the scene around one table. Hunter describes how Hogarth 'came to me when I had a gravid uterus to open and was amazingly pleased, "Good God!" says he, "how snug and compleat it lies..."'. These artistic interests and connections served him well during the production of *The anatomy of the human gravid uterus. . . .*

In order to emphasize the degree of co-operation needed to produce a classic text of anatomical illustration, we shall supplement the above remarks on William Hunter with some consideration of the other three men primarily involved: the artist, van Riemsdyk; the engravers, represented by Strange; and the printer, Baskerville.

Jan van Riemsdyk or Rymsdyk (there are other spellings) (*fl.* 1750–84). Nothing is apparently known of van Riemsdyk before Hunter employed him in about 1750. He was born in the Netherlands—'my country, the Republic of Holland'. From the style of his work, it has been suggested that he was trained, or he had been influenced, by Jan Wandelaar, the illustrator for B. S. Albinus. A plate from Jenty's *An essay...*, 1757—one of those still preserved in Philadelphia—could be used to justify this suggestion; but this picture was of a lower standard of accuracy and elegance than Wandelaar's work. Within two years or less of starting with Hunter, van Riemsdyk was working also for Smellie, preparing, as we have seen, many illustrations for *A sett of anatomical tables ... on midwifery*, 1754. He then worked for Jenty, producing illustrations for his book on general anatomy and for the obstetrical anatomy work, in both using the 'black art', namely mezzotint engravings. John Hunter also employed van Riemsdyk as an artist for his collection in the late 1750s; some of these illustrations may still be seen at the Royal College of Surgeons, in London.

Since Jenty refers knowledgeably to mezzotint colour printing, it has been suggested that he or van Riemsdyk had seen such work done for Ruysch and for Albinus in Holland by Ladmiral in the period 1736–41; there is also the possibility that Jenty or his artist knew of the inventions of LeBlon, or the development of these by the elder Gautier d'Agoty in Paris. Gautier's first anatomical publication with prints in colour was in 1745. Some of van Riemsdyk's mezzotints for Jenty resemble in their extravagance the obstetrical plates of Gautier d'Agoty.

In 1758 and 1759, van Riemsdyk was in Bristol; there are portraits in oils by him of prominent Bristol citizens, painted in the early sixties. From 1764 until 1772, van Riemsdyk was again working for Hunter and others in London.

The acknowledgements to van Riemsdyk by the authors of the three principal obstetric anatomy books to which he contributed are of interest. In *A treatise on ... midwifery*, 1752, Smellie refers to van Riemsdyk as 'a very able artist ...' surpassing, in design and anatomical exactness 'any figures of the kind hitherto made public'. In *A Sett ...*, 1754, van Riemsdyk is named as the artist for the majority of the illustrations, but is neither praised nor thanked. In Jenty's books, van Riemsdyk's name appears in the title and signatures on the illustrations. Hunter made no specific mention of van Riemsdyk in *The Anatomy of the human gravid uterus ...*, 1774; only general references such as that to 'the ingenious artists who made the drawings and engravings'.

It is perhaps not surprising that van Riemsdyk in his later life was upset by the lack of recognition for his contributions to these three obstetric atlases, contributions that have made these works reference standards in medical illustration. In his ponderous text and accompanying, unremarkable illustrations to a book on the newly opened British Museum (1759), *Museum Britannicum, being an exhibition of a great variety of antiquities and natural curiosities, belonging to ... the British Museum*, London, 1778, van Riemsdyk refers in a number of places to his mistreatment, saying that he had borne with patience and for a long time any insults and injuries, 'but', he added, 'such is the way of the world ...'. His footnote to an illustration of a stuffed Ibis, refers scathingly to *Dr. Ibis*, who has a hooked nose, long stiff legs, and shining black clothes, a person with the characteristics of this bird; this probably caricatures William Hunter. Van Riemsdyk then adds:

I flatter myself that I have been very useful as a designer, and sacrificed my talents to a good purpose, more so than any painter in my profession in this Kingdom; though I look on myself as a man that has been ill used and betrayed ... but [I] bear all things with a manly patience. On that account and this is the only reason, which I took a dislike to the anatomical studies, etc., in which I was employed, for I found no relief from those as could do me justice; I submitted, did not resist, and I fell.

Sir Robert Strange (1721–92) made an important contribution to Hunter's *The anatomy of the human gravid uterus ...*, as is stated in the author's effusive acknowledgements in the preface. Strange himself engraved only two plates; but it has been deduced that he had a role in supervising the work of other engravers.

Strange, born in Orkney, was apprenticed to an Edinburgh engraver for six years, during which time he studied anatomy in the first Alexander Monro's classes, and is said to have drawn for this anatomist. Strange enthusiastically joined the Jacobite cause when the Young

Pretender returned in 1745, and he engraved a portrait of Prince Charles. After Culloden, at which he was present, Strange left for Paris, where he stayed for some years. This may help to explain the presence of many engravers with French connections employed for the Hunter engravings. In 1750, he was working for William Hunter in London, but his Jacobite sympathies were still strong enough for him to refuse to do a portrait of the Prince of Wales. In 1760, when the Prince became King, Strange spent a period in Italy, and established for himself a new profession, that of art-dealer. He later sold a number of master-works to William Hunter, and, to judge by the works of art in the Hunterian Collection, Strange advised his friend well. In 1768, when the Royal Academy was founded, Strange was perturbed that engravers were excluded; they were finally admitted, but not until 1928.

After Hunter's book had been published, Strange spent another period in Paris, returning in 1780 to complete what has been judged his finest work—engraved portraits after Van Dyck and others. Reconciled in his later life to the Hanoverians, Strange engraved a sentimental picture of two dead royal Princes and was rewarded with a knighthood in 1787. 'Strange! Strange! Strange!' commented, rather obviously, the *Morning Herald*.

The technique that Strange used in much of his work, and possibly that used by him and some of the other engraver's for the Hunter plates, has been described by Hind (1923):

He begins with a pure etching of the principal outlines, and lighter tones of shading, and afterwards changes the character of the great part of these lines by reworking them with the graver, adding other work with the graver, taking the etched foundation as his guide.

John Baskerville (1706–75). In the second half of the eighteenth century, this printer, together with Caslon in England, Didot in France, and Bodoni in Italy, reformed typography, returning this humane art to the fundamentals of the Venetian sixteenth-century printers, and adding a new, restrained, rational elegance.

Baskerville was born near Kidderminster, which he left for Birmingham when he was a young man. A slate still exists on which is carved: 'Grave stones cut in any of the hands by John Baskervill, writing-master'. But his fortune was made after he had joined the ranks of the capitalist entrepreneurs in the burgeoning Birmingham light-metal trade; Baskerville's factory japanned tinware.

By 1750, aged forty-four years, Baskerville enjoyed the status of a rich man with ostentatious tastes. This did not satisfy him completely, and he returned to lettering. Backed by the profitability of his factory he set up a printing-shop, determined to produce 'books of consequence, of intrinsic merit, or established reputation ... at such a price, as will repay the extraordinary care and expence [sic] that must necessarily be bestowed upon them'. Baskerville was a patient man, and, with his experience of letter-shapes and with metal-working, he started from scratch, building his own presses, designing and casting his own type. Baskerville's ink, formulated from his knowledge of pigments used in his japanned goods, and his paper, obtained from John Whatman, were of the highest quality. It was more than six years before his first volume was issued, a *Virgil*, 1757. In 1760, he printed a *Book of Common Prayer* in a type 'calculated for people who begin to want spectacles, but are ashamed to use them in church'. Baskerville himself was a staunch opponent of superstition: his gravehead read: 'Stranger, beneath this cone, in unconscrated [*sic*] ground a friend to the liberties of mankind directed his body to be inhum'd. May the example contribute to emancipate thy mind from the idle fears of superstition and the wicked arts of priesthood'. It is a happy thought that Baskerville's type was sold to Beaumarchais, and used to print an authoritative edition of Voltaire. (The type punches returned to England as a gift in 1953, and are now at the Cambridge University Press.)

Hunter's obstetrical atlas was his last major production—an unusual one for Baskerville, for the text was of a technical nature, and the book depended primarily on illustration. One feels that Baskerville must have needed persuasion to print such a different sort of work. He died a month after the atlas was published.

Van Riemsdyk's anatomical drawings depicted carefully, yet with compassion, Hunter's precise dissections of women who had died during pregnancy, many in childbirth. These illustrations had been transferred accurately to the copperplates at a time when British engraving had reached a high standard of technical competence. It was entirely appropriate that Baskerville's formal, restrained, rather cold, and almost monumental typography should be used on the title-page (*Fig. 12.5*). It had been thirty years or so since Baskerville had cut gravestones; but it may not be too fanciful to regard this title-page as a memorial tablet to the subjects of the studies contained within.

As Leonardo had before him in Renaissance times so Hunter, but with a confidence entirely appropriate to the age of enlightenment, clearly saw how anatomical science was co-existent with anatomical illustration. Anatomical prints communicated detailed and precise information quickly and without language barriers. He writes in the preface to *The Anatomy of the human gravid uterus*:

The art of engraving supplies us upon many occasions, . . . with what has been the great *desideratum* of the lover of science, an universal language. Nay, it conveys clearer ideas of most natural objects, than words can express . . . [it] gives an immediate comprehension of what it represents.

From the time when this art came more generally into use, it has been much more easy both to communicate and to preserve discoveries and improvements; and natural knowledge has been gradually rising, till it is at length become the distinguishing characteristic of the most enlightened age of the world.

Anatomy had kept pace with other branches of science, most of the principal parts having been successfully illustrated.

ANATOMIA
UTERI HUMANI GRAVIDI
TABULIS ILLUSTRATA.

AUCTORE
GULIELMO HUNTER,

SERENISSIMAE REGINAE CHARLOTTAE MEDICO EXTRAORDINARIO,

IN ACADEMIA REGALI ANATOMIAE PROFESSORE,

ET SOCIETATUM, REGIAE ET ANTIQUARIAE, SOCIO.

BIRMINGHAMIAE EXCUDEBAT JOANNES BASKERVILLE, MDCCLXXIV.

LONDINI PROSTANT APUD S. BAKER, T. CADELL, D. WILSON, G. NICOL, ET J. MURRAY.

THE ANATOMY
OF THE
HUMAN GRAVID UTERUS
EXHIBITED IN FIGURES,

BY
WILLIAM HUNTER,

PHYSICIAN EXTRAORDINARY TO THE QUEEN, PROFESSOR OF

ANATOMY IN THE ROYAL ACADEMY, AND FELLOW OF THE

ROYAL AND ANTIQUARIAN SOCIETIES.

PRINTED AT BIRMINGHAM BY JOHN BASKERVILLE, 1774.

SOLD IN LONDON BY S. BAKER AND G. LEIGH, IN York-Street; T. CADELL IN THE Strand; D. WILSON AND G. NICOL,
OPPOSITE York-Buildings; AND J. MURRAY, IN Fleet-Street.

12.5   Title-page of William Hunter's *The anatomy of the human gravid uterus*, 1774.

One part however, and that the most curious, and certainly not the least important of all, the pregnant womb, had not been treated by anatomists with proportionable success.

The atlases of Smellie, Jenty, and Hunter remedied this deficiency.

102 Fetus *in utero.* Tab. XII in William Hunter, *The anatomy of the human gravid uterus...*, 1774. Engraving (private collection). 47.8 × 31.9 cm.

This drawing is of a specimen removed from a woman who died 'of a flooding in the ninth month of pregnancy'.

The first, and perhaps natural, impression is that it is a uterus opened from the front. However, closer examination of the adnexa, such as parts of the broad ligament and the ovaries (B and D), together with the Fallopian tubes (A), suggests that this is a posterior view, and this is confirmed in the text.

This was a case of placenta praevia, as the placenta (I) obviously covers over the cervix (H). Hunter explained that the placenta 'had originally stuck to the inside of the neck and mouth of the womb; but as parturition approached, the dilatation of these parts occasioned a separation, which was necessarily followed by an hemorrhage'.

The large fetal head is pleasing, as also the general 'chubbiness' of the limbs, though the fingers of the left hand are rather out of proportion. The general configuration of the umbilical cord (L) is felicitous, and it is interesting that, on the left side of the illustration, Hunter has seen fit to depict the corpus luteum.

It must be admitted that the anatomy of the vagina (G) and its surroundings is confusing and difficult to understand. This may have been due to the manner in which the specimen was removed.

It is puzzling that Hunter chose to open the uterus from the back instead of from the front, but whatever the reason, it gave his artist van Riemsdyk an opportunity to produce an unusual and beautiful anatomical illustration, probably the first to feature a placenta praevia.

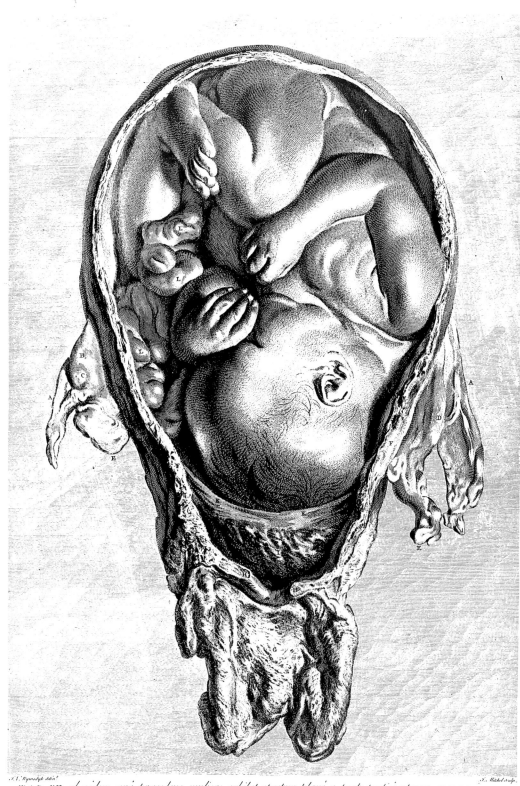

J.V. Rymsdyk delin.   J. Mitchel sculp.

T A B. XII. ab eadem, quà praecedens, muliere, exhibet apertum planè a parte postici uterum cum vagina,
quo situs Foetus, parsque inferior Placentae sub Foetus capite indicarentur. Placenta scilicet orificio
uteri interno accreverat; eoque sub finem graviditatis dilatato fatali inde divisione separata est

Pub: Nov: 15: 1774, by Dr. Hunter.

PLATE 102

Chapter 12: Selected Reading

The rise of the man-midwife

Aveling, J. H. (1967). *English midwives: their history and prospects.* (Reprint of 1872 edition, ed. J. L. Thornton.) Hugh K. Elliott, London.

Donnison, J. (1977). *Midwives and medical men.* Heinemann, London.

J. van Riemsdyk

Huffman, J. W. (1969). Jan van Riemsdyk .... *JAMA,* **208,** 121–4.

Huffman, J. W. (1970). The great eighteenth century obstetric atlases and their illustrator. *Obs. Gynec.,* **35,** 971–6.

Thornton, J. L. (1982). *Jan van Rymsdyk...* The Oleander Press, Cambridge.

Thornton, J. L. and Want, P. C. (1979). Jan van Rymsdyk's illustrations of the gravid uterus drawn for Hunter, Smellie, Jenty and Denman. *J. audiovisual Media in Med.,* **2,** 10–15.

William Smellie

Butterton, J. R. (1986). The education, naval service, and early career of William Smellie. *Bull. Hist. Med.,* **60,** 1–18.

Glaister, J. (1894). *Dr. William Smellie and his contemporaries...* J. Maclehose and Sons, Glasgow.

Johnstone, R. W. (1952). *William Smellie...,* E. & S. Livingstone, Edinburgh.

Charles Jenty

de Lint, J. G. (1916). The plates of Jenty. *Janus,* **21,** 129–35.

Thornton, J. L. and Want, P. C. (1978). C. N. Jenty and the mezzotint plates in his 'Demonstrations of a pregnant uterus', 1757. *J. audiovisual Media in Med.,* **1,** 113–15.

William Hunter

Brock, C. H. (1980). Dr. William Hunter's Museum, Glasgow University. *J. Soc. Biblphy. nat. Hist.,* **9,** 403–12.

Bynum, W. F. and Porter R. (ed.) (1985). *William Hunter and the eighteenth-century medical world.* Cambridge University Press.

Cope, Z. (1961). *The Great Windmill Street School of anatomy* In *Some famous general practitioners.* Pitman, London.

Corner, B. C. (1951). Dr. Ibis and the artists. *J. Hist. Med.,* **1,** 1–21.

Eales, N. B. (1974). The history of the lymphatic system, with special reference to the Hunter–Monro controversy. *J. Hist. Med.,* **29,** 280–94.

Fox, R. H. (1901). *William Hunter; anatomist, physician, obstetrician...* H. K. Lewis, London.

Hind, A. M. (1963). *A history of engraving and etching...* Dover, New York. (Reprint of 1923 edition).

Illingworth, C. (1967). *The story of William Hunter*. E. and S. Livingstone, Edinburgh.

Kemp, M. (ed.) (1975). *Dr. William Hunter at the Royal Academy of Arts*. University of Glasgow Press.

LeFanu, W. R. (1958). The writings of William Hunter, F.R.S. *The Bibliotheck*, **1**, 3–14.

Ollerenshaw, R. (1974). Dr Hunter's 'Gravid uterus'—a bicentenary note. *Med. biol. Illust.*, **24**, 43–57.

Oppenheimer, J. M. (1946). *New aspects of John and William Hunter*. Henry Schuman, New York.

Schumann, E. A. (1940–2). William Hunter lecturing on obstetrics and infant care. *Trans. Coll. Phys. Philadelphia*, **8–9**, 155–183.

Stevenson, L. G. (1953). William Hewson, the Hunters, and Benjamin Franklin. *J. Hist. Med.*, **8**, 324–8.

Tait, H. P. and Wallace, A. T. (1952). Dr. William Smellie and his library of Lanark, Scotland. *Bull. Hist. Med.*, **26**, 403–20.

Thornton, J. L. (1983). William Hunter (1718–1783) and his contributions to obstetrics. *Brit. J. Obs. Gyn.*, **90**, 787–94.

Thornton, J. L. and Want, P. C. (1974). William Hunter's 'The anatomy of the human gravid uterus.' 1774–1974. *J. Obs. Gyn. Brit. Comm.*, **81**, 1–10.

John Baskerville

Benton, J. H. (1944). *John Baskerville: type-founder and printer 1706–1775*. The Typophiles, New York.

Pardoe, F. E. (1975). *John Baskerville of Birmingham* . . . Frederick Muller, London.

13

British anatomical illustration 1775–1830

T HE advance of the science of human anatomy has always depended on the availability of bodies for dissection. In Britain and North America, until well into the nineteenth century, there were no legal ways to ensure an adequate supply of subjects for the teaching of anatomy.

The supply of bodies to dissecting rooms

In early modern times in Britain there was no insistence on first-hand anatomical experience for aspiring apothecaries; but the physicians and the surgeons of London, by their sixteenth-century charters, had been granted the right to acquire the bodies of persons hanged. Harvey's anatomies in front of the physicians were presumably carried out on such subjects. An Act of Henry VIII specified that the Company of Barbers and Surgeons 'maie have and take without contridiction foure persons condempned adjudged and put to deathe for feloni ... for anatomies ... to make incision of the same deade bodies for their further and better knowlage instruction in sight learnyng and experience in the sayd scyence or facultie of surgery'. Similar arrangements were made at Edinburgh and other centres. During the eighteenth century, the physicians—who were entitled to six bodies each year—gradually let slip their privileges, but the surgeons continued jealously to guard their rights; they fined surgeons who anatomized, for the benefit of their students, outside of the Barber-Surgeons' Hall. Disciplinary cases of this kind are recorded as early as 1573. In 1714 William Cheselden was rebuked:

Our Master acquainted the Court that Mr. Wm. Cheselden, a member of the company did frequently procure the dead bodies of malefactors from the place of execution and dissect the same at his own house as well during the Company's publick lectures as at other times without the word of the Governors and contrary to the Company's By-law in that behalf by which means it becomes more difficult for the beadles to bring away the Company's bodies and likewise drew away the members from the publick dissections and lectures at the Hall. The said Mr. Cheselden was thereupon called in but having submitted himself to the pleasure of the Court with a promise never to dissect at the same time as the Company had the lectures at their Hall nor without leave of the Governors for the time being the said Mr. Cheselden was censured for what had passed with a reproof for the same pronounced by the Master at the desire of the Court.

From early Tudor times to 1783, judicial hangings in London were carried out at Tyburn on 'Albion's Fatal Tree'. At each execution-day, crowds assembled to await the arrival of the condemned, brought to the west of London by cart from Newgate in the City. The methods used did not break the neck, but caused death by suffocation, and on very rare occasions a hanged person would revive on the way to burial or even in the dissection rooms, as we have seen (Chapter 11, p. 398). Each body in the eighteenth century was a commodity with a price; sometimes condemned prisoners would anticipate the hangman and sell their bodies to pay prison debts or to buy decent clothes in which to die. More usually the bailiffs or the surgeons would claim the body by right of their charters—would claim but not necessarily receive, for relatives and friends of the prisoner would travel, sometimes a great distance, to Tyburn, and would dispute for the body in order to give it decent burial. These groups of persons—called by the authorities *the mob; loose, disorderly persons; scum of the people*; and so on—often fought with the surgeons' servants and with detachments of the army called in to support the surgeons' claims. Samuel Richardson described hangings at Tyburn, followed by fights between friends of the hanged man or woman and 'persons sent by private surgeons to obtain bodies for dissection. The contests between these were fierce and bloody, and frightful to look at.'

From the middle of the eighteenth century the law regarded anatomizing as a further punishment, condemning the prisoner both to hanging *and* dissection; and this indeed terrorized many. It was reported about one man: 'he was greatly frighted lest his body should be cut, and torn, and mangled after death'. *A dictionary of buckish slang, university wit, and pikpocket eloquence*, published in London as late as 1811, has, under the heading *Ottomised*, this example of usage: 'You'll be scragged, ottomised and grin in a glass case'—that is, you'll be hanged, anatomized, and your skeleton kept in a glass case at Surgeons' Hall. The last in the series of Hogarth's paintings entitled 'the reward of cruelty' shows the anti-hero being dissected in an anatomy

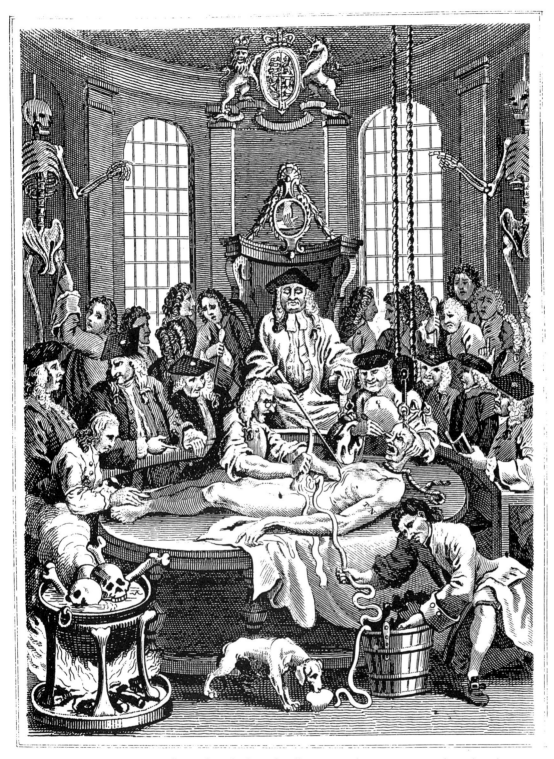

13.1   Dissection in Surgeons' Hall, London, the last of William Hogarth's 'Four Stages of Cruelty', drawn in 1751.

theatre after being hanged, a parody of the Renaissance anatomy title-page even down to the dog, who in this scene is running away with the subject's heart (*Fig. 13.1*).

From 1832, after the passing of the Anatomy Act, and until quite recent times a particular and deep anxiety of many common people was that they would die friendless and in reduced circumstances, and that their corpse would therefore suffer the indignity of providing dissecting material as if they were common criminals. Burial clubs and friendly societies were formed to ensure that members received decent burial.

In many cases, in the eighteenth century, an assembled council of surgeons would accept the corpse from their bailiffs, record its delivery, and then perform merely a symbolic, crucial incision on the chest, the body then being assigned to an anatomist for proper dissection before students in his school or hospital.

When there were comparatively few students studying at London and Edinburgh, infrequent dissections of the bodies of executed persons may have proved adequate; but with the rise of student numbers in the eighteenth century—earlier in London than in Edinburgh—the demand for more instruction in anatomy led to the start of private anatomy and surgery classes. The need for bodies in the extramural schools far outstripped any supply. The anatomy classes at the University of Edinburgh conducted by the Alexander Monros, *secundus* and *tertius*, were criticized for not providing opportunities for all students to get close to the dissected material; the private schools flourished partly because they did allow such opportunities. To meet the lack of subjects for anatomy, unscrupulous persons turned to robbing recent graves. In Edinburgh, the extramural schools were located, along with Surgeons' Hall, around Surgeons' Square; also in the vicinity was the graveyard for the old Infirmary. Students could see this burial ground from the windows of some of the anatomy rooms, and, when burials took place, they exhumed the bodies the next night. It became an expected part of attending classes for students of anatomy to assist in providing bodies. Other burial grounds were robbed in Edinburgh, and students, sometimes assisted by the anatomists themselves, ventured further afield, even going so far as to row across the Firth of Forth in order to rob the graveyards in villages on the Fife coast. 'And when at last we needs to die / the doctors cannot save / from death—they still most kindly try / to snatch us from the grave': one verse from *The Doctors*, a poem included in *Whistle Binkle: A collection of songs for the social circle*, published in Glasgow in 1832.

By the middle of the eighteenth century the schools in London and Edinburgh were emphasizing methods of anatomy teaching that included direct access to bodies by the student; by the end of that century students were expected to do the dissections themselves, assisted by their teachers. It became a prerequisite in 1820 in the Edinburgh College of Surgeons' examinations that students attend practical anatomy classes for one session, and, in 1828, for two sessions—a whole academic year. In this period—thirty years either side of 1800—the supply of bodies to the anatomy rooms was met largely by the private enterprise of loose organizations of men, who, outside the law, would during the day wander around town gossiping and keeping their eyes open for recent deaths and burials; then at night (but *not* when there was a full moon in a clear sky) they would rob the new grave, taking the bodies to the anatomy halls of the private schools and the hospitals. The grave robbers were called 'resurrectionists', or 'sack 'em up' men. One London resurrectionist kept a diary during 1811 and 1812 in which he described the daily life of a grave-robber. The men were often in league with the grave-diggers and keepers of burial grounds, and with door-keepers and attendants of the school with whom they transacted their business—the anatomists and surgeons dealt largely at arm's length through these attendants. The whole enterprise was very profitable: four guineas or more—(professional fees were naturally in guineas!)—were given for each adult body, less for 'smalls' (children less than three feet in height), babies, and fetuses. On successful days more than one corpse could be obtained. The standard time required to rob a grave was about one hour, and the highest number recorded by one gang was twenty-three bodies obtained in four nights. The total numbers taken for nine months in 1810–11—there were few entries for the summer months, when the schools were closed—was 312 adults and 47 'smalls'. The total amount of money netted was probably about 1500 guineas, to be divided between six or seven persons—a very large return for their endeavours. The work was so profitable that an 'import' trade developed in Edinburgh and London for this commodity, with bodies supplied from as far away as Liverpool and Dublin. They were shipped in barrels, sometimes packed in salt or spirits. (In the middle of the nineteenth century in the United States, bodies stolen from rural graveyards were similarly barrelled and moved to the medical schools in Virginia.) One London resurrectionist, Crouch, travelled to Edinburgh to ply his trade there, in association with the surgeon, Robert Liston. In 1825 Lizars wrote with irony that 'liberal, enlightened, and truly philanthropic public authorities of Glasgow and Newcastle have arrested in their progress *subjects* travelling through their cities, as if they were Radicals carrying death and destruction through the country'.

Throughout the years of grave-robbing there were angry responses from the authorities and the public. The legal position of the grave-robbers proved to be ambiguous: a body was not thought to be a chattel in the possession of the relatives; indeed resurrectionists, both student amateurs and the professional 'sack 'em up' men, were careful to leave the shrouds and winding-sheets behind, so that they could not be charged with larceny. Many magistrates, however, severely punished professional grave-robbers when they were apprehended; and there were cases in which even medical men were fined and imprisoned.

In parts of Scotland grave-robbery was so prevalent that it became the practice to mount a guard at the burial place for the nights following interment, that is until the corpse became unsuitable for anatomizing. Heavy iron railings called 'mort-safes', immovable by small gangs, were placed around and over the grave, but the resourceful resurrectionists tunnelled from beyond these to obtain the corpse. Iron coffins were sold. In burial grounds such as Greyfriars in Edinburgh, as one commentator described, 'there was a strange resemblance to zoological gardens, the rows of iron cages suggesting rather the dens of wild animals than the final resting-places of the dead. And, in fact, these barred and grated cells were designed as a protection against human wolves who nightly prowled about such places in quest of prey ...'. For the most part it was the graves of poor persons which were robbed; the rich could afford iron coffins and mort-safes, and could pay to have the graves guarded. The reaction of the wealthy was more to be feared.

When it became known that the grave of a well-liked person had been desecrated, the anger, belligerence, and destructiveness of crowds was turned towards the anatomists and their servants, and on the keepers of burial grounds. Doctors printed denials, and handbills were posted; the College of Surgeons of Edinburgh gave public warnings to their Fellows that grave-robbing would not be tolerated; but everyone knew that the education of medical men required training in anatomy, which could, for all practical purposes at that time, only be obtained by the dissection of resurrected subjects.

The most infamous suppliers of subjects to anatomy schools were William Burke and William Hare, two Irishmen who had come to Scotland to work as navvies on the Union Canal linking Edinburgh and Glasgow. Though arriving separately in Edinburgh, they became acquainted, and Hare and his wife acquired a lodging-house for near-destitutes, in Tanner's Yard; Burke and Helen M'Dougal, with whom he lived, lodged nearby. One of Hare's lodgers, an old man, died, November 29, 1827, owing four pounds sterling to the landlord. Burke and Hare, although they had no actual experience, had heard that corpses were marketable items. So after they had unnailed and emptied the coffin, making up the weight from the pile of tanner's bark outside their back door, they took the old man's body to the University to attempt to sell it to Alexander Monro *tertius*. A student, from whom they enquired the way, directed them instead to Robert Knox's extramural school, Number 10 Surgeons' Square, where they sold the merchandise to Knox's assistant, Paterson, and were pleased to receive £7.10s. Robert Knox (1791–1862) was perhaps the most brilliant of the extramural lecturers in anatomy and surgery in Edinburgh, and certainly the most popular; in 1825 he had more than five hundred students, whom he taught in three sessions a day, since his theatre only held two hundred. He was outspoken in contempt of creeds and persons, a radical, and a precursor of the group of Victorian scientific racists. Although his students stood up for him through the Burke and Hare affair, his courses became less successful, and he moved to Glasgow and then to London, but never achieved an equal success again. Knox published a commentary to a popular series of anatomical plates issued in Edinburgh in 1825; the illustrations were not original, but taken from the work of others, principally Tiedemann and Vicq d'Azyr.

Burke and Hare devised a plan to supply Knox's anatomy and surgery classes with further subjects by murdering people, many in Hare's lodging-house. A total of sixteen were suffocated and sold to Paterson in the next nine months; most were made drunk with whisky and then suffocated by pillows. Burke and Hare carried out their plan in a most inefficient manner, becoming known to the children of the neighbourhood, as they trundled body after body in tea-chests up to Surgeons' Square. They were nearly caught after the second murder, for this was of Mary Paterson, a young prostitute. One of Knox's students and assistants, who was later to become Sir William Ferguson, Baronet and FRS, President of the Royal College of Surgeons of England, and Surgeon to Queen Victoria, had known Mary and recognized her corpse. Moreover Mary's friend Janet Brown, and their landlady, instituted a search for the missing girl; but the enquiries came to nothing, and Mary Paterson's corpse, preserved for some months, was sketched by one of the artists attending the anatomy school. The sketch is of a beautiful woman, a sentimentalized odalisque in the smooth, romantic manner used by some Edinburgh anatomical illustrators.

The last murder was of an old woman—'Madgy or Margery or Mary M'Gonegal or Duffie, or Campbell, or Docherty'. A neighbour suspected foul play and informed the authorities: and Burke, Hare, and M'Dougal were arrested before the subject could be sold to Knox's school. Thus it came about that Knox was not called as a witness at the trial. Hare turned King's evidence, and was freed at the end of the trial, which started at 10 a.m. on Christmas Eve and continued for twenty-four hours into Christmas morning, 1828. M'Dougal received the Scots verdict of 'not proven': 'Nellie you are out of the scrape,' said Burke to her in court when the finding was given. Burke, found guilty, was hanged in public, and his corpse brought to the anatomy theatre at the University, where it was dissected before a large audience—thousands of men and women subsequently filed past the corpse. Alexander Monro *tertius* was the anatomist, and lectured for two hours, paying special attention to the brain. Later there was a pamphlet war over the shape of Burke's skull and brain: were they or were they not in accord with phrenological theory?

The activities of Burke and Hare were matters of great public interest; the verb *to burke* was coined, broadsheets were published, and rhymes were composed:

> Up the close and doon the stair,
> But and ben [in and out] wi' Burke and Hare:
> Burke's the butcher, Hare's the thief,
> And Knox the boy who buys the beef.

The anger against the doctors was directed naturally enough towards Knox, and his house was attacked; when he himself narrowly escaped, the crowd hanged and burnt his effigy. At other levels of society, the Burke and Hare case was equally significant. The use of judicial immunity for Hare, after he had turned King's evidence and provided the information on which Burke was tried, was widely discussed.

Murder for anatomical purposes was not confined to Scotland; Williams and Bishop were hanged in 1831 for murdering an Italian boy and attempting to sell his body to the anatomy department of King's College, London.

In medical education, an important consequence of the murders was to focus attention generally on the dilemma in which the medical profession found itself: there were regulations, by the medical authorities, that students should know the anatomy of the human body, knowledge only obtained by dissection. But sufficient subjects for dissection could not legally be obtained.

John Lizars, in the dedication to the King of his book. *A system of anatomical plates . . . , 1825*, regretted the obstacles that arose to the practice of anatomy, obstacles that were 'injurious to Your Majesty's subjects, both in the public services, and in all the ranks of private society'. Lizars approved of the situation in France, Germany, and Denmark, where the prosecution of anatomy was protected by their respective governments, and described the contrasting situation in Britain, where medical youth collected 'by repeated failures in their treatment of the living, that knowledge which they might have early, and safely and ably, acquired from intimacy with the dead'. Lizars was bold enough to urge the King to intervene with government and recommend the matter to the serious attention of his 'wise and liberal Ministers'. The Rt. Hon. Robert Peel MP, Secretary of State for the Home Department, was petitioned in an open letter published in Glasgow in 1829 by 'A Medical Officer in the Royal Navy,' a pupil in Charles Bell's classes at the Great Windmill Street School, London, *Reflections suggested by the murders recently committed at Edinburgh, etc.* Three of his propositions were.

I. The present state of the laws affecting that part of medical education which depends on anatomy, makes it impossible to study that science efficiently, without incurring some degree of criminality.

II. It is impossible for a surgeon, or surgeon-apothecary, to practise his profession independent of an intimate acquaintance with the structure of the human frame, and at the same time consistently with the safety of the public, his own comfort, and the security of his property.

III. When the legislature requires one thing, and necessity demands another, not only must the enactment of the former be disregarded, but, in process of time, temptations will accumulate to supply the wants of the latter by unlawful as well as by illegal means.

The author contrasted the situation in London, where dissecting rooms 'support whole gangs of hardened and unprincipled men, who, for money, will dare to breathe defiance at the state, and brave its every penalty' with that in Paris, 'where so cheap are bodies, so unrestrained is dissection, that a majority of the medical students of Great Britain emigrate thither to prosecute their professional studies, and, by way of counterbalancing the advantages derived from French anatomy and pathology, bring back with them French politics, which are republican, French morals, which are licentious, and French *Deligion*, a term there can be no occasion for me to explain or characterize'.

In 1828 Parliament appointed a Committee on Anatomy under the chairmanship of the radical, Henry Warburton, 'to inquire into the manner of obtaining subjects for dissection in the Schools of Anatomy, and into the state of the law affecting the persons employed in obtaining and dissecting bodies'. Evidence was obtained from anatomists, including Astley Cooper and Charles Bell, and from resurrectionists themselves, identified by initials, A. B., C. D., and so on. Warburton introduced a Bill to Parliament in 1829, and this passed the Commons, but was rejected by the Lords. Opposition came from the country surgeons, and from some of the private schools, for it was proposed to make it illegal to dissect in unlicensed places, restricting the practice to recognized authorities. The *Lancet* called the measure a Bill for preventing country surgeons from studying anatomy. The Bill, somewhat modified, was reintroduced in 1831, passed both Houses, and became law in 1832. From that date onwards, the resurrectionists were out of business; and grave-robbing and burking became matters of history in Britain.

Since 1832 bodies for dissection in Britain have come from two sources. The first consists of the bodies of persons who have died and whose bodies remained unclaimed by friends and relations, and who would otherwise have been buried at public expense. In 1827 in London there were 3103 buried as a charge to the parishes, and for 1108 of these there were no relatives at the grave-side for the commitment. The second source of cadavers has been from voluntary donations made by persons prior to their death. Since a body could not be bequeathed, this meant that relatives had to be willing to comply with the wishes of the deceased. An early example of such a donation was the Utilitarian philosopher Jeremy Bentham, whose body was dissected in 1831. Preceding the dissection, the orator spoke of Bentham's admiration of medical science and his recognition that 'the safe and successful practice of the healing art entirely rests on a thorough knowledge of the natural structure and function of the human body ... that there was but one method of obtaining such knowledge, viz., dissection'.

In some of the United States the bodies for the medical schools were still being supplied by resurrectionists into the middle of the nineteenth century.

As all British observers pointed out during the discussions leading up to Warburton's 1832 Anatomy Act, countries of the continent of Europe had not been short of subjects for dissection. In Leiden for example, from the eighteenth century on, the hospitals of Amsterdam had provided a supply of bodies, and in French, Italian, and German schools similar arrangements were made.

In the years immediately before the enactment of the Anatomy Act in Britain there were issued, in Edinburgh and London, a number of anatomical plate-books. With the more ready availability of subjects for dissection, the demand for such works may have lessened. As one early biographer of John Lizars pointed out: 'the superior facilities now afforded to the study of anatomy have made all such aids less necessary'.

In the fifty years either side of 1800, many prominent British anatomists were educated in Edinburgh, at the University Medical School and the co-existing, symbiotic, private schools. Anatomy was regarded, naturally enough, as a necessary foundation for a career in surgery, but many did not leave anatomy behind as they established themselves as surgeons. John Bell, perhaps the most prominent Edinburgh surgeon in his day, taught anatomy; and Charles Bell, knighted for surgery, had academic responsibilities for anatomy both in Edinburgh and London. John Lizars, sometime Professor of Surgery at the Royal College of Surgeons of Edinburgh, was known equally as the author and artist of a series of anatomical plates.

Medical men trained in Edinburgh often had previous experience of medical practice derived from a period of apprenticeship; this they supplemented by courses in the private schools and in the University. The majority did not graduate from the University, but took instead the licentiate, or diploma, examinations from the Royal Colleges. Many of those qualified returned home to practice. Such a one was Joseph Swan. He became known as surgeon and anatomist, first in his home town of Lincoln and later in London, where his work on the anatomy of the nerves received international recognition.

The Scottish Schools, particularly Edinburgh, produced so many medical men that there were not opportunities for them all to settle down in Scotland as surgeon-apothecaries (the forerunners of general practitioners) or as medical specialists. One favoured route to advancement was to become for a period a surgeon in the Royal Navy. It was possible during tours of service to accumulate enough money to tide over the lean initial years of private practice. The anatomist-obstetrician, William Smellie, is one who falls, as we have seen, into such a category; John Lizars, as we shall see, was another. An alternative route taken by some medical men was to try one's luck overseas, in the United States or in Canada for example. Alexander Ramsay had studied and had taught anatomy in Edinburgh, possibly considering himself to be a likely successor to Monro *secundus*. However he emigrated, around 1802, to the United States as an anatomist and surgeon-apothecary.

Alexander Monro *secundus* had no great difficulty in mapping a useful and profitable career, for from his early days he was groomed for his father's chair in anatomy and surgery at Edinburgh University. He succeeded Monro *primus* while still a young man.

In the remainder of this chapter we shall consider the surgeon-anatomists mentioned above — Alexander Monro *secundus*, the brothers John and Charles Bell, Alexander Ramsay, John Lizars, and Joseph Swan. To these, we have added an artist-anatomist of the same period, a remarkable individual, George Stubbs

Alexander Monro secundus (1732–1817)

In 1764, Alexander Monro *primus* (see Chapter 11) resigned his chair in favour of his youngest son, who had the same name and is now identified as Alexander Monro *secundus*. This son 'shewed a particular turn to anatomy', and was employed by his father as a dissector, as a lecturer, and as a contributor to *Medical Essays and Observations*, which Alexander Monro *primus* edited. These activities 'raised such expectations of the son, that upon the recommendation of his father with the concurrence of all the professors under whom he had studyed, and of all the students whom he had taught, the Patrons of the University appointed him colleague and successor to his father'. This was in the summer of 1754, and before the young man of twenty-one had taken his MD; he obtained this from Edinburgh University in October of the same year. Like his father, he had a further period of study in London (where he attended William Hunter's lectures), in Paris, and in Leiden (where he was acquainted with B. S. Albinus and Camper). He also went to Berlin to live and work with the elder J. F. Meckel. While there, he wrote *De venis lymphaticis valvulosis* ..., 1757, issued at Berlin, a book that went through three Berlin editions and one Edinburgh edition, all in Latin. Returning to Edinburgh in 1758, he was soon after admitted Fellow of the College of Physicians there.

His published work included public arguments with William Hunter and with Hewson, accusing them of not recognizing the priorities due to him for discoveries relating to the lymphatics (the weight of evidence, in the case of their origin and their absorbent functions at least, is in favour of Hunter and not Monro). In 1783, a more mature and original work was produced: *Observations on the structure and functions of the nervous system*, Edinburgh. Our *Plate 103* is from this book. In this Alexander Monro, MD, is described as President of the Royal College of Physicians, and Professor of Physic, Anatomy, and Surgery in the University of Edinburgh. The work is physiologically orientated, attempting, for example, to quantitate blood-flow to the head, and to explain physiologically the effects of cerebral anaemia; he argued by analogy, and mistakenly, for the presence of lymphatics in the brain, and he discussed the brain as a medium between the mind and the rest of the body. The book includes a description of the foramen by which each lateral ventricle of the brain communicates with the third ventricle. Nearly twenty years earlier Monro had noted its existence in the normal, having seen it greatly enlarged in cases of hydrocephaly, and had reported this to the Philosophical Society of Edinburgh. Monro's interest in the nervous system was maintained, for in 1793 he published: *Experiments on the nervous system* ..., Edinburgh and London, in which he argues that the nerve force is not identical with electricity.

Alexander Monro *secundus* gave lectures in anatomy in Edinburgh every year from 1759 to 1800; from 1800 to 1807 he gave a part of the course. In 1808 he was able only to give the introductory lecture, and retired that year. He was succeeded in his chair by his son, also named Alexander (1773–1859), who occupied it until 1846. It is said of the last of the Monro dynasty of Edinburgh anatomists, Alexander Monro *tertius*: 'None of his works are of permanent value, and those written when he was in the prime of life are as confused, prolix, and illogical as his senile productions'.

103 Left half of brain viewed from medial side. Tab. II from A. Monro [*secundus*], *Observations on the structure and functions of the nervous system*, 1783. Engraving (private collection). 21.2 × 26.2 cm.

In spite of the present-day trend in anatomy texts to abolish the use of eponymous nomenclature, the communication between the lateral and third ventricles remains for many the 'Foramen of Monro'.

In his text Monro commented that communication between the ventricles of the brain was known to Galen and other anatomists, such as Vesalius, Spieghel, Bauhin, Vieussens, Willis, Cowper, and Winslow. He went on to state 'A hole or passage at the upper and fore part of the third ventricle has not only been described, but painted by different authors [for example, Vesalius], under the name of vulva. A few authors [for example, Vieussens] likewise have mentioned a place [situated posteriorly near the pineal gland] under the fornix, to which they have given the name of anus, where they supposed the lateral ventricles to communicate with each other, and with the third ventricle.'

He then emphasized 'no author has *delineated* the beginnings of the passages by which the lateral ventricles can discharge their contents into the third ventricle'.

In this plate, the foramen in question (S) is seen beneath the anterior part of the fornix (P), bounded anteriorly by the anterior column of the fornix (Q). The foramen itself is, in fact, much better portrayed in smaller drawings in Tab. III, one of which clearly shows the choroid fissure and the choroid plexus extending posteriorly from the foramen.

While the pituitary gland (V) is correctly placed in the sella turcica, and the mammillary bodies (X), optic chiasm (W), and septum pellucidum (O) are easily distinguishable, there are a number of anatomical short-comings. A minor one is that, although much of the falx cerebri (L) has been cut away so as to show the medial aspect of the left hemisphere, the anterior attachment of the falx to the crista galli is not depicted. The rostrum or front part of the corpus callosum (N) appears to end in bone above the sphenoidal sinus (C); the anterior commissure (R) is positioned too high; the pineal gland (Z) is too circular, and the nearby posterior commissure (a) too large; the basilar artery (k) seems to have been added as a sort of afterthought; the aqueduct (b) is very poorly portrayed; and the spinal cord and brain stem are most oddly drawn. The gyri and sulci of the cerebral hemisphere (save the anterior part of the cingulate gyrus and sulcus) are also unrealistic.

It is of interest that Monro still termed the superior and inferior colliculi (c, d) 'nates' and 'testis', and also that he denied the existence of the communication between the fourth ventricle and the central canal of the spinal cord: 'The bottom of the fourth ventricle has no such communication with the cavity of the spinal marrow, as Dr. Haller supposed, being completely shut by its choroid plexus and pia mater'.

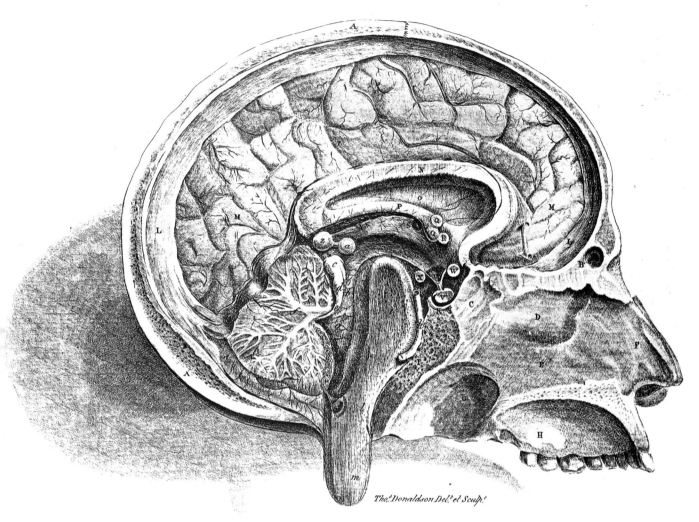

Tho.ᵈ Donaldson Del.ᵗ et Sculp.ᵗ

TAB. II

John Bell (1763–1820) and Charles Bell (1774–1842)

With the Monro dynasty occupying the University of Edinburgh chair of anatomy and surgery for a hundred and twenty-five years it was initially difficult for others to make their way in the profession from within that school. Some of the assistants became well known: John Innis (1739–77)—assistant to the second Alexander Monro—published a pocket myographia, *A short description of the human muscles* ..., 1776, which went through many editions in Edinburgh and London, and was published in the United States. Most other aspiring anatomists, however, resolved to make their way outside the University by opening private classes; during the reign of Alexander Monro *tertius* particularly these schools attracted large numbers of students. One of the remarkably able group of extramural lecturers that dominated Edinburgh anatomy and surgery during the second and third Monros was John Bell. He was the second son of an Anglican clergyman in Presbyterian Edinburgh; two brothers, George and Robert, became Professors of Law at Edinburgh, and a third was Charles, of whom more later.

Apprenticed to a surgeon, John Bell attended lectures at the University, and passed the College of Surgeons' examinations when he was twenty-three. In 1790 he opened an extramural school where he taught both anatomy and surgery. The school was in a building in a square next to the Surgeons' Hall. Bell's school flourished, and so did his practice of surgery, both privately and at the Royal Infirmary. A virulent personal attack on Bell, led by the Professor of the Practice of Medicine, Dr James Gregory, and probably motivated by partisanship to Alexander Monro *secundus*, the official teacher of anatomy and surgery at the University, caused Bell to be excluded from the Infirmary. Printed sheets were 'stuck up like a play-bill in a most conspicuous and unusual manner, on every corner of the city; on the door of my lecture rooms, on the gates of the College, where my pupils could not but pass, and on the gates of the Infirmary, where I went to perform my operations'. John Bell's cantankerous replies were printed in a massive volume: *Letters on professional character and manners* ..., Edinburgh, 1810.

In 1799, Bell retired from lecturing into private practice, and became generally recognized in Edinburgh as the foremost surgeon of his day, publishing a three-volume *Principles of Surgery* ..., Edinburgh 1801–8.

In his classes, Bell emphasized always the surgical relevance of the anatomy he was demonstrating. He criticized the methods of teaching in the University: 'In Dr. Monro's class, unless there be a private succession of murders, not three subjects are dissected in the year. On the remains of a subject fished up from the bottom of a tub of spirits, are demonstrated those delicate nerves which are to be avoided or divided in our operations; and these are demonstrated once at a distance of 100 feet!—nerves and arteries which the surgeon has to dissect, at the peril of his patient's life.' Since Monro and Bell had earlier competed for student fees, these deprecatory remarks must not be viewed necessarily as an accurate account.

With three years of teaching experience behind him, and to assist his students, John Bell prepared a text of human anatomy, the first volume of which appeared as: *The anatomy of the bones, muscles, and joints* …, Edinburgh and London [1793]. To accompany this volume there were issued: *Engravings, explaining the anatomy of the bones, muscles, and joints*, Edinburgh and London, 1794 (Bell was thirty-one years old at the time). There were 28 plates with 4 outline engravings (our *Plate 104* is taken from the 1804 edition). John Bell, who had had instruction in drawing from his talented mother, not only drew all the illustrations but also etched them, and engraved all but seven. The application of practising surgeons of that period to anatomy was remarkable. Bell was willing to devote much of his time to lecturing and dissection, compiling a museum, writing texts, and drawing specimens.

Bell's preface to his book gives a rare insight into his scientific, educational, and artistic intentions. He thus justifies his small-scale drawings, which were against the trend established by such as Cheselden, Hunter, and Albinus:

If a man were to take this fancy, that nothing of anatomy could be drawn but of the full size of life, with what high contempt must he look down upon these little plates; where I have endeavoured to represent, in this miniature form, what it must be confessed, might be more fully represented on a larger scale: and yet I am sensible, that those, who cannot understand these plates, will hardly profit even by that stately anatomical figure of full six feet high …

Bell wished to provide a straightforward text:

I have ventured, instead of setting up this rank and file of tall opaque words betwixt the reader's imagination, and my own conceptions, to make every description as simple as may be—using no hard words, but the pure names; choosing rather that my book should be plainly understood, than admired as a piece of unintelligible profound anatomy.

But 'a book of anatomy without [plates] seemed to me no better than a book of geography without its maps … or solving Euclid's problems without the help of figures or lines, by the mere force of imagination alone'. Bell attempted, he says, in his book to make drawings and descriptions correspond, but:

Even in the first invention of our best anatomical figures, we see a continual struggle between the anatomist and the painter; one striving for elegance of form, the other insisting upon accuracy of representation. It was thus that the celebrated Titian consented to draw for Vesalius: Though it is but too plain that there can be no truth in drawings thus monstrously compounded betwixt the imagination of the painter, and the sober remonstrances of the anatomist, striving for accurate anatomy, where the thing cannot be; for those figures which are supposed to be drawn truly from the anatomical table, are formed from the imagination of the painter merely; sturdy and active figures, with a ludicrous contrast of furious countenances, and active limbs, combined with ragged muscles, and naked bones, and dissected bowels, which they are busily employed in supporting, forsooth, or even demonstrating with their hands. This vitious practice of drawing from imagination merely is well exemplified in this, that anatomists have, with one consent, agreed to borrow the celebrated Torso for putting their bowels into, to explain them there; a practice which had descended from the time of Vesalius down to Cheselden, and from him to the systems of the present day.

No painter in natural history, in botany, in mechanics, nor in any thing that relates to science, would dare to draw without his subject immediately before him: but anatomists, who most of all need this clearness and truth, have been most of all arbitrary and loose in their methods; not representing what they saw, but what they themselves imagined, or what others chose to report to them:—hence the careless copying from book to book, the interpolations of anatomists, the interference of painters in a subject degrading to their higher art, the errors and mistakes of engravers, and the subjection of true anatomical drawing to the capricious interference of the artist, whose rule it has too often been to make all beautiful and smooth, leaving no harshness nor apparent blur in all his work.

This passage has been quoted at length because it is a valid criticism of much anatomical illustration. He has much softer words for some of the anatomists of his own period:

A higher taste prevails in the present age; and the splendid and noble works of Morgagni, Haller, Bidloo, and Albinus, and of Cheselden, Hunter and Cowper, are drawn truly, and from nature, and cannot be forgotten, while anatomy, and the arts depending on it, continue to be esteemed. Yet even, among those great men, we have seen an idea gradually improving, till at last it was brought by Haller to the true point.

Bell describes the methods of Albinus:

If an anatomist shall set up a skeleton, and draw it in postures resembling those of life; if he shall dissect the human body, studying and drawing it in parts; if he shall continue drawing muscle after muscle, and one part after another, till he have gone through the whole; if he shall proceed then to take these drawings and notes of individual parts, and lay them over his first drawings of the bones; if he shall try to match the parts belonging to fifty individual bodies of different sizes, of various forms, dying, some suddenly, and others slowly, some full and muscular, others emaciated and poor; what will the result of all this be, but a mere plan? It was an unlucky theory of this kind that carried the great ALBINUS, for fifteen years, through a course of labourious dissections, painful and useless to himself; but useful to all those who have to follow him: Still each drawing of his is but a mere plan, resembling no individual body, resembling in nothing the general drawing of the body; it is such a view as never is to be seen in a dissection.

Contrasted with these techniques of Albinus was the practice of Bidloo, whose illustrations are true representations of actual dissections, but in these 'the master-hand of the painter prevails almost alone . . .'

. . . in Albinus we think that we understand every muscle of the human body! but our knowledge hardly bears the test of dissection . . . In Bidloo, we have the very subject before us! the tables, the knives, the apparatus, down even to the flies that haunt the places of dissection . . . so that the dead subject and the engraving can well bear to be compared . . . [but] in respect of anatomy, they are all disorder and confusion; and one must be both anatomist and painter to guess what is meant, how the limb is laid, and what parts are seen.

Bell, having complete control of the anatomy and its representation, attempted to combine these two approaches. How well do the illustrations meet his intentions? Certainly they have the immediacy of drawings made in the dissecting rooms of late-Georgian Edinburgh. Some are quite gruesome and even perverted, with unnecessary depictions of roped, twisted bodies; others are too reminiscent of the appearance of meat on the block in a shambles. The background shading is slapdash in many places. In their context, however, they are admirable, for they were intended to be used to supplement the teacher's demonstrations, to remind the student of what he had seen, and to be a guide when the student sat down with the prosected material. It was under the Bells—John's younger brother Charles had become his assistant—that the extramural schools brought the aspiring surgeon much closer to the cadaver, allowing the student opportunities for actual dissection. As John Bell writes:

If anatomy is to be acquired in this way only, then must we understand by a school of anatomy a school of dissection: Yet those who have had the happiness of prosecuting their studies in foreign universities, or in the London schools, will hardly believe it, that there is at least one place of education much celebrated, and worthy to be so, where the study of anatomy is denied or proscribed.—Where not only is it not praiseworthy, but even dangerous to propose dissections ...

Following the successful publication on the bones, muscles, and joints, John Bell continued the work with a volume on the heart and arteries, first issued in Edinburgh and London in 1797. In this influential work, he was assisted by his brother Charles Bell, who drew the illustrations, which were then engraved professionally. Following the publication of this volume there was 'a rapid improvement in the surgery of the arteries ...'. (The sketches for this book are in the National Library of Medicine, Bethesda, Maryland, and have recently been reproduced in facsimile. The completed drawings are in the Royal College of Surgeons of England.) Two subsequent volumes in the series, both published in London, were by Charles Bell alone: on the nervous system, 1803, and on the viscera of the abdomen, on the pelvis and on the lymphatic system, 1804. At least twelve editions of the complete work were issued in the next thirty years, from London and New York.

Charles Bell was educated at the High School and at the University of Edinburgh. His mother had the most considerable part to play in his upbringing, for his father died when he was a young boy. Charles studied anatomy and surgery at his brother's extramural school, and assisted him there in dissection classes. From 1798 to 1803 he published from Edinburgh: *A system of dissections....* (Our *Plate 105* is taken from Volume 2, Plate 5, 1803.) The next year he was admitted as a Fellow of the Royal College of Surgeons. As we have seen he collaborated with John in completing *The anatomy of the human body ...*, 1797–1804. Charles's role was that of illustrator from the second volume onwards, and author of the third and fourth volumes.

John Bell's exclusion from the Royal Infirmary made prospects in Edinburgh less than good for Charles; moreover when he took over John's classes he was not successful in attracting large numbers of students. With his brother's blessing, he left for London in 1804, where he set up and remained in surgical practice for twenty-two years. He taught anatomy to medical students and artists, and in 1809 became a partner in the Great Windmill Street School established fifty years earlier by William Hunter. Bell used part of his wife's dowry to buy his share of the School.

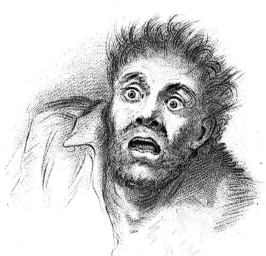

13.2 'Fear', from Charles Bell's treatise on expression. This particular figure may have been drawn, not by Bell, but by David Wilkie.

Charles Bell was, for much of his life in London, surgeon to the Middlesex Hospital, and, for a while, professor at the newly established University of London, later University College. He was a courteous man to both his students and to his patients whilst conducting bedside teaching, at which he excelled.

In 1836, he returned to Edinburgh at the age of sixty-two to take the Chair in Surgery at the University. By this time he had been knighted, on the ascent to the throne of William IV; he was internationally famous for his surgery and for work on the anatomy, physiology, and pathology of the nervous system. Bell's principal scientific contribution was to suggest that individual nerve elements acted independently and carried specific information to or from the central nervous system—a hypothesis later to be known, rather quaintly, as (Johannes) Muller's *Law of specific nerve energies*. Bell's name has long been associated with that of Magendie in a closely related discovery in physiology: the Bell–Magendie 'Law' recognized the ventral (or anterior) roots of the spinal nerves as motor and the dorsal (or posterior) roots as sensory. Bell's observations relating to such topics were printed in 100 copies of a book of 32 pages, distributed to his friends in 1811; this was entitled: *A new idea of the anatomy of the brain* ..., but the work as issued contains no clear statement on separate motor and sensory roots. The crucial experiments were made by François Magendie in 1821. Bell, in subsequent publications, including papers to the Royal Society 1821–9 collected in a book in 1830, left his readers and many others in the scientific world with the impression that the credit for recognizing these functions of the spinal roots was due to him; he distorted evidence to give this impression. It is more just to give the credit to Magendie alone.

Bell published, while in London, a number of other works mostly illustrated by himself. In 1806, his *Essays on the anatomy of the expression in painting*, was issued in London. Bell had sketched out text and illustrations for the book during his Edinburgh days. The work, one of the first to be published on this subject, was a critical and popular success, and did much to establish Bell's reputation in London (*Fig. 13.2*). Flaxman and Fuseli both used the book, and so, in a quite different way, did Charles Darwin; editions were still being published fifty years later, and copies were given as prizes at art schools. Another popular work was his volume in the series of Bridgewater Treatises. This—*The Hand: its mechanism and vital endowments, as evincing design.* London, 1833—was based, as required by the terms of the Bridgewater trustees, on a teleological explanation of form and function as 'illustrating the power, wisdom, and goodness of God'; the pre-Darwinian concepts of purpose reiterated throughout the book make for uncomfortable reading by a rationalist in the late twentieth century.

104 Muscles of the back of the neck and trunk. Plate VII, Book II of J. Bell, *Engravings of the bones, muscles and joints . . .*, second edition, 1804. Engraving (Cambridge University Library). 24.5 × 17.4 cm.

Figure I shows the muscles of the back after trapezius and latissimus dorsi have been removed. It is dissection-true, although the delineation of the muscles could be clearer. The suspensory ropes add a macabre touch that many might consider unnecessary. Muscles such as the rhomboids (64, 65), deltoid (71), infraspinatus (74), levator scapulae (63), serratus posterior superior (aaa) and inferior (114), are very well portrayed. One would expect splenius capitis (118) to be wider and cover more of semispinalis capitis (119) than it does.

With regard to the deeper-lying muscles, seen in figures II, III, and IV, the nomenclature used in the text differs somewhat from that employed nowadays, though in the case of quadratus lumborum (125), spinalis (131), multifidus (133), levatores costorum (115), and the suboccipital muscles seen in Figure IV the names are identical. Other muscles illustrated and described—such as longissimus dorsi (126), sacro-lumbalis (127), cervicalis descendens (128), transversalis colli (129), and trachelo-mastoideus and transversalis cervicis (unnumbered)—would seem to make up the modern longissimus, semispinalis, and sacrospinalis groups. Bell states 'that not even the largest drawing can make this piece of dissection perfectly easy',—sentiments with which many modern anatomists and their students will ruefully concur!

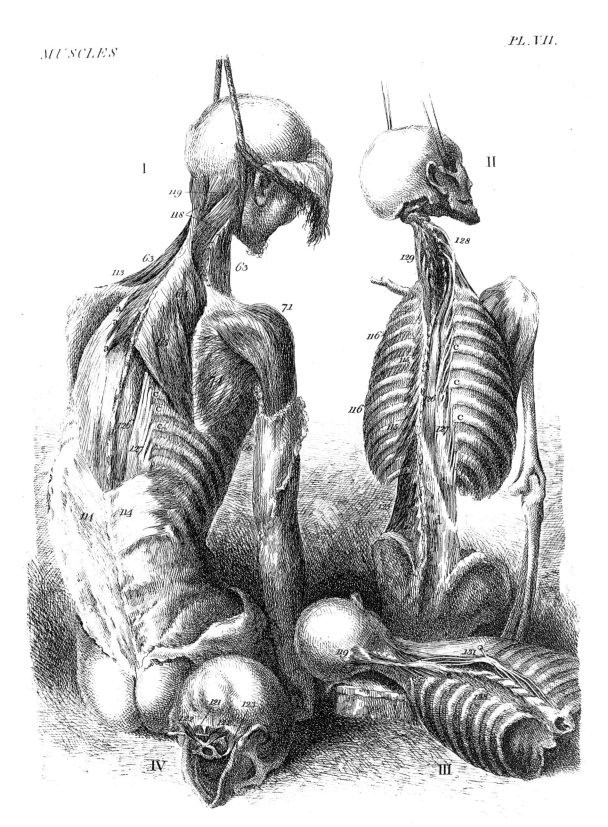

I

II

III

IV

119
118
63
113
63
71
a
a
a
125
c
c'
c''
126
127
116
114 114

128
129
116'
115
116
116
126
115 127
c
c
c
121
119 131

121 123
122

Published for Longman & Rees 1804

PLATE 104

105 Superficial dissection of face and neck. Plate V, Volume II of C. Bell, *A System of dissections . . .*, 1808. Engraving (Cambridge University Library). 32.1 × 25.5 cm.

In his text Charles Bell makes a particular point that, unlike the extremities, the neck is *not* invested with strong fascia binding down the underlying structures, but has an 'extended web of muscular fibres' (the platysma) the better to afford the head and neck 'an ease and variety of motions'.

This may explain the prominence in this illustration of the platysmal muscle-sheet (A D E) which has been deliberately left intact, obscuring as it does such structures deep to it as the external jugular vein. This emphasis is reminiscent of Cowper, some seventy-five years earlier (see *Plate 94*, p. 421).

It is interesting that, although the muscles around the mouth are both labelled and described— for example, depressor anguli oris (a), zigomaticus [*sic*] (y)—there is no recognition of the orbicularis oris as an entity, although the orbicularis oculi ('palpebrarum') is both present and labelled (T).

The size of the supraorbital nerve is rather too large, but nevertheless it seemingly supplies only a small amount of the anterior part of the scalp: it is simply termed 'frontal' in the legend.

The illustration of facial structures such as the parotid gland (O) and duct (R), facial artery and vein (d and c), and infraorbital nerve and branches of the facial nerve is clear and accurate.

The neck structures are less easy to understand and identify. From its course the nerve (M) must represent the great auricular, but it is described as being a communication from the third cervical to the facial nerve. The components of the cervical plexus depicted are also not very clear—NNN are merely termed the second, third, and fourth cervical nerves. The occipital veins behind the ear are rather too large.

As was usual in his day, Bell considered the hypoglossal nerve to be the ninth cranial nerve (the vagus, glossopharyngeal, and accessory nerves were thought to be parts of the eighth) and so the descendens hypoglossi (I) is here termed the 'descendens noni'. It would appear that the normal configuration of the ansa cervicalis was fully appreciated.

This drawing is an exceptionally faithful rendering of how the anatomy of the area concerned would appear during the course of a dissection, and so achieves Bell's stated aim of conveying to the viewer a 'presential reality of form'. He intended this and his other drawing, to be helpful in informing students (particularly surgical students) what they should observe during their own dissections.

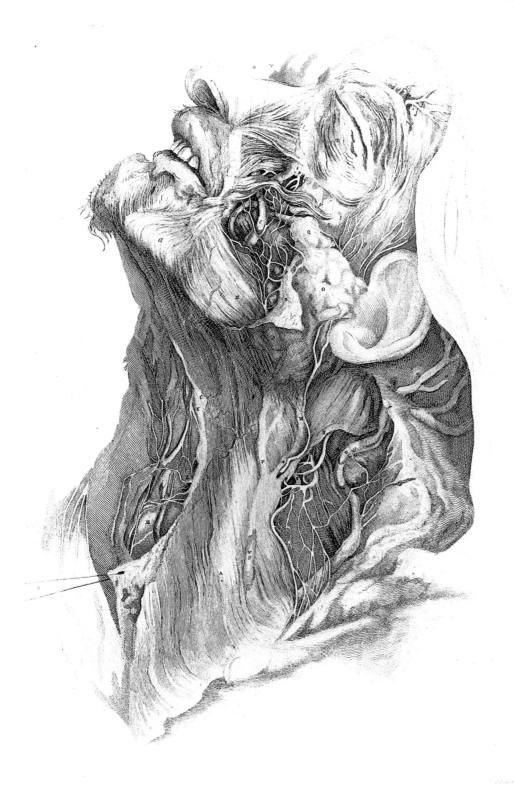

PLATE 105

Alexander Ramsay

This Scottish-trained anatomist died in the State of Maine in 1824, when he was said to be seventy years of age. His place of birth has been variously given as London and as Edinburgh; he was undoubtedly of Scottish descent. After studies in London, Dublin, and Aberdeen, he

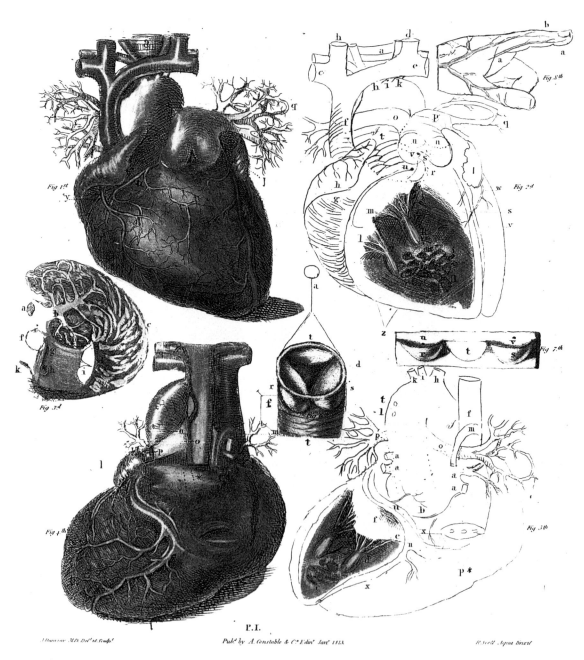

13.3 The heart, from Alexander Ramsay's atlas, 1813.

became one of the private teachers in anatomy in Edinburgh, lecturing and supervising dissection from an establishment in Surgeons' Square. He published an *Anatomy of the heart, cranium, and brain* . . . , Edinburgh and London, 1813, a revision of a shorter book issued the previous year. In the introduction he wrote: 'The plan I followed in this treatise, I originally adopted in my lectures in Surgeons' Square . . .'. The illustrations were drawn and engraved by Ramsay himself (*Fig. 13.3*). The dedication was to Sir Joseph Banks, President (*de facto* President for life) of the Royal Society. A letter by Banks, printed in the book, congratulates Ramsay for:

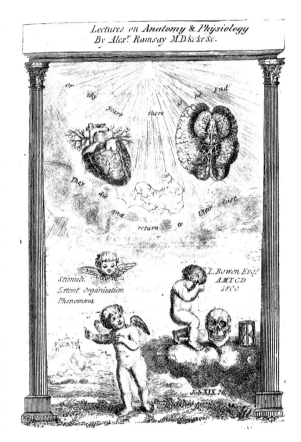

weaving into the texture of anatomical studies, opinions deduced from facts, which cannot fail to give to the minds of your pupils a disposition to recollect their Creator, and to adore his benevolence, in the course of those studies, which are to make them able to be themselves benefactors of their species.

Anatomists have often been considered by those established in authority to have reprehensible leanings to atheism; and indeed Robert Knox, the most popular lecturer in anatomy in Surgeons' Square about that time, was known as a free-thinker.

In 1801 or 1802 Ramsay went to the United States of America. He lectured in anatomy in the 'colleges of New York, Dartmouth and Brunswick'. Dartmouth Medical School had been established a few years earlier in 1798; Yale's was not opened until 1810. In these American seminaries, he says, 'I successively taught, by invitation, when I visited that Con-

13.4 Engraving to accompany Ramsay's lectures in anatomy and physiology, 1800.

tinent, with a view of investigating the human frame, under the varieties of climate, government and police [i.e. constitution]'. Perhaps he had intended to stay only a few years, but he spent much of the rest of his life there. His anatomical dissections at Dartmouth were conducted on bodies sent to him in barrels of rum.

Ramsay made Fryeberg, a village in Maine, of some seven hundred and fifty persons his base. His collection or museum of anatomical specimens there he valued at $14 000. He founded at Fryeberg an institution which he hoped would become a medical academy to rival others in New England. At various times he sought money for this scheme, petitioning the State unsuccessfully, and travelling to Britain. In America, like others at this time, he ventured from

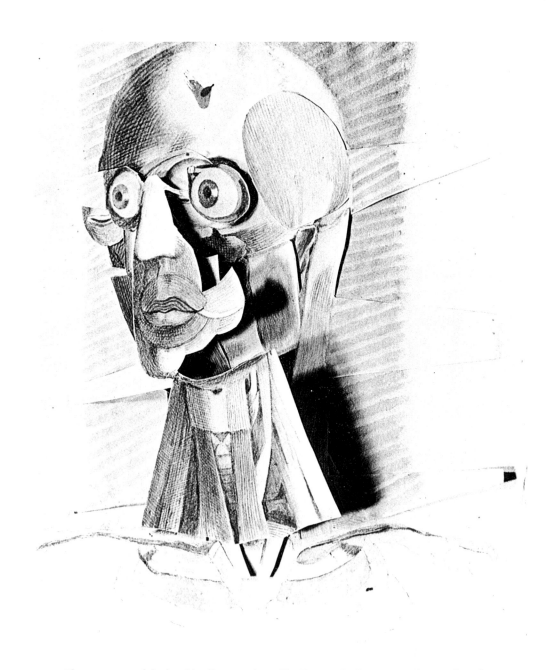

13.5   Flap anatomy of the head by Ramsay, from The Francis A. Countway Library of Medicine, Boston.

town to town advertising his lectures.[1] From *Fig. 13.4*, it can be seen that 'moral anatomy' was as alive in the English-speaking world early in the nineteenth century as it had been in the Netherlands in the seventeenth and eighteenth, and in Italy in the sixteenth. Ramsay's journeys, lecturing and soliciting for money for his institution, took him into the Southern States and also north into Canada, to Montreal and other cities.

Particularly remarkable are the complex flap-anatomies that Ramsay devised for these lectures. Some of the original drawings, paintings and constructions are to be found in The Francis A. Countway Library of Medicine in Boston. The layered flaps showing the anatomy of the head and neck are derived from Albinus' atlas (*Fig. 13.5*). Those of the upper limb (*Plate 106*) are elegant and straightforward. How Canano would have appreciated these representations!

Concerning this restless, gifted anatomist and draughtsman, whose plans for a major medical institution at Fryeberg failed, Kelly and Burrage wrote:

According to some, he was a compound of personal deformity, immense learning, uncontrollable temper, and inordinate vanity. According to others, he was a wonderful dissector, an unapproachable lecturer on anatomy, and a man who once known could never be recalled without unfailing reverence and deep affection.

[1] Public lectures in anatomy based on demonstrations of dissections were also known in England at the time, in smaller country towns as well as in the larger cities.

106
Muscles of the upper limb, four drawings, Alexander Ramsay manuscript folios, *c.*1810–20 (Countway Library, Boston, Mass.).

The four illustrations that compose this plate represent the anatomy of the posterior aspect of the upper extremity. On the verso of each of the original folios there is a drawing of the structures concerned, annotated in Ramsay's handwriting.

The illustrations, developed as teaching aids, were designed to be placed successively one over the other.

The first drawing is of the skeleton of the right arm, with the scapula rather poorly represented in outline. There is also a small drawing of the bones of the elbow region showing the supinator muscle. In the main drawing the humerus, particularly the shaft and distal portion, is very ugly, and the styloid processes of the ulna and radius are absent.

The second drawing consists mainly of muscles and tendons with, in places, the bones showing through 'window' cut-outs. The muscles seen in the upper arm include a small portion of subscapularis, teres major, coraco-brachialis, brachialis, and medial head of triceps, while in the forearm are the long and short radial extensors and their tendons, supinator, flexor digitorum profundus (most medially), and, in the mid-line between the radius and ulna, parts of the flexor pollicis longus and pronator quadratus. Adductor pollicis and the dorsal interossei are seen in the hand, together with the tendons of extensor digitorum cut across just proximal to the fingers.

In the third drawing (which is incorrectly numbered 2d) further muscles have now been added. These include teres minor, long and lateral heads of triceps, anconeus, abductor pollicis longus (with extensor pollicis brevis), extensor pollicis longus, and extensor indicis.

The last drawing (incorrectly labelled 3d) constitutes the final 'layer' of muscles, which include the deltoid, infraspinatus, and teres minor in the shoulder region, while in the forearm are shown extensors digitorum and digiti minimi, then extensor carpi ulnaris, and a thin and displaced brachioradialis.

It seems most likely that these drawings were done in reverse order to that given above, using dissections of progressively increasing depth. If this were so then the choice of muscles to be illustrated in any particular plate would be a difficult one to make, and, once made, exactly what to cut out for the 'windows' could have presented another problem.

The anatomical correctness of each individual drawing varies from plate to plate—the drawing of the bones are, oddly enough, the least well done. One might have expected the posterior interosseous artery and nerve to be included in our second drawing, as in illustrations of the flexor aspect of the forearm the anterior interosseous artery is there shown.

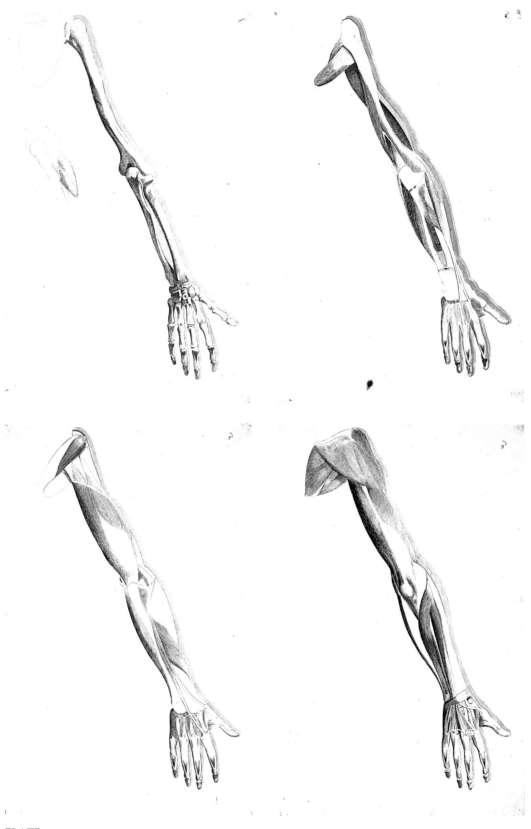

PLATE 106

John Lizars (1787–1860)

Lizars was one of the protagonists in the interminable and acrimonious squabbles amongst the surgeons when Edinburgh was at its zenith as a medical centre. He was the son of Daniel Lizars, an Edinburgh publisher and engraver. (Daniel Lizars had engraved, for instance, plates for Charles Bell, including our *Plate 105*.) After attending the High School, John Lizars became a pupil of John Bell, receiving his diploma in 1808. Like so many surgeon apothecaries, he enlisted as a naval surgeon, serving under Napier and others during the Peninsular War. In 1815 he became a Fellow of the Royal College of Surgeons of Edinburgh and a partner to John Bell and Robert Allan in their extramural school, lecturing there on anatomy and physiology. When this partnership dissolved, he taught from No. 1 Surgeons' Square; in 1828, he moved to the Brown Square School. As Chambers described, for five days each week, throughout the academic year, he gave a morning lecture on anatomy, an anatomical demonstration, and an afternoon lecture on surgery, 'besides which he had a large class of practical anatomy—a department, the conducting of which was then a much less easy or safe matter than it now-a-days proves to us, who have merely to receive bodies under the peaceful operation of the anatomy act'. The average attendance at his classes was about a hundred and fifty students. He also carried on at this time a private surgical practice, with mixed success.

During his period as an anatomy teacher, to assist his students, he issued a series of five folio paper-bound volumes of plates, with accompanying octavo text. These parts, issued 1822–6, were intended to be bound together to make a book of 101 plates: *A system of anatomical plates of the human body* ... In later editions (in 12 parts) the plates could be obtained plain or coloured; the text was published in folio, to be included within the one binding (*Fig. 13.6*). The name of the publishing firm appearing on the original parts was John's father, Daniel Lizars, and the engraver of all the plates was his brother, William Home Lizars (1788–1859)—an artist who had studied alongside the Scottish painter, David Wilkie. W. H. Lizars took over his father's firm; he continued to be in demand as an engraver, becoming known for particular engraving techniques.

Although W. H. Lizars is identified at the foot of his brother's plates as an engraver, the printed page shows no plate marks, as it would if it were a true copper-engraving printed by an intaglio process. In this latter, the engraved lines contain ink, the surface being wiped clean; paper has to be forced by a heavy press into these grooves, creating at the same time a 'blind' impression of the copperplate itself. Lithography, in use for anatomical illustration in the 1820s, is a planographic process; it creates no plate marks on the printed page. Some have mistakenly thought the Lizars plates to be lithographs. The *Gentleman's Magazine*, quoting the *Edinburgh Philosophical Journal* described, in 1821, a 'New style of engraving on copper in *alto relievo*, invented by Mr W. H. Lizars'. The essential elements of this process, probably used for printing his brother's anatomical plates, were as follows: the drawing to be reproduced was made on a copperplate using blackened turpentine varnish. The plate was acid-treated, which etched away unvarnished copper, leaving the drawing in relief. The surface was then inked, taking care not to let the ink into the etched parts, and then printed in a letterpress in a similar manner to a relief woodcut. The article praised lithography (so much cheaper than engraving) and also wood *engraving* (printed along with type), but suggested that W. H. Lizars's new method might have something to recommend it. This is not the place to enter into a history of relief metal printing.

Except for Lizars, such methods have rarely been used in anatomy books. (William Blake, professional engraver as well as poet, produced in the years preceding 1820 a number of wonderful illustrated printed books prepared by himself and his wife, Catherine, from metal relief plates. *The Songs of Innocence*, 1789, was the first book they printed in this manner.)

The collection of Lizars's plates was dedicated to George IV, and this dedication continued to be printed even after 1830, when King George was dead. As mentioned earlier, he urged the King to use his influence to ensure legitimate access by students to dissection subjects. In a late issue of these plates, there is a footnote in the dedication: 'Such appeals as these have fortunately led to the passing of the Anatomy Act, a short time ago.'

The book was costly to produce, for the engravings or etchings were, as usual, time-consuming, and the colouring was done skilfully and painstakingly by hand; the fifteen plates of the brain were printed in sepia, and bear a similarity to those of Vicq d'Azyr. As

13.6   Title-page of John Lizar's *A System of Anatomical Plates*.

Chambers put it in his note on this anatomy book: 'It was a noble attempt, in the prevailing difficulty of procuring subjects, to assist students with substitutes; and the engravings of this splendid work, which were executed with great care and at much expense, were made chiefly from original dissections.' The sale of the book in its various forms was reported to be immense. Robert Knox, in his disparaging way, held other opinions as to the value of these engravings, calling them 'huge misrepresentations of nature'.

John Lizars produced a number of other books—on ovariectomy; on club-foot; on tobacco; *A system of practical surgery*, Edinburgh 1838; but the anatomical plate-book was his most successful work. Lizars became Professor of Surgery to the College of Surgeons of Edinburgh, taking the position after competition with James Syme, who then became a most bitter enemy. Lizars, a blunt, irascible man of some eccentricity, seems however to have maintained cordial relations with his fellow surgeon at the Royal Infirmary, Robert Liston—no mean feat. Lizars is said in one biography to have died suddenly, in 1860, 'not without suspicion of laudanum'.

107 Contents of the orbit. Plate X, Part IX in J. Lizars, *A system of anatomical plates of the human body* ..., [1825]. Engraving (private collection). 42.8 × 27.2 cm.

This plate comprises four drawings of the eye and other orbital structures. Although these are identified by letters and numbers, the book itself does not contain an explanatory list; one was, however, available in octavo letterpress. Fig 2 is a frontal view of the orbit with the eyeball in position, surrounded by the orbicularis oculi. Above the eyeball are seen the levator palpebrae muscle (L) and the tendon of the superior oblique (O) passing through its pulley.

The upper drawing, Figure 3, is of a dissection, viewed from the left side, where the medial wall of the right orbit has been removed. The trigeminal ganglion (G) is seen giving rise to the ophthalmic, maxillary, and mandibular nerves, although it is doubtful if the foramen rotundum could in fact be seen from this particular viewpoint.

The nerves entering the orbit, namely the optic (2), oculomotor (3), trochlear (4), abducent (6), and frontal (f) are clearly shown; having regard to the size of the other nerves the trochlear is too thick.

The lacrimal gland in the upper part of the orbit is seen receiving the lacrimal branch of the ophthalmic nerve, and the frontal nerve divides into its supratrochlear and supraorbital branches. Other orbital structures include fat, levator palpebrae superioris (L), and the superior oblique (O) muscles, the latter being positioned too inferiorly.

In a superior view of the right orbit, in the lower drawing, the levator muscle and attached upper eyelid are swung over to the left. The muscle is represented as being narrower than it is, and its origin seems to lie below the optic nerve. Behind the muscle a circular structure represents, confusingly, the left internal carotid artery.

The lacrimal gland, its nerve, and also the frontal nerve have been swung to the right. The superior oblique muscle (its tendon of insertion also a little too narrow) has been detached from its origin and retracted to the left; presumably the posteriorly situated curved white structure is meant to be the trochlear nerve (hardly the muscle origin!); but if so it is again too thick, and in any case it does *not* enter the muscle thus.

The abducent nerve (6), which supplies only the lateral rectus muscle (a), has undergone a remarkable reduction in size where it is seen immediately prior to entering the muscle. The

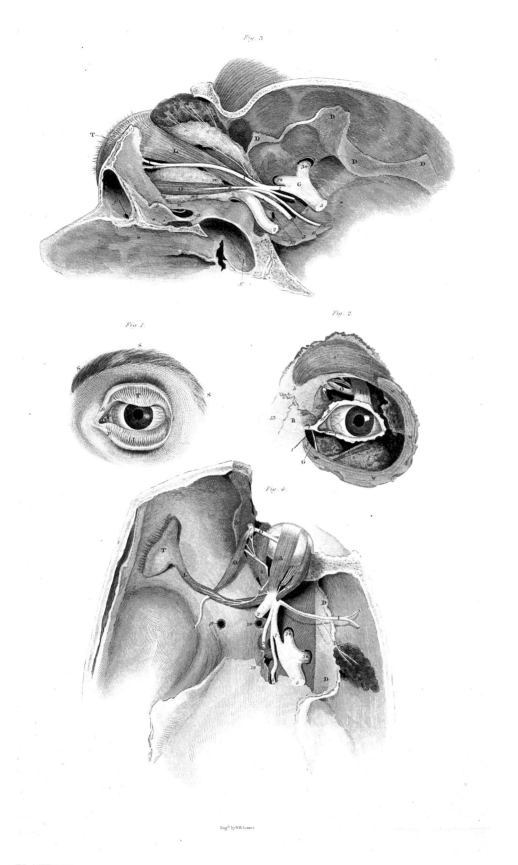

Fig. 3.

Fig. 1.

Fig. 2.

Fig. 4.

Eng.d by W.H.Lizars

PLATE 107

superior, medial, and lateral rectus muscles are shown as though arising from the optic nerve itself, and the third and sixth nerves, together with the ophthalmic and optic, seem all to fuse together. The portrayal of this area is not very helpful in understanding the anatomy involved, though in a subsequent illustration the delineation of the nerves is considerably improved. Either Lizars was not quite sure of the origin of the muscles moving the eyeball, which seems unlikely, or was unable to overcome the admittedly difficult task of accurately portraying them.

Joseph Swan (1791–1874)

Alexander Monro *secundus* had used simple and compound microscopes to investigate the structure of nerves. Joseph Swan, in a work on the nervous system, expressed his gratitude to Monro *tertius* for 'assiduous instructions in minute [that is, detailed] anatomy whilst he was a student in the University of Edinburgh'. In the same book, Swan states: 'For various reasons minute anatomy should be anxiously cultivated; by the man who would understand the groundwork of his profession, it ought to be considered a subject of intense interest and the utmost importance ...'.

Joseph Swan was born into a family some of whom had practised surgery in the city of Lincoln for many years. He was apprenticed to his father, Henry Swan, surgeon at the Lincoln County Hospital, and then continued his education in Edinburgh, where he heard the lectures of Monro *tertius* and attended the demonstrations of Andrew Fyfe. He went to London, where, at Guy's and St Thomas's Hospitals, he was a pupil of the younger Henry Cline. Astley Cooper 'gave him the first impulse towards scientific researches'. He was made a Member of the Royal College of Surgeons of London in 1813, aged twenty-two, and soon followed his father by becoming surgeon to the Lincoln County Hospital. While there, he continued his anatomical investigations; to assist him, Astley Cooper sent him each Christmas a hamper, labelled 'glass with care', containing a well-preserved cadaver for dissection. Abernethy showed similar 'public spirited liberality ... towards him, when an entire stranger'. (This was some twenty years before the Anatomy Act ensured an easier supply of subjects.) Encouraged by successes of prize essays for the Royal College of Surgeons in 1817 and 1819 on the pathology of nerves, Swan wrote an essay: *A minute dissection of the nerves of the medulla spinalis* [that is, the spinal cord] *from their origin to their terminations and to their conjunctions with the cerebral and visceral nerves, authenticated by preparations of the dissected parts*, 1825; and a similar work on the cranial nerves, 1828.

In 1827, he moved to London, to a house in Tavistock Square; he converted its billiard room into an anatomy theatre. He was a retiring bachelor, and his practice as surgeon was not extensive; but he continued to anatomize and to publish books for the rest of his life, the most remarkable being one summarizing his 1825 and 1828 prize dissections: *A demonstration of the nerves of the human body*, London, 1830. This work was in very large folio, and consisted of an introductory text and 25 illustrated plates of nerve dissections. A quarto edition appeared, dated 1834. The work went through a second London edition, prepared by Swan: 1865, folio. A French translation was issued in 1838. Each plate was accompanied by an unlettered and unnumbered outline plate and descriptive letterpress. In the Preface, Swan wrote: 'The sympathetic and the nerves of the thoracic and abdominal viscera form an important feature in each subject ... The consideration of this division of the nervous system is [together with the vagus] most difficult and perplexing to the student....' The origins, distribution, and ramifications of the sympathetic, satisfactorily described in earlier anatomies only by Eustachius, became in the late eighteenth and nineteenth centuries a test of skill and persistence in dissection—the work of Walter being a notable early German example (see *Plate 82*, p. 361). The labour was, however, not sufficiently rewarding, for individual variation made the detailed description of any one dissection somewhat arbitrary and of limited value. The illustrations of Swan are to some extent open to this criticism. The artist for all the plates was E. West, and the engravers were J. Steward (for plates 1–9 dated July and September 1830) and W. and E. Finden (for plates 10–25 dated January and December 1833). William Finden (1787–1852) and his brother Edward (1791–1857) were for a time the most successful of the firms of engravers in Britain, at a period before the two techniques of lithography and of wood-engraving dominated book illustration. William Finden's success in engraving Smirke's illustrations to *Don Quixote* led the brothers to establish a workshop, eventually employing many pupils. The works that appeared above their names were carried out by these pupils and assistants under their direction; the elaborate finishing touches that gave each plate an apparent authenticity were by one of the Findens themselves. Their engraving for the Swan neuroanatomy was carried out at a time when they were working also on Lodge's *Portraits* (1821–34) and the illustrations to the life and works of Byron (1833 onwards). They were then also illustrating and publishing their succession of bound annuals and keepsakes—sentimental books directed to the growing market of the English bourgeoisie. The fortune acquired in this way was mostly lost when the Findens over-extended themselves with their *Royal Gallery of British Art* ... (1838–40). They received large sums for the engraving of single large plates: £2000 was paid for engraving Sir Thomas Lawrence's portrait of King George IV, and £1470 from the Art Union for a plate engraved after a crucifixion scene—the Art Union sold copies suitable for framing and displaying in middle-class sitting-rooms.

108 Nerves of the neck and thorax. Plate II in J. Swan, *A demonstration of the nerves of the human body*, 1830. Engraving (Cambridge University Library). 49.0 × 23.0 cm.

It should be stated at the outset that, consistent with the general belief of the early nineteenth century, Swan considered there to be nine pairs of cranial nerves, which he termed: olfactory; optic; common oculo-muscular [oculomotor]; superior oblique oculo-muscular [trochlear]; three-fold or fifth; abducent oculo-muscular; auditory or soft portion of the seventh; facial or hard portion of the seventh; vagus or eighth; glossopharyngeal or associate of the eighth; and hypoglossal. In addition the very first sentence in the book states 'The sympathetic extends from the sixth nerve of the brain [abducent] to the extremity of the sacrum', a view which oddly was still generally accepted as fact in those days.

Following this illustration in the book is a line-diagram where the structures are labelled and numbered for identification, though the employment of both capital and lower-case letters, as well as numbers, is not ideal, particularly as use was made only of numbers 1–25.

Irrespective of the names (or numbering) applied to nerves, their anatomical appearance in drawings should be consistent with their anatomy. It is therefore perplexing to discover that in this plate, making reference to the line-diagram, the cervical nerves, as depicted from above downwards, are considered cervical 1 to 7. Thus the descendens cervicalis arises from C1 and C2; the phrenic predominantly from C3; C4 and C5 join together; and the very large C8 apparently is absent. This is, of course, incorrect; but it came about because Swan termed the first cervical nerve the 'suboccipital'; thus the true second cervical became his first, and so on down.

This aberration apart there is a great deal to admire in this plate. The descendens hypoglossi and descendens cervicalis join to form a (very large) ansa cervicalis, seen anterior to the carotid artery and supplying branches to the strap muscles. A branch of dubious authenticity descends from the ansa to join the phrenic nerve near the diaphragm.

The large superior cervical sympathetic ganglion (overlain by and posterior to the upper part of the vagus) and the middle cervical ganglion (below the inferior thyroid artery) and their branches are excellent—in particular the cardiac branches of the latter. A small inferior cervical ganglion is largely hidden behind the thyro-cervical trunk, but its medial portion can just be seen at the anterior border of the artery.

The vagus nerve is very prominent, as are both its recurrent branch (hooking around the ligamentum arteriosum) and its cardiac branch, descending between the parent trunk and the carotid artery. Proximally, though less easily seen, are laryngeal and pharyngeal branches. Just behind the upper part of the vagus, overlain by the occipital artery, the 'accessary' [sic] nerve is seen cut short.

The typically intimate relationship of the inferior thyroid artery with elements of the autonomic system is admirably portrayed.

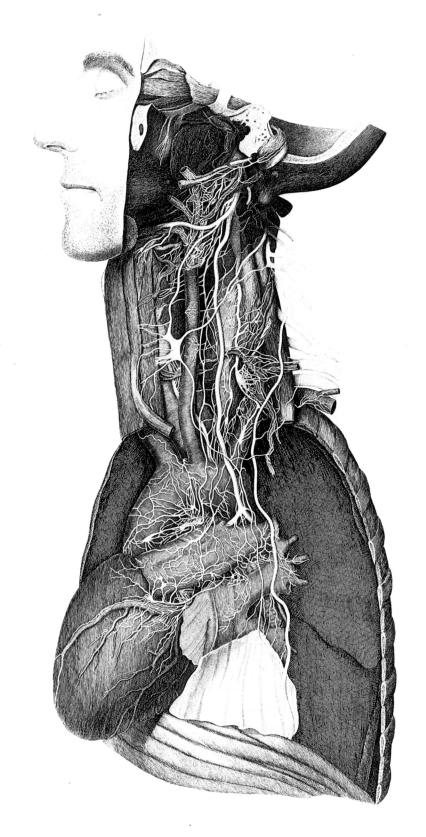

PLATE 108

The cardiac ganglia and plexus lie between the arch of the aorta and the pulmonary trunk, while the pulmonary plexus is seen as a network on the left pulmonary artery and veins.

It is of interest to compare this plate with the similar one drawn by Scarpa (see *Plate 86*, p. 379) some thirty-six years earlier; for example, the origin of the phrenic nerve and the configuration of the middle cervical ganglion.

An artist-anatomist: George Stubbs (1724–1806)

The British artists of the late eighteenth century realized the importance of anatomy: the Royal Academy of Arts appointed William Hunter as Professor of Anatomy in 1769, and the Society of Artists had John Hunter to lecture them the next year. But only George Stubbs—elected to the Academy, and at one time President of the Society—had a serious interest in anatomy for its own sake. (For an unknown reason, Stubbs refused to submit a diploma painting, and thus never became an Academician.) Indeed Stubbs could be considered as one of the few major artists who devoted a substantial amount of time to the first-hand study of scientific anatomy. His dispassionate and closely observed recordings of dissections he himself had carried out may be compared with those of Leonardo da Vinci. The purposes and methods of the two artists, and the range and scale of their achievements in this field, were quite different; but they may both be regarded as true anatomists. There may indeed have been a direct influence of Leonardo on Stubbs's final anatomical work, for some anatomical sketches of Leonardo became more generally known when the Windsor notebooks were rediscovered, widely noted by William Hunter, and, as we have seen, published in 1796 by John Chamberlaine, Keeper of the King's Drawings and Medals; Stubbs's major work on human anatomy was done 1795–1806. Stubbs is on record as having called Leonardo an excellent anatomist, from which it may be taken that he had either seen this book or the actual sketches.

George Stubbs was born in Liverpool, the son of a leather-seller and processor. He was, from his early boyhood, interested in drawing and in the study of animal and human anatomy. For the most part he was self-taught. From 1745 to 1753 he was in York receiving commissions for portrait paintings, and working at anatomy. In the mid-1750s the loosely-organized medical school at York—a city lying half-way between London and Edinburgh—was second only to schools in those two cities. York Hospital had recently (1740) been established by John Burton, MD (Rheims), and others. Burton had been educated at Cambridge, and at Leiden under Boerhaave, and had set himself up as a physician and man-midwife; but his career was interrupted for eighteen months when he was imprisoned in London as a suspected party to the 1745 Jacobite rebellion. Burton was caricatured unjustly as 'Dr Slop' in Laurence Sterne's *Tristram Shandy*. The Reverend Jacques Sterne, uncle of the writer, who lived near York, had denounced Burton as a traitor and Jacobite in 1745. When he was freed, he returned to York, and re-established his practice, and began to put into book form his experiences in midwifery. The work—*An essay towards a complete new system of midwifery theoretical and practical*, London—was published in 1751, and contained eighteen small plates drawn and etched and engraved by George Stubbs. Burton hurried through this publication in order to have precedence over Smellie's anticipated *Treatise on the theory and practice of midwifery ...*, which in the event began publication the next year. Stubbs's illustrations are of pelvic bones, the uterus and adnexa, the placenta, fetuses *in utero*, and obstetrical instruments. Some of the illustrations were made 'after nature' from women who had died in labour, possibly one or more 'resurrected' from the grave, for Stubbs was said to have a 'vile renoun' in York because of grave-robbing for anatomical studies. The illustrations are not to be compared with the work that van Riemsdyk did for Smellie, Jenty, and Hunter. Stubbs's drawing is scientifically and artistically inferior, and the etching is unaccomplished. He probably realized that his work would not stand comparison with such illustrators, and kept his name from appearing anywhere in the book. He had had to learn how to etch and engrave from relatively unskilled workmen, a house-painter and a clock maker.

While in York, Stubbs studied human anatomy with the York Hospital surgeon, Charles Atkinson; he was soon employed to lecture on this subject to students.

After a short visit to Italy in 1754 Stubbs went back to Liverpool; but in 1756 he began his most important work in the anatomical sciences in an isolated farmhouse at Horkstow, in Lincolnshire. The work was on the anatomy of the horse, and, with the active help of a patroness, Lady Nelthorpe, and others, numerous horse cadavers were procured, injected, and dissected. He spent sixteen months on the project. (The most important previous work on the anatomy of the horse was by Carlo Ruini: *Dell'anotomia et dell'infermatà del cavallo*, Bologna, 1598 (*Fig. 13.7*). The style of the illustrations to this book was derived directly or indirectly from those of Vesalius' *Fabrica*.)

Many of the methods Stubbs used, both for dissection and drawing, were based on those of Albinus. While in Lincolnshire undertaking the immense labour required for this work—one horse was studied for eleven weeks—he maintained himself, his common-law wife, Mary Spencer, and their infant son by portraits painted for Lady Nelthorpe. When Stubbs brought the finished anatomical drawings to London in 1758 he tried unsuccessfully to persuade Charles Grignion and other professional engravers to prepare the plates. Stubbs then turned to the labour of engraving the 24 plates himself, and the work this time was of the highest quality (*Fig. 13.8*).

Letters from the Dutch anatomist Camper, written in 1771 and 1772, express admiration for Stubbs's work: 'The myology-neurology and angiology of men have not been carried to such perfection in two ages as these horses by you ... I am amazed to meet in the same person so great an anatomist, so accurate a painter and so excellent an engraver'. Camper, who had studied with, and illustrated for, William Smellie, and who illustrated his own anatomical works, recognized that Stubbs had had before him 'the scheme of the great Albinus'—a man with whom Camper had disputed politely concerning anatomical illustration. Stubbs combined some of the anatomical talents of Albinus with the artistic capabilities of Wandelaar. Stubbs's *The anatomy of the horse* ... was advertised in 1765 for subscription at four guineas; it was addressed to comparative anatomists and to gentlemen, so that they could give 'proper instructions to the more illiterate practitioners of the veterinarian art into whose hands they may accidentally fall'. It was published for the author in 1766, at five guineas, and was a great success, serving to make Stubbs generally known to the artists of London, and to the nobility and gentry of the country. What better way to gain renown in polite circles at that time than to write useful works, illustrated by beautiful plates, about this noble animal! Stubbs then began his most active and popular period as a painter of portraits, of wild and domestic animals, and so on. He did no more sustained work on scientific anatomy, as far as is known, for thirty years or so. Stubbs however retained his interest in anatomy after the publication of *The anatomy of the horse*.... One evening he heard of the death of a tiger in Pidcock's Menagerie at Exeter Change in the Strand, and hurrying down, purchased for three guineas the specimen to dissect. Thus, in 1795 when he was seventy-one years old and when his popularity was beginning to wane, he took up anatomy again, starting work on a very large and extraordinary project which was to occupy him for the remainder of his life. The

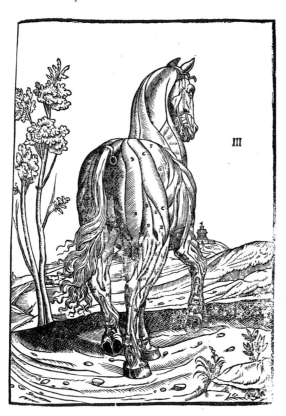

13.7   Dissection of the horse. Woodcut from Ruini, 1598.

work—*A comparative anatomical exposition of the structure of the human body with that of a tiger, and common fowl ...*—was advertised in 1802, and began to appear in parts in 1804; our *Plate 109* is from this work. Only two parts were actually issued by Stubbs, and one appeared posthumously in 1806; the remainder of the work was published, perhaps not exactly in the form Stubbs had intended, in 1817.

What motivated Stubbs to take up this work, in which human anatomy, principally the anatomy of muscles and bones, was compared with that of two other vertebrate species? Stubbs produced paintings, exceptionally fine ones, for both William and John Hunter—paintings of a moose, for instance, for William, and of a rhinoceros for John. He cannot have been unaware of their museums of comparative anatomy—John's museum in Leicester Square was opened to interested gentlemen in 1788. A further association that may have turned Stubbs's ideas towards comparative anatomy was his contacts with various members of the Lunar Society, a convivial group of scientists, engineers, industrialists, and like-minded persons in the Birmingham area. He was a portrait painter for Josiah Wedgwood, and experimented with him, using fired ware as a basis for enamel paintings. He also painted Erasmus Darwin, and they very likely discussed natural history during the sittings; it is possible that ideas on the correspondence of structure between vertebrates stem partly from that early evolutionist, the grandfather of Charles Darwin. Certainly, inhibitions of religion would not have hindered speculation by either Stubbs or Darwin.

It is fortunate that so many of Stubbs's complete drawings still exist, both for *The anatomy of the horse*—a parcel of working drawings for these was also discovered in 1963 in a cupboard at the Royal Academy; and also the later *A comparative anatomical exposition* .... The sheets of drawings for this work, accompanied by 669 pages in four volumes of manuscript by Stubbs (the text to the illustrations), were sold at auction when Mary Spencer died in 1817; they were subsequently donated in 1863 by Dr John Green, along with his entire library, to help found the Free Public Library at Worcester, Massachusetts. The 125 pages of drawings were brought once more to general attention when they were found during re-cataloguing in 1957. They have been exhibited and reproduced a number of times since then. In 1980, with the financial assistance of Mr Paul Mellon, these drawings and the accompanying text were acquired by the Yale Center for British Art, New Haven. Working sketches of the dissections have not survived; only the

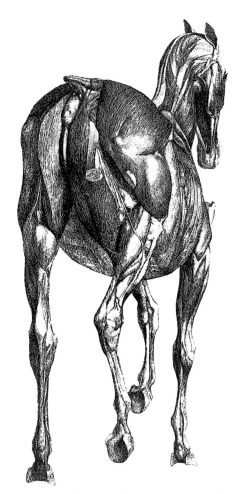

13.8 Engraving from Stubbs's *The Anatomy of the Horse*, 1766.

generalized final drawings, each highly shaded and finished. Some of the skeleton and muscle figures of the human subjects were placed in postures unusual in anatomical illustration; these were designed to show equivalences with natural postures in the tiger and the fowl. One drawing, for instance, shows a side view of a human skeleton crawling in what has been called the pronograde position. Ackerman's *Repository*, April 1811, described a Stubbs skeleton: '... in it a great number of copper and annealed iron wires ... This not only retains the posture it is placed in, but it cannot be put into an unnatural position.'

From these drawings, carried out in the ten years preceding his death in 1806 at the age of eighty-one, Stubbs completed the engraving of 15 plates. The precise engraving is most accomplished, especially when it is remembered that Stubbs was in the eighth decade of his life. As a man of forty or so years, Stubbs had spent six years engraving 18 plates for his book of horse anatomy; he was only slightly slower with his last work. The engraved line, used by itself in the work on the horse, was replaced by stippling, a technique in which dots rather than lines were used, and which well reproduced the original pencil shading of the drawings. F. Bartolozzi (1727–1815) was chief exponent of this technique. (In 1788 Stubbs's print on his favourite topic, *A horse frightened by a lion*, had been prepared using etching, stipple, and mezzotint combined.)

The day before Stubbs died, as Mary Spencer wrote, 'he as usual walked eight or nine miles; and returned in very good spirit'. Before he died, probably of a coronary occlusion, '... he sayed to his surronding friends "perhaps I am going to die", but continued he "I fear not death, I have no particular wish to live. I had indeed hoped to have finished my Comparative Anatomy eer I went, but for other things I have no anxiety"'.

Stubb's straightforwardness of observation when painting wild and domestic animals and gentlemen, their families and servants was also characteristic of his anatomical studies. His human anatomical drawings were done at about the same time as those of John and Charles Bell; where the talented amateur work of the Bells expressed with moralizing fervour the unpleasantness of dissected corpses, Stubbs gave his skeletal and muscle figures a lively poise, as if one could penetrate through an undissected form to the muscle and bones beneath the living skin.

109 Skeleton of striding man. Tab. III in G. Stubbs, *A comparative anatomical exposition ...*, 1804. Engraving (Wellcome Institute Library). 50.7 × 38.1 cm.

This is a stipple-engraving of a human skeleton unusually posed as a striding figure—so to speak the 'bare bones' of the nude human figure illustrated in another of Stubbs's drawings.

Its very unusualness has a great visual impact on the viewer; but from an anatomical standpoint it has numerous drawbacks.

In the skull the ascending mandibular ramus is very wide, the zygomatic bone too 'heavy', and the configuration of the pterion unusual. There is very little curvature of the cervical vertebral column, and the posterior arch of the atlas is shown rather thicker than it should be.

In the upper limb the head of the left ulna is too massive, as, indeed, is the whole bone. Much the same fault exists with regard to the radius, which, in addition, is devoid of a styloid process. The bones composing the index finger are too long, and the carpal bones, particularly in the left hand, are very poorly portrayed.

TAB. III.

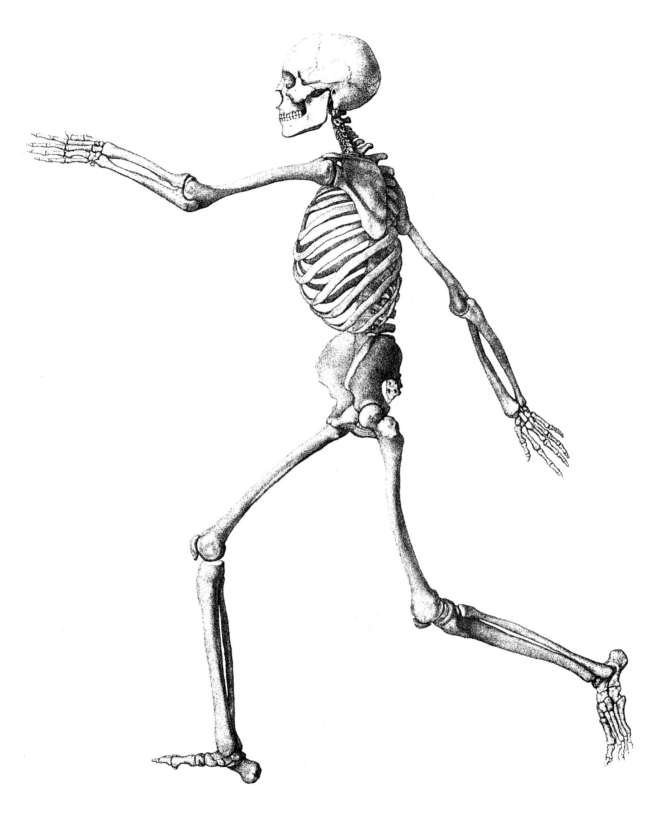

PLATE 109

The costal margin reaches to too low a level, almost to the iliac crest. The entry of the lower part of the vertebral column into the pelvic girdle region is placed too anteriorly, and the lower part of the sacrum is certainly too vertical.

The head of the left femur is very large, having regard to the size of the acetabulum, and the depiction of the long bones of the lower limb in general leaves much to be desired: for example, the two femora are dissimilar, and the right tibia little short of disastrous. Oddly, the skeleton of the foot is very good.

It is perplexing to compare the short-comings of Stubb's numerous human skeletal drawings with his excellent figure-studies. His human muscle plates are few, and mainly concerned with the more superficial muscles, as one might expect from an artist's natural concern with external form. It may be that accurate delineation of the bones of the skeleton did not rank very high in his priorities; this may explain why they are disappointing, coming from a man of such great artistic talent—one, moreover, who had had considerable experience in the study of human anatomy.

Chapter 13: Selected reading

The supply of bodies to dissection rooms

Bailey, J. B. (1896). *The diary of a resurrectionist 1811–1812*. . . . Swan Sonnenschein, London.

Barzun, J. (1974). *Burke and Hare: The resurrection men.* . . . The Scarecrow Press, Metuchen, NJ.

Biddiss, M. D. (1976). The politics of anatomy: Dr Robert Knox and Victorian racism. *Proc. roy. Soc. Med.*, **69**, 245–50.

Breeden, J. O. (1975). Body snatchers and anatomy professors. . . . *Virginia Mag. Hist. Biog.*, **83**, 321–345.

Forbes, T. R. (1981). 'To be dissected and anatomized'. *J. Hist. Med.*, **36**, 490–2.

Lawrence, C. (1988). Alexander Monro *Primus* and the Edinburgh manner of anatomy, *Bull. Hist. Med.*, **62**, 193–214.

Linebaugh, P. (1977). The Tyburn riot against the surgeons. In D. Hay *et al.*, *Albion's fatal tree*. . . . Penguin, Harmondsworth.

Rae, I. (1964). *Knox the anatomist*. Oliver and Boyd, Edinburgh.

Richardson, R. (1987). *Death , dissection and the destitute*. Routledge and Kegan Paul, London.

Roughead, W. (1948). *Burke and Hare*, Notable British Trials Series. W. Hodge, London.

Wolf-Heidegger, G. and Cetto, A. M. (1967). *Die anatomische Sektion in bildlicher Darstellung*. S. Karger, Basle.

Surgeon-anatomists

Altschule, M. D. (1975). Pionieres in der medizinischen Abbildung, [Reproductions, *inter alia*, of Ramsay's anatomical illustrations]. *Du*, **10**, 16–59.

Amacher, P. (1970). Charles Bell. *Dict. sci. Biog.*, **1**, 583–4.

Anderson, R. G. W. and Simpson, A. D. C. (1976). *Edinburgh and medicine*. Royal Scottish Museum, Edinburgh.

Behrman, S. (1960). John Lizars. ... *Brit. med. J.*, **2**, 1665–6.

Chambers, R. (1971). *A biographical dictionary of eminent Scotsmen*, revised T. Thomson, 1870. (Reprint.) Georg Olms, Hildesheim.

Comrie, J. D. (1932). *History of Scottish medicine*. For The Wellcome Historical Medical Museum, London.

Cope, Z. (1966). *The private medical schools of London (1746–1914)*. In *The evolution of medical education in Britain*, (ed. F. N. L. Poynter) Pitman, London.

Cranefield, P. F. (1974). *The way in and the way out: François Magendie, Charles Bell and the roots of the spinal nerves*. Futura, Mount Kisco, NY.

Creswell, C. H. (1926). *The Royal College of Surgeons of Edinburgh ...* Oliver and Boyd, Edinburgh.

Cummings, F. (1964). Charles Bell and The anatomy of expression. *Art Bulletin*, **46**, 191–203.

Drake, F. S. (1872). *Dictionary of American Biography*. [Ramsay]. James R. Osgood, Boston.

Finlayson, C. P. (1974). Alexander Monro (*secundus*). *Dict. sci. Biog.*, **9**, 482–4.

Guthrie, D. (1965). *Extramural medical education in Edinburgh. ...* E. & S. Livingstone, Edinburgh.

Jack, G. *et al.* (1982). *The Royal Society of Edinburgh: 100 medical fellows elected 1783–1844*, (ed. by S. Devlin-Thorp). Scotland's Cultural Heritage, Edinburgh.

Kelly, H. A. and Burrage, W. L. (1920). *American medical biographies*. [Alexander Ramsay]. Norman, Remington, Baltimore.

Loudon, I. S. L. (1982). Sir Charles Bell and the anatomy of expression. *Brit. med. J.*, **285**, 1794–6.

Miles, A. (1918). *The Edinburgh school of surgery before Lister ...* A. and C. Black, London.

Moore, N. (1975). *Alexander Monro, textius*. Dick. nat. Biog., **1**, 1395.

Shepherd, J. A. (1969). *Simpson and Syme of Edinburgh* [see for Lizars]. E. and S. Livingstone, Edinburgh.

Shryock, R. H. (1960). *Medicine and society in America, 1660–1860*. New York, University Press, New York.

Turner, A. L. (1937). *Story of a great hospital: The Royal Infirmary of Edinburgh 1729–1929*. Oliver and Boyd, Edinburgh.

Who was who in America ... 1607–1896 [Ramsay]. (1963). Marquis Who's Who, Chicago.

Stubbs

Doherty, T. (1974). *The anatomical works of George Stubbs*. David Godine, Boston.

Egerton, J. (1976). *George Stubbs: anatomist and animal painter*. The Tate Gallery, London.

[Egerton, J.] (1984). *George Stubbs 1724–1806*. The Tate Gallery, London.

14

New methods in anatomical illustration

IN THE first fifty years (1450–1500) following the invention of printing, initial letters of chapters, paragraphs, and so on were specially treated in books. Initials were sometimes added to a printed text by hand or, if printed, coloured by hand. This was in imitation of hand-copied books. A somewhat later technique was to have initials cut on wooden blocks which, though placed in the same pattern with the type, were separately inked in different colours. Similar ways of adding colour to the printed page were used in association with woodcut illustrations.

Another technique, occasionally found in medically-related illustrations, was to colour the printed black-and-white woodcut impressions by using various stencils, one for each colour; some copies of the *Fasciculo de medicina*, Venice, 1493 show this technique. It was a small step from there to impress the page more than once, using complementary and successive blocks, inked with different colours. In Germany, tinted prints were obtained using coloured paper, one wood-block printing the outline drawing, usually in black, with a second block inked in white gouache to print highlights. This German method of colour-printing was exploited by Dürer and others. The Italian method was to use some three or four blocks. Areas of colour washes could be added to outlines, the white highlights being the original paper showing through where the wood had been cut away on all the blocks. In this way, white and darkly-coloured areas were juxtaposed; the process was called 'chiaroscuro' (that is, light–dark). The process was developed by Ugo da Carpi (1480–1533), and used by him to reproduce the wash drawings of such Italian masters as Raphael and the early mannerist, Parmigianino.

The earliest true colour-printed medical illustrations were in Gaspare Aselli's posthumous work describing his discovery of the lacteal vessels in animals—*De lactibus, sive lacteis venis . . .*, 1627. These were chiaroscuro prints, with a printed black background and superimposed brick-red 'washes'. White highlights (unprinted areas) among the red washes and black outlines, together with hatched shading, emphasized the three-dimensional structure of the parts shown. Chiaroscuro woodcut printing continued through to the eighteenth century, but was little used in technical or applied art, since it was more suitable for the reproduction of sketches and drawings—*broad impressions* would describe both technique and effect—and was therefore unsuitable for the precision and unambiguity necessary for good anatomical illustration.

Sometimes individual engraved plates, printed not in black but in a single coloured ink, sepia for example, were inserted in a book whose text, lettering, and other illustrations were printed in black. But most multi-coloured book illustrations of anatomy in the period up to 1820 are hand-coloured engravings. True colour-prints could, however, also be obtained from etched and engraved copperplates; but the techniques were time-consuming, required great skill, and were expensive. For instance, if the plate was inked using padded stumps or 'dollies' (hence printing *à la poupée*), then it was possible to ink parts of the plate with different pigments, and to print different colours in one impression. Alternatively, the page could be impressed by many plates successively, care being taken that each plate was carefully positioned (that is, registered). If shading techniques—mezzotint, aquatint, etc.—were used then the resultant effect imitated colour washes. Such techniques were found to be especially suitable for reproducing landscape illustrations, but were less used and perhaps less suitable for precise technical work, though anatomical illustrations of the brain were produced in this way for Vicq d'Azyr in the 1780s (see later in this chapter).

A substantial modification of multiplate coloured engravings which was used for anatomical illustration was invented in the eighteenth century. This technique exploited ancient knowledge that new colours can be produced when different pigments are mixed together (for example, blue and yellow mixed to make green), and the new knowledge of colours that stemmed from Newton's work with prisms in 1710—sunlight could be split into component colours by a glass prism. Three plates were made, designed to be inked red, blue, and yellow, so that when the page was printed by each in turn the colours would superimpose to give (theoretically) all possible colours. Each of the plates was prepared using a mezzotint technique, so that gradations of shading in each colour could be obtained; shades of grey and black could also be added by a further plate inked black. Three-colour (or four, with black) printing of this type was invented by Jacob Christian LeBlon, and developed, particularly for anatomical illustration, by Ladmiral and the Gautier family. Similar techniques are employed today in colour photo-reproduction.

J. C. LeBlon (1667–1741) was born in Frankfurt-on-Main, but started work on colour-printing in Amsterdam, continuing in London, where by 1720 he had established a printing-house to exploit his invention. He emphasized the Newtonian basis of his prints, and so persuaded a number of influential persons to back him. The venture failed, each print selling for about half what it cost to produce. The prints were most often touched up by small areas of hand-painting, varnished, framed, and hung in the houses of those not wealthy enough to afford oil-paintings. LeBlon escaped his creditors and started again in Paris, but with limited financial success. In 1737 LeBlon had obtained a copyright to publish an anatomy book based on coloured illustrations; but at his death he had made no progress with the project.

A follower of LeBlon was Joanne Ladmiral (1698–1773); born in France, his principal work in colour-printing was done in the Netherlands, and published from Leiden between 1736 and 1741. Like Wanderlaar, Ladmiral worked both for Ruysch and for B. S. Albinus. For the former he illustrated two works on the dura mater of the brain, and one on the vessels of the human penis injected with coloured wax—an example of Ruyschian art. Included in the work he did for Albinus was a colour mezzotint print, using four plates, of specimens of skin from coloured and from white persons.

The Gautier family

Jacques Fabien Gautier (1711–85) was trained by LeBlon, and took up his master's project to print a complete anatomy in colour, He was granted the copyright in 1745, and from this date a succession of anatomical, surgical, and natural-history coloured plates were produced, some life-sized. The copyright recognized Gautier's claim to have invented the method of printing in three colours and black; but LeBlon had also used this technique. It may be noted that the independent Gautier did not accept Newton's theories of colour; his opinions were discussed sympathetically by Goethe when he attacked the Newtonian theory.

The bibliography of J.-F. Gautier's publications is complex; we may note the following:

An early work, *Myologie complètte* [sic] *en couleur et grandeur naturelle ...*, 1746, combined two publications that had appeared the previous year. Gautier's roles were those of artist, engraver, printer, and publisher; his anatomical collaborator for the work was G. J. Duverney, anatomist at Le Jardin du Roi,[1] who made and displayed the dissections. The original issue was published under Duverney's name. As in many of Gautier's illustrations, the background was dark green in colour; this forms a neutral background to the colours of the dissected anatomical parts, much as green drapes and clothing are used in present-day operating theatres.

In 1748 Gautier produced and published *Anatomie de la tête en tableaux imprimés. ...* The

---

[1] The scientific activity of this institution extended beyond botany to other sciences, with chairs in botany, chemistry, anatomy, and medicine. The Jardin du Roi, first organized in 1635, was renamed the National Museum of Natural History in 1793, with medical sciences ceasing to be represented in 1855.

anatomical collaborator was again Duverney. The eight plates were as large as life, and show the vessels, the brain, and other parts of the head and neck.

Gautier's *Anatomie générale des viscères, et de la neurologie, angiologie et osteologie du corps humain* ..., 1754 included three large folded pages which when joined together complete a full-sized figure of a woman, whose face is turned to show a winsome, erotic smile. Gautier's anatomist for this particular figure was Mertrud. The work was dedicated to the French King, and Gautier is named as a member of the Academy at Dijon and 'Pensionnaire de Sa Majesté'.

A series of twenty plates were issued in 1759, *Exposition anatomique*. ... This was distributed from Marseilles and Amsterdam, as well as Paris. These pages also may be joined together to make nine full-length figures. Included as a single sheet was one figure of a woman squatting, with her uterus opened to show the contained fetus, a realistic re-creation of the squatting figures shown in medieval manuscripts and in the printed versions of Ketham's anatomy (see *Plate 8*, p. 43).

In 1773, J. F. Gautier, who had by now taken the title 'Dagoty' or 'D'Agoty', issued, again from Paris, a work on sexual anatomy, a subject that had continually fascinated him: *Anatomie des parties de la génération de l'homme et de la femme*. ... Some of these pages again make up complete figures.

Gautier edited *Observations sur l'histoire naturelle* ..., 1752–5, one of the earliest French scientific journals. The basis of this enterprise was more than fifty colour-printed plates prepared by his firm, some of which were of anatomical subjects. Assisting the founder of the firm were his family. At least three of his sons were involved in colour-printing, and they continued to publish after their father's death. The anatomical work was continued by Armand Eloi Gautier Dagoty. He published from Nancy, *Cours complet d'anatomie* ..., 1773. The first of the fifteen plates showed male and female nudes, pictured for similar reasons to those of Vesalius when he included a naked man and a naked woman in his *Epitome*. Most of the illustrations in the *Cours complet* ... were after Albinus; in general the work by this son was 'cooler', less extravagant than that of his father.

The colour mezzotint process was used by the Gautier family for anatomical illustration for more than twenty-five years. The work, though well thought-out and generally accurate, was not outstanding either scientifically or didactically when compared with the illustrations available, in the mid-1700's, in the atlases of Albinus, Haller, Cheselden, or the British obstetrical anatomists. Gautier's pictures seem to us to be in the tradition of the early *gravida* illustrations and the figures of Berengario and Charles Estienne—often attracting attention through sexual emphasis: dissected parts were placed within a 'living' body, usually possessing a lively face, whose expression is sometimes quizzical, sometimes erotically inviting, sometimes serene, always with a romantic and elegant hair-style. In one of Gautier's plates there are two naked women, one standing with emphatic breasts and dissected pregnant uterus, the other sitting at her feet with open thighs so disposed as to exhibit her external genitalia. Such erotic figures may have also played a useful role in the sex education of physicians and others; they may be contrasted in their romantic extravagance of feeling with the matter-of-fact illustration in William Smellie's work (1754) of the female external genitalia, an illustration that was often torn out by nineteenth-century bowdlerizers. (Most previous illustrations of this area, such as those of Leonardo or Vesalius, were remarkably inaccurate.) The Gautier figures could, within the confines of anatomy, be quite tender, as in a fine plate in *Anatomie générale* ... of a new-born child, asleep but dissected, lying close to the recently-delivered mother, whose uterus has been opened for display. Whether the introduction of such confusing and conflicting emotions into scientific anatomical illustration is appropriate remains questionable. There is no doubt however as to the originality of these anatomical paintings.

110 Superficial muscles of the head and neck. Planche 2 from J. F. Gautier, *Myologie complètte en couleur ...*, 1746. Coloured mezzotint (Wellcome Institute Library). 39.8 × 32.2 cm.

This plate portrays the muscles of the right side of the head and neck. There is a list of identifying symbols given on the opposite page of the book.

The muscles are well drawn, though in a rather artificial manner. The anterior belly of the digastric muscle is shown *attached* to the hyoid bone rather than bound down to it by fascia. The thyroid cartilage appears to possess no inferior cornu, and neither the sterno-thyroid nor thyrohyoid muscles are attached as they should be to the oblique line of that cartilage. The orbicularis oculi (20) is turned outwards to show a rather artificial levator palpebrae superioris (21). The superior and inferior oblique muscles of the eyeball are well illustrated, as are the tendons of the recti muscles. On the face the masseter muscle (26) and the buccinator (D), with the parotid duct piercing it, are excellently drawn. Many of the small facial muscles are not portrayed; but these had been illustrated in a preceding plate.

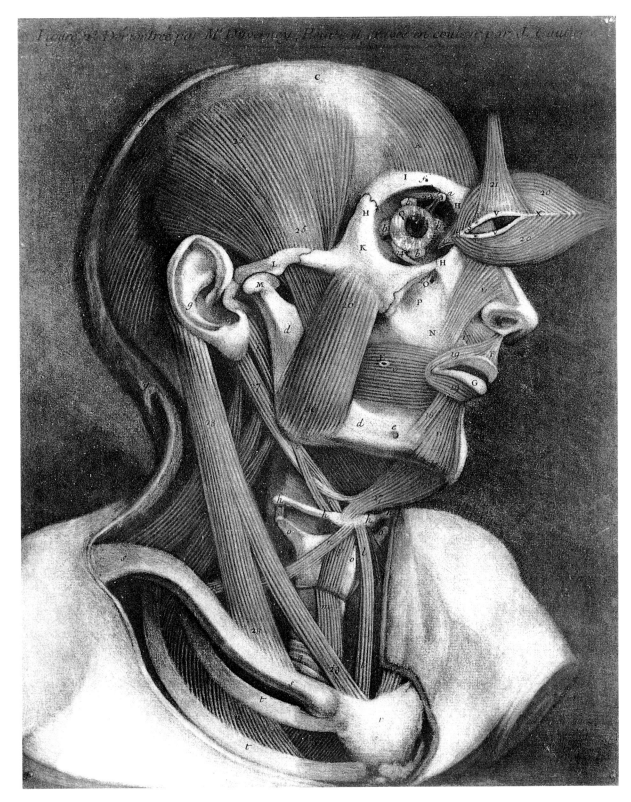

PLATE 110

111 Partially dissected females and fetus, a composite of planches VII and VIII from Jacques Gautier D'Agoty *Anatomie des parties de la génération de l'homme et de la femme* ... 1773. Mezzotint. (Wellcome Institute Library.) 63.8 × 22.0 cm.

This purported anatomical illustration, originally on one side of a sheet folded across the middle, is at once both disturbing and macabre. By no stretch of the imagination could it have been of much help either in presenting or in explaining human anatomy, rather it verges on gratuitous impudicity.

Anatomical detail is very difficult to discern, and that which can be made out is in the main but second-rate. The best is the musculature depicted in the upper figure where sternomastoid, sternohyoid (too thin), temporalis ('muscle crotophite'), mylohyoid, deltoid, rectus abdominis, and external oblique (cut) can all be distinguished. Just visible are the thyroid gland and cartilage, also the epigastric arteries in the left rectus sheath.

The portrayal of a baby's head presenting at the vulva of its dissected mother is grotesque.

In the other main figure the uterus (b) has been opened to reveal the placenta; the bladder lies anteriorly. Little can be recognized inside the opened trunk of the fetus save for its lungs and heart. It is still attached to the umbilical cord, which presumably connects through the mother's vagina to the placenta *in situ*.

Subsidiary figures include an isolated post-partum uterus, with ovaries and Fallopian tubes and opened vagina; detached placentae with amnion, chorion, and umbilical cord; a fetal heart with major blood vessels; and lower left, another fetal heart with a thymus gland placed above it.

The question as to whom the illustrations in this book were addressed is a perplexing one. When coupled with other illustrations produced by Gautier—such as those in his *Exposition anatomique des maux vénériens* ... (often bound with his *Anatomie* ...) one concludes they were probably aimed more at prurient-minded lay-persons than at anatomists.

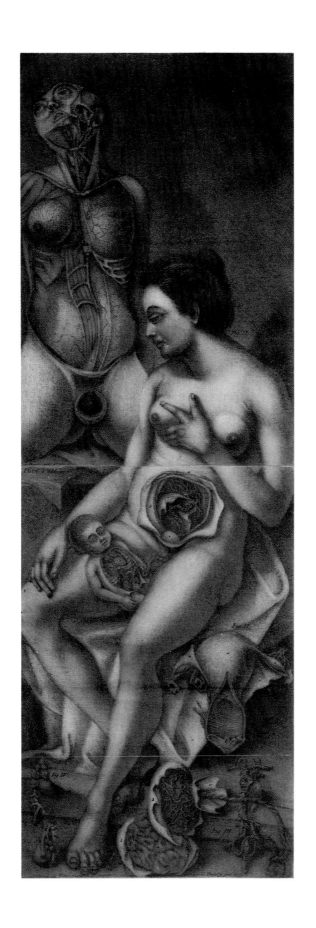

Félix Vicq d'Azyr

Vicq d'Azyr (1748–94), the son of a Normandy doctor, was educated first in Caen and then in Paris, where he obtained his medical doctorate in 1774. Even before this date, while a senior student, he had started a free, public course in the anatomy of humans and animals. Owing to the envy of established teachers, or to the crush of hopeful listeners, or for some other cause he was forced to abandon the course; but his interests in comparative anatomy continued for the rest of his life. Indeed, a later appointment was as anatomist at a new veterinary school established at Alfort, near Paris—the 1760s and 1770s were times when the economic usefulness of a sound scientific base to agricultural France was well recognized. Vicq d'Azyr's administrative success in containing an epizootic in the *Midi* was thought to be due to the effective employment of quarantine, slaughter of sick animals, and the use of sulphur, sulphuric acid, and gunpowder as disinfectants. Like some other investigators—Robert Koch, Louis Pasteur, and William Osler spring to mind—Vicq d'Azyr was convinced that veterinary and human medicine can be mutually beneficial to each other.

In anatomy, Vicq d'Azyr was among the first to emphasize the comparative method, comparing in the laboratory analogous organs and functions in a series of animals (see, for example, his *Système anatomique. Quadrupèdes*, Paris, 1792). Along with contemporaries, including J. Blumenbach and L. J. M. Daubenton, Vicq d'Azyr emphasized organization as the characteristic of living things. Later French scientists, particularly Bichat, used systemization and classification to uncover principles of *general anatomy*, although the emphasis of these later scientists was not on the organ but on the tissue as the fundamental principle.

In 1778 Vicq d'Azyr was appointed permanent secretary of the *Société royale de médecine*, a body he had helped to form. From this position, he was able to bring some influence to bear on an extensive reorganization of the structure of medical practice and education. This took place both immediately before and after the events of 1789. Before the Revolution Vicq d'Azyr had close connection with the Royal Household; he was Marie Antoinette's personal physician. In 1790, in the name of the Royal Society of Medicine, he presented to the Constitutional Assembly 'a new plan or constitution for medicine in France'. One of the reforms suggested was that the education of medical students should start out in the same way whether they were destined to practice internal medicine as physicians or to operate as surgeons. Such reforms were taken up and presented to the Convention by A. de Fourcroy in 1794. In that year, Vicq d'Azyr died at the age of forty-six, after a fever acquired, it was said, by attending the Festival of the Supreme Being.

Vicq d'Azyr was a thoughtful, melancholy man: 'mon philosophe', said Marie Antoinette. With some justification he feared he would be apprehended as a royalist sympathizer.

It is Vicq d'Azyr's contributions as a neuroanatomist to which we now turn, especially noting his publication: *Traité d'anatomie et de physiologie* ... Paris, Amb. Didot, L'ainé, 1786. This single volume, the first part of which is devoted to the brain, was intended as the first of a series on the whole of anatomy and physiology. It represents Vicq d'Azyr's scholarly and critical review of previous work, and includes the results of his own investigations. His laboratory approach was partly quantitative: studies on brain weight in relation to body weight. His precise, close observations lead him to recognize the morphology of some cerebral gyri and sulci. For example he pictured the Rolandic, or central, fissure before Rolando. The tracts of white matter were of particular interest to him: he described the mammillothalamic tract which passes to the anterior group of nuclei in the thalamus; this was later called by Vicq d'Azyr's name, though he was not the first to recognize it.

The illustrations to this 1786 volume helped to make Vicq d'Azyr internationally known. The plates were much admired, being often copied by later authors. Robert Knox's reproductions of Scarpa's *Engravings of the ... nerves ...*, Edinburgh, 1832, included supplemental plates from Soemmerring—on the base of the brain, and from Vicq d'Azyr—on the thalamus, corpora quadrigemina, etc. As Secretary of the Parisian Royal Society of Medicine, Vicq d'Azyr presented the introductory *éloges* for both Scarpa and Soemmerring.

These coloured aquatints may be seen as remarkable examples of sophisticated intaglio technique, giving the impression of a painting in water-colours. Most were printed using pale-coloured inks, with additional colour added by hand. Vicq d'Azyr's artist and engraver was Angélique Briceau, later to become Mme A. Allais. The thirty-four original plates were accompanied by parallel outline engravings, which was, as we have seen, a common practice at that period.

The six-volume *Œuvres de Vicq-d'Azyr ...*, Paris, 1805, and *Planches pour le traité de l'anatomie du cerveau*, Paris, 1813 do not include all the original illustrations; some of the replacements inserted in these later editions are less than satisfactory.

The plates by Vicq d'Azyr and Angélique Briceau may be compared with the (somewhat earlier) plates of Gautier d'Agoty *père*. The former appear to be precise, highly-finished water-colour drawings, which accurately represent a somewhat idealized appearance of actual anatomical structures. The Gautier plates, in contrast, are remarkably freely sketched; they were, perhaps consciously, made to resemble oil-paintings. They are more diagrammatic, forceful, and emotional, highly mannered and individualistic, in contrast to the neo-classicism of Vicq d'Azyr–Briceau. Both sets of illustrations were made using intaglio techniques to achieve a colourful picture, but the use of an aquatint method in the one, and a three-colour-and-black mezzotint process in the other, produced quite different results.

112 Base of brain. Volume 1, Pl. 17, from F. Vicq d'Azyr, *Traité d'anatomie et de physiologie ...*, 1786. Engraving (Countway Library, Boston). 32.0 × 24.3 cm.

Vicq d'Azyr's brain illustrations, according to Meyer (1971) were at that time unrivalled in their quality and accuracy as well as in their comprehensiveness. The illustration we have chosen is primarily concerned with the origins of the cranial nerves. These stand out pleasingly from the rest of the drawing.

With regard to the olfactory tract one notes that three central roots are present—racines interne et courte; interne et longue; externe et longue. At least two of these were known and illustrated by Casserio, over one hundred and fifty years before Soemmerring described and illustrated the third in 1778. Close by these roots is seen stippling representing the anterior perforated substance, the first time that this had been either described or illustrated.

The origin of the oculomotor nerves, seemingly arising from the stippled area (posterior perforated substance) behind the ball-like mammillary bodies, gives little impression that they in fact emerge from the quite deep fossa between the cerebral peduncles.

The thin trochlear nerves can be seen just in front of the large trigeminal nerves. The abducent pair, passing over the pons, are perhaps a shade too thick. However, the facial and stato-acoustic nerves, and the filaments going to form the glossopharyngeal, vagus, cranial accessory, and hypoglossal nerves are excellent. They are superior to those illustrated by Soemmerring when he introduced his new cranial nerve classification some eight years earlier.

The patterns of the rather faint gyri and sulci are not so impressive—indeed Rolando dissmissed Vicq d'Azyr's illustrations of the cerebral convolutions as speaking more for the artist's ability than for that of the anatomist.

Although he discovered (but did not name) the locus ceruleus, Vicq d'Azyr's name is nowadays best known with regard to the mammillothalamic tract—the bundle of Vicq d'Azyr. However, the basics of this had already been described by Pourfour du Petit (1710) and Santorini (1724): Vicq d'Azyr's contribution was essentially to refine and add to their descriptions, and to illustrate this tract in his Figure 2, Table 25.

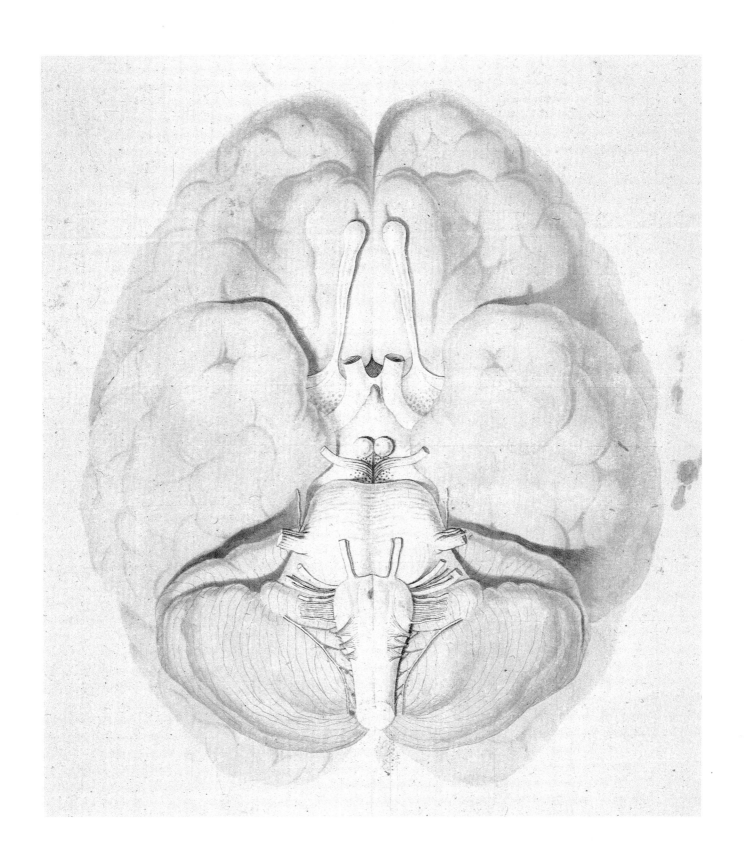

The origins of lithography

At the end of the eighteenth century a Bavarian, Alois Senefelder, invented a new printing process that depended on quite a different principle from that of the two processes then available, relief and intaglio, processes that had been in existence at least since the fifteenth century. The new method was called stone or chemical printing, or polyautography; from 1804 the word 'lithography' has been used to designate this method of printing, in which the ink lies on the surface rather than on projecting reliefs or in depressed grooves. The process is described as planographic, rather than relief or intaglio printing.

Senefelder, 1771–1834, was a struggling playright who wished to distribute copies of his plays, but could not afford to have them printed in the usual way: so he turned to experimentation, becoming obsessed with the technicalities of *relief* printing on stone. He, like others before him, discovered that a waxy mark made, for example, by a crayon on a limestone that was then wetted, would protect that part of the stone from an acid wash; the unwaxed part would be etched away, leaving a relief which could be selectively inked and printed. Senefelder himself described his new key discovery, made in 1798, in these words:

I took a cleanly polished stone, inscribed it with a piece of soap, poured thin gum solution over it and passed over all a sponge dipped in oil colour. All the places marked with the fat [the soap] became black at once, the rest remaining white. I could make as many impressions as I pleased; simply wetting the stone after each impression and treating it again with the sponge produced the same result each time (from : *A Complete Course in Lithography*, London, 1819; German edition, 1818).

He outlined the fundamental principle of this surface, or planographic, printing:

... the reason why the ink, prepared of a sebaceous matter adheres only to the lines drawn on the plate [stone], and is repelled from the rest of the wetted surface depends entirely on the mutual chemical affinity, and not on mechanical contact alone. [The wetted surface was lipophobic, the waxy crayon lines drawn on the stone, lipophilic. The ink was lipid in nature.]

The stones that Senefelder used proved remarkably suitable to this purpose. They came from the Kellheim region, about a hundred kilometres north of Munich. He and his successors subsequently exploited metal, as well as stone, surfaces, using zinc and aluminium. (The techniques of offset lithography need not concern us here.)

In 1799 Senefelder copyrighted his invention in Bavaria, and made an agreement with a business-like, but honourable, printer of Offenbach-on-Main, J. A. André, to divulge his secret: 'how to print music and pictures from stone'. Senefelder travelled to London, obtained a patent in 1801, and set up a press in association with J. A. André's brother. A press was founded in Paris the next year under the direction of a third André. Senefelder, in Munich within a few years of his invention, was responsible for a large volume of lithographic printing for the government.

From 1816 or thereabouts there was intense exploitation of the lithograph for commercial use in the German-speaking world, in London, and, particularly, in Paris. The first extensive use of lithography for printing anatomical illustration was in Paris from 1821 onwards.

The French lithographic atlases: Cloquet, Bourgery, Bonamy and Beau, and Hirschfeld

A principal centre for lithography in its earliest days was, naturally enough, Senefelder's in Munich. Other places where lithographic presses were active were Offenbach-on-Main and Berlin. Within a few years, the centre shifted to France, with the establishment of a lithographic printing-shop by Charles Philibert, Comte de Lasteyrie (1759–1849).[2] He had visited Munich in 1812 and again in 1814 specifically to learn lithographic techniques. In 1815 he set up a lithographic press in Paris. It was used as a copy-centre for Government administrative departments, producing facsimiles of important and historical documents. Lasteyrie's press also printed music scores, maps, biological illustrations, book illustrations, and individual art prints. In 1816 a second litho-shop was functioning under Godefroy, or Gottfried, Engelmann (1788–1839); he had moved his press from Mulhouse in Alsace. Within a few years there were other presses in Paris; medical publishers utilized a number of different lithographic firms to produce the plates for anatomical multi-volume atlases. Lasteyrie, as we have seen, was soon involved in such publishing. Between 1823 and 1826 his establishment produced, in the short period of some thirty-odd months, lithographs of some of Mascagni's plates that Antommarchi had bought to Paris after the death in 1818 of his patient Napoleon Bonaparte (see Chapter 10).

At about the same time *Jules Cloquet* and A. Béchard, Parisian anatomists, conceived, on a grand scale, a human anatomical atlas in the form of a compilation of plates. Mostly the plates were to be original, some were to be taken from the best work of 'the most exact of other authors'. In the event, plates of the gravid uterus, for example, were copies from William Hunter, Loder, Soemmerring, and Tiedemann. Plates from Haller, Walter, Mascagni (on lymphatics), Charles Bell, Scarpa, and others were also reproduced by lithography in Cloquet's book.

Béchard had to drop out, but Cloquet persevered with his plan. The first of five volumes was issued in 1821, the last in 1831. A total of 300 plates in large folio containing more than 3000 figures were finally produced, of which a little more than half were 'drawn from nature', and the remainder copied. The artists for the original illustrations were Jules Cloquet and his sister Lise, 'une artiste extrêment habile'. It may be noted that Cloquet's plates were themselves copied. Edward Mitchell, for instance, engraved twenty-four of Cloquet's muscle plates, and published them in Edinburgh in 1832.

This vast work by Jules Cloquet (1790–1883) was *Anatomie de l'homme ou description et figures lithographiées de toutes les parties du corps humain*, Paris, Comte de Lasteyrie, 1821–31. It was supervised throughout by Cloquet, but many others were, of course, involved. By the time the third volume, on neurology, was published in 1828 Engelmann and others also contributed

[2] In the first years of the century, Frédéric André had issued a number of fine lithographs from his press in Paris.

lithographic plates. Different publishers issued the volumes as they appeared. For the third, fourth, and fifth volumes, a Dr Drosart and a Monsieur Bompard, *fils*, edited the text from Cloquet's notes. He had as prosector Dr Pailloux, who, in Cloquet's absence, directed the artists. P. Feillet, Dubourjal, and particularly Haincellin were responsible for most of the original plates. (Some copies were bound into three 'Tomes', as was the case with the Wellcome copy from which our *Plates 113 and 114* were taken.) The atlas was reissued in quarto rather than folio, 1825–36, with some relatively minor additions, including sections on histology.

Cloquet's father, J. B. A. Cloquet, was an artist, an art teacher, and an engraver who had illustrated and engraved Egyptian scenes in the context of Napoleon's campaigns. The father, before his death in 1828, had seen his son's great work through to the fourth volume. Cloquet's doctoral thesis on hernia, 1817, was illustrated by the author, the engravings being made by his father. This work was reissued two years later, in 1819, with lithographic plates actually made by Jules Cloquet himself. Indeed, he had started his career as apprentice to his father, and only moved to medicine after work as a wax-modeller in the Paris medical faculty. His brother Hippolyte, three years older than Jules, completed Vicq d'Azyr's large survey of anatomy, and later published a two-volume human anatomy—a much less grand effort than Jules's. Jules Cloquet lived to a great age, honoured, moving in aristocratic circles, renowned throughout Europe and America. He published other works, including a treatise on acupuncture; the technique was of fashionable interest in Paris, having been brought to notice by French expansionist enterprises in South-East Asia. He also wrote a biography of his friend Lafayette, soldier, libertarian, and patriot of both France and the United States.

Cloquet's wonderful atlas was in accord with the high romantic view of anatomy which he outlined right at the beginning of the first volume:

Dans l'étude de cette belle et vaste science, on droit sans cesse suivre la méthode analytique, séparer, diviser, isoler les parties par la dissection.

In 1829, another young anatomist, only two years after his medical doctorate, decided that he too would produce an atlas of the whole of anatomy. Cuvier, the great comparative anatomist, gave *Jean-Baptiste Marc Bourgery* (1797–1849) encouragement in this project, but warned him that it could well turn out to be the work of a lifetime. Nevertheless Cuvier congratulated him on his plans and on his good fortune in having enlisted the help of Nicolas-Henri Jacob (1782–1871) as the artist for the project: 'Courage donc! et marchez droit devans vous sans vous laisser arrêter par aucun obstacle.' A first volume appeared in 1831/2, the text of the eighth and last volume is dated 1854, the separate title page for the plates, 1844. The work was *Traité complet de l'anatomie de l'homme comprenant la médecine operatoire ... avec planches lithographiées d'après nature par N.-H. Jacob*, Paris, C. A. Delaunay. There were re-issues, including a complete set in 1866–71 with additional plates and altered text; in this way, the title-pages to the volumes and the plates themselves may have different and various dates.

Bourgery had indeed carried his work through to completion, and, as Cuvier had predicted, it occupied many years of his life. Bourgery covered the whole of anatomy, with original plates and text, including a volume on surgical anatomy and a last volume on embryology, microscopic anatomy, and *anatomie philosophique*. These volumes serve as fine summaries of anatomical knowledge and ideas current in Paris during the middle of the nineteenth century. On the plate at the end of the work, Bourgery wrote feelingly: 'Plate 60 and the last of the eighth and last volume'. Jacob had stayed the course; Cuvier had been correct in congratulating Bourgery on his collaborator.

Bourgery's other collaborators should be mentioned. The office of the publisher of the early volumes was described as being situated close beside the School of Medicine, in the *Librarie Anatomique*—a bookshop specializing in anatomy, indicating the importance attached to this subject in Paris in the 1830s. The printer for some of the volumes was a member of the Didot family; we have earlier had occasion to note this family. The many lithographers, that is the artists responsible for transferring the artists' drawings to stone, include Mme C. A. Jacob Hublier, whose fine work for the last volume is particularly notable. The commercial lithographic establishments included Bénard and Frey and Lemercier. Among the academic contributors was the great experimental physiologist Claude Bernard; he jointly authored and co-edited a number of volumes, for example the one on operative surgery in the 1867–71 reissue. Bourgery had the assistance of many prosectors, among whom was Ludovic Hirschfeld, whose many contributions are usually noted beneath the plates simply as *Ludovic*; we shall note his work later in this section.

It is Nicolas-Henry Jacob who should be particularly recognized as the most important collaborator, as Bourgery himself stated plainly. In the reissue of the sixth volume, the joint authorship of Bourgery and Bernard is noted, along with the contributions of N.-H. Jacob, who was now entitled *professeur-dessinateur-anatomiste*. Indeed some of the plates indicate that Jacob directed the prosection. He had studied for a period with Jacques-Louis David, the neoclassical artist of the French Revolution. As artist and lithographer Jacob had been involved in the early days of that printing technique, putting the artistic work of Restoration salons on stone for a number of leading lithographic establishments. To the first volume of Bourgery's atlas, Jacob contributed a frontispiece showing a slightly absurd, romantically-posed family—all modestly naked. The child, man, woman, and old man serve to indicate the ages of human life, a theme well-liked also in Renaissance times. During much of his work for Bourgery, Jacob was *Maître de dessin* at the veterinary school at Alfort. He also contributed to other medical projects, including lithographs for Dupuytren, printed at the lithographic presses in the *Ministère de la Marine*. His pupil J.-B. Leveille assisted in the production of the plates in the later volumes of Bourgery's atlas. Cuvier, reporting favourably to the Institute on Bourgery and Jacob's work, emphasized the importance of illustration to biomedical science: 'On peut dire que sans l'art de la gravure, l'histoire naturelle et l'anatomie, telles qu'elles existent aujourd'hui auraient été impossible'; the invention of lithography he thought particularly significant in this context.

Before Bourgery and Jacob had completed their work, yet another multi-volume anatomical atlas began publication in Paris. This work, *Atlas d'anatomie descriptive du corps humain*, was by *Constantin Louis Bonamy*, the anatomist, and *Émile Beau*, the artist. The four volumes appeared at intervals: 1844, 1847, 1850, with the last volume delayed until 1866. There were in all 251 lithographic plates. Beau stayed with the project until the end; Bonamy, for the last two volumes, also had as collaborator Paul Broca (1824–80), who later became well-known for his work on cerebral localization, defining an area on the left cortex, damage of which in right-handed persons was associated with aphasia. By 1850 Bonamy was Professor of Anatomy at *L'école préparatoire de médecine* at Toulouse. The lithographers included Artus, Lemercier (who was also used by Bourgery), and Auguste Bry.

By the time the last volume of Bonamy's atlas was issued, and when Bourgery's atlas was being reprinted, the second edition of an illustrated anatomical work using lithography appeared in Paris. This was an impressive large quarto book with 92 plates: Ludovic Hirschfeld, *Traité et iconographie du système nerveux*, Paris, Victor Masson *et fils*, 1866 (first edition 1853). As we have previously noted, the author had been Bourgery's prosector. The artist and lithographer was J.-B. Leveille, N.-H. Jacob's pupil, and a technical contributor to Bourgery's atlas. The lithographic printers and publishers of Hirschfeld's and Bonamy's atlases were the same—respectively Lemercier (used also by Bourgery) and Masson.

Ludovic Hirschfeld (1816–76) had been born in a ghetto in Central Europe. In Paris he was a protégé of Bourgery, who saw him through medical school. He became *Chef de Clinique* at the Hôtel Dieu, and taught both anatomy and surgery. Later he was appointed Professor of Anatomy in Warsaw. He still often continued to sign himself simply as Ludovic.

Each of these four atlases—Cloquet, Bourgery, Bonamy, and Hirschfeld—contained coloured plates, but they used different methods, the first two being hand-coloured, the last two being colour-printed. At least one of Bourgery's volumes could be obtained uncoloured. The technique of colour-printing using lithography had continued to develop during the fifty years after Senefelder's invention, overcoming technical difficulties of obtaining precise registration of successive prints. Engelmann was one of those who patented colour-printing processes in the 1830s. Hullmandel obtained similar patents in London in 1837. By mid-century, the number of stones used, each inked with a different colour, could be as many as nine or more for the printing of facsimiles. (As a very early example we may refer to facsimiles of medieval miniatures printed at the Lithographic Institute in Vienna *c*.1820.) It should be noted that, in the completed chromo-lithograph, the colours were achieved by using, on separate stones, the actual final coloured inks, not by superimposing three colours, which was the mezzotint method that Ladmiral, LeBlon, and Gautier d'Agoty had employed. (The techniques of modern photographic colour-separation for offset lithography are also essentially similar to the latter method. Engelmann's patented technique again employed a process of over-printing with three primary colours and black.) Senefelder himself as early as 1808 produced lithographs in two colours.

The fifty years after 1821 saw the production of many large, detailed anatomical lithographs. The three complete atlases listed above contain together many hundreds of plates. During this period in the Paris School students had unsurpassed access to dissection. A plentiful, inexpensive supply of bodies was available, since every person dying in the large state-run hospitals in the city was a potential subject—grieving friends and relatives could not oppose a post-mortem examination. Anatomical lectures were conducted in large amphitheatres with easily obtained admission; both public and private instruction in anatomy was readily available, given as the body was dissected by the student himself. Foreign students flocked in large numbers to Paris, and benefited from these arrangements for the study of anatomy.

It has been suggested that anatomical atlases flourished when oportunities for dissection were scarce; when cadavers were available then there was less need for book illustration. This hypothesis would not seem to be true in Paris from 1820 to 1870. This was a period when dissection flourished *and* when anatomy books were produced in profusion. The demand for such books must have been great; and lithography was able to provide the new illustrations more quickly and cheaply than engraving. From 1820 on there were competing companies ready to print both lithographs and text, and there were publishers ready to issue the books and booksellers ready to sell them. It would be interesting to know whether the entrepreneur who put up the money for the venture—the publisher?—made significant profits. Presumably some publishers profited, since companies would take on a project to produce a new anatomical atlas while still completing a previous one. Certainly artists and lithographers were employed from decade to decade, sometimes establishing companies that worked on more than one of these mammoth projects. As the years went by, the principal anatomist involved often began to employ prosectors, and even left to the experienced artist the responsibility of determining how a particular dissected part should be shown.

These large atlases would not have been bought by many students, nor were they appropriate for use as dissection manuals. They were volumes which most probably found their place on the bookshelves of the studies of doctors and those of other bourgeois, to be used as reference material. And, as with all such reference books, they may well have remained on those shelves unconsulted for long periods. Copies of these atlases brought into the sale rooms nowadays are often in very good condition, as are many of those held in rare-book collections in medical libraries. They do not give the appearance of having been much used. Still, it remains true that to have these atlases available meant that a surgeon, an anatomist, or any other enquirer could most often find answers to their anatomical queries in these beautiful collections of plates. We must confess that we have been tempted to think, quite anachronistically and improperly, how amazed and delighted Eustachio, Vesalius, or Albinus would have been by the great anatomical atlases of Cloquet, Bourgery, and Bonamy.

113 Side view of male and female skeletons. Tome 1, planche 55, première partie, from J. G. Cloquet, *Anatomie de l'homme* ... 1821–31. Lithograph (Wellcome Institute Library). 45.0 × 29.0 cm.

In this plate, the male skeleton on the left is that of a thirty-eight-year-old five feet six inches tall sea captain, who was said in life to be 'good-looking and regularly proportioned'. The skeleton is shown gesturing to a female skeleton on the right, that of a twenty-two-year-old five feet one inch tall female, who was 'beautiful and elegant in life'. The pose was chosen so that the viewer could compare the differences in dimensions and configuration of male and female skeletons. The relative positioning of the skeletons is pleasing, and has considerable impact; it does appear, though, that the female was somewhat flat-footed.

The plate's appeal is more aesthetic than anatomical: the skulls convey to the viewer a too-smooth textural 'feeling', as do the female scapula and hip-bone; both the pelvic girdles are tilted too far backwards, particularly in the female; and the male eleventh rib and cartilage are rather too long. The tibiae are proportionately too long with regard to the femora, and the skeletal height is too great for the femoral length. All the teeth appear to have the same morphology.

It is interesting that the positioning of the patellae with regard to the knee-joint is similar in both female limbs, even though the right leg is flexed at the knee-joint. One wonders why the right forearm was so pronated in the female; presumably this may have been to depict the anatomy differently, but it results in an awkward positioning.

The skeletal sexual differences between a 'typical' male and a 'typical' female that may be seen in a lateral view include the following: the male skull is larger and the mandible more massive (the male also usually possesses a larger mastoid process, but this cannot be distinguished in this plate); the heads of the male humerus and femur are larger than the female, as are the femoral and tibial condyles, while the femoral shafts are longer and thicker; the male greater sciatic notch is narrower, and the sacrum is less curved. In addition, the long bones of the limbs are generally considerably heavier.

Most of the above differences are shown in this most attractive, not to say touching, skeletal illustration.

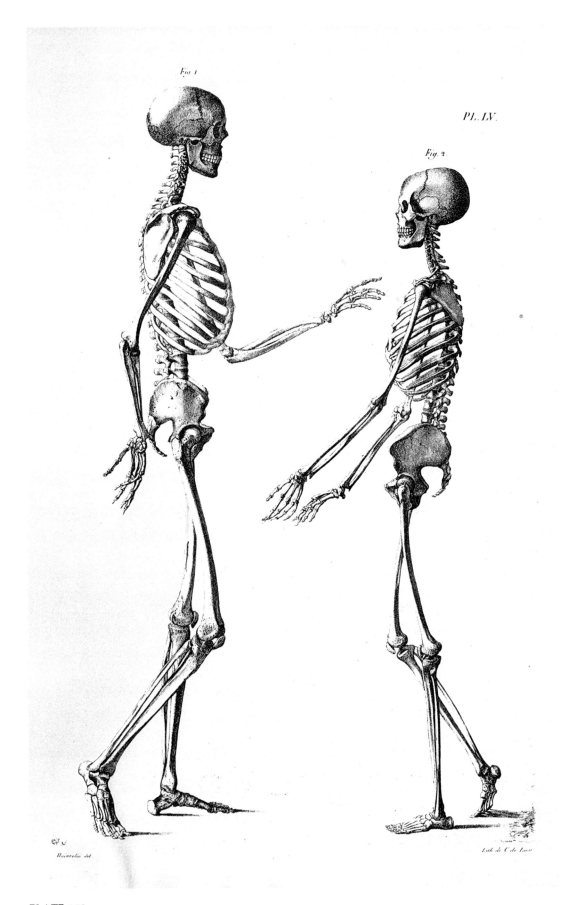

Fig. 1

Fig. 2

Pl. LV.

PLATE 113

114 Sagittal section through the skull. Tome 2, Planche 153, troisième partie, from J. G. Cloquet, *Anatomie de l'homme ...*, 1821–31. Lithograph (Wellcome Institute Library). 32.0 × 26.9 cm.

This is essentially concerned with the nerves in the orbit: the cerebral hemispheres and upper part of the mid-brain have been removed.

The dissections and illustrations of the cranial nerves contained in this volume are quite excellent; the plate chosen is, in fact, one of the simplest. Although the terminations of the motor nerves to the eye muscles are not shown they are referred to in the accompanying text. For example, the abducent (38) supplies the 'muscle droit externe' [lateral rectus]. The portrayal of the trigeminal ganglion is better than the rather miserable origin of the fifth nerve itself from the pons. The maxillary and mandibular divisions, being of no further concern in this illustration, are shown exiting via the foramina rotundum and ovale respectively. The ophthalmic nerve divides into the lacrimal, naso-ciliary ('branche nasale'), and frontal, the latter then dividing into the supraorbital and supratrochlear nerves.

The oculomotor nerve with its upper and lower divisions and the long and very slender trochlear nerve are well portrayed.

The ciliary ganglion, shown receiving filaments from both the naso-ciliary nerve and the nerve to inferior oblique (from the oculomotor), gives off six 'wriggly' short ciliary nerves; the naso-ciliary nerve is seen giving ethmoidal and infra-trochlear (32) branches.

The quality of production of Figure 1 and the clarity and accuracy of the anatomy it portrays are alike excellent; few modern illustrations are better.

The lower figure is unhappily less good, being rather stereotyped, and the too-close association of the lateral geniculate body (3) to the inferior colliculus (2) should be noted; in the text, also, the lateral geniculate body is considered as a lateral portion of the inferior colliculus.

Fig. 1.

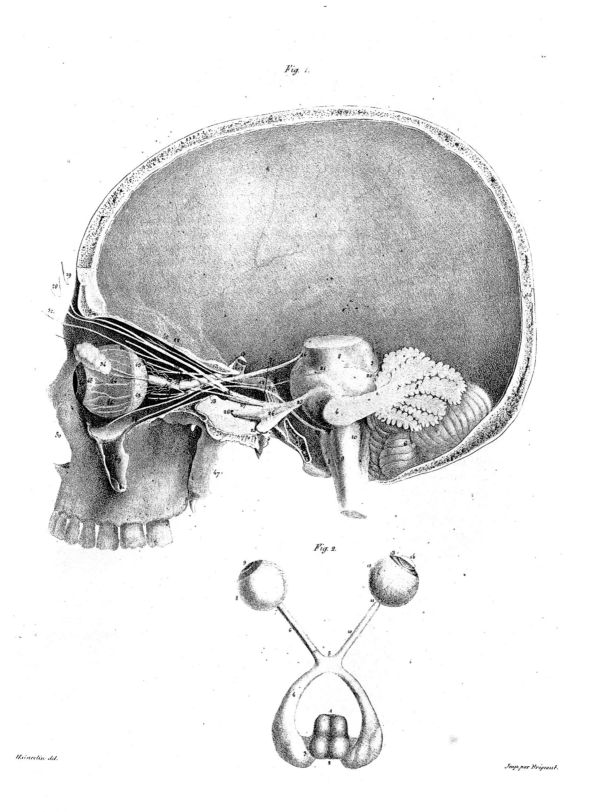

Fig. 2.

Usincelin del.

Imp. par Brigeaut.

PLATE 114

115 Disarticulated skull. Volume 1, Planche 30, from J.-M. Bourgery, *Traité complet de l'anatomie de l'homme. ...* 1831. Lithograph (Wellcome Institute Library). 30.1 × 22.5 cm.

This is one of the first illustrations of the 'exploded' disarticulated adult skull.

Such a preparation (this one by M. Morand, dentist) is extremely difficult to draw, and here much of the anatomy, particularly of the facial skeleton, including the ethmoid bone, is confusing. Elsewhere in the book the frontal bone (save in the fetus) is shown as a single bone; but in this drawing it is in two halves, that is, the metopic suture is present. The very small letters, many difficult to identify, refer to the bones themselves, not to particular parts of them.

The upper three cervical vertebrae were deliberately portrayed as being well separated, the better to show their anatomical features.

Some of the separated sutural articulations, such as the coronal and squamosal, are well displayed; but others, like the fronto-maxillary, are less well defined.

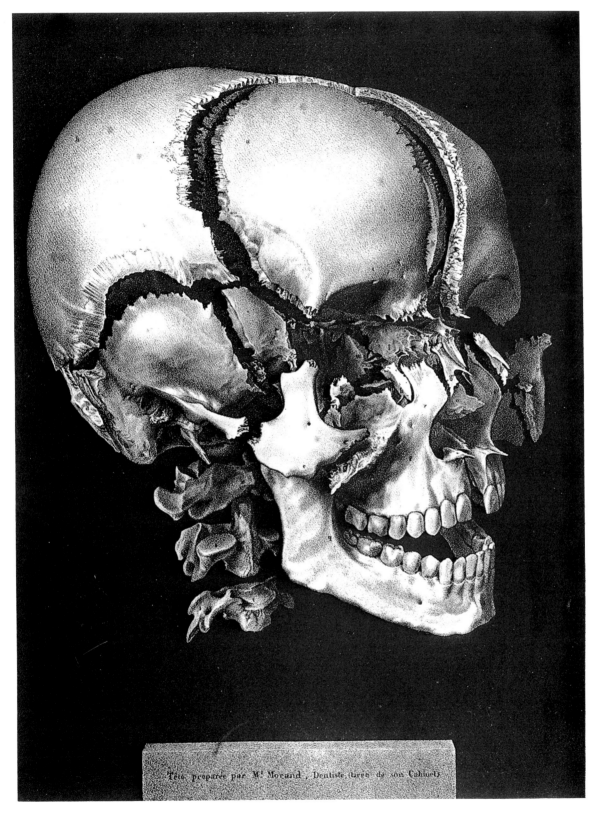

Tête preparée par M.ʳ Morand, Dentiste (tirée de son Cabinet)

PLATE 115

116 Superficial dissection of vessels, nerves, and muscles of the axilla and neck. Volume 6, Planche 6 from J.-M. Bourgery, *Traité complet de l'anatomie de l'homme ...*, 1839. Lithograph (Wellcome Institute Library). 40.3 × 30.5 cm.

This plate is coloured in the original. In places the muscles have been removed and a 'perimysial' outline is substituted; for example the anterior belly of the digastric and the sternomastoid muscle.

The anatomy of the neck region is reasonably easy to follow, but for some reason the arm is rendered 'transparent', lifted up and then cut off—a most confusing way to present what is in effect a well-organized area. It is strange that so much trouble should be taken to so little effect; for one thing it makes it impossible to show the radial nerve—the largest nerve in this region. Most identifying numbers lie 'on' the structures to which they refer, but four are 'off' them (in the black surround); then white indicator lines travel to the structures concerned, but these lines are so faint as to be virtually invisible.

The submandibular gland (B) is too closely associated with the parotid (A), and almost appears to be part of it: it should also be positioned more over the mylohyoid and digastric muscles than it is here. The axillary artery and vein, the brachial artery, the thoraco-acromial vessels, axillary lymph glands, and the median and musculo-cutaneous nerves are readily identifiable.

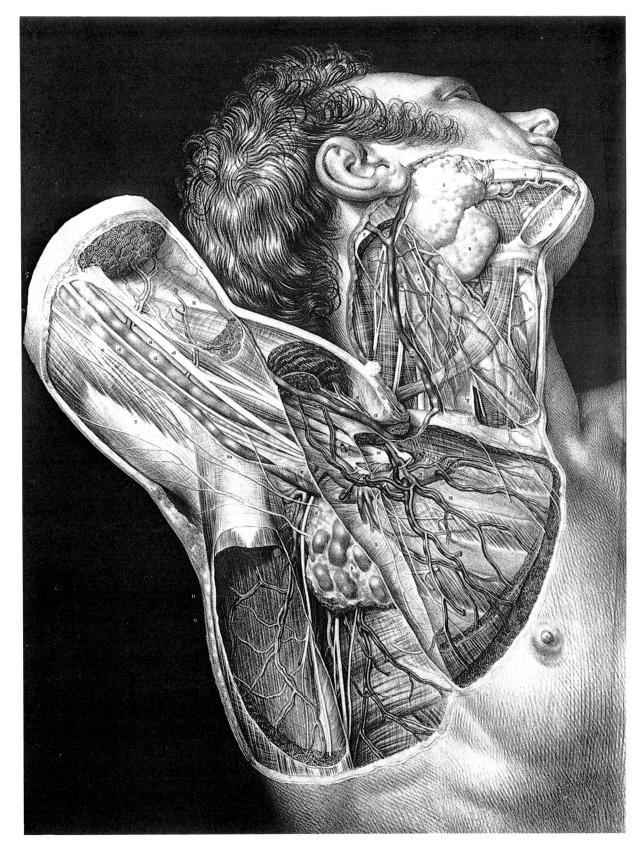

PLATE 116

117 Lymph nodes, vessels, and thoracic duct. Livraison 36, Pl. 51–2 from C. Bonamy and E. Beau, *Atlas d'anatomie descriptive* ..., 1847. Lithograph (Wellcome Institute Library). 31.4 × 15.2 cm.

This illustration, on a folded sheet, shows a male figure, thorax and abdomen widely opened, with all viscera and the diaphragm removed so as to reveal the posterior abdominal wall with certain blood-vessels either in place or cut short.

The main intent is to portray the thoracic duct, its tributaries, and its termination. Reference numbers are placed on the side of the plate, but the indicator lines are so faint as to be almost useless in many cases.

The upper part of the thighs show the superficial inguinal glands, with Cloquet's gland on the medial side of the femoral vein (deep to where the inguinal ligament would be). Lymph vessels and nodes alongside the external iliac vessels lead to a plethora of para-aorti lymph nodes and plexuses. It is curious that no internal iliac nodes and lymph vessels are depicted.

The thoracic duct, with a peculiar plexiform arrangement at mid-thoracic level, is shown arising, but only in part, from a rather poorly defined cysterna chyli; the lower bulbous part is termed 'citerne de Pecquet', named after the seventeenth-century French lymphologist who discovered it.

After crossing over to the left side, anterior to the hemiazygos vein, the thoracic duct is shown opening into the junction of the left subclavian and left internal jugular veins. Here it appears rather large—would that it were always so easy to find in a dissection as would appear from this drawing!

The duct is shown receiving intercostal lymphatics; many intercostal lymph glands are shown, particularly on the left side, where the subcostalis muscles have been removed.

The relatively sparse musculature in this illustration serves well as a frame for the lymphatic presentation. It is a good, clear, no-nonsense illustration, which does not contain so many lymph vessels that the overall arrangement is obscured.

It is of interest to compare this plate with that of Mascagni, some sixty years earlier ((*Plate 89*, p. 393).

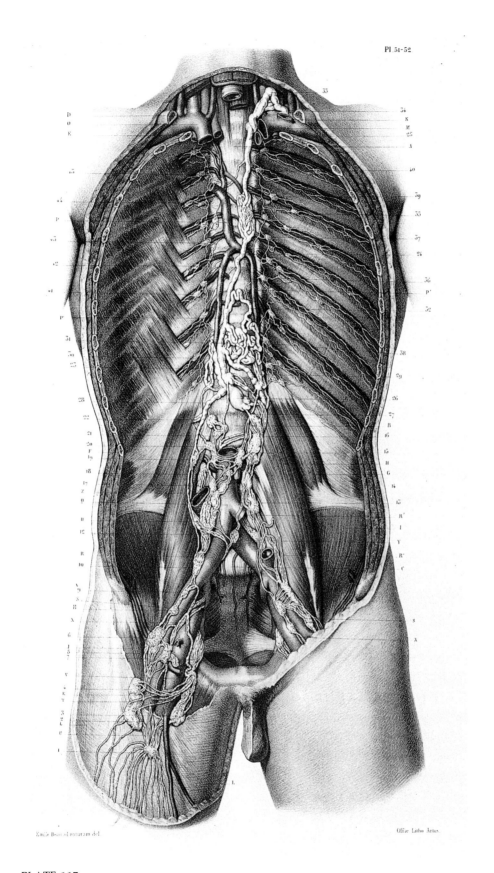

Pl.51-52

Emlis Beau ad naturam del.

Offic Litho Artes.

PLATE 117

118 Coeliac ganglion and associated autonomic plexuses. Planche 70 from L. Hirschfeld, *Traité et iconographie du système nerveux ...*, 1866. Lithograph (private collection). 19.7 × 16.0 cm.

The liver has been lifted up antero-superiorly by hooks placed in the gall-bladder and ligamentum teres. Most of the stomach and parts of the pancreas and of the portal and splenic veins have been removed, so as to reveal the coeliac plexus and ganglia. The 'nodules' of the latter are well portrayed, as is the very clear distribution of autonomic fibres to the various surrounding organs and along the blood-vessels. The density of the fibres lying on the aorta and on the branches of the superior mesenteric artery and the inferior mesenteric artery is excellently brought out. Less felicitous features are the manner in which the vagus nerves feed into the coeliac plexus and the configuration of the pancreas, which has no uncinate process and a very unusual relationship of its body and tail to the splenic vessels. The gastroduodenal artery is far too small, particularly in relation to the left gastric artery. However, it is gratifying to see branches of the left portal vein and left hepatic artery supplying the quadrate lobe of the liver, which, because it lies to the right of the fissure for the ligamentum teres, was for many years erroneously considered to belong to the right lobe of the liver.

PL.70.

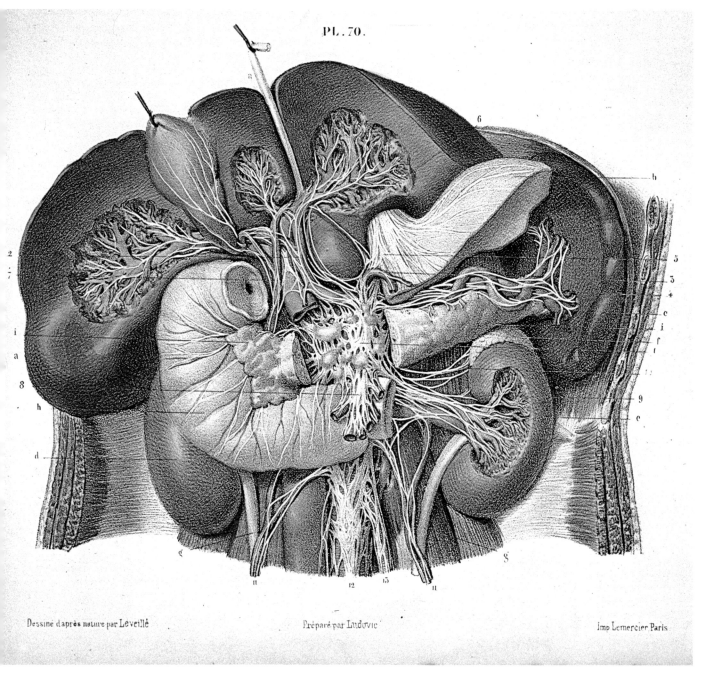

Dessiné d'après nature par Léveillé   Préparé par Ludovic   Imp Lemercier Paris

PLATE 118

German lithographic monographs: Tiedemann, Arnold, and Kilian

The early lithographic presses in Germany were put to various tasks, including the printing of music, topographical views, facsimiles (Dürer's drawings were often copied), and maps and plans. For the first years after its invention the technique was apparently not used to reproduce significant anatomical illustration. An early German example of such use was F. Tiedemann, *Tabulae arteriarum corporis humani ...*, Karlsruhe, Christian Friedrich Muller, 1822 (supplemental plates were issued in 1846). The printer was well established as a lithographer, and worked here directly under this anatomist's supervision.

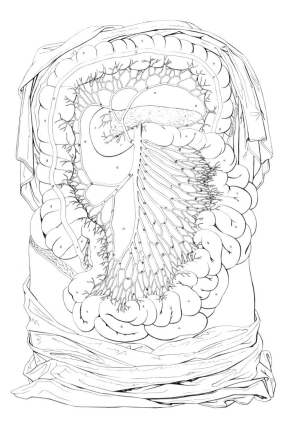

14.1 Outline diagram of distribution of the superior mesenteric artery from F. Tiedemann, *Tabulae arteriarum*, 1822.

Friedrich Tiedemann (1781–1861) a protégé of Soemmerring, taught at Heidelberg, and researched particularly in the physiology of digestion and in neuroanatomy, where he established the value of the embryological and comparative approach. His systematic atlas of the arteries was on a grand scale, the thirty-eight illustrations mostly life-sized, on pages approximately 73 × 53 cm. Each semi-naturalistic lithograph was accompanied by a corresponding outline plate. The artist was a fellow professor, Wilhelm Jacob Roux. Tiedemann in his preface states that only Haller, Camper, Scarpa, and Soemmerring have illustrated the arteries accurately, and he reminds us that Haller took his anatomy largely from children, Camper only showed the arteries of the arm and pelvis, Scarpa only those of the arm and leg, and Soemmerring only the arteries of the organs of sense. He thus justifies his work on this atlas.

Tiedemann's plates were widely copied; Robert Knox translated the text of the author's scholarly notes and reissued them along with the lithographic plates re-drawn to quarto size. This reproduction was published in Edinburgh in a number of editions in the 1830s. Other authors, including, as we shall see, Richard Quain, benefited greatly from Tiedemann's work. To reproduce one of these very large plates at the page-size of our book would not do them justice; so we have illustrated an outline plate, much reduced in size, as a text figure (*Fig. 14.1*). A pupil of Tiedemann's at Heidelberg was (*Philipp) Friedrich Arnold (1803–90)*. He held chairs successively at Zürich, Freiburg-im-Breisgau, and Tübingen. He then returned to Heidelberg for the remainder of his academic life, retiring at the age of seventy years. His fields of study included work on the brain and the special senses, particularly the ear. His dissertation on this latter subject, printed in 1826, apparently attracted little attention; but a subsequent publication, *Über den Ohrknoten*, 1828, with three plates, made his discoveries more widely known. A further work, published in 1832, was in the Soemmerring tradition, and was intended to establish a definitive anatomy of the ear. In 1834 his major atlas on neurology appeared: *Icones nervorum capitis* ..., Heidelberg, *sumptibus auctoris* [at the expense of the author], 1834. The large illustrations to this book were produced by lithography, and, as was common, the plates were in two states, one detailed and unlettered and the other lettered but in outline only. It is to be noted that the work is in Latin; at this late date most publications in anatomy were in the vernacular. Arnold obviously intended his work for an international audience; in 1834 the German language had not yet become a standard medium for the exchange of scientific ideas. Certainly by the time Arnold's students (for example Bischoff, von Kölliker, or Bilharz) came to publish their own seminal work, their writings would have been more easily understood internationally in the German than in the Latin tongue.

Arnold's *Icones* ... was dedicated to the memory of the Englishman Thomas Willis, the Frenchman Vicq d'Azyr, and the German J. C. Reil (1759–1813), this last a prominent neurologist, who in his last years had become an exponent of *Naturphilosophie*. The lithographic plates are signed by F. Wagner. In 1860 the atlas was reissued, again from Heidelberg, in an amended form with most of the plates re-drawn on the stone to a larger page-size; this time the artist was Max Wieser, who, in a smoother manner, attempted to emphasize a three-dimensional appearance.

Arnold's illustrations on neurology are incorporated into the first *fasciculus* of *Tabulae anatomicae* ..., published in Zürich and Stuttgart, 1838. The publishers indicated, in the preliminary material to this fascicle, that the book was to be completed in ten parts, and that subscribers paying for nine would receive the tenth free. Subscriptions could be placed at named booksellers in London, Paris, Petersburg, and Utrecht. Arnold's later publications included a handbook of human physiology (1836–42), written with his older brother, Wilhelm Arnold, and a text on human anatomy, 1845–51.

Hermann Friedrich Kilian (1800–1865). Contemporary with Arnold's *Icones* ... was an atlas devoted to obstetrics that included many anatomical illustrations: H. F. Kilian, *Geburtshulflicher Atlas* ..., Dusseldorf, Arnz [1835–8]. The 48 large plates were reproduced by lithography.

Kilian's education was nothing if not cosmopolitan. His schooling from the age of ten was in Petersburg, where his father was personal physician to the tsar, Alexander I. He studied medicine in Lithuania, at three German universities, and in London, Edinburgh, and Paris. He wrote a doctoral dissertation at Edinburgh on the origin of the glossopharyngeal nerve. He continued to wander from medical centre to medical centre—Strasburg, Munich, Vienna, and Budapest. He then held academic positions in the medical school in Petersburg. After a period in Paris and elsewhere he settled in Bonn, and specialized in obstetrics. His scientific work related to the fetal and new-born circulation, and his medical contributions were in the field of pelvic skeletal deformities.

In his lithographic atlas, Kilian takes and modifies illustrations from previous (engraved) plates, including some from the obstetrical atlas by Smellie. His own plates relate to the practice of obstetrics—detailing various forceps, or illustrating Caesarean section, or the manual removal of the placenta—but others deal, for instance, with the relevant anatomy of the uterus and adnexa and of the normal fetus in *utero*. Our plate (*Plate 120*) shows one of five figures that together comprise a two-page illustration portraying aspects of the fetal circulation. Accompanying our back view of a dissected fetus, there is a coloured outline (with a colour key), a front view, showing dissected blood-vessels, and two dissections of the fetal heart. These figures summarize Kilian's work on the fetal circulation.

The first figure in this book is made up of three plates; these are often to be found pasted on one page and folded into the large folio volume. When opened out they form one figure approximately 140 cm in height. This life-size figure pictures the same skeleton that had been prepared and illustrated by Soemmerring thirty-eight years previously (see *Plate 84*, p. 369). It will be remembered that this was made originally to show the ideal form of the female bones of a woman aged twenty years (see p. 366). Kilian added two other life-sized views of this skeleton to his atlas, showing it both from the side and from the back. Soemmerring had originally prepared his plate to complement Albinus' view of his so-carefully-prepared male skeleton. Both his predecessors' illustrations were trumped by Kilian's life-sized lithograph of the female skeleton!

119 Dissection of the cranial nerves. Tabula sexta from F. Arnold, *Icones nervorum capitis* ..., 1834. Lithograph (Wellcome Institute Library). Page size 41 × 27 cm.

This drawing is one of a series of dissections designed to show the origin and course of the cranial and cervical nerves. While this is a well-executed plate, it has to be admitted that the structures were more clearly defined in the later edition (1860).

A few criticisms may be made. The thalamus appears to be concave in its centre, and the termination of the optic tract, the lateral geniculate body, is not differentiated from the rest of the thalamus. One also notes that the medial surface of the cerebral hemisphere immediately anterior to the parieto-occipital sulcus is lacking a blood-supply. The trochlear nerve, winding round the brain stem, is too thick, and the cut mylohyoid muscle is *much* too thick. The origin of the hypoglossal nerve, from spread-out wispy rootlets, leaves something to be desired; in fact, the origin of this nerve is shown much better in a previous drawing, but is there not

TABULA SEXTA.

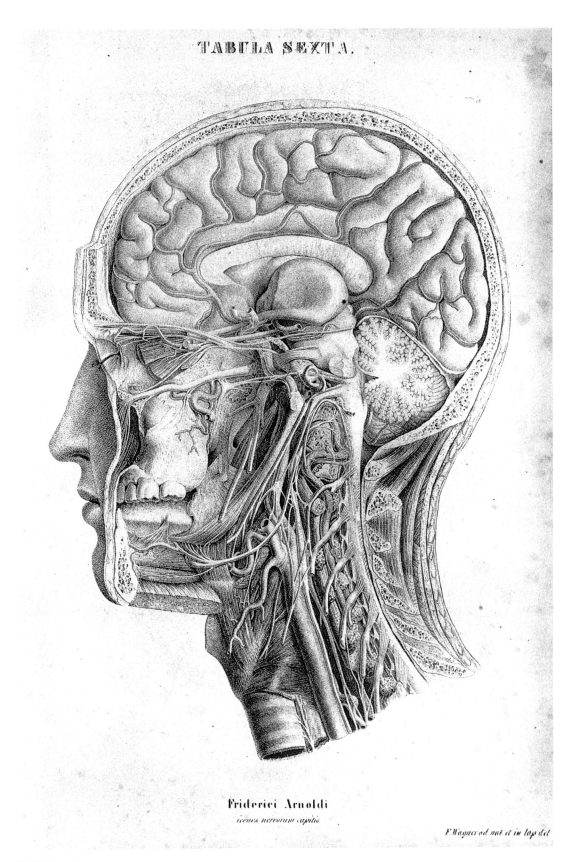

Friderici Arnoldi
icones nervorum capitis

F. Wagner ad nat. et in lap. del.

PLATE 119

identified. The superior thyroid artery is larger than is usual; the structure parallel to it inferiorly, which appears to be an artery arising either from the common carotid ('arteria carotis primitiva') or the origin of the external carotid, in fact is the external laryngeal nerve.

None the less, the plate as a whole amply repays close study. The portrayal of the facial nerve curving in its canal around the superior (anterior) semicircular canal; the distribution of the hypoglossal nerve; the origin of the greater (superficial) petrosal nerve, and the joining to it of the deep petrosal nerve from the sympathetic plexus on the internal carotid artery—all these are rarely so well depicted. Arnold is also credited with the discovery of the otic ganglion, but this is not shown here.

120 New-born baby with back cut away. Tab. XXIX, figure 2 from H. F. Kilian, *Geburtshulflicher Atlas* . . ., [1835–8]. Lithograph (Wellcome Institute Library). 34.0 × 20.2 cm.

This plate portrays a new-born baby dissected so as to illustrate essentially the fetal circulation from the posterior aspect—a most unusual presentation. As was common in those days, the baby possesses a lot of hair!

On the opposite page in the book there is a drawing of a dissection of the thorax and abdomen, this time viewed more conventionally from the front.

The plate is rather diagrammatic in presentation; the liver is swivelled anteriorly so as to show the umbilical vein (a), the ductus venosus (e), and the cut inferior vena cava (c). Superiorly the two not very accurate brachiocephalic veins (h) join to form the superior vena cava (i), which receives the stub of the azygos vein.

The left lung is collapsed; both it and the right drain into the left atrium (k) by pulmonary veins. Inferior to the atrium is seen the coronary sinus and the left ventricle, while superiorly are seen the bronchi, pulmonary arteries, and aorta. Because one rarely sees a dissection such as this it is difficult to be dogmatic; but perhaps the aorta should be higher than it is shown here.

There is no text in the book from which to check the labelling; in fact, this plate is but one of seven, out of a total of forty-four, which bear identifying letters. Presumably (e) is the caudate lobe of the liver; but, if so, it is difficult to understand why its texture is different from that of the rest of the liver.

This is a most interesting drawing, mainly because of the decision to show the anatomy from the back. Yet one wonders why, once embarked on such a course, the anatomy was not depicted exactly as it would appear in such a dissection—the portrayal of the liver and associated structures is confusing, not least the relation of the cut and tied portal vein (b) to the gall-

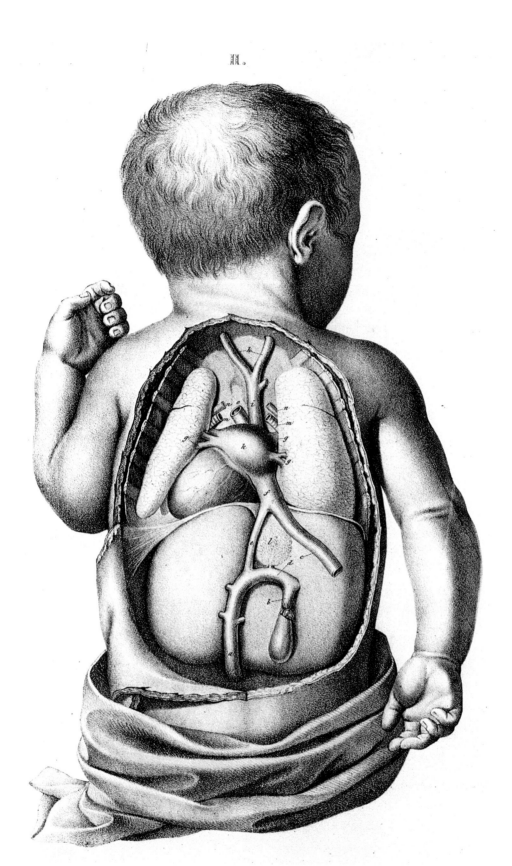

PLATE 120

bladder and the 'dangling' inferior vena cava. The whole gives the impression of being semi-diagrammatic rather than an anatomical presentation, so to speak, 'from the life'.

Early English lithography

We have seen that Senefelder, the inventor of lithography, set up in London a lithographic press in 1801, having obtained a patent for '... printing on paper, linen, cotton, woolen and other articles'. It was soon taken over by Philipp André. The intended commercial uses for printing fabrics proved unsuccessful at that time, but a publication of original artwork by Benjamin West, Fuseli, and others was issued in lithography in 1803: *Specimens of polyautography*. Neither this nor a similar publication in 1806–7 was a success. The press then passed to the Quartermaster-General's Office at the Horse Guards, which used it to print rapidly and accurately a vast number of maps, plans, circulars, and forms needed by the British Army. A sketch made in the field at Corunna, 1809, was printed ten days later.

In 1824 a London lithographic printer, C. Hullmandel, issued a technical manual: *The art of drawing on stone. ...* He also published maps, drawn by J. Wyld and others, and, as we shall see, he collaborated in the lithographic printing of anatomical atlases.

Lithographic atlases from University College, London

Before 1828 any man wishing to study medicine at a university and obtain a medical degree in England would have had to attend Oxford or Cambridge. But Jews, Roman Catholics, dissenters, or atheists would have had to assent to the doctrines of the Established Church to obtain admission. Such persons often went to the Scottish universities or to universities abroad, particularly to Leiden. This did not mean that London, by far the largest city in Britain, did not cater for medical students. There were private schools and, by 1800, formally constituted medical schools based at major voluntary hospitals: at The London Hospital in Whitechapel and St Bartholomew's Hospital in Smithfield, and at Guy's and St Thomas's Hospitals on the south bank in the Borough; others were added early in the century. Private schools included the Great Windmill Street School, founded in 1767 by William Hunter, which finally closed its doors in the 1830s. The study of anatomy, particularly after the passing of the 1832 Anatomy Act, formed a major part of medical students' studies at all these institutions; anatomy dissecting rooms and theatres were to be found in both private and public institutions. The career as a medical student of John Keats, poet, as outlined in his notebooks, in the early 1800s is typical of the training most men received in London.

A number of men who had studied at Edinburgh conceived and founded in the 1820s a University in London. Among these were Thomas Campbell the poet, Whig politician Henry Brougham (Lord Vaux), and William Birkbeck, MD, of the Glasgow and the London Mechanics'

Institutions. Another person deeply and effectively involved was Isaac Lyon Goldsmid, financier and reformer. From the first, medical and law schools were considered to be fundamental to the enterprise. Students were to be eligible for admission regardless of belief. Fees were to be low; no expensive residences were to be provided. Women, however, were not at first allowed to attend.

The inaugural lecture of the University of London was given in 1828 by the newly appointed Professor of Surgery, Charles Bell. He, it will be recalled, had left Edinburgh to establish himself in London as a surgeon, anatomist, physiologist, and illustrator. Another Edinburgh man was appointed as Professor of the Nature and Treatment of Disease, namely John Conolly. Later, in 1834, the rumbustious Robert Liston arrived from Edinburgh to become Professor of Surgery. Other charter professors came from overseas: John Meckel from Halle in Germany, and the Glasgow-trained G. S. Pattison from the United States. The naming of the professorships was, it appears to us now, a somewhat arbitrary affair, and indeed professors were at first left to arrange among themselves what subjects they actually taught. The first class of medical students lived through, and participated in, many contentions between the professors, and also between the teaching staff and the administration. Pattison, perhaps too devoted to fox-hunting, was an early casualty; he was dismissed and returned to the United States. J. Richard Bennett was appointed as Adjunct Professor of Anatomy, but died in 1831. Nevertheless, the Medical School at the University of London prospered, and by the 1834/5 session there were 390 students passing through the anatomy department. Students who qualified from this school entered practice with an exceptionally wide undergraduate experience in anatomy and surgery; internal medicine was in these early days less emphasized.

The University of London, founded on non-sectarian lines, provoked a Tory reaction, leading to the foundation in 1828, under Royal patronage, of a college adhering firmly to the established Anglican Church; King's College opened in 1831. The former University of London then became known as University College. Through various stages of association, the two colleges collaborated in examinations, at first very much at arm's length; other institutions later joined in this confederation, known collectively as the University of London. (We shall refer from this point on to the institution founded in Gower Street as University College, regardless of date.)

Jones Quain (1796–1865) became the professor responsible for anatomy at University College in 1831. He had been born in Cork, and attended the protestant Trinity College, Dublin, graduating in medicine in 1820. He studied for a long period in Paris, returning to London in 1825 to join one of the private medical schools, the Aldersgate School. P. M. Roget, doctor, lexicographer, and genius, was also a lecturer in the school. Three years later Quain published *Elements of descriptive and practical anatomy . . .*, London, 1828. This was extraordinarily popular, remaining in print, under various eminent editors, for nearly a century. The illustrations to this book were small wood-engravings, undistinguished and few in number. Jones Quain resigned after only a few years in the anatomy chair, and from 1836 lived in London and Paris until his death in 1865. He began a major project before his resignation: the production of a folio anatomical atlas of lithographic plates to compete with those of Mascagni, Cloquet, and others. The first volume was on the musculature; it was published in 1836: *The muscles of the human body; in a series of plates with references and physiological comments*, London, Taylor and Walton. The rest of the body was dealt with in separate publications—vessels 1837, nerves 1839, viscera 1840, and bones and ligaments 1842. These four later volumes were co-authored by Jones Quain and Erasmus Wilson.

William James Erasmus Wilson (1809–84) acquired his medical training through apprenticeship and by attending the private Cripplegate and Aldersgate schools. At the latter place he came under the notice of Jones Quain. In 1830 he passed the licenciate examinations of the Society of Apothecaries, and in 1831 became a member of the Royal College of Surgeons. He then joined the anatomy department at University College, working under Jones Quain and assisting him in the mammoth task of completing the lithographic atlas. Wilson's name may be seen on a number of the plates as *W. J. E. Wilson invt.*, the plates were designed by him, although actually drawn by another. The artists employed were principally J. Walsh and W. Bagg. In the 1837 volume Wilson is named as William J. E. Wilson, but in the 1842 volume he is designated Erasmus Wilson, a name he later used consistently. On the title-pages, he is stated to be Consulting Surgeon to the St Pancras Infirmary, and Lecturer on anatomy and physiology in the Middlesex Hospital Medical School. Before joining the Middlesex he had tried to establish, without much success, a private school, Sydenham College, in the Bedford Square area. In later years Wilson became a prominent citizen: dermatologist, President of the Royal College of Surgeons, Knight, and public benefactor. In this last role he was the principal financial mover in bringing the obelisk, called popularly *Cleopatra's needle*, to London, where it still stands on the Embankment. His fortune, made one assumes as a dermatologist and not as the co-author of an anatomical plate-book, amounted to more than £200 000. Wilson's other illustrated work was a magnificent atlas of dermatology, *Portraits of diseases of the skin*, London, 1855, in which he again employed W. Bagg to put into final form the drawings he himself had made as the cases presented themselves.

The faculty at the medical school of University College included other men who were both capable doctor-scientists and capable artists. The most distinguished of these were Charles Bell, already noted, and Robert Carswell. Carswell had stayed for a number of years in Paris, studying morbid anatomy under P. C. A. Louis and others, and making drawings illustrating diseased structures. In 1828 he was appointed as Professor of Morbid Anatomy at University College, but was allowed to remain in Paris to complete this work. Eventually two thousand drawings were produced, a selection of which formed his *Pathological anatomy: Illustrations of the elementary forms of disease*, 1835–1838, the lithographs being made by Carswell himself. Another artistically-minded professor was John Marshall, trained at University College, and Professor of Surgery there from 1866. He was lecturer in artistic anatomy at the South Kensington School of Art,

Professor of Anatomy at the Royal Academy (a successor to William Hunter), and author of a popular *Anatomy for Artists*, 1878.

Jones Quain had obtained his medical qualification from Trinity College, Dublin. His younger brother, *Richard Quain* (1800–87) took a different route into medicine, being apprenticed to a surgeon in Cork, and then finishing his studies in London under his brother at the Aldersgate School and in Paris under the British private lecturer in anatomy, Richard Bennett, to whom he became an assistant. When Bennett was appointed to University College, Richard Quain moved there with him. Bennett died shortly after, and Quain was eventually appointed, in 1832 as Professor of Descriptive Anatomy, a position he held until 1850.

His brother Jones Quain was Professor of General Anatomy from 1831 to 1836. Richard Quain had a stormy career as a surgeon at University College Hospital, but advanced to become Professor of Clinical Surgery in 1848.

THE

ANATOMY OF THE ARTERIES

OF THE HUMAN BODY

WITH ITS APPLICATIONS TO PATHOLOGY AND OPERATIVE SURGERY

IN

LITHOGRAPHIC DRAWINGS

WITH

PRACTICAL COMMENTARIES

BY RICHARD QUAIN F.R.S.

PROFESSOR OF ANATOMY IN UNIVERSITY COLLEGE LONDON AND SURGEON TO UNIVERSITY COLLEGE HOSPITAL

THE DRAWINGS FROM NATURE AND ON STONE BY JOSEPH MACLISE ESQ. SURGEON

WITH AN OCTAVO VOLUME OF LETTER-PRESS

LONDON
PRINTED FOR TAYLOR AND WALTON
BOOKSELLERS AND PUBLISHERS TO UNIVERSITY COLLEGE
UPPER GOWER STREET
MDCCCXLIV

14.2 Title-page of Richard Quain's *The anatomy of the arteries*, 1844.

He married a widow, a viscountess, became surgeon to Queen Victoria, and died a wealthy man, leaving most of his money to University College for studies in English and the natural sciences.

In 1848, Richard Quain edited, with William Sharpey, Professor of Physiology, the fifth edition of his brother's *Elements of anatomy*. His major contribution to anatomy, however, was a very large lithographic atlas, *The anatomy of the arteries of the human body with its applications to pathology and operative surgery in lithographic drawings with practical commentaries*, London, Taylor and Walton, 1844 (*Fig. 14.2*). The work was based on the findings of the dissection of nearly a thousand subjects. The artist for these 87 drawings, imperial folio, 'the figures the size of life', is acknowledged on the two title-pages—'drawn from nature, and on stone, by Joseph Maclise, M.R.C.S.'. In the text, Maclise was referred to as a friend and former pupil. It was a great advantage, Quain stated in thanking him profusely, to have the assistance of an anatomist and surgeon able to draw with spirit and effect.

Like Tiedemann before him, Quain pointed out the excellencies and disadvantages of previous atlases of the arteries by Haller and Scarpa. He praised Tiedemann for his very valuable systematic and clear delineations, but pointed out that they did not show the veins and nerves in connection with the arteries. Moreover they gave less emphasis than they should have done to variations and anomalies. Quain stated:

… difficulties which have often occurred in the performance of those surgical operations where the larger arteries are concerned have arisen, in great part, from want of a significant acquaintance with the differences in anatomical disposition to which these vessels are subject …

Two years after the publication of Richard Quain's *Anatomy of the arteries …*, 1844, surgeons were able to extend their repertoire to ligating arterial aneurisms, as anaesthesia had made possible more prolonged delicate operations. During the second half of the nineteenth century, formerly inaccessible parts of the body came under the surgeon's knife. The first surgical operations under anaesthesia in England were undertaken in 1846. That year an amputation was performed at University College Hospital by the surgeon Robert Liston, who, some reports say, remarked after the operation 'This Yankee dodge, Gentlemen, beats mesmerism hollow.' It may now in retrospect be seen to have been appropriate that Joseph Lister was present as a medical student at this operation, for with later developments in anaesthesia and antisepsis and asepsis every part of the human body became accessible to the surgeon.

Richard Quain and Joseph Maclise's very large hand-coloured lithographs were to be obtained also unbound and loose in a portfolio for £12. 10s. Experience has shown us that this format is a much more satisfactory form for ready consultation. A volume of this size is almost impossible to bind or to manage. The lithographic impressions were taken on to thin paper, which was then mounted on one of a heavier weight. An accompanying explanation of the plates was issued as an octavo volume, the text of which was written with the assistance of Richard Quain, M.B., a cousin of Jones and Richard Quain. This cousin later became a highly successful physician and a baronet.

We turn now to *Joseph Maclise* (c.1815–c.1880), anatomist and surgeon, and general practitioner in the Bloomsbury area. No doubt encouraged by the success of his contributions to Richard Quain's *The anatomy of the arteries*, Maclise published a volume of thirty-five lithographic anatomical plates, many hand-coloured: *Surgical anatomy*, London, John Churchill, 1851. For a second edition, 1856, some plates were re-drawn and others added. There were also editions published in the United States. The preface stated that the object of the work was 'to present to the student of medicine and to the practitioner removed from the schools, a series of dissections demonstrating the relative anatomy of the principal regions of the body'. Maclise's personality showed through in other remarks, the definitive voice of a scientific surgeon: the nomenclature of descriptive anatomy remained 'a barbarous jargon, barren of all truthful signification, inconstant with nature, and blindly irrespective of the *cognitio certa ex principiis certis exorta* [certain knowledge arising from definite and determined principles]'. Everything done in anatomy must be re-examined:

It must be now by the broad clarion sounds of laws and systems, not by the narrow piping notes of isolated particulars and dislocated phenomena, that we can ever hope to wake to attention again her [Science's] slumbering ear ... Dissection has done its work. The iron scalpel has already made acquaintance with not only the greater parts, but even with the infinitesimals of the human body ...

He considered microscopy to have merely 'drawn forth demonstrations of objects as little in respect to practical importance as they are in regard to physical dimensions'. And then he had a go at physiology. William Sharpey, physiologist and histologist, was probably in Maclise's mind when he was making these criticisms. Sharpey had succeeded to Jones Quain's chair at University College, and Maclise had possibly resented the change in direction in the anatomy department.

Maclise presented a finely written justification for anatomical illustration, which, since it is central to the subject of our book, we wish to quote in full:

The forms, especially of organic bodies, cannot be described without the aid of figures. Even the mathematical strength of Euclid would avail nothing if shorn of his diagrams ...

An anatomical illustration enters the understanding at once in a direct passage, and is almost independent of the aid of written language. A picture of form is a proposition which solves itself. It is as an axiom encompassed in a frame-work of self-evident truth. The best substitute for Nature herself, by which we may teach the knowledge of her, is an exact representation of her form.

Mr. Liston could draw the same anatomical picture mentally which Sir Charles Bell's handicraft could draw in presential reality of form. Camper and Scarpa were their own draughtsmen.

He continued:

If there may be any novelty now-a-days possible to be recognised upon the out-trodden tract of human relative anatomy, it can only be truthful demonstrations well planned in aid of practice. Under this view alone may the anatomist hope to add anything new to the beautiful works of Cowper, Haller, Hunter, Scarpa, Soemmering and others.

Of the illustrations of this work I may state, in guarantee of their anatomical accuracy, that they have been made by myself from my own dissections, first planned at the London University College, and afterwards realized at the École Pratique, and School of Anatomy, adjoining the Hospital La Pitié, Paris, a few years since. As far as the subject of relative anatomy could admit of novel treatment, rightly confined to facts unalterable, I have endeavoured to give it.

Finally Maclise summarized the importance of thinking in anatomical terms when a surgeon examines a patient:

The surface of the living body is perused by the surgeon as a map explanatory of the relative position of the organs beneath; and to aid him in this respect the present dissections have been made. We dissect the dead body in order to furnish the memory with as clear an account of the structures of its living representative as if this latter, which we are not allowed to analyse, were perfectly translucent, and directly demonstrative of its component parts.

The drawings of Maclise for Quain's *Anatomy of the arteries* and for his own *Surgical anatomy* are indeed done, as Quain wrote, with spirit and effect. These figures of anatomical dissection seem lifelike; in many plates the figure is shown as a torso, or a bust, or as a full- or half-length figure. The faces seem to be a gallery of portraits, perhaps of visitors to the 1851 Great Exhibition. They are mostly young men with fine hair—bearded, clean-shaven, or moustachioed, with or without sideburns; occasionally there are remarkably handsome black men. Many appear god-like. This is indeed 'high' art, only incidentally of an anatomical subject (*Fig. 14.3a and b*). If the analogy is not too far-fetched, Maclise's drawing may be compared with the work in different media of the English Romantic poets or of the composer Berlioz. The same comparisons have been made in relation to the work of the Victorian artist Daniel Maclise (1806–70), Joseph Maclise's older brother. They remained close, travelling in Italy together, and sharing houses in Bloomsbury and Chelsea.

The brothers were born in Cork, the sons of a Presbyterian Cork woman and a Scotsman, Alexander MacLeish or Maclise—other spellings were used. Alexander was a soldier and an artisan. Daniel's drawing ability was recognized as a young man. He attended art school in Cork, and came to wider notice in that city when he sketched Walter Scott from life. Lithographed, the work circulated widely. Daniel Maclise ventured to London in 1827, and attended the Royal Academy school. Commissions for the new Houses of Parliament took him years to execute. His portraits included one of Dr Quain, presumably Jones Quain. Daniel's work was intensely serious. It was art on a lofty, often historical, theme, unsullied by vulgar incidents—the 'Meeting of Wellington and Blücher', the 'Death of Nelson', and so on—although there is a strange 'fairy' painting, 'Undine'. Daniel Maclise, realist and romantic, friend

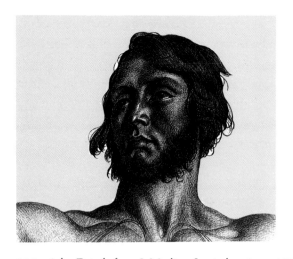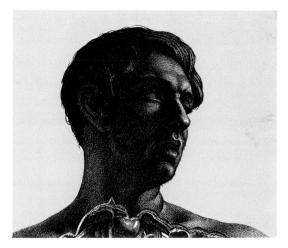

14.3 a & b   Details from J. Maclise, *Surgical anatomy*, 1851.

of Dickens and Thackeray, anticipated to a degree the English Pre-Raphaelites. Joseph Maclise, realist, as any anatomical illustrator must be, nevertheless draws perhaps the most romantically noble dissected figures that have been produced. Their faces and their bodies, even when laid open, have the dignity of Daniel's figures. They are even more handsome and noble than the labourers in Ford Maddox Brown's painting entitled 'Work' (1852–65). Yet the subjects of these dissection pictures were almost certainly acquired from hospitals or workhouses; they were the bodies, unclaimed by relatives or friends, of persons who had died young and destitute.

G. *Viner Ellis* is the last of the University College anatomists of whom he shall take note. In 1867, his *Illustrations of dissections of the human body*, London, James Walton, was published. The title page of the octavo text volume describes Ellis as Professor of Anatomy, and continues: 'The drawings are from nature and on stone by Mr. [G. H.] Ford, from dissections by Professor Ellis, and form a separate volume in imperial folio'. The method of reproducing the illustrations was colour-printed lithography; Bonamy and Beau's and Hirschfeld's near-contemporrary atlases were printed in a similar manner. The printer, known also for artistic, non-technical chromo-lithography was W. West. Ellis acknowledged 'the difficulties attendant on the printing in colours of such complicated figures, and ... the successful way in which they have been overcome by Mr. West'. The dates printed under some of the plates indicate the great labour involved. The first mentioned is 1 March, 1863; the work continued through to 6 September 1867, with from four to seven being done each year. Help in the preparation of the specimens from students and demonstrators was acknowledged. Some figures closely resemble the plates drawn by Maclise for Richard Quain's book on the arteries, 1844. Was this due to the use of the same preserved specimens, or were Ellis and Ford making use of the earlier illustrations? Ford's style of illustration was influenced by Maclise, just as that anatomist had been influenced by Jones Quain's artists, W. Bagg and Fairland. Ellis had been trained at University College, and was, like Wilson, demonstrator to Richard Quain.

The school of anatomy at University College, London, in the first thirty-five years of its existence, produced a remarkable series of illustrated anatomical lithographic plates, useful alike to students, as in J. Quain's *Elements of anatomy*, and to practising surgeons, as in R. Quain's *Arteries*, J. Quain's and Wilson's *Anatomical Plates*, Maclise's *Surgical anatomy*, and Ellis's *Dissections*. Early in the same period Charles Bell, who remained only a short time at University College, produced work on the hand and on expression. During this period also Carswell and Marshall were productive in the fields of morbid anatomy and in art anatomy respectively.

Physiology, embryology, and histology advanced particularly through the influence of William Sharpey and the school he founded. (The admiration of the physiological histologist Edward Schafer for his teacher was so great that he adopted his name, and became Sharpey Schafer.) This aspect of University College may be noted, but cannot be considered here, nor can the clinical work in the Dispensary attached to the College or of University College Hospital, which, in 1834, opened its doors across the street as the North London Hospital.

121 The male urethra. Plate 26 from J. Quain, *The viscera of the human body ...*, 1840. Lithograph (private collection). Page size 46.2 × 30.6 cm.

Apart from the drawing by Leonardo, this is one of very few illustrations appearing in an anatomical textbook (or notebook) featuring a penis in the erect position. It seems not unlikely that here it was drawn thus so as to conform to available page-space.

The two larger figures portray the bladder, prostate, and penis laid open to show the course and certain salient features of the urethra. These include the *veru montanum* (Fig. 1.10), with the openings of the ejaculatory ducts alongside; the navicular fossa (Fig. 1.21); Cowper's gland and duct (Fig. 1.14 and Fig. 2.17); and the narrow external urethral meatus (Fig. 2.25). One may consider that it would have been better to have kept the identifying numbers the same in all the drawings.

The text makes it clear that the prostatic portion is the widest part of the urethra, but this is far from being shown as the case in Figure 1. The interrelationship of the vasa deferentia (Figs 3.2 and 4.5), the seminal vesicles (Figs 3.3, 4.4, and 2.12) and the ejaculatory ducts (Figs 2.13 and 4.6) do not suggest that in fact the (coiled) duct of the seminal vesicle joins the vas deferens to become the ejaculatory duct. Indeed one could be excused for thinking that, as portrayed in Figure 3, the two vasa join together.

In Figure 2 it appears as though the penile urethra lies between the erectile tissue of the corpus spongiosum and the thick fibrous envelope of the corpus cavernosum, instead of being wholly surrounded by the former.

Apart from the above minor criticisms, this plate is a straightforward and informative one, particularly when it is studied in conjunction with the excellent accompanying text.

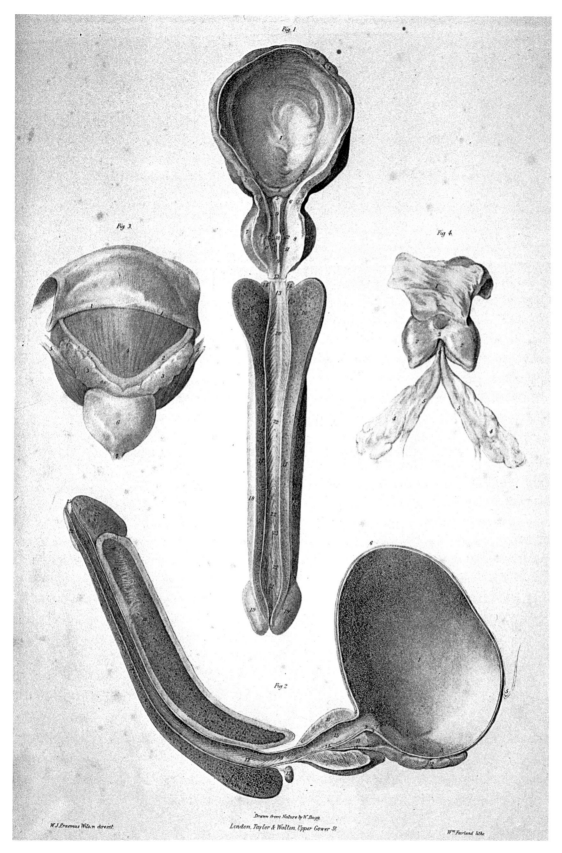

Fig. 1

Fig. 3

Fig. 4

Fig. 2

Drawn from Nature by W. Bagg.

W. J. Erasmus Wilson direxit.

London, Taylor & Walton, Upper Gower St.

W.ᵐ Farland litho.

PLATE 121

122 Distribution of the left internal iliac artery. Pl. 59 from R. Quain, *The anatomy of the arteries of the human body ...*, 1844. Lithograph (private collection). 48.9 × 64.4 cm.

This is an unusual dissection, where the left leg and buttock have been removed by cutting through the superior pubic ramus, somewhat to the left of the midline, and disarticulating the left sacroiliac joint—a modified hindquarter amputation.

Small letters and numbers are placed on various structures for identification purposes, but photographic reduction renders the majority of these almost invisible.

It is a masterful and arresting drawing, with the inclusion and positioning of the hand supplying essential balance to the pose: this is brought out if the hand is covered up. The stark reality of the anatomical dissection is softened by the inclusion of drapes—that over the leg, with its stitched border, is more realistic than that covering the abdomen.

The viscera displayed include the globular bladder, behind which are seen the fundus of the uterus, the Fallopian tube and fimbria (drawn forwards), the round ligament of the uterus, and the ovary (lifted up by a hook). The ureter, after passing deep to the sigmoid mesocolon and over the (cut) external iliac artery, can be seen entering the bladder after being 'encircled' by the uterine artery. Behind the bladder are the vagina and rectum, while antero-inferior to the cut pubic bone is the left crus of the clitoris.

The mode of origin of the branches of the internal iliac artery is subject to much variability; the pattern shown here is a common one, and need not be commented on as such.

One may note the umbilical artery becoming obliterated after giving off a small superior vesical branch; the very tortuous uterine artery, shown giving branches which anastomose with the ovarian artery, seen wriggling downwards over the internal iliac artery; the cut internal pudendal artery, dividing into posterior labial and deep and dorsal arteries of the clitoris (though its inferior rectal branch is not featured); the various branches to the ureter; and the vaginal artery supplying also the bladder neck.

All of these, and many others, are excellently portrayed in this visually most attractive plate.

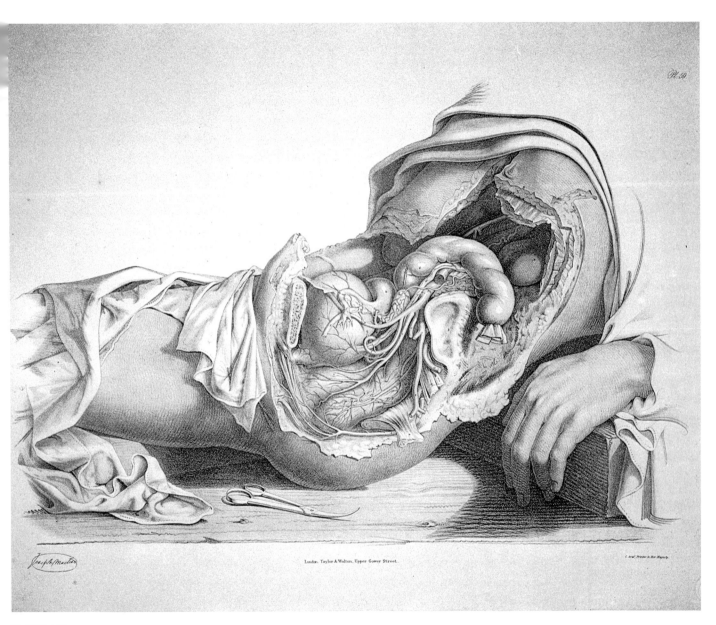

Pl. 59

Joseph Maclise

London. Taylor & Walton, Upper Gower Street.

C. Graf, Printer to Her Majesty.

PLATE 122

123 Contents of the axilla in the male and female. Plate X from J. Maclise, *Surgical anatomy*, 1856. Lithograph (private collection). 44.5 × 32.5 cm.

In the 1851 edition the forerunner of this plate featured the male and female figures without any overlapping, the former to the left of the latter, and much more of their bodies was shown; that plate as a whole was somewhat reminiscent of Estienne, in that there was a great deal of drawing but little anatomy. The identification lettering was very faint, and one's conviction that a more close-up view would better achieve the author's intent was strong.

For the second edition, 1856, all the plates were redrawn, and it is from this edition that our *Plate 123* has been taken; this is indeed a close-up compared to the earlier plate.

Apart from the axillary tail of the mammary gland (not shown) the contents of the male and female axilla differ very little. This is borne out in this illustration, although the female is portrayed as possessing many more lymph nodes—a dubious distinction, in fact.

In his commentary Maclise termed the female mammary gland 'a plus-fully developed organ'. He also discussed operations on the axilla for 'morbid growths' or abscesses, and in doing so pointed out that 'as the coracoid process points to the situation of the [axillary] artery in the axilla, so the coraco-brachialis muscle, C, marks the exact locality of the vessel as it emerges from the region; the artery ranges along the inner margin of both the process and the muscle, which latter, in fleshy bodies, sometimes overhangs and conceals it'.

The anatomy that is presented in the plate is realistic, though it is difficult to understand why (L), the median nerve (in the male drawing) is so differently portrayed in the female drawing.

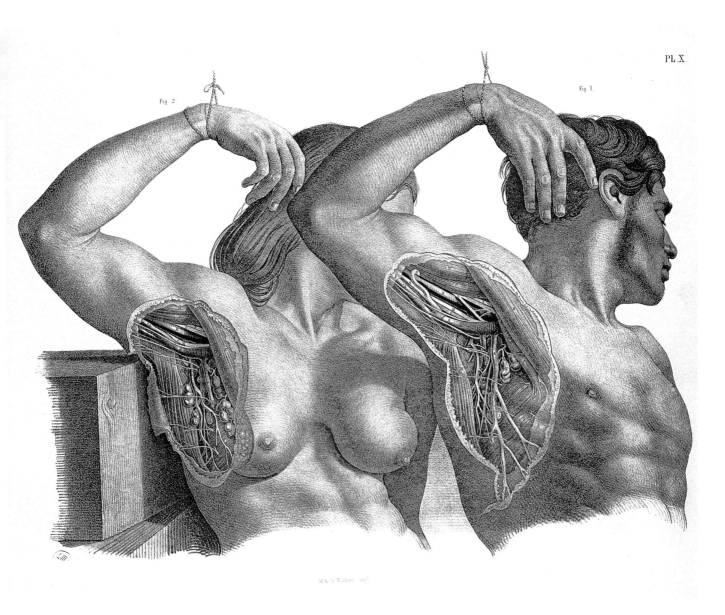

Fig 2.

Fig 1.

PLATE 123

124 Arterial system in the thorax and abdomen. Plate XXIV from J. Maclise, *Surgical anatomy*, 1856. Lithograph (private collection). 45.2 × 27.1 cm.

This plate is taken from the 1856 edition. Although the hand-coloured plate in the edition of 1851 presents better definition of the structures to the naked eye, it nevertheless photographed much less well in black and white than that in the later edition.

Much interest lies in the commentary that accompanies the plate. This is based on the premise that the arterial system 'assumes, in all cases, somewhat of the character of the forms upon which they are distributed, or of the organs which they supply'. In this sense Maclise equates the aorta with the central vertebral column; the coronary arteries with the left and right sides of the heart; the intercostal arteries with the ribs; the inferior phrenic arteries with the two sides of the diaphragm; the hepatic and splenic arteries with right and left viscera (ditto the renal and gonadal arteries); the superior mesenteric artery with the mid-gut and part of the hindgut; the leftward inclined inferior mesenteric with the rest of the hindgut; and the external iliac arteries with the lower extremities.

However, in this respect the commonest form of the origin of the three branches of the aortic arch presented Maclise with some difficulty. He met this by pointing out that often the right subclavian and right common carotid arteries arise separately, or, alternatively, that the left subclavian and left common carotid may sometimes arise from a common truck. One gets the impression that Maclise would have preferred the latter to be the commonest pattern, so that he could then correlate it with the branches of the terminal part of the aorta, namely the two common iliac arteries which divide into internal and external iliacs. He also pointed out the correspondence beween the two brachiocephalic veins being formed by the junction of the internal jugular and subclavian veins with the formation of the common iliac veins by the junction of the external and internal iliac veins. In both cases the largest veins then join again, one forming the inferior, the other the superior, vena cava.

In the plate the origins of the coronary arteries are correctly situated, but the 'sprouting' of the bronchial arteries from the aorta is very awkward. The inferior phrenic arteries more often arise directly from the aorta than from the coeliac trunk, though the latter is not uncommon, and is depicted here.

The right ureter (V) is far too sinuous, and both it and the left one appear rather dilated.

Overall this illustration, if a trifle stylized, portrays the anatomy extremely clearly. It is interesting to compare the pelvic distribution of the internal iliac artery, here in the male, with that of the female pictured in our *Plate 122*: both, of course, were drawn by Joseph Maclise.

PL. XXIV.

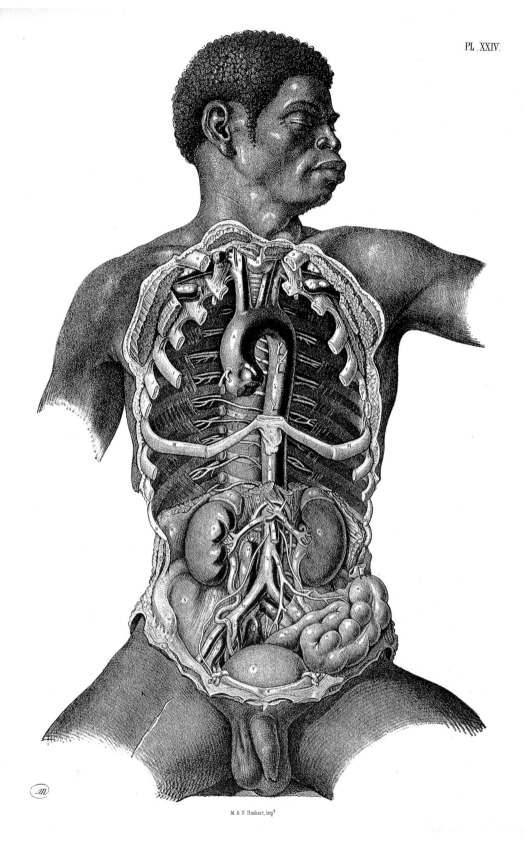

M & N Hanhart, Imp.t

PLATE 124

125 Dissection of the side of the head. Plate XXIII from G. V. Ellis, *Illustrations of dissection of the human body*, 1867. Lithograph (Wellcome Institute Library). 43.1 × 30.3 cm.

In this illustration the right orbit has been widely opened from above and laterally, and the zygomatic arch cut and turned down, together with the masseter muscle. The dissection shows the Gasserian ganglion, the proximal portions of the ophthalmic, mandibular, and maxillary divisions of the trigeminal nerve, and the distribution of the latter to the face.

It is an unusual presentation, that is accurate and of exceptional clarity; and the undissected parts are more pleasantly presented than is usual.

One might have expected the nerve to the masseter to be featured; but there is no sign of this, unless the small twig seemingly arising from the buccal branch of the mandibular nerve is, inaccurately, supposed to represent it. But the quality of the dissection surely invalidates any supposition of such an error.

Those muscles of facial expression that are shown, and the branches of the facial nerve to them, are pleasingly drawn; and indeed, if, as stated in the preface, Ellis's plates are illustrative of the method of dissection that was practised by University College medical students of that time, one can only believe that they profited greatly from them. This particular plate is dated November 1864; but the book was not published until 1867, some nine years after Gray's anatomy was first issued.

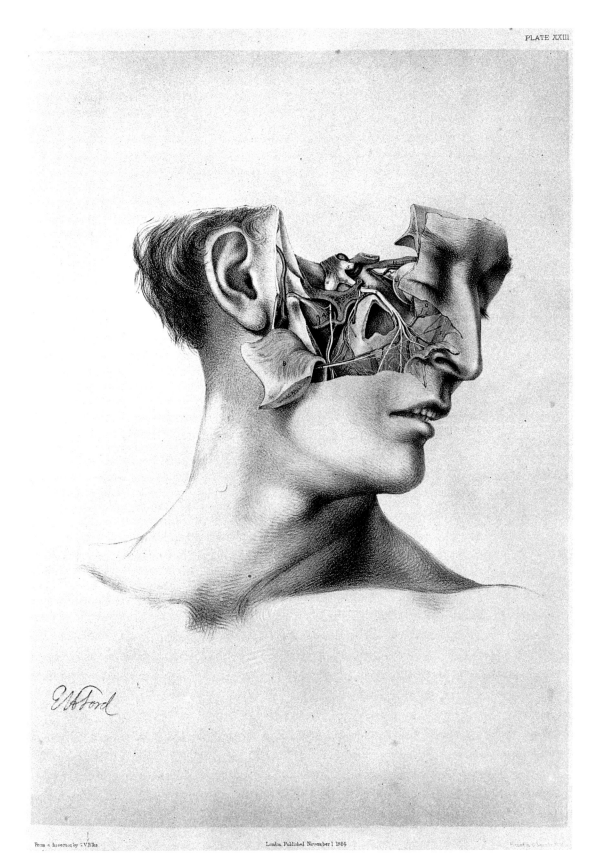

PLATE XXIII

From a dissection by G.V.Ellis   London, Published November 1 1864

PLATE 125

A Russian lithographic atlas

Nikolay Ivanovich Pirogov (or *Pirogoff*), 1810–81, was educated at Moscow's medical school, graduating before he was nineteen. His doctorate was obtained in 1832, by which time he was working at the University in the city of Tartu in Estonia. (This city was called at that time Dorpat, since when it has been named Yuriev (until 1918), and, more recently, Tartu.) The university, originally founded in the seventeenth century by the Swedish King Gustavus Adolphus, was remarkable for its observatory, its botanical garden, and, after 1836, not least for the work done there by Pirogov. That year he was appointed Professor of Surgery, and was assiduous in the pursuit of surgical anatomy, both normal and pathological. Our *Plate 126* is taken from the German reprint, *Chirurgische Anatomie der Arterienstämme und Fascien*, 1860, of an atlas published by Pirogov 1837–40. A proficient linguist, Pirogov had studied surgery in Germany, at Berlin and Göttingen, before taking up his appointment in Tartu. A number of his books were published first in the German language. The artist for this lithographic plate was F. Schlater, and the lithographer C. Schmiedel. The revised 1860 edition, prepared by Julius Szymanowski, was published from Leipzig and Heidelberg.

The virtue of Pirogov's atlas lies in its dedication to surgically useful anatomy, which our *Plate 126* exemplifies, and in the unusual dissections pictured. One of these shows the stump of the neck looked at from above. Pirogov's further unusual and independent studies in anatomy, carried out at Tartu from 1835 to 1840, and in Petersburg from 1841 to 1856, were published in Latin in eight parts: *Anatome topographica sectionibus ...*, Petersburg, J. Trey; 1852–9. This atlas contained a text based on cross-sections of frozen corpses, a technique apparently invented by P. de Riemer in the Netherlands in 1818, and also, independently, by Pirogov, and published by him in this atlas. The technique enabled him to investigate the relationship of structures as they actually exist in a body undisturbed by dissection. Pirogov's dedication to his work has been widely noted: it has been said that he made 12000 autopsies while Professor at the Medical-Surgical Academy in Petersburg.

The son of an army officer, Pirogov served also in the field of military surgery. His most influential period was perhaps during the Russo-Turkish War, the Crimean War. He was present at the siege of Sevastopol, 1854–5. Pirogov was employing ether under war conditions as early as 1847, and during the siege of Sevastopol anaesthetics were given under his direction at the front. He was responsible for establishing women's corps of nurses in the Russian army; later he became a great supporter of women's education. He introduced new methods of haemostasis, employed antiseptics, and introduced plaster casts into surgery. He recommended small pavilions, rather than large hospitals, to control the spread of wound and surgical infections—as Florence Nightingale and James Simpson were also advocating.

Pirogov summarized his experiences of field surgery in a book published in German in 1864, *Grundzüge der allgemeinen Kriegschirurgie*, Leipzig. A rewritten Russian edition was issued from Dresden in two volumes in 1865–6.

Pirogov's designation of war as a traumatic epidemic reflects both medical and psychological realities. We believe that Florence Nightingale, who was helping to organize nursing services for the other side in the Crimean War, would have concurred with this remark. His originality, perseverance, practicality, and scientific inquisitiveness were coupled with immense surgical experience in peace and war.

After returning from the Crimea, Pirogov resigned his professorship at Petersburg and spent periods as an educational administrator, working from time to time in war surgery: he was consulted when Garibaldi was wounded; he visited the front for the Red Cross during the Franco-Prussian War, 1870; and participated in the second Russo-Turkish War, 1877.

Ambrose Paré, John Hunter, and Nikolay Pirogov—surgeons all—were men of similar great accomplishments.

126 Dorsum and sole of foot. Taf. 50, figures 1 and 2. From N. I. Pirogoff, *Chirurgische Anatomie der Arterienstämme und Fascien*, 1860. Lithograph (Wellcome Institute Library). 20.6 × 22.9 cm.

The first figure shows the fascia of the dorsum of the foot, with a rather stylized origin of the long saphenous vein, and also the terminal branches of the superficial peroneal nerve. The fascia of the lower leg has been incised so as to display the tendons of tibialis anterior (D), extensor hallucis longus (B), and extensor digitorum longus (C), together with the deep peroneal nerve alongside the anterior tibial artery. The rather large malleolar branch of the peroneal artery is seen laterally. Further portions of the continuation of the anterior tibial artery as the dorsalis pedis artery are seen through further incisions in the fascia; but it is not so much an anatomical display of the artery and its branches and termination, as an indicator of its position and course.

The second figure features the three portions of the plantar aponeurosis, split in places so as to reveal the abductor muscle of the big toe in one case and the cut portion of the flexor digitorum brevis together with the medial plantar artery and its venae commitantes in the other. The artery is termed simply 'arteria plantaris'—there is no depiction of the tibial artery dividing into medial and lateral plantar arteries.

Both these figures are short on topographical anatomy, but they were primarily designed for surgeons, to convey information as to where the superficial arteries—and nerves—could be found in operations on the foot, and in this context would have proved valuable.

Fig.1.

Fig.2.

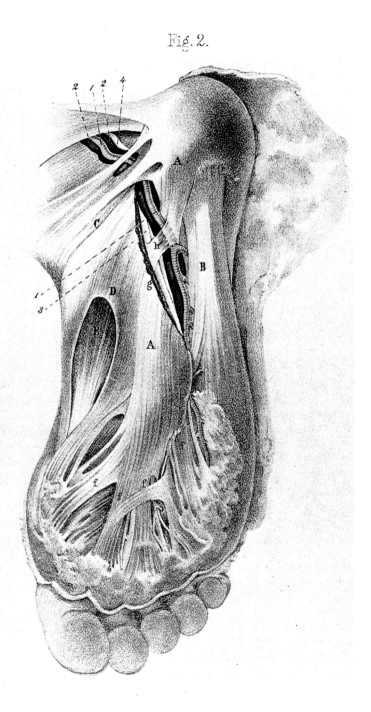

PLATE 126

Chapter 14: Selected reading

The Gautier D'Agoty family

[Franklin, C.] (1977). *A catalogue of early colour printing.* . . . Colin and Charlotte Franklin, Culham, Oxford.

Lilien O. M. (1985). *Jacob Christoph LeBlon 1667–1741: Inventor of three-and four-colour printing.* Hiersemann, Stuttgart .

Prevost, M., *et al.* (ed.) (1981). *Jacques Gautier d'Agoty. Dict. biog. française,* **15,** 847.

Vicq d'Azyr

Bayle, A. L. T. and Thillaye, A. J. (1855). *Vicq. d'Azyr* Biog. méd. **2,** 718–20.

Coury, C. (1970). *The teaching of medicine in France.* . . . In *The history of medical education,* (ed. C. D. O'Malley) University of California Press, Berkeley.

Huard, P. and Imbault-Huart, M J. (1976). Felix Vicq d'Azyr. *Dict. sci. Biog.,* **14,** 14–17.

Meyer, A. (1971). *Historical aspects of cerebral anatomy.* Oxford University Press, London.

Schiller, F. (1965). The rise of the 'enteroid processes' in the 19th century. . . . *Bull. Hist. Med.,* **39,** 326–38.

The origins of lithography

Godfrey, R. T. (1978). *Printmaking in Britain.* . . . Phaidon, Oxford.

Griffiths, A. (1980). *Prints and printmaking.* British Museum, London.

Johnson, W. McA. (1977). *French lithography.* . . . Agnes Etherington Art Centre, Kingston, Ontario.

Man, F. H. (1971). *Homage to Senefelder.* . . . Victoria and Albert Museum, London.

Twyman, M. (1970). *Lithography 1800–1850.* Oxford University Press, London.

French lithographic atlases

d'Amat, R. (ed.) (1961). *Les médecins Cloquet, J.-B.-A. Cloquet. Dict. biog. française,* **9,** 25–6.

Cloquet, G. (1910). *Jules Cloquet, sa vie—ses œuvres* . . . Jules Rousset, Paris.

Prevost, M. and d'Amat, R. (ed.) (1954). J.-B.-M. Bourgery. *Dict. biog. française,* **6,** 1482.

German lithographic monographs

Anon. (1952). Arnold, Ärtze. *Neue Deutsche Biog.,* **1,** 383–4.

Clarke, E. and Dewhurst, K. (1972). *An illustrated history of brain function.* Sandford Publications, Oxford.

Kahle, E. (1977). H. F. Kilian. *Neue Deutsche Biog.,* **11,** 605–6.

Meyer, A. (1971). *Historical aspects of cerebral anatomy.* Oxford University Press, London.

Lithographic atlases from University College, London

Bellot, H. H. (1929). *University College London 1826–1926*. University of London Press, London.

Dictionary of National Biography (compact edn) (1975). Biographies of G. V. Ellis, D. Maclise, J. Quain, R. Quain, E. Wilson by various authors, Oxford University Press, London.

Forman, M. B. (1934). *John Keats's anatomical and physiological notebook*. Oxford University Press, Oxford.

Hadley, R. M. (1959). The life and works of Sir William James Erasmus Wilson 1809–1884. *Med. Hist.*, **3**, 215–47.

Lawrence, S. C. (1988). Entrepreneurs and private enterprise: the development of medical lecturing in London, 1775–1820. *Bull. Hist. Med.*, **62**, 171–92.

Ormond, R. (1972) *Daniel Maclise 1806–1870*. Arts Council, London.

Smith, G. E. (1929–30). Obituary notice: Sir George Dancer Thane. *J. Anat.*, **64**, 364–7.

Pirogov

Mikulinsky, S. R. (1974). Nikolay Ivanovich Pirogov. *Dict. sci. Biog.*, **10**, 619–21.

15

The evolution of illustration in modern anatomy texts

THE production of multiple identical (or nearly identical) illustrations by means of the printing press was, we argued earlier in this book, an essential step in the development of anatomical science. Various reproductive methods have been used to print the black-and-white or coloured illustrations for anatomy books—woodcut, metal-engraving in all its varieties, lithography, and wood-engraving. Each technique has virtues and limitations when used in anatomical illustration; some of these we have indicated in earlier chapters. In the later nineteenth century and in the twentieth century photographic methods, including colour-separation techniques, have been employed to prepare relief, intaglio, and planographic printing surfaces. In more recent years the computer has been used to modify images, however generated. There are now virtually no limitations on printing accurately, and at relatively moderate cost, any coloured or uncoloured drawing, painting, or photograph.

Faced with such extraordinary opportunities, publishers—particularly those on the continent of Europe—responded by issuing comprehensive atlases, many with plates taken from water-colour drawings.

The photographers, blockmakers, and printers who worked in Vienna and Munich for Pernkopf before and after the Second World War, had their remote counterparts in the men who cut wood-blocks in Venice in the sixteenth century, and those who printed those blocks for Vesalius and Oporinus in Basle. But at the centre of any scheme to issue a book of scientific anatomy there remains, in twentieth-century Vienna and Munich as in Renaissance Padua and Venice, the anatomist and his collaborator, the artist. These two were, and are, shackled together in a laborious, time-consuming, and inevitably expensive enterprise. Without them, nothing.

Many of the artists we shall mention in this chapter were anatomists, or had spent so many years in the dissecting room that they became as knowledgeable as their professional collaborators. Both anatomist and artist were, as always, influenced by the traditions and the styles around them, each dependent on chronology and geography for the ways in which anatomical structures were presented and drawn. It would be possible, for instance, to compare the evolution, through many editions and decades, of Gray's English anatomical textbook (first edition 1858) and Spalteholz's German hand-atlas (first edition 1895–1903). We have however only space to indicate a few of the directions that anatomical illustration has taken during this period. We have, perforce, to say nothing of interesting atlases from France, Italy, or many other European countries. And, as throughout this book, we have limited ourselves to aspects of the European tradition, and have not considered the remarkable textbooks of anatomy issued elsewhere in the world.

We outline first those aspects of Gray's *Anatomy* that allowed it to establish itself in the mid-nineteenth century, and then to continue to mutate for the next hundred years or more. After consideration of an anatomical monograph—on the skeleton, by Frazer, a follower of Gray—we describe the German and Austrian school of anatomical illustration, and its translocation by Max Brödel to North America. We mention the work of Grant and his artists in Toronto, and that of Netter in New York, as following Brödel's lead. Finally we consider the photographic anatomical atlas, using that of McMinn and Hutchings as the type example.

Henry Gray (1827?–1861)

In the English-speaking world, for more than a century, one book symbolized anatomy: Henry Gray's *Anatomy descriptive and surgical* was first published in London by John W. Parker and Son, 1858, and in Philadelphia by Blanchard and Lea, 1859. The current edition in England is the thirty-seventh, 1989. There have been separate US editions, the book evolving differently there; the present American edition is the thirtieth, 1984/85.

What kind of illustrated anatomy was to be found in Gray's textbook? In this, as in Vesalius' *Fabrica*, text and illustration are closely related. The illustrations in Gray, however, for the most part showed the details of an area, often in keyhole, semi-diagrammatic representation. Little attention was paid to three–dimensional appearance. In the older tradition of Vesalius and his successors the bones, muscles, vessels and so on were commonly shown *in situ* in the whole body. Gray was content to picture detailed descriptive anatomy. At least in the early editions variations and anomalies were not emphasized. Nor was there any attempt to picture an Albinian 'ideal' or 'perfected' anatomy. The text and illustrations rather constituted a pragmatic anatomy, useful for reference by students, by anatomists, and, particularly, by surgeons. The wood-engravings, originally all uncoloured, faithfully represented the relative sizes and positions of anatomical structures, but not their actual appearance in the dissecting room.

It is difficult to take much pleasure in looking at these illustrations, except the pleasure of seeing something useful. Anatomists, by reference to these wood-engravings and the accompanying text, can readily confirm, say, the number, size, and distribution of the branches of an artery or nerve. A surgeon can find, in an efficient way, the disposition of structures in a potential operative field.

In 1858 wood-engraving was probably the ideal medium for reproducing at low cost these small diagrams. Our *Plate 127* shows, somewhat enlarged, a figure as it appeared in the original edition. This figure has proved so useful in demonstrating the distribution of the oph- thalmic and other nerves of the orbit that, in various modified forms, it is to be found in many, perhaps all, editions of Gray—both English and American—right up to the present time. Jones Quain's *Elements of anatomy*, 1844, had included an even smaller wood-engraving of many of the same anatomical structures (*Fig. 15.1*), and this was in turn derived from an illustration by Arnold. Such similarities may have been the basis for the accusation by one hostile reviewer (*The Medical Times and Gazette*, 1859) that Gray was guilty of blatant plagiarism:

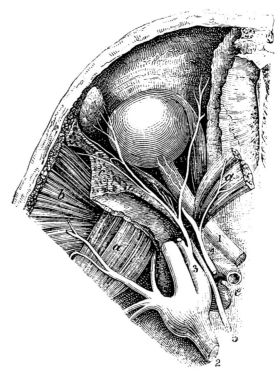

15.1   Wood engraving of orbit from Jones Quain's *Elements of anatomy*, 1844.

Mr. Gray has published a book that was not wanted, and which, at any rate, ought not to have been dedicated to Sir Benjamin Brodie. It is low and unscientific in tone; and it has been compiled, for the most part, in a manner inconsistent with the professions of honesty which we find in the preface ... A more unphilosophical amalgam of anatomical details and crude surgery we have never met with ...

... those who will take the trouble to compare the plan of the book with that of Quain, and will examine the two books together ... must admit that the interests of the profession demand a full exposure.

... an example of debased compilation and unscrupulous assumption.

However the *Lancet* thought the illustrations 'perfect' and the text 'scientifically excellent', and the *British Medical Journal* considered the work 'far superior to all other treatises on anatomy'.

The objectives of Gray's *Anatomy* and Quain's *Elements of anatomy* were originally similar, but these two most popular anatomy books developed along different lines during the following fifty or so years. That of Quain, even by 1864, had become a two-volume work, and by the time of its last edition in 1920 was a multi-volume handbook dealing *in extenso* with histology, embryology, and other aspects of general anatomy. Gray's work remained and remains a single, albeit thick, volume.

The semi-diagrammatic figures in Gray and other textbooks built on similar principles have been compared with the figures constructed on blackboards with coloured chalks during the course of traditional anatomical lectures. But the printed diagrams, now often in colour, are much *less* sophisticated than blackboard figures. These later are built up gradually, the visual presentation being developed in time and accompanied by explanatory talk. (The diagram in a book is without ontogeny.) Ideally the illustrated anatomical lecture occurs in parallel with examination of the relevant parts of a cadaver prepared according to a dissection manual. It used to be that all students carried out the dissections themselves; now more commonly prosections prepared in advance by teachers are demonstrated.

In the English-speaking world Gray's text has been used by many students and teachers alike to reinforce knowledge of particulars of topographical anatomy learned from lectures and demonstrations. It would indeed be foolish to attempt to read Gray as a *book*, from cover to cover. For such a pattern of anatomical instruction there seems to be no need for the student to have available the type of anatomical atlases typified by those of Mascagni, Cloquet, or Richard Quain and Erasmus Wilson.

There are however losses, both aesthetic and practical. The older tradition of showing anatomical details in a recognizable human body enabled the anatomical artist to call on the tradition of figure-drawing and painting, and to benefit in this way from the long-standing artistic obsession in Europe with the nude. The illustrations in Gray and other similar texts ignore that tradition. Moreover, these down-to-earth, practical illustrations have certain didactic deficiencies not unrelated to such considerations. They make little attempt to show the parts in the context of the whole body—local arteries are pictured in relation to other nearby structures, but the origin of these vessels may not be pictured. From Vesalius through to the lithographic atlases of the nineteenth century one can comprehend in many illustrations the general and the particular distribution of the arteries of the body at a glance. Gray only made perfunctory attempts to do this.

The approach of Gray and Jones Quain answered the needs of contemporary British—and American—medical students. In the Scottish universities, in the newer London colleges, and in the private schools much emphasis was placed on anatomy. Detailed knowledge was required in the Colleges of Surgeons' examinations which many students sat. Cynics might suggest that only anatomy had then a sufficient corpus of factual knowledge; physiology, pharmacology, and the aetiology, classification, and treatment of disease were subjects resting on the shifting sands of uncertain opinion. Honest examiners could, however, remain confident in passing or failing students on the basis of their knowledge of anatomy. And yet, except for innovators in medical science or in surgery, a detailed knowledge of anatomy was hardly required in the day-to-day work of physicians or general practitioners. It would be possible to illustrate this point by reference to Osler's *Principles and Practice of Medicine*, first issued at the end of the nineteenth century, in which knowledge of anatomy plays a minor role.

Gray's text was designed primarily for students preparing for rigorous examinations in anatomy, but also for surgeons. The first major operation under anaesthesia in England was carried out, as we have seen, in London in 1846 by Liston of University College. He could amputate a leg in less than a minute. But speed became less paramount when a patient was rendered unconscious by anaesthetics. It was then possible carefully to dissect in areas previously unexplored by a surgeon's knife—but not unexplored by that of the anatomist. When antisepsis and asepsis were added later in the century regions such as the abdomen and the brain became for the first time accessible to non-heroic, careful surgeons. Gray's text, as it evolved through successive editions, incorporated the special, surgically-relevant anatomy of these areas. In the 1940s, with open-chest anaesthesia, chemotherapy, and antibiotics, the technology of intrathoracic surgery, first of the lung, and then of the heart was developed—and the relevant applied anatomy was introduced into Gray's text. The lung segments were identified, became important to thoracic surgery, and were incorporated as coloured diagrams into anatomy books.

Gray's *Anatomy* was originally a product of St George's Hospital and its Medical School. The 363 drawings were by Henry Vandyke Carter, formerly Demonstrator in Anatomy there. They were taken from dissections made by Gray and Carter. The St George's surgeons Timothy Holmes and T. Pickering Pick edited, or assisted in editing, many editions from the first through to the sixteenth, 1858–1905. Gray himself was associated during the whole of his brief professional life with St George's, first as a student, 1845, and after as house surgeon, 1850. He was Demonstrator (1852) and Lecturer (1853) in Anatomy in St George's.

While still a student, Gray wrote on the embryology of the retina and optic nerve, and compared it with the development of the membranous labyrinth and auditory nerve. In 1852 a paper on the embryology of the thyroid and adrenal glands and the spleen, which he called collectively ductless glands, was also published in the *Philosophical Transactions* of the Royal Society; this work shows Gray to have been a forward-looking embryologist, histologist, and physiologist. He was elected FRS that year, and received encouragement in further research on the spleen, which resulted in a definitive work in 1854: *The structure and use of the spleen*.

A second edition of Gray's textbook, with further illustrations, this time by J. G. Westmacott, was issued in 1860. Gray died, in his mid-thirties, in January of the following year of confluent smallpox, caught by looking after his sick nephew. The original publishers, Parker and Son, retired from business after the 1860 edition: the book was taken over by Longman's, who remain the English publishers one hundred and twenty-five years later.

J. Ernest S. Frazer (1870–1946)

Even the details contained in a 'late-model' Gray are insufficiently elaborated for a detailed review of the human anatomy of any particular medical or surgical subspecialty. Separate monographs on various aspects of brain anatomy are obviously required for neurosurgery. (Of course, these also rely heavily on sources other than naked-eye anatomy.) Equally, but perhaps less obviously, the presentation of the skeleton in any all-inclusive text, such as Gray's, is lacking in the details required on occasion by orthopaedic surgeons, rheumatologists, and others treating patients with musculo-skeletal problems. As a fine example of such a monograph, we show figures from J. E. Frazer *The Anatomy of the Human Skeleton*, London, J. and A. Churchill, first published in 1914 (*Plate 128*). Frazer, educated at St Bartholomew's Hospital, initially developed a career as a surgeon, and he retained his surgical interests. But, recovering from a severe illness—a septicaemia following a wound acquired while conducting a post-mortem— he turned his career towards anatomy. He taught at St George's and King's College, before moving to St Mary's Hospital Medical School. He was in charge of the anatomy department at St Mary's from 1911 to 1940. His work on embryology was substantial: *A Manual of embryology* was published in 1931. His most lasting contribution was his monograph on the human skeleton.

The illustrations in this book, drawn by Frazer himself, are proportionately accurate. They use colour to create remarkably clear diagrams, but there is little attempt to make them look 'lifelike'. The text is similarly precise and clear. Frazer's intention was expressed in his preface. It was to induce the student—and this surely means any inquirer—

... to think of the bones as they exist in the body rather than as they lie on the table before him, and to do this I have laid stress—because he must use the prepared specimens—on the meaning of small details and on the relations of the bone ... in other words, each part of the skeleton has been used as a peg on which to hang a consideration of the neighbouring structures, in the hope that this may afford a new point of view to the reader and enable him to grasp the intimate connection between them.

127 Nerves of the orbit, from above. Figure 252 from H. Gray, *Anatomy descriptive and surgical*, 1858. Wood-engraving (Cambridge University Library). 11.0 × 7.0 cm.

The anatomical illustrations in the first edition of Gray's anatomy, when compared with many of those that preceded or were contemporary with it, were certainly on the small side, none of them exceeding 20 cm; the majority of them were very much smaller.

They were primarily designed to portray up-to-date anatomy of small areas: this being the aim they were not required to be works of art in their own right.

In the illustration chosen it is interesting to note the 'Casserian' ganglion. This labelling error

252.—Nerves of the Orbit. Seen from above.

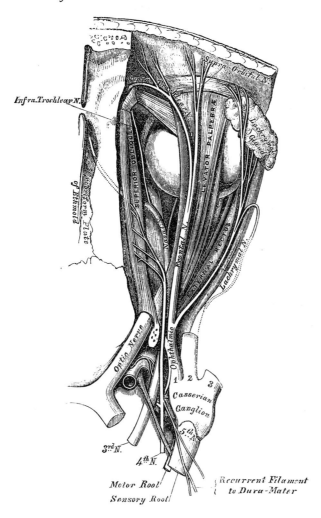

PLATE 127

is repeated in a number of other illustrations in the book, but the ganglion is correctly referred to as 'Gasserian' in the text. The nasal nerve (naso-ciliary nerve) is shown as being much more substantial than it should be. It is seen giving off a long ciliary branch to the eyeball, then an (unlabelled) ethmoidal branch, and then terminating as the infratrochlear nerve.

The frontal nerve and its two terminal branches need no comment, but the fourth or trochlear, here supplying the superior oblique muscle via four separate branches, presents some odd features. For instance, it is erroneously shown giving off a meningeal branch, and also a medial branch which disappears deep to the oculomotor (third) nerve. This may possibly represent a communication with the sympathetic plexus on the internal carotid artery. If the nerve joining the ophthalmic nerve is meant to arise from the trochlear, then this is in agreement with present-day belief. The text further describes the trochlear nerve as giving a branch which assists in forming the lacrimal nerve, indicated in the drawing by the dotted lines. Nowadays, this is considered to be a very occasional branch.

The motor root of the trigeminal nerve is well in evidence, but the abducent nerve is absent, even though one would have expected to see it on the medial surface of the external (lateral) rectus muscle.

Although Gray's black-and-white illustrations possess little aesthetic quality in themselves, and the book was originally not well-received in some quarters, the fact that it has now seen, in England alone, thirty-seven editions over some one hundred and thirty years entitles it, together with its drawings, to an honourable place among anatomy textbooks.

128 Upper portion of the right femur. Figure 118 from J. E. Frazer, *The anatomy of the human skeleton*, 1914. Halftone (Cambridge University Library). 20.2 × 3.8 cm.

These four drawings epitomize Frazer's stated objective of using each part of the skeleton 'as a peg on which to hang a consideration of the neighbouring structures...'.

This plate is an excellent example of the enviable ability of Frazer to convey his wide knowledge of human bones in an accurate and detailed manner, albeit one easily comprehensible. The description of the drawings on the facing page, in addition to providing further identification of the many structures illustrated, also further informs the viewer by means of 'observations'. For example, with regard to the first figure, 'observe that the gluteus minimus is attached only to the outer ridge of the trochanter, but its tendon is continuous below with an aponeurotic sheet, the ilio-trochanteric band, which covers the bursa in front and reaches the bone internal to it'.

Frazer's own careful and innovative illustrations, over two hundred of them, admirably complement his detailed yet lucid text, and make his book a treasure for students seeking to understand human skeletal anatomy. Seventy-five years later it still has no rival in its field.

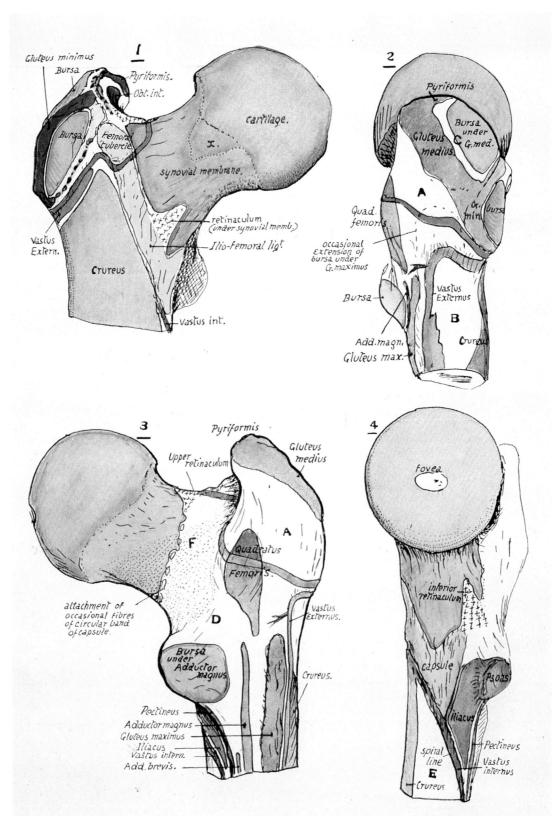

FIG. 118

Later developments in Germany and Austria: Spalteholz and Pernkopf

Jones Quain and Gray exemplify a British tradition. Whether the approach was system-by-system, regional, or topographical, these anatomy texts used semi-diagrammatic figures to illustrate details rather than the whole. Attempts to portray anatomy life-sized, so much a concern in previous decades, had been abandoned.

A somewhat different approach can be discerned in illustrations produced in Germany and Austria at the turn of the century and for the next fifty years or so. In this, more attention is paid to giving the parts of the body a lifelike appearance. Shading is used, even in what are undoubtedly diagrams, to show the parts in a smoothed, rounded, three-dimensional way. This approach is based, it should be remembered, on abstraction rather than realism, since it depicts imagined rather than actual preparations. No part of any corpse ever seen on the dissecting table resembles these illustrations.

Early elements of this approach may be seen in the atlas produced by *Werner Spalteholz* (1861–1940), *Handatlas der Anatomie des Menschen*, Leipzig, S. Hirzel, 1895–1903. This work was as influential in the teaching of human anatomy on the Continent as Gray's less precisely illustrated text was in the English-speaking world. The *Handatlas* soon appeared in other languages—English, Italian, Russian, French, and Spanish. It continues to be published to this day. Our *Plate 129* may be compared with Frazer's diagram (*Plate 128*): the former conveys directly the actual appearance of the bony and ligamentous structures of the knee-joint; Frazer indicates diagrammatically the relationships of the upper end of the femur, placing the burden of constructing the actuality of these relationships on the student.

The development of such quasi-realistic illustrations may be seen in a succession of German-language anatomical atlases from 1870 onwards. *Carl Heitzman* (1836–96) drew the illustrations himself for his *Atlas der Descriptiven und topographische Anatomie des Menschen*, Vienna, W. Braumuller, 1870. They were reproduced as wood-engravings. *Figure 15.2*, taken from the 1887 American edition, is a didactically useful display of the salivary glands, shown semi-diagrammatically, but placed in the context of a supposed dissection. A later, and in the event final, edition of this work was published in two volumes in 1902–5 under the editorship of E. Zuckerkandl. New illustrations were added, the original drawings for which are still extant; these may be compared with the resulting wood-engravings. The engraved lines have failed to reproduce well the shading and highlights present in the original drawings.

The updating and revision in 1902–5 of Heitzmann's formerly popular atlas was in competition with a new atlas by *Carl Toldt* (1840–1920), Professor at the University of Vienna: *Anatomischer Atlas für Studierende und Ärzte*, Vienna, Urban and Schwarzenberg, 1896–1900. Most of the original drawings in this were by Fritz Meixner; photographs were taken of these drawings and transferred to the end-grain of the wood, and engravings made with the burin. The engraver, F. X. Matolony, respected the intentions of the artist; his original blocks lasted through twenty-five editions.

A few years later, *Johannes Sobotta* (1869–1945), Professor at Würzberg, was the author of yet another atlas: *Atlas der descriptiven Anatomie des Menschen*, Munich, J. F. Lehmann, 1904–7. The drawings were by Karl Hajek. They were reproduced photographically by halftone; this preserved the shading and highlights of the original, so imparting an aura of reality and authenticity. Multiple plates added colour to the final print.

It was the atlas by *Eduard Pernkopf* (1888–1955) which brought this type of anatomy to a sort of culmination. The work, supervised by Pernkopf, Director of the Anatomical Institute in Vienna, was started in 1933, continued as well as it could be during the war years, and was completed twenty-two years and nearly nine hundred illustrations later: it was published

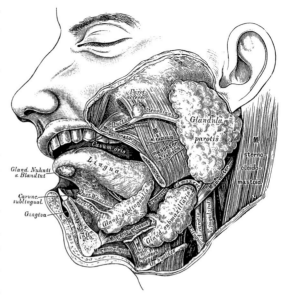

15.2 The salivary glands from C. Heitzmann, *Anatomy descriptive and topographical*, New York, 1887.

as *Topographische Anatomie des Menschen*, Munich. Urban and Schwarzenberg, 1937–60. The group of at least eight artists, using water-colour as their medium, adopted, if not a similar style, certainly a similar approach. Their work was admirably printed using halftone photographic methods. Colour was used boldly, even garishly in places. Black-and-white photographs of such plates present to eyes accustomed to Gray and others like him a more modern appearance; colour serves to heighten the unreal abstraction of these hyper-real illustrations, such as our *Plate 130*. Arteries, veins, bronchi, muscles, and so on are not coloured like this either in life in the operating theatre or in the dissection room of the anatomical institute. Yet in spite of this, some aspects of this plate *are* lifelike: the fibres of the diaphragm can be clearly seen as they arch upward to form the dome. The undoubted visual impact of this plate may result from a tension between diagram and picture.

Pernkopf's work has rightly been immensely popular, being published in several languages, and republished in both the larger and smaller forms.

129 Knee-joint menisci and ligaments viewed from the front. Volume I, figure 255 from W. Spalteholz, *Hand-atlas of human anatomy*, 1907. Lithograph (Cambridge University Library). 12.0 × 11.3 cm.

One drawback of Spalteholz's *Hand-atlas*, apart from the rather small size of many of the illustrations, is that the plates tend to be cluttered with too many identifying legends and lines: this distracts the viewer from the anatomy itself, quite apart from the fact that tracing the indicator lines to their various destinations is often a difficult and painstaking task.

This plate, of the right knee-joint with the patella and retinacula removed and the joint flexed to the right angle, has been chosen in part because of the relative paucity of legends and lines, but primarily because it is such a simple, clear, and accurate drawing. What labelling exists is in accord with the BNA nomenclature introduced in 1895.

The two cruciate ligaments and the medial and lateral collateral ligaments and their attachments are shown. The essentially fibrous nature of the menisci is well brought out, which emphasizes the point that the term 'cartilage' commonly applied to them is misleading.

Many of Spalteholz's plates, including this one, have formed the basis for illustrations in numerous anatomy texts, even to the present day. As Franklin Mall of Johns Hopkins pointed out in the preface to this second English-language edition, the *Hand-atlas* rapidly became a favourite choice of students of anatomy, not only at Johns Hopkins medical school but in many places throughout the world. It is sad that some later editions were so poorly produced as to besmirch its well-deserved and honourable reputation.

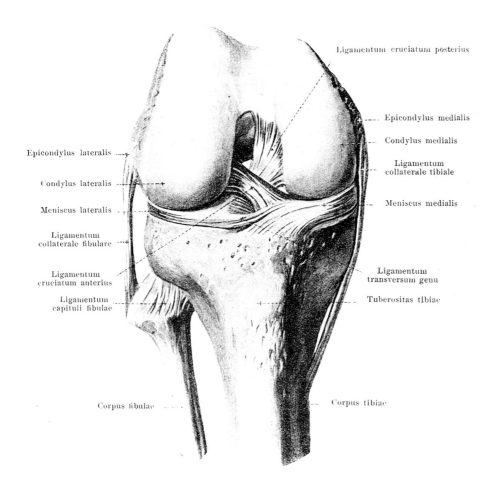

Ligamentum cruciatum posterius

Epicondylus medialis

Condylus medialis

Ligamentum collaterale tibiale

Meniscus medialis

Epicondylus lateralis

Condylus lateralis

Meniscus lateralis

Ligamentum collaterale fibulare

Ligamentum cruciatum anterius

Ligamentum capituli fibulae

Ligamentum transversum genu

Tuberositas tibiae

Corpus fibulae

Corpus tibiae

PLATE 129

130 Thoracic structures after removal of the heart. Volume I, Tafel 71, Abb. 81 from E. Pernkopf, *Topographische Anatomie des Menschen*, 1943. Halftone (Urban and Schwarzenberg). 19.7 × 18.7 cm.

This double-page plate is equally a feast of colour and of anatomy—almost too much of both. It must surely have been based on a considerable number of separate dissections, and the anatomy displayed is commendably accurate and clear.

The vagal and sympathetic trunks, their branches, and associated ganglia are excellently portrayed, as also are the bronchial arteries, the thoracic duct, and the grouping of the lymph nodes. The left recurrent laryngeal nerve is accurately shown hooking around the ligamentum arteriosum, although the latter is depicted as a somewhat stylized cord.

There are, perhaps, a few minor anatomical short-comings. On the left side a sizeable nerve (unlabelled) is found descending anterior to the suprascapular artery and vein. The only nerve that does this (apart from the very much more superficial supraclavicular nerves) is the nerve to the subclavius muscle: if this in fact is the nerve represented here it is surely much too large, being equal in size to the suprascapular. It is also interesting to note that the left inferior thyroid, superficial (transverse) cervical, and suprascapular arteries are shown arising separately from the subclavian—a configuration, though not uncommon, that is less usual than their origin from a thyro-cervical trunk.

Even allowing for distortion caused by retraction of the lungs it is difficult to equate the pattern of the bronchi shown here, particularly those of the left inferior lobe, with present-day knowledge of broncho-pulmonary segmental anatomy. The cut lower portions of the phrenic nerves and pericardiaco-phrenic vessels are clearly seen, but the superior epigastric vessels are, oddly, not featured.

Minor criticism apart, the overall quality of this plate is quite superb, and is a fine example of what can be achieved by close co-operation and understanding between artist and anatomist. Most of the later anatomical atlases present the anatomy shown here by means of a number of separate drawings, each centred on specific systems or structures. While this approach may render a particular 'portion' of anatomy more easily comprehensible, it often results in the complex interrelationship of structures being more difficult to appreciate. Like those of a number of anatomical atlases, however, the plate is too heavily labelled, and the strong colours make the indicator lines difficult to trace.

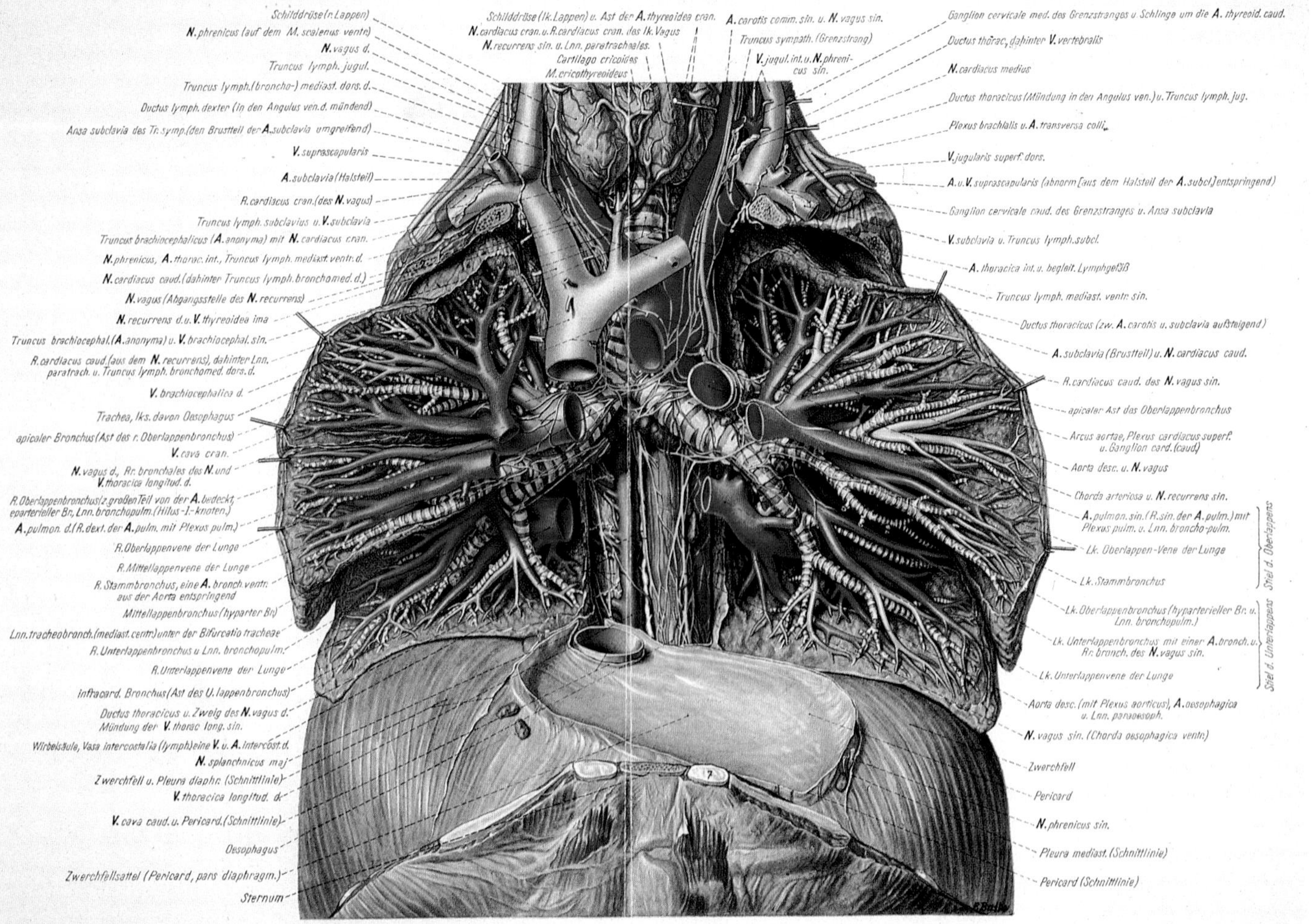

Schilddrüse (r. Lappen)
N. phrenicus (auf dem M. scalenus ventr.)
N. vagus d.
Truncus lymph. jugul.
Truncus lymph. (broncho-) mediast. dors. d.
Ductus lymph. dexter (in den Angulus ven. d. mündend)
Ansa subclavia des Tr. symp. (den Brustteil der A. subclavia umgreifend)
V. suprascapularis
A. subclavia (Halsteil)
R. cardiacus cran. (des N. vagus)
Truncus lymph. subclavius u. V. subclavia
Truncus brachiocephalicus (A. anonyma) mit N. cardiacus cran.
N. phrenicus, A. thorac. int., Truncus lymph. mediast. ventr. d.
N. cardiacus caud. (dahinter Truncus lymph. bronchomed. d.)
N. vagus (Abgangsstelle des N. recurrens)
N. recurrens d. u. V. thyreoidea ima
Truncus brachiocephal. (A. anonyma) u. V. brachiocephal. sin.
R. cardiacus caud. (aus dem N. recurrens), dahinter Lnn. paratrach. u. Truncus lymph. bronchomed. dors. d.
V. brachiocephalica d.
Trachea, lks. davon Oesophagus
apicaler Bronchus (Ast des r. Oberlappenbronchus)
V. cava cran.
N. vagus d., Rr. bronchales des N. und V. thoracica longitud. d.
R. Oberlappenbronchus (z. großen Teil von der A. bedeckt, eparterieller Br., Lnn. bronchopulm. (Hilus-1.-knoten.)
A. pulmon. d. (R. dext. der A. pulm. mit Plexus pulm.)
R. Oberlappenvene der Lunge
R. Mittellappenvene der Lunge
R. Stammbronchus, eine A. bronch. ventr. aus der Aorta entspringend
Mittellappenbronchus (hyparter Br.)
Lnn. tracheobranch. (mediast. centr.) unter der Bifurcatio tracheae
R. Unterlappenbronchus u. Lnn. bronchopulm.
R. Unterlappenvene der Lunge
Infracard. Bronchus (Ast des U. lappenbronchus)
Ductus thoracicus u. Zweig des N. vagus d. Mündung der V. thorac. long. sin.
Wirbelsäule, Vasa intercostalia (lymph.) eine V. u. A. intercost. d.
N. splanchnicus maj.
Zwerchfell u. Pleura diaphr. (Schnittlinie)
V. thoracica longitud. d.
V. cava caud. u. Pericard. (Schnittlinie)
Oesophagus
Zwerchfellsattel (Pericard, pars diaphragm.)
Sternum
Schilddrüse (lk. Lappen) u. Ast der A. thyreoidea cran.
N. cardiacus cran. u. R. cardiacus cran. des lk. Vagus
N. recurrens sin. u. Lnn. paratracheales.
Cartilago cricoides
M. cricothyreoideus
A. carotis comm. sin. u. N. vagus sin.
Truncus sympath. (Grenzstrang)
V. jugul. int. u. N. phrenicus sin.
Ganglion cervicale med. des Grenzstranges u. Schlinge um die A. thyreoid. caud.
Ductus thorac., dahinter V. vertebralis
N. cardiacus medius
Ductus thoracicus (Mündung in den Angulus ven.) u. Truncus lymph. jug.
Plexus brachialis u. A. transversa colli
V. jugularis superf. dors.
A. u. V. suprascapularis (abnorm [aus dem Halsteil der A. subcl.] entspringend)
Ganglion cervicale caud. des Grenzstranges u. Ansa subclavia
V. subclavia u. Truncus lymph. subcl.
A. thoracica int. u. begleit. Lymphgefäß
Truncus lymph. mediast. ventr. sin.
Ductus thoracicus (zw. A. carotis u. subclavia aufsteigend)
A. subclavia (Brustteil) u. N. cardiacus caud.
R. cardiacus caud. des N. vagus sin.
apicaler Ast des Oberlappenbronchus
Arcus aortae, Plexus cardiacus superf. u. Ganglion card. (caud.)
Aorta desc. u. N. vagus
Chorda arteriosa u. N. recurrens sin.
A. pulmon. sin. (R. sin. der A. pulm.) mit Plexus pulm. u. Lnn. broncho-pulm.
Lk. Oberlappen-Vene der Lunge
Lk. Stammbronchus
Stiel d. Oberlappens
Lk. Oberlappenbronchus (hyparterieller Br. u. Lnn. bronchopulm.)
Lk. Unterlappenbronchus mit einer A. bronch. u. Rr. bronch. des N. vagus sin.
Lk. Unterlappenvene der Lunge
Stiel d. Unterlappens
Aorta desc. (mit Plexus aorticus), A. oesophagica u. Lnn. paraoesoph.
N. vagus sin. (Chorda oesophagica ventr.)
Zwerchfell
Pericard
N. phrenicus sin.
Pleura mediast. (Schnittlinie)
Pericard (Schnittlinie)

Abb. 81. Darstellung der Gebilde des retrocardialen Mediastinum sowie des intrapulmonal sich verästelnden Bronchial- und Gefäßbaumes von ventral her. Nach Entfernung der dorsalen Partie des Herzbeutels wurde die Präparation der im retrocardialen Mediastinum befindlichen Gefäße und Nerven vervollständigt, der Lungenflügel seitwärts herübergedrängt und das Parenchym derselben zum großen Teil unter fortlaufender Präparation der in den Lungen sich verästelnden Gebilde entfernt.

Max Brödel and the North-American tradition

Max Brödel (1870–1941) as a pupil at the Leipzig Academy of Fine Arts worked in his vacations during the late 1880s as illustrator to both the physiological and anatomical institutes in that city. He worked in physiology for the great Carl Ludwig, and in anatomy for both Wilhelm His sr. and the young Spalteholz. A visiting anatomist from the United States, Franklin P. Mall, researching embryology with His, recognized Brödel's potential. Mall, on his return to Johns Hopkins in Baltimore to become Professor of Anatomy in the new medical school, extended an invitation to the artist to join in this new venture. Brödel took up his appointment in 1894, and worked first in the gynaecology department and later for a number of surgeons. In 1910 a Department of Art as Applied to Medicine was founded specifically to keep him at Johns Hopkins. More than two hundred students were trained there during the next thirty years.

Our *Plate 131* is one of two completed drawings that Brödel made after his retirement. He had often been called on to contribute illustrations to ear, nose, and throat surgery, and he continued independently and privately to explore the structure of the human ear. The figure stands alone, without text; it explains itself to those who have relevant elementary knowledge. It was based on observations of wet and dry specimens made over a period of months, and, in particular, on the study of serial sections in different planes. Using a *camera lucida* he reconstructed from the sections accurate three-dimensional models, and it was from these that his drawings were modified and corrected to prepare the final picture. One thinks here of the painstaking work in presenting 'perfected' anatomy by Jan Wandelaar in the eighteenth century under B. S. Albinus' direction. In Brödel's drawing of the ear, anatomist and artist were one and the same person. Many of the strictures we might have expressed as to the validity of the German school of realist, three-dimensional artists are silenced when we look at such a Brödel illustration.

The work done by Brödel shows that he developed and refined in Baltimore the ideas of anatomical illustration current in Leipzig and Vienna during his apprentice years. His work equals that of the best illustrators of the Toldt and Pernkopf atlases. As with them, so with Brödel, one feels at first glance the presence of the parts illustrated. He had the ability to place the observer alongside himself, as it were, within the structures he illustrates. His knowledge of physiology, embryology, and histology was based on his apprentice work with His and Carl Ludwig, and complemented his profound knowledge of gross anatomy. In this way some of his illustrations are of the small world of microanatomy; they are so drawn that they make plain the functions of the structures illustrated. At Johns Hopkins, moreover, he rapidly became adept at illustrating surgical technique, and for the remainder of his life produced such work for Howard Kelly, Harvey Cushing, William Halstead, Samuel Crowe, and others. Thomas S. Cullen (1945) quotes Brödel's rigorous, intellectual, and austere approach to a new subject:

The artist must first fully comprehend the subject matter from every standpoint: anatomical, topographical, histological, pathological, medical, and surgical. From this accumulated knowledge grows a mental picture, from which again crystallizes the plan for the future drawing. A clear and vivid mental picture always must precede the actual picture on paper. The planning of the picture, therefore, is the all-important thing, not the execution.

J. C. Boileau Grant, 1886–1973

Grant was a Scot by birth and education. Graduating from the University of Edinburgh in 1908 with awards in anatomy, he kept to this subject for the remainder of his life save for the war years, 1914–18. He taught anatomy at Edinburgh and Durham before becoming, in 1919, Professor of Anatomy at the University of Manitoba in Winnipeg, Canada. In 1930 he moved to Toronto, and remained head of the anatomy department there until 1956.

In 1937 Grant published the first edition of *A method of anatomy*, Baltimore, Williams and Wilkins. This has been appreciated for more than half a century, particularly by those weak students of anatomy who can discern little order in the messy dissections they themselves have attempted, and who cannot interpret the abstracted illustrations of Gray and his like. Grant's diagrams make sense even to those whose grasp of three dimensions is defective. The diagrams in *A method of anatomy* are similar to sketches made on the blackboard by an experienced anatomy teacher while instructing a small group of students in the dissecting room. The sketches, as Grant explained, were intended 'to anticipate a question, to solve a difficulty, to offer an explanation or otherwise speed comprehension'. Many figures in Grant's *Method* show how much information Grant and his artist were able to include in one small diagram.

A method of anatomy was immediately popular, and, in answer to requests, Grant produced a more formal atlas: *An atlas of anatomy*, Baltimore, Williams and Wilkins, 1943 and subsequent editions. The principal textual matter of this book is in the form of short numbered paragraphs calling attention to salient and significant points. These observations interpret, but do not describe exhaustively, the structures shown in the plates. As we have seen, Frazer had used this device in his monograph on the skeleton. There are also similarities in this approach to some of the continental European hand-atlases. But such similarities are most obvious in the style of drawing. A number of figures in Grant's *Atlas* demonstrate the German–American style of anatomical illustration, which is not surprising, for many artists were directly or indirectly influenced by the work of Max Brödel; many drawings are by Dorothy I. Chubb, for instance, and she was trained by Brödel himself in Baltimore.

Work such as this done at the University of Toronto for their medical faculty led to the formation there of a Department of Art as Applied to Medicine; Nancy Joy and Elizabeth Blackstock (who drew our *Plate 132*) are other illustrators of this school who collaborated with Grant in the production of his *Atlas*. In the Preface to the two-volume first edition Boileau Grant described in some detail how the illustrations were prepared:

In the execution of these illustrations the following preliminary steps were taken: each specimen was posed and photographed; from the negative film so obtained an enlarged positive film was made, usually one third larger than it would appear when reproduced; with the aid of a viewing box the outlines of the structures on the enlarged film were traced on tracing paper; and these outlines were scrutinized against the original specimen, in order to ensure that the shapes, positions and relative proportions of the various structures were correct. The outline tracing was then presented to the artist who transferred it to suitable paper, and having the original dissection beside her, proceeded to work up a plastic drawing in which the important features were brought out. Thus, little, if any, liberty has been taken with the anatomy; that is to say, the illustrations profess a considerable accuracy of detail.

Frank H. Netter

Born in New York in 1906, Netter as a young man studied drawing and painting at the National Academy of Design and the Art Students' League. During the depression years of the 1930s he became a successful commercial artist, accumulating sufficient funds to put himself through college and medical school in New York, graduating MD in 1931. He continued to work at illustration during his student and intern years, preparing medical illustrations for faculty members and for drug companies. After postgraduate training at Bellevue Hospital he set himself up as a surgeon in private practice, but still continued to draw professionally. When faced with growing and persistent demand on his illustrative abilities, Netter eventually decided to leave the practice of surgery behind and concentrate on serving medicine as an artist. Netter relates an episode that helped assure him of the correctness of his decision. When approached in his clinical office by a drug company to execute five medical drawings, a task he was not keen to take on, he decided to ask six times his usual price—$300 each, rather than $50. He therefore told the advertising executive that he would require $1500. The executive deferred a decision: he eventually called back to confirm that the company would pay $1500—for *each* of the illustrations!

After the years of the Second World War Netter became the most widely known medical illustrator in North America, largely through years of productive labour for the CIBA drug company. This company published, from 1953 on, ten volumes: *The CIBA collection of medical illustrations*, starting with the one on the nervous system. All the hundreds of coloured illustrations in these volumes were conceived and painted by Netter. A minority of them are academic anatomical figures; most illustrate physiology, pathology, and clinical medicine and surgery.

The factual backbone of the collections is general accepted information. 'Clinical significance has been the guiding principle. In many instances certain anatomic structures are either deliberately omitted or deemphasized in order to stress points that have broader clinical application' (Netter). He is bold enough to have taken on the task of *pictorializing* the whole core of medical knowledge, and has been willing to persist in this endeavour through decades of intense, dedicated labour. This is the way he works: first he studies the subject—as A. W. Custer writes in his introduction to *The Artist* in the preface to the 1968 CIBA collection: 'No drawing is ever started until Dr. Netter has acquired a complete understanding of the subject matter, either through reading or by consultation with leading authorities in the field'. A pencil sketch is then made at about twice the size of the final illustration, and transferred, when completed, to illustration-board; the picture is then coloured, often using water-colour and gouache. Production artists complete the process. Each volume of the CIBA Collection has an accompanying text by authoritative editors and their collaborators.

Frank Netter's style of drawing has long been widely known in the health professions. It starts from the same premises as those of the Brödel Schools at Johns Hopkins and Toronto. But to these are added many of the attitudes, techniques, and styles of 1930s and 1940s commercial art. The line, shading, and colour are certainly not as refined as those of Brödel. For didactic reasons many of the paintings are, as we have seen in the quotation from Netter above, exaggerated and coarsened.

At their best Netter's pictorial diagrams represent accurately the then-current ideas in medical knowledge; but this gives them a somewhat ephemeral status; those made thirty or more years ago are, naturally enough, unreliable guides to the present state of medical science. New and revised editions are issued from time to time to accommodate such considerations. Illustration of anatomy—the structure of the body—is not so subject to change, although, as we have seen, interpretation of the functions of a particular tissue or organ may influence, by subtle emphasis, the way in which drawings are made. To look at Netter's pictorial diagrams in the context of contemporary science imposes a considerable burden of interpretation on the viewer; it is more straightforward to look at his workmanlike anatomical plates, researched and drawn with great care. We have selected one for reproduction here (*Plate 133*). Are we prejudiced against Netter's style of anatomical illustration in thinking that the work of this remarkable, productive, and influential medical artist cannot bear comparison with that of the twentieth-century masters of the German and American schools, or the best of earlier centuries? 'He has been called the *Dean of Medical Illustrators* and *Medicine's Michelangelo*, and he more than merits both titles': this editorial comment in the *Medical Times*, 1981, seems to us quite wrong. There is no doubting the zeal and application with which Frank Netter has applied himself to interpreting modern medicine to the health professions through the medium of his art; but the anatomical illustrations are scientifically and aesthetically pedestrian.

131 Dissection of human ear. Figure 2 from M. Brödel, *Three unpublished drawings*, 1946. Halftone (W. B. Saunders). 19.5 × 14.8 cm.

The anatomy of the ear, and the relationships of the middle- and inner-ear components in particular, are difficult to illustrate, not least because of their encasement in bone.

This, the second of the ear drawings published posthumously, is signed by Brödel and dated 1941, the year of his death. It is an antero-lateral view of a section through the right ear, with the internal auditory meatus laid widely open so as to show the position and course of the facial nerve and the cochlear and vestibular components of the stato-acoustic nerve. The distal portion of the facial nerve (cut) is seen in the facial canal—it must be said that it seems rather a tight fit!

The postero-lateral part of the bony Eustachian tube is shown alongside the tunnel containing the tensor tympani muscle, the tendon of which is depicted curving laterally to its insertion on the malleus.

The interrelationship of the promontory of the middle ear and the first part of the cochlea of the inner ear is very clear, but the sectioned continuation of the cochlea is not too easy for a student to comprehend, even with the help of the arrows. However, the communication between the scala vestibuli and scala tympani at the helicotrema or apex of the cochlea is excellently displayed.

The weakest features are the portrayal of ghostly semicircular canals and the configuration of the stapes, which appears too massive for such a tiny delicate bone.

Perhaps one of the most attractive features of this plate—as is the case with most of Brödel's drawings—is the impression of three-dimensionality that it evokes in the viewer.

602   THE EVOLUTION OF ILLUSTRATION IN MODERN ANATOMY TEXTS

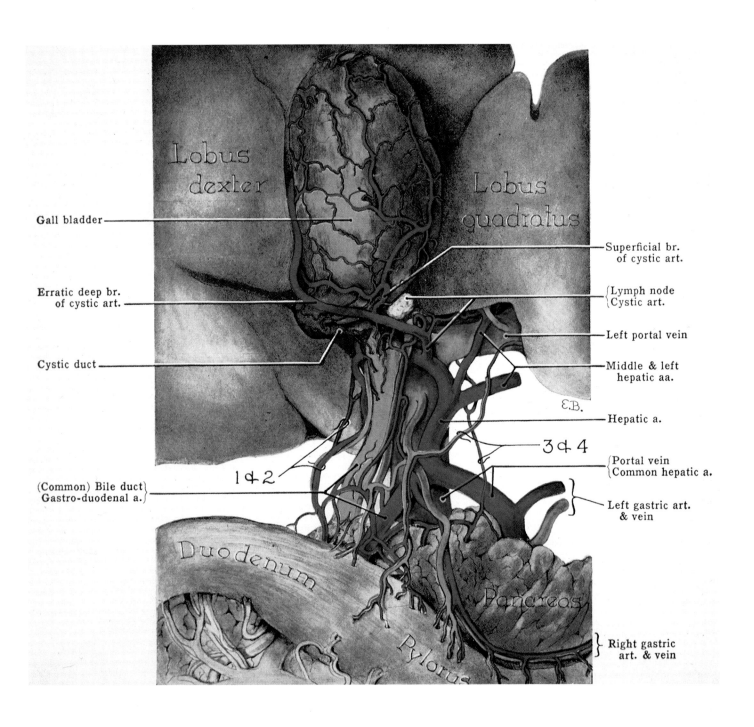

Gall bladder

Erratic deep br.
of cystic art.

Cystic duct

(Common) Bile duct⎱
Gastro-duodenal a.⎰

Lobus dexter

Lobus quadratus

Superficial br.
of cystic art.

⎰Lymph node
⎱Cystic art.

Left portal vein

Middle & left
hepatic aa.

E.B.

Hepatic a.

3 & 4

⎰Portal vein
⎱Common hepatic a.

1 & 2

⎱Left gastric art.
⎰& vein

Duodenum

Pancreas

Pylorus

⎱Right gastric
⎰art. & vein

133 Nerve-supply of mouth and pharynx. Volume 3, section 1, Plate 27 from F. H. Netter, *The CIBA collection of medical illustrations*, 1959. Colour photo-engraving (The Curtis Publishing Company). 21.0 × 15.0 cm.

As is generally the case with Netter's anatomical illustrations, this plate is a clear, informative, and, for the most part, accurate presentation. The latter should occasion no surprise when one considers the numerous eminent anatomists consulted during the work's gestation period.

The main criticism that may be levelled at it concerns the labelling technique employed. To follow the more than fifty indicator lines is a difficult and tedious task, calling alike for good eyesight and perseverance. To eliminate some of these lines and their captions, for example many of those referring to the larger arteries, would help to reduce the clutter. It might also allow the submandibular ganglion to be identified.

Some minor anatomical criticisms may be made. The phrenic nerve is shown arising from only the fourth and fifth cervical nerves; the external laryngeal nerve is portrayed as being the same size as the internal (and the former supplies too much of the pharyngeal constrictor musculature); labelling the buccal branch of the mandibular nerve as the 'buccinator nerve' is misleading—it doesn't supply the buccinator muscle, only pierces it; the superior cervical sympathetic ganglion is surely too small, especially when compared with the middle one; the otic ganglion would be hidden behind the mandibular nerve instead of lateral to it, as is suggested here; and the nerve to the thyrohyoid is too long. None the less, this is a valuable learning aid to understanding the nerve-supply of a complex anatomical area.

It is of interest to compare the technique and impact of this plate with those of Swan (*Plate 108*, p. 511) and Arnold (*Plate 119*, p. 555).

Since the above comments were written, we have received a new book: *Atlas of human anatomy*, Frank H. Netter, CIBA–GEIGY Corporation, Summit, NJ, 1989. This brings together, in one volume, most of the anatomical plates from the CIBA collection, many updated and revised, though without the original accompanying text. There are also a number of new plates, the atlas containing 514 plates in all.

Our *Plate 133* has been revised, and appears in Netter's *Atlas*... as his plate 65.

It is gratifying to note that the phrenic nerve now receives a contribution from the third cervical nerve; the submandibular ganglion is labelled; the otic ganglion has been banished; the 'buccinator nerve' has become 'buccal nerve (V3)'; and the nerve to thyrohyoid has been shortened appropriately. The too-small superior cervical sympathetic ganglion is no longer labelled.

The legends, now in lower case, are much easier to read; but, alas, the number of indicator lines has only been reduced from fifty-six to fifty-two. The overall attraction of the new plate, however, is greater than the old—it is better in every way.

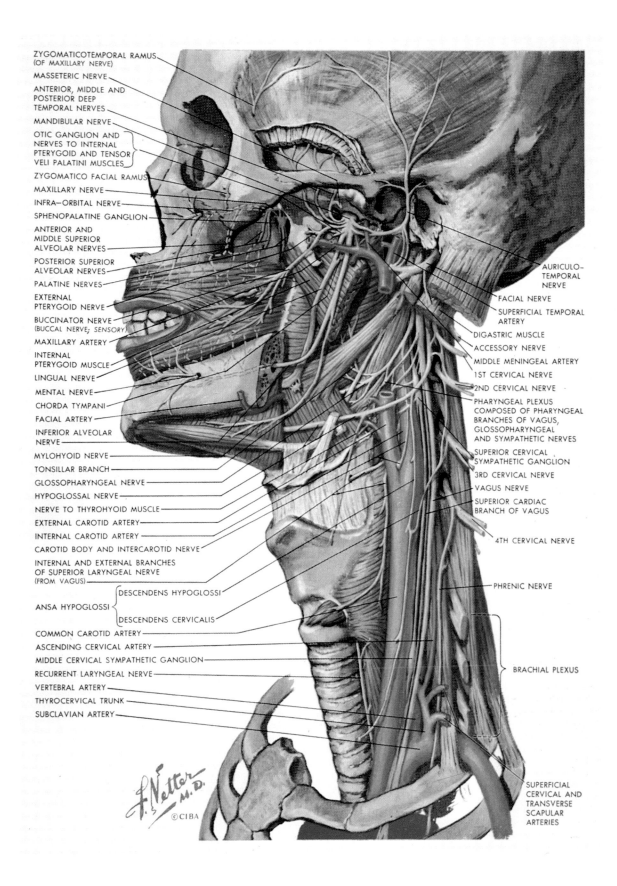

ZYGOMATICOTEMPORAL RAMUS
(OF MAXILLARY NERVE)

MASSETERIC NERVE

ANTERIOR, MIDDLE AND
POSTERIOR DEEP
TEMPORAL NERVES

MANDIBULAR NERVE

OTIC GANGLION AND
NERVES TO INTERNAL
PTERYGOID AND TENSOR
VELI PALATINI MUSCLES

ZYGOMATICO FACIAL RAMUS

MAXILLARY NERVE

INFRA—ORBITAL NERVE

SPHENOPALATINE GANGLION

ANTERIOR AND
MIDDLE SUPERIOR
ALVEOLAR NERVES

POSTERIOR SUPERIOR
ALVEOLAR NERVES

PALATINE NERVES

EXTERNAL
PTERYGOID NERVE

BUCCINATOR NERVE
(BUCCAL NERVE; SENSORY)

MAXILLARY ARTERY

INTERNAL
PTERYGOID MUSCLE

LINGUAL NERVE

MENTAL NERVE

CHORDA TYMPANI

FACIAL ARTERY

INFERIOR ALVEOLAR
NERVE

MYLOHYOID NERVE

TONSILLAR BRANCH

GLOSSOPHARYNGEAL NERVE

HYPOGLOSSAL NERVE

NERVE TO THYROHYOID MUSCLE

EXTERNAL CAROTID ARTERY

INTERNAL CAROTID ARTERY

CAROTID BODY AND INTERCAROTID NERVE

INTERNAL AND EXTERNAL BRANCHES
OF SUPERIOR LARYNGEAL NERVE
(FROM VAGUS)

DESCENDENS HYPOGLOSSI

ANSA HYPOGLOSSI

DESCENDENS CERVICALIS

COMMON CAROTID ARTERY

ASCENDING CERVICAL ARTERY

MIDDLE CERVICAL SYMPATHETIC GANGLION

RECURRENT LARYNGEAL NERVE

VERTEBRAL ARTERY

THYROCERVICAL TRUNK

SUBCLAVIAN ARTERY

AURICULO-
TEMPORAL
NERVE

FACIAL NERVE

SUPERFICIAL TEMPORAL
ARTERY

DIGASTRIC MUSCLE

ACCESSORY NERVE

MIDDLE MENINGEAL ARTERY

1ST CERVICAL NERVE

2ND CERVICAL NERVE

PHARYNGEAL PLEXUS
COMPOSED OF PHARYNGEAL
BRANCHES OF VAGUS,
GLOSSOPHARYNGEAL
AND SYMPATHETIC NERVES

SUPERIOR CERVICAL
SYMPATHETIC GANGLION

3RD CERVICAL NERVE

VAGUS NERVE

SUPERIOR CARDIAC
BRANCH OF VAGUS

4TH CERVICAL NERVE

PHRENIC NERVE

BRACHIAL PLEXUS

SUPERFICIAL
CERVICAL AND
TRANSVERSE
SCAPULAR
ARTERIES

F. Netter M.D.
©CIBA

Photographic atlases

The dissecting-room appearances of anatomical structures have been reproduced by photography for more than a century. What need is there then for an artist? Photography should be able to eliminate at least one of the intermediate steps between the reality of the dissected part and the reproductive illustration. The camera lens, recording accurately and objectively, should be able—should it not?—to replace the subjective, distorting hand and eye of the artist. To respond to such queries it is necessary to know what distortions and unrealities are introduced when constructing an anatomical illustration.

First of all it should be remembered that most gross anatomical research has been conducted on cadavers. From Renaissance times anatomy has been carried out on such subjects. Inevitably artefacts arise, even if the body has been obtained and dissected shortly after death; the reference point for anatomy is not a dead corpse, but a walking, talking, living person. So the structures discovered by dissection must be transposed to an imagined living state. Nowadays information obtained during surgical operations, from radiographs, scanning technology, endoscopy, and the like may be used to bridge the gap between the dissected cadaver and the living body.

Because of autolysis and the action of micro-organisms a cadaver decays. Without preservation there is a limited period during which dissection can be carried out; the classic illustrated anatomical texts in the sixteenth and seventeenth centuries were prepared on the basis of such fresh subjects. With modern preservation methods a cadaver may be kept for long periods. Many anatomical institutes have prosected material that has been acquired over decades. We have seen in Leiden specimens in preserving fluid prepared by B.S. Albinus more than two hundred years ago. But preservation alters, at the very least, the texture and appearance of tissues, creating thus certain artefacts.

If dissection is carried beyond the tissues beneath the skin then there is a danger that displacement will alter the relative positions of structures. For instance the position of the stomach in normal individuals was variously and uncertainly pictured in the seventeenth, eighteenth, and even nineteenth centuries. Advances were made when Pirogov and others perfected cross-sectional anatomy of frozen cadavers, when radiographs after barium swallows were introduced, and when CT and other scans were used to 'section', as it were, the living subject.

Other distortions than displacement can be caused by dissection. When dissecting the finer autonomic nerves in a preserved cadaver care must be taken not to create threads of connective tissue, under the misapprehension that they are unmyelinated fibres. Robert Lee's wonderful dissections of the nerves to the uterus, made in mid-1800s, were declared, erroneously, by a Royal Society commission to be artefactual. In the subsequent dispute, Lee was vindicated— the repercussions led to the resignation of the President of the Royal Society.

Bearing in mind these considerations we can see that a photograph of any particular dissection may well record the preconception held by the anatomist performing the dissection as to what that particular part *should* look like. The more complete the knowledge of the anatomist the fewer mistakes in presentation.

The photographer has in front of him a 'reality', created by the knowledge and techniques of current anatomy. The way a photographer looks at an anatomical presentation is determined by his training, experience, and imagination. A realistic, or recording, photograph of a landscape, for example, or of a nude figure, made in the early years of this century, can be recognized as different from those of the present time. A photographer, as much as a draughtsman, painter, or engraver, cannot record objectively and dispassionately, no matter how hard he tries, when taking a photograph of an anatomical specimen. A photographer eliminates confusing highlights and shadows from the dissection, arranging a large number of variables—lighting, contrast, and so on, to emphasize particular elements of the dissected presentation, and so create an instructive image. A photographer taking a single shot makes particular compromises so as best to accommodate the insoluble problem of representing depth on a plane surface.

It can be seen that a photograph can never be an impartial, objective record of 'true' anatomy. Anatomist and photographer should together make almost all these difficult decisions. Indeed an artist can create approaches to 'truths' in anatomy that are beyond the reach of a photographer. An artist can generalize in one illustration the knowledge gained by investigating a structure in a number of different ways: Brödel, for example, in his drawing of the ear (*Plate 131*), used information gained by investigating its structures with the naked eye and the microscope, using a battery of techniques—dissection of the temporal bone, serial sectioning, and so on. It is doubtful that a single photograph could lead the viewer into an understanding of the structure of the ear such as is obtainable by studying Brödel's drawing.

What then are the virtues of photographs of anatomy? To explore these we have chosen as type-example a superb atlas prepared at the Anatomy Department of The Royal College of Surgeons of England, mostly from preserved specimens accumulated there in their collection over many years: R. M. H. McMinn and R. T. Hutchings, *Colour atlas of human anatomy*, London, Wolfe Medical Publications, 1977.

This book, first published from London, proved to be an international success. It owed this to the care and thought that had gone into the selection of specimens and their photography, to the fine colour-printing, done in the Netherlands, and to the experience of the authors as anatomical educators. Just as Gray's *Anatomy* had, a century before, become a pattern followed by others, the success of their work naturally enough led to the production of other photographic atlases of human anatomy, each produced with a particular readership and purpose in mind.

Photography had of course been used to illustrate anatomy for a hundred years preceding McMinn's and Hutchings's book, most successfully perhaps in the remarkable collections of stereoscopic photographs of the period around 1900. The disadvantages of these were many; it was difficult to store and preserve the complementary pairs of photographs, the viewing stand was cumbersome to use, and it was impossible to survey the collection quickly—a book is, at least to our generation, the easiest way yet devised to scan through multiple pages of text or illustration. Yet if one is patient enough to use these stereoscopes, the three-dimensional affect is remarkable, if somewhat artificial. The dissection illustrated has neither the flat appearance of an ordinary photograph, nor does it appear as to the naked eye. One seems to be looking at an anatomical diorama, as in a museum display.

The Preface to the *Colour atlas of human anatomy* contains a clear, succinct summary of the anatomist's and photographer's intentions:

We believe it is helpful to show body structures as they actually exist in suitably prepared specimens of the kind that students see in the dissecting room and meet in examinations. In this way we hope to bridge the gap between the description of the textbook and the reality of the body.

The same purposes could have been expressed almost in the same words by many anatomists of the past, say, in the nineteenth century in Edinburgh or at University College, London.

In McMinn's and Hutchings's *Colour atlas* the reference point, as in earlier centuries, is the cadaver, not the living body. The student, it is noted in this preface, is confronted by a disparity between the appearance of the dissected body and the figures of his classical textbook, in which arteries are red and veins blue. But there is also disparity between the appearance of arteries and veins in the cadaver and that in the living body; the arteries, seen by a surgeon, are pulsating, the veins collapsed or full, and the glistening tissues multicoloured. Anatomy students often experience difficulty in distinguishing between arteries and nerves in the cadaver. Appropriate to their positions at the Royal College of Surgeons of London, McMinn and Hutchings made sure, by careful dissection, arrangement, and lighting that the parts present an appearance of reality not too dissimilar to what the surgeon sees when she or he exposes that part. But this appearance, photographed in these plates, is a construct of the authors. That the end result is a photograph does not ensure absolute fidelity to the 'real' situation; its truthfulness, as always, rests in the knowledge, hands, and eyes of the anatomist and artist—and in the eyes of the beholder.

Two other perennial preoccupations of earlier anatomists are seen also in this photographic atlas, namely the question of labelling; and the difficult decision to be made regarding size—should the anatomical parts in the illustration be pictured life–size or smaller or larger? The first dilemma was resolved in the book (but not featured in our *Plate 134*, which is from copies of the original photographs) by imposing numbers on the coloured photographs, with a key placed on the page nearby. There is no text accompanying the photographs, save a few short notes under the key, which comment for example on difficult anatomical relationships, or on surface markings, or the functional significance of particular ligaments.... Concerning the second dilemma, the question of size, McMinn and Hutchings argue:

When a student is dissecting or being asked to identify a structure in an examination, when a physician is examining a patient, or when a surgeon is operating, they direct their gaze at any one time on to a fairly small area, and the size of the printed page has been carefully chosen so that the illustrations could be made approximately life-size.

McMinn and Hutchings, in the last paragraph of their Preface, indicate that an illustrated atlas whose primary purpose is to instruct and inform can achieve more:

We would like to think that this book may be regarded as something more than an aid to academic learning and the passing of examinations. The human body is indeed 'fearfully and wonderfully made', and we hope our attempt at exercising some degree of photographic artistry to display the interior of the body will lead to a wider appreciation of the fact that beauty of form is not limited to the exterior.

The pictures of the bones, in particular, show how well they have succeeded in their attempt.

134 Muscles of the back of the forearm. (Courtesy of R. M. H. McMinn and R. T. Hutchings.) Colour photographs. 25.0 × 22.0 cm in the printed book, 1977.

While the cliché 'the camera cannot lie' may have some validity, everyone knows that any particular photograph may well present a distortion of the original subject. For instance, retouching or air-brushing can produce an image quite different to that seen by the eyes of the observer.

In this atlas, however, the authors point out that 'the camera has an all-embracing eye'; and indeed their photography faithfully records the appearance of the structure of the body. In this plate, for example, photograph B features an anomaly present in only ten per cent of bodies, namely extensor digiti medii, a muscle separated from extensor indicis, and one whose slender tendon, in this instance, extends to the extensor expansion of the middle finger: it may, on occasion, send slips to both the middle and index fingers.

With an appropriately dissected specimen and this photograph before them, students should have no difficulty in identifying the muscles of this region. They will no doubt note the origin of the dorsal interossei muscles from contiguous metacarpal bones, the arrangement of the slips from the tendons of extensor digitorum on the dorsum of the hand, the insertions of the tendons of the radial and ulnar wrist extensors, and the angulation of the tendons of extensors digiti minimi and pollicis longus. In short, these photographs are excellent anatomical learning aids.

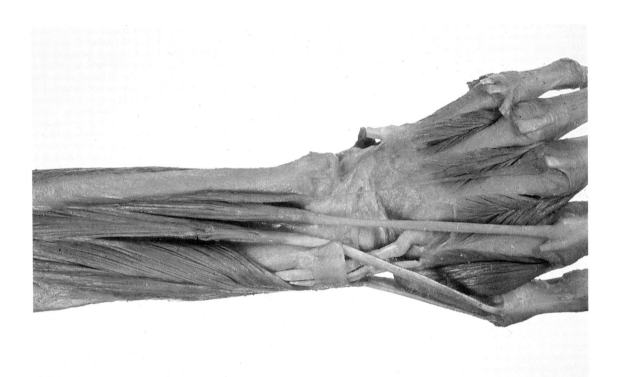

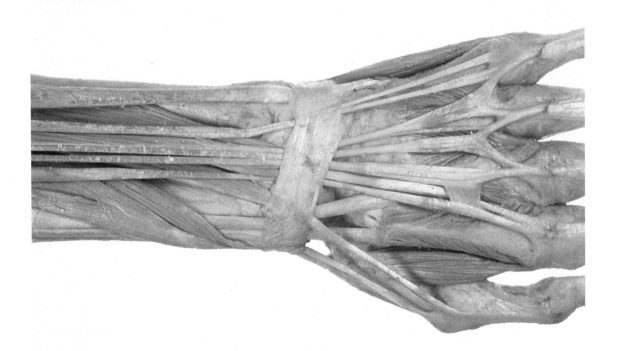

Chapter 15: Selection reading

Henry Gray

Brockbank, W. (1958). The centenary of a false prophesy: a warning to reviewers. *Med. Hist.*, **2**, 67–8.

Erisman, F. (1959). The critical response to Gray's Anatomy (A centennial comment). *J. med. Educ.*, **34**, 589–91.

New England Journal of Medicine (1959). Editorial, One hundred years' of Gray's Anatomy. *New Eng. J. Med.*, **261**, 1249–50.

Poynter, F. N. L. (1958). Gray's Anatomy: the first hundred years. *Brit. med. J.*, **2**, 610–11.

Williams, W. C. (1972). Henry Gray. *Dict. sci. Biog.*, **5**, 514–15.

J. E. S. Fraser

British Medical Journal. (1946). Obituary, J. E. S. Frazer *Brit. med. J.*, **1**, 664.

Lancet (1946). Obituary, John Ernest Sullivan Frazer. *Lancet*, **1**, 635.

The later development in Germany and Austria

Anon. (1977). *The Urban and Schwarzenberg Collection of medical illustrations since 1896.* Urban & Schwarzenberg, Baltimore.

Max Brödel

Cullen, T. S. (1945). Max Brödel, 1870–1941 ... *Bull. Med. Library Assoc.*, **33**, 5–29.

Hodge, G. P. (1982). Student days at Johns Hopkins: Evelyn Erickson Sullivan. *J. Biocommun.*, **9**, 18–22.

Papel, I. D. (1986). Max Brödel's contributions to otolaryngology.... *Amer. J. Otology*, **7**, 460–69.

J. C. B. Grant

Canadian Medical Association Journal (1973). Obituary, Dr. John Charles Boileau Grant. *Can. med. Assoc. J.*, **109**, 1028–9.

F. H. Netter

Anon. (1981). Frank Netter: the man, the artist, the surgeon. *Med. Times*, **109**, 31–3.

Brass, A. (1984). Frank H. Netter, M.D. *Med. J. Australia*, **141**, 880.

16

Some themes of the book

THE structure of the major parts of the body—the brain, the kidney, the hand, and so on—is appropriate to the way they function. This is the case also for the minute parts; at the level of fine structure, cell organelles show a fitness for the molecular reactions with which they are associated. The development of evolutionary biology has provided the theoretical basis for understanding the relationships between structure and function, and molecular biology has uncovered more clearly some of the ways in which these relationships have come into being.

The unity of form and function in the body was appreciated by the naturalists of the classical world, who discussed the relationship teleologically, in terms of purpose and divine intent. For Aristotle and Galen, as for the investigators in early modern times, all structures have been put in place by the Creator in order to carry out a particular useful function in the best possible way. It is thus that Galen's book *The usefulness of parts*, composed between AD 165 and AD 175, discussed physiological anatomy; that Harvey's physiological work on the circulation is named *Exercitatio anatomica de motu cordis . . .* ('An anatomical disputation concerning the motion of the heart', 1628); and thus that the anatomist, physiologist, and surgeon Charles Bell wrote a Bridgewater treatise in 1838 on *The hand: its mechanism and vital endowments, as evincing design.* Even the title of Vesalius' *De humani corporis fabrica...*, 1543 implies a functional anatomy: not only the structure of the human body but the way it works, its living functions.

It is nevertheless possible to study anatomy, as Galen did in *On procedures in anatomy*, without making the relationship between structure and function the central theme. In this way, anatomy is studied for its own sake, investigated primarily for itself, and not secondarily as a basis for understanding physiology.

While progress has not been uninterrupted, it is obvious that more is now known about anatomy than was known, say, in Renaissance times: the figure of the lungs in Dryander's 1537 *Anatomiae* and that of the skeleton in Berengario's 1521 *Commentaria* are obviously inferior to those in modern textbooks. It should be remembered, however, that until the post-Vesalian consolidation of printed illustration, knowledge of the structure of the human body was conveyed primarily by words, not by drawings. While a history of anatomical illustration is not therefore at all times coincident with a history of anatomy, after 1550 or thereabouts the best illustrations document the progress of the science.

Thus in retrospect we can see that the anatomical knowledge conveyed by illustration becomes refined, more precise and more accurate. This does not mean that representations shown in anatomy books are uninfluenced by contemporary circumstance, by social, economic, artistic, technical, and cultural conventions, emphases, inhibitions, and restraints. These factors, in addition to anatomical knowledge, determine the form a particular illustration will take. Comparisons may be made, for example, between the woodcut skeleton in Berengario, 1521, which resembles a Dance of Death figure; the mannerist skeleton-man of Vesalius' *Fabrica*, 1543; the neo-classical copper-engraved skeletons of Albinus, 1734; and the romantic lithographs of male and female skeletons approaching each other in Cloquet's *Anatomie...*, 1825. The detailed impersonal illustrations in Frazer's *Anatomy of the skeleton*, 1914, represent another approach to the bones: an approach which requires a reader to construct a three-dimensional image by imagining the surrounding structures. The illustrations mentioned differ in anatomical accuracy and sophistication; but they also differ in many other ways, not all related to the subject of anatomy itself.

The earliest known anatomical pictures, those drawn before the advent of printing, accompanied collections of texts of medical significance, but in no way had they the same purpose as a modern illustrated text. The anatomy of the compilations, often derived from Galenic sources, was explained textually rather than by figures. Many of these manuscript illustrations fall into one of three categories: first, representation of body structures within a figure of a human being, which itself, in one persistent convention, was placed in a squatting, or frog-like, stance; second, outlines of organs removed from the body—the heart, the stomach, and so on (these were diagrammatized to a greater or lesser extent); and third, purely diagrammatic schemata of body systems—particularly the eyes, and the male and the female urogenital tracts. The figures were copied, and mis-copied, from manuscript to manuscript.

The originals from which squatting figures stem are not known; they may have had more relevance to structures seen by dissection. In extant manuscripts, the anatomy shown in these frog-like figures has but a distant relationship to the realities of the human body. They are symbols of anatomy, not anatomical illustration. The figures of individual organs are simplified sketches, but are occasionally quite naturalistic. The diagrammatic schemata are potentially more informative as to the contemporary state of anatomy; are they derived from earlier diagrams, possibly even from a series illustrating Galenic texts? The eye diagrams of Islamic medicine are notable examples in this tradition.

In the fifty or so years after 1500, there were extraordinary advances in anatomical illustration. This may be seen by comparing any manuscript or printed illustration circulating prior to 1500 to any of Vesalius' illustrations in the *Fabrica*, 1543. The necessary conditions for such dramatic advances were wide-ranging.

First, in order to draw anatomical figures in a representational rather than a diagrammatic or symbolic manner, an artist surely should be competent in representing the living naked person. This ability was developed, first by sculptors and then by draughtsmen, during the fifteenth century. Apprentices had copy-books of their masters to follow; studies of long-known or recently excavated classical sculptures were made. Toward the end of this period, life drawing became a standard practice; moreover many artists began to attend, and even perform, dissections in order to find out what lay beneath the skin to give the body its external shape. Pollaiuolo and others drew fighting nude men to demonstrate their newly-acquired artistic ability. In the sixteenth century *écorchés* were constructed in wood to show the appearance of flayed men. These wood sculptures became known to many students in the academies, where dissections were also performed to supplement their anatomical studies of the skeleton and of naked men.

Secondly, by 1500 human dissection had been long established as a valid practice in the medical faculties of the universities of Europe. Not that it was a frequent, or even a regular, event in all.

Thirdly, a shift from manuscript to printed duplication of an author's work had almost been completed by 1500. In the first fifty years or so of printing more than 30 000 different works, of all kinds, had been printed; medicine was well represented in this *incunabula* period, mostly by contemporary authors, although, of course, these relied heavily on classical authors. In 1500 humanists were already at work establishing a canon of Greek texts, including those on anatomy; they continued to do so to midcentury and beyond. It was not, however, until more than seventy years after the invention of movable type that illustration was used to convey significant information regarding anatomy—or indeed, regarding any descriptive science or technology. The potential of printed illustration was then realized. About 1540 copiously illustrated books on anatomy, and on botany, began to be produced. There was a similar development in cartography, and, to a less clear extent, in engineering and in military technology and strategy: the multiple production of nearly-identical illustrations was so much more useful than textual material for conveying complex, yet precise, descriptive information. Even at a time when nomenclature was not standardized, anatomists could confirm, criticize, and modify an illustration, and publish their own, which more correctly portrayed that part of the human body.

Fourthly, by the sixteenth century, the business of printing, publishing, and distributing books was carried out by a network of international enterprises. Correctable information contained within printed illustrations became more or less simultaneously available to scholars across Europe. Academic books were often published in many editions. Large sums of money were invested to produce these new illustrated texts. Many of the publishers were themselves humanists.

The use of illustrations as an aid to understanding has been, from medieval times, regarded with suspicion. Guy de Chauliac in the fourteenth century criticized Henri de Mondeville's use of figures. Sylvius in Paris, following the publication of Vesalius' *Fabrica*, used much the same arguments; protesting the disrespect shown to Galen, he urged the Emperor Charles V to punish Vesalius. The fearsomely knowledgeable Edinburgh anatomist, Robert Knox, discusses the same questions in the mid-nineteenth century:

There are persons who indiscriminately censure and condemn anatomical drawings and engravings, rating them as dangerous and bad; and I well remember the time when I was one of these persons, because I had seen them substituted for actual dissection—a destructive practice and which, if persisted in, must necessarily prove ruinous to the reputation of the person as a surgeon...

The sixteenth-century masters of the woodcut produced many of their prints in the form of single leaves. These could be pinned to a wall, or inspected on a table. Some of the prints were of popular medical interest, recording, say, multiple births, or the birth of babies with gross malformations. Skeletons were portrayed personifying Death, and these representations were sometimes no worse than contemporary skeletons shown in popular anatomy prints. Some illustrations of anatomy were printed in the same manner, as single sheets, with explanatory text surrounding the figure. Vesalius and Calcar together in 1538 produced six large sheets in this format, and Vesalius' *Epitome* issued five years later had eleven plates with surrounding letterpress that could be used in this way; but it had, in addition, a title-page, and pages of unillustrated text. The earlier six sheets were probably treated by purchasers as collections and handled unbound; this may account for the extreme rarity of complete sets. A very few copies of the *Epitome* have been preserved in sumptuous bindings.

Anatomical illustrations are however more characteristically included within a bound book. If the intention was to instruct or to convey the results of research, then a text, of greater or lesser length, formed an integral part of the publication. In Berengario's *Commentaria*, 1521, there were only twenty illustrations amidst hundreds of pages of text. In 1538 in a Greek edition of the works of Galen, in thick folio volumes of text, there were just two pages of figures (one of a skull, the other showing skeletons), and these were placed in a Latin appendix on the bones. During the next hundred years however, illustration played a much more prominent role. Indeed many original books of anatomy from the eighteenth century onwards have been bound collections of plates, the text being restricted to the naming of structures. Modern atlases of anatomy sometimes use this format.

Berangario's *Isagoge* is a small book that can fit inside a coat pocket. The *Fabrica* or Estienne's *De dissectione* are sizeable folio volumes, but easy to carry from bookcase to reading desk. Reference to the illustrations of their pages is quite convenient. The same cannot be said for anatomical 'elephant' folios. Albinus' magnificent atlas of the bones and muscles, and Richard Quain's lithographs of the arteries, are huge, heavy volumes or portfolios. (Consulting atlas after atlas at The Wellcome Institute Library, the authors decided that their future research in libraries lay with duodecimal books!) Yet such extremely large volumes are trumped by the collected plates of Mascagni; two persons are needed to carry them safely to a table for consultation. The table has to be conference-sized to accommodate assembling the plates to form a full-length figure. The passion for reproducing anatomical structures life-sized, on a scale of one to one, coincided with an ambition to picture the anatomy of the whole body. The end results are cumbersome, and indeed useless: the leaves are inconvenient to turn, their edges split and crack; the binding inevitably breaks. One cannot sit to study the plates, but must walk around them, leaning over the table to check detail, just as one has to when studying a dissected cadaver. In the last hundred years or so, anatomists and publishers have abandoned these obsessions. Modern atlases still from time to time boast that their diagrams or photographs of anatomical details are life-sized; but they no longer attempt to reproduce the whole body on one plate.

With notable exceptions, the most important being Leonardo, a survey of scientific anatomical illustrations is a survey of anatomical *books*. We have to ask questions about these books: how were the figures produced? by whom and at what cost? and to whom were the books addressed?

Up to and including the works of Berengario, Estienne, and Vesalius, the illustrations in printed anatomy books were woodcuts. Sometimes these figures were of great refinement, as in the 1493 *Fasciculo*, and of great power and sophistication, as in the 1543 *Fabrica*. Others used imagery that had a more direct and simplified impact, as in Berengario's muscle-men or Dryander's dissections of the head. Draughtsmen, and those that actually cut the wood-blocks, had developed great artistic and technical competence by the 1550s. Woodcuts had the additional advantage that the blocks could be placed in the same forme as the movable type of the text, the two being printed together on the page. It is therefore not surprising that woodcuts were at this period by far the commonest medium used for anatomical and other technical illustration. But there was also a particular advantage in an available alternative technique—copperplate engraving. The line could be more delicate, with detail represented to a finer level. By the early 1540s, copperplates had begun to be used to illustrate anatomy. In 1545 the Vesalian woodcuts were copied successfully using copper-engraving. By 1600, and then for two hundred years, copperplate engraving was the predominant medium for printing anatomical figures. There were disadvantages. Text had to be run through the press separately. Properly prepared wood-blocks could last for centuries, standing up to many impressions, but copperplates were more easily worn down; the engraving had then to be touched-up, which coarsened the printed image. Moreover, copper was expensive, and so were the costs of engraving, for this took great care and a long time. If the image were complex and detailed, as was inevitable in most anatomical illustrations, then many weeks could pass in the production of a single plate. Short cuts were developed to produce an intaglio plate, specifically the technique of etching; but the painterly qualities of an etched plate were less suited to technical and scientific illustration than was an engraved plate. Other modifications of the intaglio print, such as the eighteenth century aquatint, mezzotint, and stipple engraving were but seldom used in anatomy illustration, for the same reason.

In the early 1800s an entirely new printing technique—lithography—was exploited. From 1820 to 1900 many of the most impressive anatomical plate-books were printed in this way.

Two other techniques were common in the nineteenth century. First, copper gave way to other metals, principally steel, for intaglio printing. This harder metal lasted through many more print-runs. Secondly, wood-blocks came again into their own, this time as wood-*engravings*, not woodcuts. The smaller, detailed close-up figures of regional anatomy, as in Gray's textbook, were printed this way. The technique was unsuitable for large illustrations in which the whole body was figured.

From the end of the nineteenth century, other printing techniques have come into being and have been used to reproduce illustrations. Many use planographic methods that ultimately derive from lithography. Photography is at the basis of most of these techniques, supplemented now by digitalization of the image.

Turning to the questions: by whom and at what cost were these illustrated anatomical works produced?

We have considered illustrations that recorded knowledge of anatomy, not anatomical pictures used primarily for other purposes. (Ruysch's displays of 'moral anatomy' barely managed to find a place in our book.) It is not surprising, then, that professional anatomists themselves were the originators of so much of the work we have chosen. At some periods and in some places books with anatomical figures have originated not with anatomists but with enterprising publishers. This may have been the case in the early days of printing in the German-speaking countries, when serious encyclopaedic compilations of knowledge included what were, for the time, good illustrations of anatomy. Certainly, three centuries later, after the invention of lithography, publishers began to take a major role in initiating illustrated anatomical texts. But Canano, Casserio, Haller, Hunter, and Mascagni probably each decided to produce an illustrated anatomy book, and determined what structures should be illustrated. They were responsible for the initiation and execution of their projects. Not that they all achieved their object. Canano never completed publication of his work, Casserio died before the illustrations he had caused to be made were issued, and Mascagni overreached himself—his magnificent and somewhat absurd illustrations were not printed in his lifetime.

In the best work, the anatomist who initiated the project very soon established a working relationship with a competent and patient artist, as did Albinus with Wandelaar, Soemmerring with Koch, Bourgery with Jacob, and McMinn with his photographer and colleague, Hutchings. The actual relationship between Vesalius and Calcar and other artists who worked with him is not apparent, though we can more easily conceive Vesalius directing the artists than his uncritically accepting their work. This latter situation however may have existed in the Bidloo–Lairesse partnership, for Bidloo—a good anatomist—may have allowed some of Lairesse's illustrations to be printed even though he knew certain details were inaccurate.

In some instances the anatomist was his own artist. At best, as in the work of Cowper (for his *Myotomia*), Camper, the Bells, or Scarpa, this is an ideal situation. Although many anatomists have very highly developed topological and topographical senses, and some have abilities in design, few have the technical ability, training, or experience to be able to produce an illustration good enough for general publication. *Mutatis mutandis*, few artists have initiated work on scientific human anatomy; a larger number have produced works of artistic anatomy. We think of Stubbs and his comparative anatomy, in which human anatomy takes its place (Stubbs had been a teacher of anatomy for a while). And, of course, of Leonardo; his anatomical notebooks, because they were private and pre-Gutenberg in spirit and execution, could not be reproduced satisfactorily save in facsimile. So Leonardo's work on anatomy only became generally available four hundred years after his death.

The relationship between anatomy and surgery has from the earliest times been exceptionally close, for obvious reasons. It must however be remembered that detailed anatomy was of limited usefulness until the late nineteenth century and after, when anaesthesia and antisepsis opened up all parts of the body to operating surgeons. A surgeon who only lanced abscesses, amputated limbs, cut for stone, couched cataracts, and dressed wounds and sores required but a limited knowledge of anatomy. But there was an emphasis on anatomy, not wholly explained, in London in the period 1700 to 1850, a period when the works of Cowper, Cheselden, and Quain and Maclise, for example, provided practical and useful anatomy illustrations for surgeons, and those of Hunter and Smellie for obstetricians. John Bell and Lizars are but two of many who established a parallel tradition of excellence in surgery, anatomy, and anatomical illustration in Edinburgh. Similar developments occurred in surgical and obstetrical anatomy in Germany (Kilian's work, for example), Italy (Scarpa), France (Jules Cloquet), and Russia (Pirogov) . . .

The physicians have less commonly contributed to the anatomical literature. In seventeenth-century England, Thomas Sydenham, as reported by John Locke, deprecated the intense interest in anatomy, asking what use its finer points were to the sick patient. However his contemporary,

Thomas Willis, also a physician, with much help from his friends, produced a work on cerebral structure and function which included fine anatomical illustrations drawn by the polymath Christopher Wren.

Since about 1850 anatomical atlases and illustrated textbooks have most often been written by professional anatomists not by practising doctors: Gray's *Anatomy*, the great Austrian and German contributions from Spalteholz, Pernkopf, and others, McMinn's and Hutchings's photographic atlas, and so many others. But the old relationship between anatomy and surgery continues, a new pattern emerging in which artists, working alongside surgeons, have achieved the recognition so often denied to their predecessors for the work they do in illustrating surgically-relevant anatomy. Max Brödel, Tom Jones, Frank Netter, and the artists of the Johns Hopkins and Toronto Schools of Art as Applied to Medicine have significantly advanced anatomical illustration in recent times, particularly in relation to operative surgery.

The anatomist has almost always been granted full recognition in any anatomy publication; the anatomical illustrator sometimes. But persons who are responsible for transferring the artist's drawing to the printed page are not often acknowledged. On occasion the engraver and lithographer, and, less often, the wood-cutter and printer may be noted. Vesalius complained of the cost of employing Venetian craftsmen who cut the wood-blocks for his *Fabrica*. But he fully recognized, as he certainly should have done, the seminal contribution of his Basle printer and publisher, the humanist and scholar Oporinus, whose subtle layout of text and figures on the page was a major element of this innovative publication.

The technology and economics of preparing and printing drawings and paintings determine the form that a text book or atlas will take to a much greater extent than has yet been fully recognized. These technical considerations must be analysed specifically and in detail in a number of examples before any valid generalization can be made. (Such matters can only form a small part of our anthology of plates.) The change-over from woodcut to engraving soon after 1550, the elaboration of engraving techniques in the late eighteenth century, the switch to lithographic methods from the 1820s, the employment of wood- and steel-engraving in the second half of the nineteenth century, and the influence of photographic methods in association with offset lithography—these are themes within our book, noted, but not developed in detail.

Similar lacunae exist in respect to our final question: To whom was the work directed? Ideally we should be able to answer it in respect of each book that we have mentioned. Reference to statements of intent in the preface or in the body of the work is sometimes helpful; more usually the question remains open.

Leonardo made his drawings largely for his own purposes, not for distribution. Fifty years later Eustachio presumably spent his or another's money in having copper-engravings made from a series of fine anatomical drawings. For whom did he intend the prints? And what were the circumstances that led Canano, Eustachio's contemporary, to abandon his projected illustrated monograph on the muscles? Berrettini, Martinez, and James Douglas also carried

622   SOME THEMES OF THE BOOK

their work to near-completion, but, for unknown reasons, failed to see their work in print. Cheselden did finish his *Osteographia*, and sold copies from his own house, but the costs of production were great, the work sold poorly, and he probably failed to recoup his expenses. (Cheselden's small format textbook: *Anatomy of humane bodies . . .*, however remained profitable through many editions and many years.) Another important work that probably was not a financial success was William Hunter's *Anatomy of the human gravid uterus*. This was started in 1750, but the work was not published until 1774. Hunter employed a well-known artist, incurred additional expenses to have the plates engraved, and had his work printed by the most fastidious printer in England. The fine atlases of Cheselden and Hunter were bought, in very small numbers, by well-off physicians, surgeons, and gentlemen, not by medical students. It is possible medical men and the middling classes of French society bought Cloquet's and other lithographic atlases produced in the first half of the nineteenth century. We know that Gray's *Anatomy*, designed with surgeons in mind, became for more than a century a profitable commodity, the premier English and American textbook of anatomy for medical students, surgeons, and others. In the twentieth century, the chief illustrated textbooks of anatomy in Germany—for example those issued in Vienna and Munich by the Urban and Schwarzenberg firm—differed from Gray's in many respects. Their illustrations were realistic, highly coloured paintings of anatomy, produced over many years by the publisher's in-house artists, directed closely by academic authorities under contract. Gray's were, for many years, diagrammatic wood-engravings, sometimes in later editions coloured in a subdued manner, from sketches made by surgeon-anatomists. To explain these differences we would need to take into account many factors— social, economic, educational, and professional—in the medical and publishing worlds of Germany, Britain, and the United States. This is beyond the intended purpose of this anthology.

In an obituary of Sir George Dancer Thane (*Journal of Anatomy*, 1929–30) Eliot Smith addressed the problem of plagiarism in text books of anatomy. He pointed out that Jones Quain's *Anatomy* was translated into German in an edition that served, in turn, as an unacknowledged basis for Rauber's text. Editions of Rauber's *Lehrbuch* were translated, again without reference to Quain, into various languages, and formed the substance of a treatise in France by Poirier and Charpy. Many English anatomy texts owe their descriptions of the muscles to that in Rauber, itself derived from Quain. Eliot Smith wrote: 'the time is not yet ripe for a candid history of these translations and retranslations. The practice of piracy in textbooks of anatomy, both in former times and today, would provide an illuminating theme for an essay an human nature!' Only an anatomist of the old school could today write such an essay. We have from time to time noted the recriminations and complaints of anatomists who have regarded themselves as victims of plagiarisms: Vesalius fulminated against anatomists and booksellers in many countries. Bidloo named William Cowper as an intellectual criminal; James Yonge exposed John Browne as a thief; and so on.

We have argued that the spread of information by way of printed illustrations has contributed significantly to the development of anatomy. Such figures are not produced in an ahistoric void, but rely on descriptions and illustrations of former times. Anatomists have, through four centuries, used such information to make anatomy clearer and more accurate. This is admirable; it is the way descriptive science develops. Any survey of anatomy will demonstrate the persistence of convention in anatomical illustration. The representation of an articulated complete skeleton newly inserted into the second edition of McMinn and Hutchings, 1988, is in an ancient tradition. Representations of the nerves of the orbit in many late-nineteenth- and in twentieth-century texts have many common features; there is, after all, a limited number of ways these structures can be pictured satisfactorily.

Piracy and plagiarism occurs in anatomy when unacknowledged copies are made of the work of others, when anatomists claim for themselves credit for the knowledge, intelligence, imagination, and hard work of others. Winslow with propriety acknowledged Eustachio's plates reprinted in his textbook; Cowper and his publishers, with foolish deceit, failed to recognize publicly that the plates in his book belonged to the anatomist Bidloo and his artist Lairesse. Winslow cannot be censured; Cowper should be.

There are much less clear cases. Valverde was generous in acknowledging his debt to Vesalius; Geminus was mean. Vesalius had blanket condemnation for both, and for others who based their work on the figures in his *Fabrica*. (To create a set of new anatomical figures not based on Vesalius was a difficult option—as Casserio, his successors, and their artists found.) Vesalius was distressed and angered by infringement of his unenforceable 'copyright'. Such legal questions remained even when full acknowledgement was made.

Vesalius was most probably the only begetter of the *Fabrica*; but of the others involved, only one—the printer-publisher Oporinus—received acknowledgement. Indeed the illustrations, which were its extraordinary achievement, remain unattributed. We now regret Vesalius' failure to acknowledge his collaborators.

Gross anatomy is essentially a descriptive account of the structures of the human body derived from exploratory dissection. The account given may be ordered in a number of ways—system by system, regionally, and so on. The account, which for centuries has included pictorial representation, is verifiable. (Variation in anatomical structure occurs; but the pattern of variation may be described, enumerated, and verified.) Such a restricted definition of anatomy excludes morphology, embryology, and many other sciences; but it is applicable to anatomy from an early period. The definition implies that the practice of anatomy is a scientific pursuit.

Building on knowledge passed on from classical times, and using the technique of dissection, anatomy started to develop rapidly as a descriptive science in the later fifteenth and in the sixteenth centuries. We argue that this development was hastened by, and was even dependent upon, the communication of the results of investigation by printed illustration. The bases of a number of other descriptive sciences were similarly constructed during the same period, specifically botany and cartography.

In the sixteenth century anatomists held prominent positions in universities, engaged in bitter disputations that could be resolved by reference to natural phenomena, and, above all, applied themselves systematically to close and detailed dissection and observation, the results of which they communicated in words and in pictures. Anatomy for a century or more came to be at the centre of scientific enquiry, and anatomical illustration came to be central to anatomy.

The biological experimental sciences were underdeveloped at a time when the basic content of anatomy had already been established. Experimental physics and chemistry also developed at this later date. Anatomy, with botany and cartography, was among the earliest of modern sciences; it preceded by decades the growth of quantitative, experimental sciences.

Anatomical illustration is a useful art, requiring the same precision as architectural or engineering drawing. But the subject matter is more complex, less rigidly organized, and in this way resembles topographical recording. Just as Turner drew the ports and harbours of Britain on commission, and for his own purposes, so creative artists have made images of the landscapes of the human body—Leonardo, Pietro da Cortona, Lairesse, Stubbs ... But the constraints of anatomical topography are the greater: what the anatomist seeks to demonstrate determines what the artist shall include.

It is impossible to record the appearance of a building or landscape without including the artist's response to what he sees; this response has all the ambiguities derived from that particular artist's personality, experience, and place in society. How much more complicated the response will be when the subject matter is a human body! Artists make use of the nude to explore object and response. But anatomical illustration is not life, but death, drawing; there is a superimposed outrage, suppressed maybe with familiarity, when a cut is made, and when the dissection is carried down to the deeper layers. Some anatomical artists have conveyed the apprehensions of the dissecting room, and some have exploited the macabre, even perverse, side of anatomy. In order to exorcize this horror, the dissected figure is often shown standing in a quiet landscape, where all seems indifferent to the figure in agony. Other anatomical illustrations are merely diagrams, removed both from the living and the dead.

We can look closely at a map of the body and concentrate on the whereabouts of a particular branch of the femoral artery; but if we step back, we can see more. One of our book's secondary purposes is to extend experience and to disturb indifference.

Index

Page references in **bold** indicate plates; references in *italic* indicate figures.